MALIGNANT LYMPHOMAS AND HODGKIN'S DISEASE:
EXPERIMENTAL AND THERAPEUTIC ADVANCES

DEVELOPMENTS IN ONCOLOGY

F.J. Cleton and J.W.I.M. Simons, eds., Genetic Origins of Tumour Cells. ISBN 90-247-2272-1
J. Aisner and P. Chang, eds., Cancer Treatment Research. ISBN 90-247-2358-2
B.W. Ongerboer de Visser, D.A. Bosch and W.M.H. van Woerkom-Eykenboom, eds., Neuro-oncology: Clinical and Experimental Aspects. ISBN 90-247-2421-X
K. Hellmann, P. Hilgard and S. Eccles, eds., Metastasis: Clinical and Experimental Aspects. ISBN 90-247-2424-4
H.F. Seigler, ed., Clinical Management of Melanoma. ISBN 90-247-2584-4
P. Correa and W. Haenszel, eds., Epidemiology of Cancer of the Digestive Tract. ISBN 90-247-2601-8
L.A. Liotta and I.R. Hart, eds., Tumour Invasion and Metastasis. ISBN 90-247-2611-5
J. Bánóczy, ed., Oral Leukoplakia. ISBN 90-247-2655-7
C. Tijssen, M. Halprin and L. Endtz, eds., Familial Brain Tumours. ISBN 90-247-2691-3
F.M. Muggia, C.W. Young and S.K. Carter, eds., Anthracycline Antibiotics in Cancer. ISBN 90-247-2711-1
B.W. Hancock, ed., Assessment of Tumour Response. ISBN 90-247-2712-X
D.E. Peterson, ed., Oral Complications of Cancer Chemotherapy. ISBN 0-89838-563-6
R. Mastrangelo, D.G. Poplack and R. Riccardi, eds., Central Nervous System Leukemia. Prevention and Treatment. ISBN 0-89838-570-9
A. Polliack, ed., Human Leukemias. Cytochemical and Ultrastructural Techniques in Diagnosis and Research. ISBN 0-89838-585-7
W. Davis, C. Maltoni and S. Tanneberger, eds., The Control of Tumor Growth and its Biological Bases. ISBN 0-89838-603-9
A.P.M. Heintz, C.Th. Griffiths and J.B. Trimbos, eds., Surgery in Gynecological Oncology. ISBN 0-89838-604-7
M.P. Hacker, E.B. Double and I. Krakoff, eds., Platinum Coordination Complexes in Cancer Chemotherapy. ISBN 0-89838-619-5
M.J. van Zwieten, The Rat as Animal Model in Breast Cancer Research: A Histopathological Study of Radiation- and Hormone-Induced Rat Mammary Tumors. ISBN 0-89838-624-1
B. Löwenberg and A. Hagenbeek, eds., Minimal Residual Disease in Acute Leukemia. ISBN 0-89838-630-6
I. van der Waal and G.B. Snow, eds., Oral Oncology. ISBN 0-89838-631-4
B.W. Hancock and A.H. Ward, eds., Immunological Aspects of Cancer. ISBN 0-89838-664-0
K.V. Honn and B.F. Sloane, Hemostatic Mechanisms and Metastasis. ISBN 0-89838-667-5
K.R. Harrap, W. Davis and A.H. Calvert, eds., Cancer Chemotherapy and Selective Drug Development. ISBN 0-89838-673-X
C.J.H. van de Velde and P.H. Sugarbaker, eds., Liver Metastasis. ISBN 0-89838-648-5
D.J. Ruiter, K. Welvaart and S. Ferrone, eds., Cutaneous Melanoma and Precursor Lesions. ISBN 0-89838-689-6
S.B. Howell, ed., Intra-arterial and Intracavitary Cancer Chemotherapy. ISBN 0-89838-691-8
D.L. Kisner and J.F. Smyth, eds., Interferon Alpha-2: Pre-Clinical and Clinical Evaluation. ISBN 0-89838-701-9
P. Furmanski, J.C. Hager and M.A. Rich, eds., RNA Tumor Viruses, Oncogenes, Human Cancer and Aids: On the Frontiers of Understanding. ISBN 0-89838-703-5
J. Talmadge, I.J. Fidler and R.K. Oldham, Screening for Biological Response Modifiers: Methods and Rationale. ISBN 0-89838-712-4
J.C. Bottino, R.W. Opfell and F.M. Muggia, eds., Liver Cancer. ISBN 0-89838-713-2
P.K. Pattengale, R.J. Lukes and C.R. Taylor, Lymphoproliferative Diseases: Pathogenesis, Diagnosis, Therapy. ISBN 0-89838-725-6
F. Cavalli, G. Bonadonna and M. Rozencweig, eds., Malignant Lymphomas and Hodgkin's Disease: Experimental and Therapeutic Advances. ISBN 0-89838-727-2

MALIGNANT LYMPHOMAS AND HODGKIN'S DISEASE: EXPERIMENTAL AND THERAPEUTIC ADVANCES

Proceedings of the Second International
Conference on Malignant Lymphomas,
Lugano, Switzerland, June 13–16, 1984

edited by

FRANCO CAVALLI
Division of Oncology, Ospedale San Giovanni
Bellinzona, Switzerland

G. BONADONNA
Istituto Nazionale, per lo Studio e la Cura dei Tumori
Milano, Italy

MARCEL ROZENCWEIG
Bristol-Myers Company
Pharmaceutical Research & Development Division
Syracuse, NY, USA

1985 **MARTINUS NIJHOFF PUBLISHING**
a member of the KLUWER ACADEMIC PUBLISHERS GROUP
BOSTON / DORDRECHT / LANCASTER

Distributors

for the United States and Canada: Kluwer Academic Publishers, 190 Old Derby Street, Hingham, MA 02043, USA
for the UK and Ireland: Kluwer Academic Publishers, MTP Press Limited, Falcon House, Queen Square, Lancaster LA1 1RN, UK
for all other countries: Kluwer Academic Publishers Group, Distribution Center, P.O. Box 322, 3300 AH Dordrecht, The Netherlands

Library of Congress Cataloging in Publication Data

```
International Conference on Malignant Lymphoma
    (2nd : 1984 : Lugano, Switzerland)
    Malignant lymphomas and Hodgkin's disease.

    (Developments in oncology)
    Includes bibliographies and index.
    1. Lymphomas--Congresses.  2. Lymphomas--
Treatment--Congresses.  3. Hodgkin's disease--Congresses.
4. Hodgkin's disease--Treatment--Congresses.
I. Cavalli, Francesco.  II. Bonadonna, G., 1934-
III. Rozencweig, Marcel.  IV. Title.  V. Series.
[DNLM: 1. Hodgkin's Disease--congresses.  2. Lymphoma--
congresses.  W1 DE998N / WH 525 I602 1984m]
RC280.L9I47  1984       616.99'446       85-5146
ISBN 0-89838-727-2
```

ISBN 0-89838-727-2 (this volume)

Copyright

PRINTED IN THE NETHERLANDS

Contents

IV. Clinico-pathologic correlations

V. Special clinical entities

X

VIII. Treatment of childhood lymphomas

Preface

Malignant lymphomas remain a fascinating research topic for clinicians as well as basic scientists. Rapidly increasing technical sophistication, expanded knowledge and broader implications of new findings underline the need for a forum to integrate the latest developments in the multiple areas involved in the challenging study of lymphoid malignancies. This volume includes contributions of renowned experts and is based on a selection of papers presented at the Second International Conference on Malignant Lymphomas that was held in Lugano, Switzerland, in June 1984. Updated information is provided on various experimental fields including cell biology, immunology, genetics and cell biochemistry. Particular attention has been given to special clinical entities such as the lymphomas associated with the Acquired Immune Deficiency Syndrome. Recent advances in the treatment of Hodgkin's disease, non-Hodgkin's lymphomas and childhood lymphomas are highlighted with emphasis on growing experience with new therapeutic approaches including monoclonal antibodies and bone marrow transplantation.

The contents of the volume reflect and translate numerous avenues of exploration. While there might be some unavoidable overlap, most appear essentially complementary. The intent of the Program Committee of the Second International Conference on Malignant Lymphomas was to promote further interactions between all those who are devoting major efforts to elucidate the nature of these diseases or their optimal therapy. This volume will hopefully amplify this objective.

The Editors wish to thank the contributors for delivering the manuscripts on schedule. Timely publication of this volume would not have been possible without the enthusiastic editorial assistance of Judi Schurig. The help of the Medical Writing Department, Bristol-Myers Pharmaceutical Research and Development Division is also acknowledged.

The Editors

Acknowledgements

The Second International Conference on Malignant Lymphomas, on which this volume is based, was organized with the very active collaboration of C. Berard, R. C. Young, S. Rosenberg, H. Rappaport and J. E. Ultmann. The Conference was supported in part by grants from the Swiss Group for Clinical Cancer Research (SAKK), the Lega Ticinese Contro il Cancro and the Swiss League Against Cancer. Major support was also obtained from Bristol-Myers, Eli-Lilly, Essex Chemie, Farmitalia Carlo Erba, Hochst-Pharma, Hoffman-LaRoche and Kyowa Hakko Kogyo. We also acknowledge the support of Asta-Werke, Bayer, Beecham, Ciba-Geigy, Lundbeck/Leo, Max Ritter, Pharmacia, Sandoz, Sanofi, Serona, Unimed and Upjohn.

I. Immunopathology

1. The cell of origin of Hodgkin's disease

C.W. BERARD
St. Jude Children's Research Hospital
Memphis, Tennessee, USA

Since the detailed descriptions by Sternberg [1] and Reed [2], Hodgkin's disease has been recognized as a form of lymphoreticular malignancy with distinctive clinical and pathologic features [3]. The neoplastic cells of the disorder, i.e., the Sternberg-Reed cells and their mononuclear counterparts referred to as 'Hogdkin's cells', are considered to be malignant on the basis of their characteristic aneuploidy and clonality (by marker chromosomes) [4, 5]. Unique to Hodgkin's disease is the fact that such cells are distributed amidst a background of diverse cytologic types, all of which are apparently benign and 'reactive'. Principal among them are lymphocytes, bland histiocytes, eosinophils, plasma cells, fibroblasts, endothelial cells, and 'stromal' cells. Hodgkin's disease is thus a peculiar cancer in which the malignant cells only rarely comprise more than a small fraction of the bulk of the tumefaction. For this same reason, within the overall spectrum of Hodgkin's disease, there is marked histologic diversity on the basis of which Jackson and Parker first proposed a subclassification of limited usefulness [6–9]. Far superior is the scheme later put forth by Lukes and Butler [10, 11] and subsequently popularized as the Rye subclassification [12].

Despite marked advances in the clinical management of Hodgkin's disease in the last two decades, the exact nature of the neoplastic cells remains uncertain. On purely morphologic grounds Sternberg-Reed cells and 'Hodgkin's cells' were considered by many observers to be derived from 'reticulum cells' [4] or histiocytes [13], a cytogeneologic theory for which there is still no firm proof. With increasing knowledge of the functional components of the immune system and their anatomic compartments [3], it has become abundantly clear that Hodgkin's disease is somehow related to the cell-mediated arm of the body's defense apparatus. Patients with Hodgkin's disease, even of limited stage and favorable histology, have demonstrable defects in cell-mediated immunity when subjected to sensitive testing [4]. Moreover, in sites of 'early' or partial involvement, microscopic foci of Hodgkin's disease preferentially involve the thymic-dependent paracortical regions of lymph nodes. Similarly, microscopic and thus presumably 'early' lesions in the spleen are also localized to the T-cell-dependent periarterial lymphoid sheaths [14]. In short, Hodgkin's disease appears to follow pathways of spread which mimic the circulatory pattern of normal T-lymphocytes [15, 16]. An alternative candidate cell of origin to the reticulum cell or 'histiocyte' emerged when these observations were coupled with the discovery that small T-lymphocytes, when stimulated by mitogens or antigens, can transform to large cells with vesicular nuclei, large nucleoli, and abundant cytoplasm, i.e., cells resembling to some degree Sternberg-Reed cells and 'Hodgkin's cells' [17]. It was hypothesized [18] that the malignant cells of Hodgkin's disease are neoplastically transformed T-lymphocytes, perhaps expressing neoantigens (? viral) to which the background cells, including normal T-lymphocytes, are mounting an immunologic response. Additional luster was provided to this provocative suggestion by the observation that Sternberg-Reed cells and 'Hogdkin's cells' in suspension frequently have tightly adherent to them numerous small lymphocytes later proven to be T-cells [3, 19]. Subsequent studies, however, have failed to provide any evidence supporting an origin of the malignant cells from the T-lymphocyte lineage [3, 19, 20].

With the advent of immunoperoxidase techniques, the initially startling discovery was made that Sternberg-Reed cells and 'Hodgkin's cells' in histologic sections contain intracytoplasmic immunoglobulin [21, 22]. The notion that they might be neoplastic B cells was dispelled when it was shown that the immunoglobulin within individual malignant cells was not only polyclonal [23–24] but also demonstrably of exogenous origin [26]. Some support for derivation of the malignant cells from the mononuclear phagocyte system, including 'reticulum cells', has come from in vitro studies of cell lines established from human tissues involved by Hodgkin's disease [27–30]. From the pattern of reactivity of monoclonal antibodies raised against another presumptive 'Hodgkin's cell' line, it was recently proposed that Sternberg-Reed cells and 'Hodgkin's cells' are neoplastic counterparts of a heretofore not-yet-described, minute, but distinct cell population demonstrable in normal lymphoid tissue and bone marrow [31]. One monoclonal antibody appeared initially to be highly selective, reacting only with Sternberg-Reed cells, 'Hodgkin's cells', and their unidentified normal equivalents. Subsequently, however, the same monoclonal antibody has been shown to react with the cells of a number of disorders including Lennert's lymphoma, malignant histiocytosis, and angioimmunoblastic lymphadenopathy [32].

The bulk of current evidence favors the concept that Sternberg-Reed cells and 'Hodgkin's cells' originate from an antigen-presenting cell of the mononuclear phagocyte/reticulum cell lineage [27–30, 33]. A prime candidate, on the basis of immunologic, histochemical, and ultrastructural studies [34–

36], is the interdigitating reticulum cell. Such cells are antigen-processing cells selectively localized to the thymic-dependent compartments of the immune system. Like Sternberg-Reed cells and 'Hodgkin's cells', interdigitating reticulum cells bind T helper/inducer lymphocytes [36, 37], possess abundant Ia determinants [20, 36], and lack, or only weakly express, hydrolytic enzymes normally associated with monocytes and macrophages [35, 36]. The major obstacle to this hypothesis has been the failure to demonstrate cross-reactivity between the normal and neoplastic cells with antisera prepared selectively against one or the other. So, the cell of origin of Hodgkin's disease remains an unknown, but the saga to date has been fascinating and the tools of modern molecular biology should soon yield an answer to the greatest mystery in neoplastic hematopathology.

References

1. Sternberg C (1898). Über eine eigenartige unter dem Bilde der Pseudo Leukamie verlaufende Tuberculose des lymphatischen Apparates. Z Heikunde (Berlin) 19:21–90.
2. Reed DM (1902). On the pathological changes in Hodgkin's disease, with especial reference to its relation to tuberculosis. Johns Hopkins Hosp Rep 10:133–196.
3. Mann RB, Jaffe ES and Berard CW (1979). Malignant lymphomas – a conceptual understanding of morphologic diversity. Amer J Pathol 94:103–192.
4. Kaplan HS (1972). Hodgkin's Disease. Cambridge, Mass.: Harvard University Press.
5. Rowley JD (1982). Chromosomes in Hodgkin's disease. Cancer Treat Rep 66:639–643.
6. Jackson H Jr (1937). The classification and prognosis of Hodgkin's disease and allied disorders. Surg Gynecol Obstet 64:465–467.
7. Jackson H Jr (1939). Hodgkin's disease and allied disorders. N Engl J Med 220:26–30.
8. Jackson H Jr and Parker F Jr. (1944).Hodgkin's disease. II. Pathology. N Engl J Med 231:35–44.
9. Jackson H Jr and Parker F Jr (1947). Hodgkin's Disease and Allied Disorders. New York: Oxford University Press.
10. Lukes RJ, Butler JJ and Hicks E (1966). Natural history of Hodgkin's disease as related to its pathologic picture. Cancer 19:317–344.
11. Lukes RJ and Butler JJ (1966). The pathology and nomenclature of Hodgkin's disease. Cancer Res 26:1063–1981.
12. Lukes RJ, Craven LF, Hall TC et al. (1966). Report of the nomenclature committee. Cancer Res 26:1311.
13. Rappaport H (1966). Tumors of the Hematopoietic System. Atlas of Tumor Pathology, Section 3, Fascicle 8. Washington, D.C., Armed Forces Institute of Pathology.
14. Berard CW (1975). Reticuloendothelial system: An overview of neoplasia. The Reticuloendothelial System. Baltimore: Williams and Wilkins.
15. Gowans JL (1968). Lymphocytes. Harvey Lectures 64:87–119.
16. Gowans JL and Knight EJ (1964). The route of recirculation of lymphocytes in the rat. Proc R Soc Lond (Biol.) 159:257–282.
17. Anagnostou D, Parker JW, Taylor CR et al. (1977). Lacunar cells of nodular sclerosing Hodgkin's disease. An ultrastructural and immunohistologic study. Cancer 39:1032–1043.
18. Order SE and Hellman S (1972). Pathogenesis of Hodgkin's disease. Lancet 1:571–573.

6

19. Aisenberg AC and Wilkes BM (1982). Lymph node T cells in Hodgkin's disease: Analysis of suspensions with monoclonal antibody and rosetting techniques. Blood 3:522–527.
20. Poppema S, Bhan AK, Reinherz EL et al. (1982). In situ immunologic characterization of cellular constituents in lymph nodes and spleens involved by Hodgkin's disease. Blood 59:226–231.
21. Garvin AJ, Spicer SS, Parmley RT and Munster AM (1974). Immunohistochemical demonstration of IgG in Reed-Sternberg and other cells in Hodgkin's disease. J Exp Med 139:1077–1083.
22. Taylor CR (1974). The nature of Reed-Sternberg cells and other malignant 'reticulum' cells. Lancet 2:802–807.
23. Landaas T, Gordal T and Halvorsen TB (1977). Characterization of immunoglobulins in Hodgkin's cells. Int J Cancer 20:717–722.
24. Papadimitriou CS, Stein H and Lennert K (1978). The complexity of immunohistochemical staining pattern of Hodgkin and Reed-Sternberg cells – demonstration of immunoglobulin, albumin, alpha-1-anti-trypsin and lysozyme. Int J Cancer 21:531–541.
25. Poppema S, Elema JD and Halie MR (1978). The significance of intracytoplasmic proteins in Reed-Sternberg cells. Cancer 42:1793–1803.
26. Kadin ME, Stites DP, Levy R and Warnke R (1978). Exogenous immunoglobulin and the macrophage origin of Reed-Sternberg cells in Hodgkin's disease. N Engl J Med 299:1208–1214.
27. Kaplan HS and Gartner S (1977). 'Sternberg-Reed' giant cells of Hodgkin's disease: Cultivation in vitro, heterotransplantation, and characterization as neoplastic macrophages. Int J Cancer 19:511–525.
28. Roberts AN, Smith KL, Dowell BL and Hubbard AK (1978). Cultural, morphological, cell membrane, enzymatic, and neoplastic properties of cell lines derived from a Hodgkin's disease lymph node. Cancer Res 38:3033–3043.
29. Ford RJ, Mehta S, Davis F and Maizel AL (1982). Growth factors in Hodgkin's disease. Cancer Treat Rep 66:633–638.
30. Olsson L. Phenotypic attributes of the malignant cell in Hodgkin's disease. New Perspectives in Human Lymphoma. The Univ. of Texas, M. D. Anderson Hospital and Tumor Institute. (In Press).
31. Stein H, Gerdes J, Schwab U et al. (1983). Evidence for the detection of the normal counterpart of Hodgkin and Sternberg-Reed cells. Hematol Oncol 1:21–29.
32. Stein H, Gerdes J, Lemke H, et al. Immunological classification of Hodgkin's disease and 'malignant histiocytosis'. New Perspectives in Human Lymphoma. The Univ. Of Texas, M.D. Anderson Hospital and Tumor Institute. (In press).
33. Resnick GD and Nachman RL (1981). Reed-Sternberg cells in Hodgkin's disease contain fibronectin. Blood 57:339–342.
34. Peiper SC, Kahn LB, Ross DW and Reddick RL (1980). Ultrastructural organization of the Reed-Sternberg cell: Its resemblance to cells of the monocyte-macrophage system. Blood Cells 6:515–523.
35. Beckstead JH, Warnke R and Bainton DF (1982). Histochemistry of Hodgkin's disease. Cancer Treat Rep 66:609–613.
36. Kadin M (1982). Possible origin of the Reed-Sternberg cell from an interdigitating reticulum cell. Cancer Treat Rep 66:601-608.
37. Borowitz MJ, Croker BP and Metzger RS (1982). Immunohistochemical analysis of the distribution of lymphocyte subpopulations in Hodgkin's disease. Cancer Treat Rep 66:667–674.

2. Hodgkin's disease:
Further information derived from cell lines

H. BURRICHTER [1], M. SCHAADT [1], C. KORTMANN [2],
W. HEIT [3]. E. SCHELL-FREDERICK [1], H. STEIN [4] and V. DIEHL [1]
[1] *Medizinische Universitätsklinik I, Köln, and* [2] *Medizinische*
Hochschule Hannover, and [3] *Universitätsklinik, Ulm, FRG, and*
[4] *Nuffield Department of Pathology, Oxford, UK*

Histologically, Hodgkin's disease (HD) is characterized by a striking cellular pleomorphism with a low percentage of Hodgkin (H) and Sternberg-Reed (SR) cells, which represent the tumor cell population, admixed with non-malignant cells, e.g., polymorphonuclears, macrophages, B-cells and T-cells. Aneuploidy and clonal development of H and SR cells confirm their neoplastic nature. However, chromosome markers that are specific for HD have not been identified in freshly sampled tumors. The reasons for the presence of non-malignant cells surrounding H- and SR-cells are still unknown. This admixture has been regarded as a type of graft-vs-host reaction.

Etiologically, HD has been described as a chronic immunologic disorder [1]. Granuloma formation suggests interaction between the tumor cells and the host. Impairment of immunologic response in HD was already suggested in 1902 [2]. Several abnormalities of T-lymphocytes *in vitro* are well established [3]. While many authors consider the impairment of T-cell function to be inherent in this cell population [4], there is evidence that the impaired function is at least partially mediated by soluble factors [5-7].

Our experiments were carried out with five cell lines representing HD tumor cells and established between 1978 and 1982 [8, 9]. They reveal the production by H and SR cells of biologic mediators that interfere with immunologic response and hematopoietic regulation. This report updates these observations and summarizes new cytogenetic findings.

Materials and methods

Establishment, maintenance and characteristics of Hodgkin cell lines L 428, L 428 KS, L 428 KSA, L 540 and L 591 have been described in detail [8, 9]. Cell lines were kept for 3 days in RPMI 1640 medium without fetal calf serum (FCS). Cell-free supernatants were centrifuged (450 g/20 min), passed through a millipore filter (0.22 m) and adjusted to pH 7.2.

The ability of colony-stimulating factor (CSF) to enhance *in vitro* growth of colony forming units was determined in semi-solid agar cultures, according to a modification of the method described by Bradley and Metcalf [10] and Heit [11]. Interleukin 1 (IL 1) activity was tested with a human lymphocyte co-stimulator assay [12]. The technique for mitogenic stimulation is reported elsewhere [13]. T-cells were separated by Ficoll hypaque density centrifugation. The rosetting of sheep erythrocytes (SRBC) was performed according to Jondal et al. [14]. Inhibition of migration of granulocytes was evaluated according to Nelson et al. [15].

For cytogenetic techniques, colcemid ($0.1–0.5\ \mu g/ml$ medium) was added to a cell suspension, containing 5×10^5 cells in 2 ml medium, 30 minutes or 2 hours before cell harvest. After separation from the supernatant by centrifugation at 1000 rpm, cells were treated with hypotonic KCl solution (0.075 M) at room temperature for 20 minutes. Procedures for fixation, dropping on ice-cold slides, air drying and staining (by a modified GAG banding technique) were performed as described [8, 9]. About 100 metaphases per cell line were analysed.

Results

1. *IL 1*. (Table I): Conditioned media (CM) from cell-lines, except L 428 KSA, were capable of replacing accessory cells in the promotion of concanavalin A (Con A) induced lymphoproliferation of monocyte-depleted human blood lymphocytes. Under serum-free conditions, kinetic studies revealed measurable IL 1-like activity in Hodgkin cell cultures 24 hours after seeding. IL 1-like activity is heat stable (56 °C) for 30 min and resistant to alkaline pH (up to pH 11). The molecular weight is in the range of 13–25 KD. Functional and biochemical properties would be in line with properties of human IL 1 [16].

Table I. IL 1 like activity in Hodgkin cell-line conditioned medium

H$_3$ Thymidine relase; 120 cpm = ×	
T-cells	×
T-cells + Con A	246 ×
T-cells + Macrophages [a]	0,4 ×
T-cells + CM HD-lines [b][c]	2,4 ×
T-cells + Con A + Macrophages [a]	431 ×
T-cells + Con A + CM HD-lines [b][c]	438 ×

[a] Irradiated.
[b] L 428, L 428 KS, L 540, L 591.
[c] CM = conditioned medium.

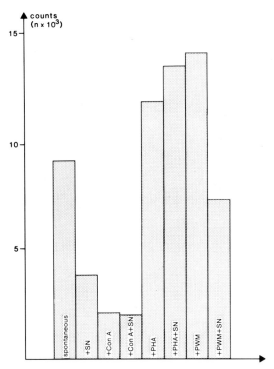

Figure 1. Influence of Hodgkin cell-line (L 428 KSA) supernatants (SN) on spontaneous and PWM induced B-cell proliferation. Mean, n = 5.

Table II. In vitro release of colony stimulation factors by Hodgkin derived cell-lines

Source of CSF[a]	Colonies per 10^5 cells	Colony morphology (P.ox., N.esterase) – day 10 –
L 428	122 (155–126)	> 80% P.ox [b]
L 428 KS	154 (144–162)	> 80% P.ox [b]
L 428 KSA	178 (162–192)	> 90% P.ox [b]
L 540	132 (128–138)	N.T.
L 591	32 (20–44)	N.T.
Standard CSF (I)[c]	178 (174–178)	> 90% P.ox [b]
Standard CSF (II)[c]	162 (160–164)	> 80% P.ox [b]
Ø CSF	Ø (Cluster [++])	

[a] 100 μl CSF/plate was assayed.
[b] Peroxidase pos.
[c] Standard CSF I: Conditioned medium (CM) (human fetal liver cell cultures)
      Standard CSF II: CM of human fetal heart culture.

10

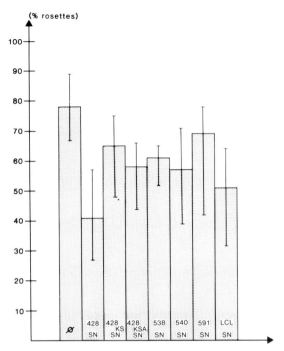

Figure 2. Influence of Hodgkin cell-line supernatants (SN) on E-rosetting capacity of T-lympho-cytes (LCL = lymphoblastoid cell-line). Mean, n = 10.

2. *CSF.* (Table II): Supernatants from cultures of all Hodgkin cell lines (L 428, L 428 KS, L 428 KSA, L 540, L 591) contained significant amounts of CSF [17]. L 428 KSA CM achieved higher activity than standard fetal liver CM. Peroxidase staining was positive for 80–90% of the colonies indicating release of g-CSF. Low concentrations of CSF for eosinophils were present. Hogdkin cell line CM induced myeloproliferation in cord blood suspension cultures and in fetal or adult bone marrow cultures. Constant and constitutively CSF production was confirmed by time-course experiments over a period of 50 days. Short-term production of CSF is widely independent of FCS concentration in the cultures. HD-line CSF has a molecular weight of about 40–60 KD and is heat stable (56 °C).

3. *Suppression of Pokeweed-induced B-cell proliferation.* (Fig. 1): Incubation of T-lymphocytes with L 428 KSA-conditioned medium and subsequent stimulation with Con A or PHA did not affect the stimulative capacity of T-lymphocytes. However, spontaneous and Pokeweed-induced B-cell proliferation was significantly suppressed.

4. *E-rosette inhibiting activity.* (Fig. 2): Most T-lymphocytes (70–80%) from healthy adults can bind SRBC at 4 °C- This capacity is significantly

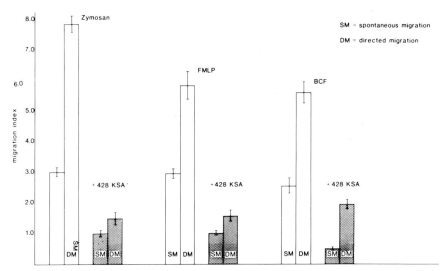

Figure 3. Migration of granulocytes after peincubation (30 min) with supernatants of Hodgkin cell-lines (FMLP = Formyl-methionyl-leucyl-phenylalanin) (BCF = Bacterial chemotactic factor).

impaired when T-lymphocytes and SRBC are incubated overnight in 30% CM (v/v) from L 428 cultures. Binding of SRBC was reduced from 78% to 41%. Suppression was marginal when CM of other cell lines were tested (L 428 KS: 65%, L 428 KSA: 58%, L 538: 61%, L 540: 57%, L 591: 69%).

5. *Migration inhibiting factor (MIF).* (Fig. 3): Serum-free supernatants from L 428 KSA reproducibly inhibit granulocyte migration. This effect is cell-directed. The extent of inhibition of both spontaneous and directed neutrophil migration varies among supernatants, but is always at least 33% and commonly 50% or higher. Inhibition persists after dialysis. Reduced cell-directed migration is observed towards bacterial chemotactic factor,

Table III. Band regions involved in the formation of marker chromosomes

Cell line, patient	1 p 22	2 q 33	7 q 22–36	11 q 21/23	14 q 32	15 p 12	21 q 21
L 428		+	+	+	+		+
L 439	+	+	fra			+	+
L 538/540	+	+	+7	+		+	
L 591			+		+		
KM 4			+				

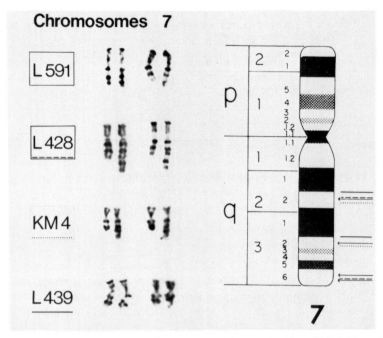

Figure 4. Two pairs of chromosomes 7 from three cell-lines and patient KM 4. Normal chromosomes 7 on the left of each pair. Arrows indicate the breakpoints and fragile sites.

serum-opsonized Zymosan and the synthetic tripeptide n-formyl-methionyl-leucyl-phenylalaline (FMLP). Supernatants from L 428 also exert this inhibitory activity, but those from L 428 KS and L 591 do not.

6. *Cytogenic findings.* Chromosome studies were performed in four Hodgkin-derived cell lines over several years. An attempt was made to differentiate within specific chromosomes the band regions that are involved in the formation of markers and coincide in different cell lines (Table III). The chromosome region most frequently affected by rearrangements was the long arms of chromosome 7, from q22 to q36 (Fig. 4). Cell line L 428 is characterized by a duplication of the segment 7q22 to 7q36. L 591 shows a smaller duplication from 7q32 to 7q36, whereas in L 439, fragile sites were demonstrated in bands 7q22 and 7q32. We also observed a duplicated chromosome 7 segment (7q22 to q32) in bone marrow metastases of a patient who developed secondary myeloid leukemia after Hodgkin's disease (Fonatsch and Holldack, unpublished).

Other structural chromosome abnormalities were found in our four Hodgkin's cell lines (Table III). A break in 2q33 occurred in L 428, L 439 and L 538/L 540, followed by a loss of long arm material without translocation in L 428, and associated with translocations in the other lines. The following chromosome aberrations were also observed. Identical deletions in chromosome 1 – del [1] (p22) – in L 439 and L 538/L 540; deletions in 11q21/23 in L 428 and L 538/L 540; 14q$^+$ chromosomes with breakpoint in 14q32 in L 428 and L 591; rearranged chromosomes 15 (breakpoint in 15p12) in L 439 and L 538/L 540; and identical deletions in chromosomes 21 – del [21] (q21) – in L 428 and L 439.

Discussion

Despite extensive investigation, there is no consensus about the origin and nature of the malignant cells in Hodgkin's disease. Establishment of five cell lines representing the *in vitro* counterparts of the *in vivo* malignant H and SR cells enabled us to perform cytochemical, immunologic, virologic and cytogenetic studies. Their *in vitro* behavior is consistent with findings in freshly sampled H and SR cells. The histogenic source of the H and SR cells could not be determined. The cell lines presented markers also found on T-cells, B-cells, granulocytes and macrophages [8]. Some markers are detected in *all* cell lines (positivity with monoclonal antibodies Ki 1, HD 5/6, TAC, ANAE-positivity, lack of phagocytosis or immunoglobulins, CSF production). Other characteristics are less consistently observed (OKT 11-, OKT 8-, 3C4-, TO 15- positivity, presence or absence of EBV or C3 receptors). Furthermore, the marker spectrum can be modified by culture conditions, such as FCS concentration, nude mouse passage or TPA exposure. It is possible that there is no consistent marker pattern of *in vivo* H and SR cells and that surface or functional characteristics are dependent on the microenvironment.

Further experiments were carried out to define functional activities and mediators produced by HD cell lines. Results clearly indicate the generation of mediators involved in immunologic responses and regulation of hematopoiesis. All cell lines produced significant amounts of CSF, which induces proliferation and differentiation of progenitor cells. In addition, when activated lymphocytes release CSF, it is capable of inducing macrophages to produce secondary mediators such as interferon, prostaglandins and IL 1 [18].

IL 1-like activity is generated by all Hodgkin cell lines (with the exception of L 428 KSA, a TPA-induced line), as demonstrated by a monocyte-depleted lymphocyte co-stimulation assay [12]. IL 1 may serve as a non-specific signal in T-cell activation. Non-immunologic effects include induction of hypothalamic fever [19] and potentiation of fibroblast growth [18].

Pokeweed-induced proliferation of B-lymphocytes was suppressed after incubation with L 428 KSA conditioned medium. This might correspond to observations of impaired B-cell function in patients with HD [20].

T-lymphocytes of patients with HD show decreased binding of SRBC [5].

14

This phenomenon is due to an inhibitory, low-density lipoprotein isolated from the spleen in HD patients [7]. The relationship between this mediator and the observed E-rosette-inhibiting activity in culture supernatants needs to be investigated.

MIF, which influences motility of normal granulocytes, is present in sera of patients with lymphoproliferative disorders. MIF activity could be demonstrated in culture supernatants of L 428 KSA.

Freshly biopsied H and SR cells were reported to produce IL 1 [21] and a growth-promoting activity for fibroblasts [22]. This demonstrates that the production of lymphokines and monokines in HD is not only a matter of culture conditions. These factors might influence immunologic cooperation and regulation *in vivo* by distubring the immunologic network. Various *in vivo* manifestations of impaired immunity have been described and *in vitro* abnormalities in T-lymphocytes are well established. Whether these factors and activities account for these abnormalities is under investigation. One could speculate whether mediator production can influence the cytologic and histologic composition and admixture of non-malignant cells in HD lymph nodes and whether certain clinical features are due to some of the described factors.

All our cell lines were derived from patients who underwent chemotherapy with alkylating agents (COPP). Therefore, chemical mutagenesis in all or some of the marker chromosomes cannot be ruled out. Further cytogenetic investigations, in combination with DNA recombinant techniques, will help clarify whether those chromosomal regions, which are nonrandomly involved in marker formation in both our Hodgkin-derived cell cultures and in directly prepared bone marrow, correspond to hot spots that are specifically vulnerable and characteristic for Hodgkin's disease.

Acknowledgements

We thank Ms. Boie, Ms. Lux, and Ms. Helbing for skillful technical assistance, and Ms. Koester and Mr. Grassen for the preparation of the manuscript. This work was supported by Deutsche Forschungsgemeinschaft and by Stiftung Deutsche Krebshilfe.

References

1. Kaplan HS (1981). On the biology and immunology of Hodgkin's disease. Hematology and Blood Transfusion 26:11–23.
2. Reed DM (1902). On the pathological changes in Hodgkin's disease with especial reference to its relation to tuberculosis. Johns Hopkins Hosp Rep 10:133–196.
3. Twomey JJ and Rice L (1980). Impact of Hodgkin's disease on the immune system. Semin Oncol 7:114–125.

4. Kaplan HS (1980). Hodgkin's disease: Unfolding concepts concerning its nature, management and prognosis. Cancer 45:2439–2474.

5. Fuks Z, Strober S, King DP and Kaplan HS (1976). Reversal of cell surface abnormalities of T-lymphocytes in Hodgkin's disease after *in vitro* incubation in fetal sera. J Immunol 117:1331–1335.

6. Goodwin JS, Messner RP, Bankhurst AD et al. (1977). Prostaglandin-producing suppressor cells in Hodgkin's disease. N Engl J Med 297:963–968.

7. Bieber MM, King DP, Strober S and Kaplan HS (1979). Characterization of an E-rosette inhibitor (ERI) in the serum of patients with Hodgkin's disease, as a glycolipid. Clin Res 27:081A.

8. Diehl V, Kirchner HH, Burrichter H et al. (1982). Characteristics of Hodgkin's disease – derived cell lines. Cancer Treat Rep 66:615–632.

9. Schaadt M, Diehl V, Stein H et al. (1980). Two neoplastic cell lines with unique features derived from Hodgkin's disease. Int J Cancer 26:723–731.

10. Bradley TR and Metcalf D (1966). The growth of mouse bone marrow cells *in vitro*. Austr J Exp Biol Sci 44:287–300.

11. Heit W, Rich IN and Kubanek B (1981). Macrophage-dependent production of erythropoietin and colony-stimulating factor. Hematology and Blood Transfusion 27:73–78.

12. Kortmann C, Burrichter H, Monner D et al. (1984). Interleukin-1-like activity constitutively generated by Hodgkin derived cell lines. 1. Measurement in a human lymphocyte co-stimulator assay. Immunobiology 166:318–333.

13. Schaadt M, Diehl V, Kalden JR et al. (1978). Langzeitauswirkungen der Splenektomie auf den immunstatus von Hodgkin-Patienten in Abhängigkeit von der Therapieform. Med Klinik 73:1381–1386.

14. Jondal M, Holm G and Wigzell H (1972). Surface markers on human T- and B-lymphocytes. J Exp Med 136:207–215.

15. Nelson RD, McCormack RT and Fiegel VD (1978). Chemotaxis of human leucocytes under agarose. In: Gallin JI and Quie PG (Eds.) Leukocyte Chemotaxis, pp 25–42.

16. Oppenheim JJ, Stadler BM, Siraganian RP et al. (1982). Lymphokines: Their role in lymphocyte responses. Properties of interleukin 1. Fed Proc 41: 257–262.

17. Burrichter H, Heit W, Schaadt M et al. (1983). Production of colony-stimulating factors by Hodgkin cell lines. Int J Cancer 31:269–274.

18. Farrar JJ and Hilfiker ML (1982). Antigen-nonspecific helper factors in the antibody response. Fed Proc 41:263–268.

19. Murphy PA, Simon PL and Willoughby WF (1980). Endogenous pyrogens made by rabbit peritoneal exudate cells are identical with lymphocyte-activating factors made by rabbit alveolar macrophages. J Immunol 124:2498–2501.

20. Ruehl H, Enders B, Bur M and Sieber G (1981). Impaired B-lymphocyte reactivity in patients with Hodgkin's disease and non-Hodgkin's lymphomas. Blut 42:271.

21. Ford RJ, Mehta S, Davis F and Maizel A (1982). Growth factors in Hodgkin's disease. Cancer Treat Rep 66:633–638.

22. Newcom SR and O'Rourke L (1982). Potentiation of fibroblast growth by nodular sclerosing Hodgkin's disease cell cultures. Blood 60:228–237.

3. Origin and biologic function of Reed-Sternberg cells

R. I. FISHER[1], S. E. BATES[1], D. J. VOLKMAN[2], V. DIEHL[3],
T. T. HECHT[1] and D. L. LONGO[1]
*From the [1] Medicine Branch, National Cancer Institute and
[2] National Institute of Allergy and Infectious Diseases, Bethesda,
Maryland, USA, and [3] Medizinische Hochschule, Hannover, FRG*

For many years it has been well known that untreated patients with Hodgkin's disease of all stages had significant impairment of their cellular immune response, as manifested *in vivo* by impaired delayed hypersensitivity skin tests, and *in vitro* by decreased E rosette formation as well as decreased T-cell proliferation in response to mitogens or antigens. Abnormalities of cellular immunity were always more pronounced in patients with advanced stages of disease. In contrast, significant abnormalities of humoral immunity have not been detected. These early studies have been reviewed in detail [1, 2].

The mechanism of the immune suppressor has been more difficult to define. Although the number of peripheral blood E rosette forming cells is reduced, the deficit in cellular immunity cannot be attributed simply to a reduced number of circulating T-cells. Studies with heterologous and monoclonal antibodies against T-cell antigens have revealed normal numbers of circulating T-cells, except in patients with very extensive disease [3, 4]. Increased suppressor monocyte activity [5, 6], increased suppressor T-cell activity [7, 8], and increased circulating soluble suppressor substances [9, 10] have all been implicated as causes of the depressed cellular immunity. However, those studies have not provided full explanation for the abnormalities of cellular immunity. Although the increased suppressor monocyte activity was originally thought to be mediated by prostaglandins [5], subsequent studies have demonstrated that increased prostaglandin production accounts for only a small proportion of the immunologic suppression [11, 12]. Studies using monoclonal antibodies to identify helper and suppressor T-cell subsets have failed to reveal significant imbalances in helper to suppressor ratios [4].

Thus, studies that revealed increased suppressor T-cell activity [7, 8] cannot explain the immunosuppression on the basis of altered numbers of suppressor cells. Studies conducted in our laboratory have demonstrated that the effector T-cells from untreated patients with Hodgkin's disease are highly sensitive to the suppressive effects of two normal immunoregulatory cells, i.e., suppressor monocytes and suppressor T-cells [13, 14]. This qualitative difference in the response of T-cells to suppressor cells may partially explain this defect in T-cell effector function.

Furthermore, one can never be certain whether the effects observed in these assays are the result of Hodgkin's disease or a potential cause of the development of Hodgkin's disease in a given patient. In that regard, we have demonstrated that many of the abnormalities of cellular immunity persist in patients cured of Hodgkin's disease by combination chemotherapy, and are not detected in long-term disease-free survivors of another malignant lymphoma treated with similar combination chemotherapy [15]. The persistent T-cell abnormalities may be either a permanent immunologic deficit acquired with the development of Hodgkin's disease or an inherent genetically determined characteristic of the patient who develops Hodgkin's disease.

Obviously, the abnormalities in various assays do not provide a simple explanation for the immunologic deficit. Studies of peripheral blood lymphocytes may not accurately reflect the status of the immune system in other sites. Therefore, research now emphasizes improvement of our understanding of the immunologic function of the malignant cell in Hodgkin's disease, and the relationship of that cell to depressed cellular immunity. These studies have been made possible by the development of a long-term tissue culture line of Reed-Sternberg cells. Reed-Sternberg cells stimulate a mixed lymphocyte reaction, function as accessory cells for mitogen induced human T-cell proliferative responses, and present soluble antigens to T-cells in a genetically restricted fashion. Based on these characteristics, Hodgkin's disease may be defined as a malignant tumor of antigen-presenting cells.

The L428 Hodgkin's disease cell line

Attempts to determine the origin and biologic function of the malignant Reed-Sternberg cell in Hodgkin's disease have been hampered by the inability to obtain long-term tissue cultures lines of Hodgkin's disease cells. In 1978, Diehl and colleagues established a cell line termed L428, derived from the pleural effusion of a patient with nodular sclerosing Hodgkin's disease [16]. This cell line now has been extensively analyzed and there is convincing evidence that the L428 cell line is a long-term culture of Hodgkin's disease cells. The morphology of these cells is identical to that of Reed-Sternberg cells or their mononuclear counterparts. When injected intracranially into nude mice, these cells produce a tumor infiltrate resembling Hodgkin's disease. The cells are aneuploid with characteristic chromosomal abnormalities and lack EBV-associated antigens. The L428 cells

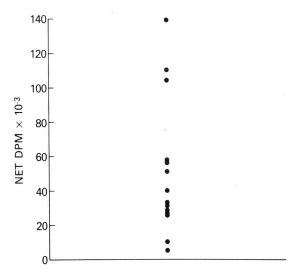

Figure 1. MLC response of normal donor peripheral blood MNL when stimulated by L428 cells. 2×10^5 MNL were cultured with 1×10^4 radiated L428 cells. Each dot represents the proliferative response of a different normal donor.

do not express any of the cell surface markers that define mature T-cells, B-cells, or monocytes. They lack cell surface immunoglobulin, complement receptors, Fc receptors, and do not rosette with sheep erythrocytes; however they do express significant amounts of Ia-like antigens and have multiple dendritic processes [3]. In addition, the L428 cells are not phagocytic, and stain weakly for nonspecific esterase and acid phosphatase. These characteristics are all present on Reed-Sternberg cells in fresh tissue sections [17].

L428 cells are potent stimulators of human primary mixed lymphocyte cultures

We have demonstrated that the cell line termed L428 is a potent stimulator of the primary human mixed lymphocyte reaction [18]. Significant proliferation occurred when mononuclear leukocytes (MNL) obtained from normal donors were stimulated with radiated L428 cells at responder:stimulator ratios varying from 200:1 to 20:1. Proliferative responses occurred between days 3 and 6 of the cultures, with maximal proliferation on day 5. Under optimal culture conditions, the mean net proliferative response of 14 normal donors was $51,000 \pm 10,600$ dpm. Moreover, there was also great variation in the proliferative responses to L428 cells of responder MNL obtained from random normal donors (Fig. 1). This was expected in view of varying degrees of histoincompatability between donors and L428 cells.

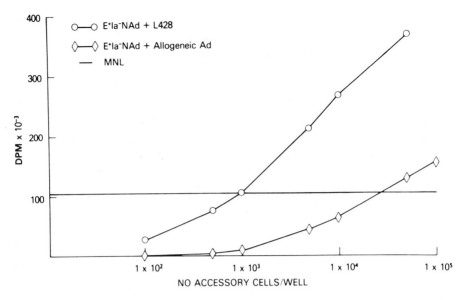

Figure 2. Dose response curve of L428 cells as accessory cells. 2×10^5 MNL or 2×10^5 E$^+$Ia$^-$NAd cells (T-cells) plus varying numbers of radiated L428 cells are cultured for 72 hours with 10 µg/ml concanavalin A. Also shown is the result of adding varying numbers of radiated allogeneic adherent cells to the E$^+$Ia$^-$NAd cells under identical conditions.

The MLC response between normal donors and the L428 cells was totally abrogated by concentrations of monoclonal anti-Ia antibodies which had no effect on the mitogen-induced proliferative response of the same MNL. Antigen processing by responder monocytes or Ia-positive cells was not required for the MLC. The cells that proliferated in response to stimulation by the L428 cells were T-cells, primarily of the helper subset. No IL 1 activity could be detected in concentrated supernatants of L428 cultures after stimulation of L428 cells by mitogens, phorbol esters, or muramyl dipeptide, or in the MLC. All of these cultures contain fetal calf serum. However, the L428 cells are capable of producing IL 1 when stimulated with LPS in the absence of fetal calf serum. These results, with the exception of the IL 1 data, are similar to results obtained when other antigen-presenting cells such as monocytes, dendritic cells or Langerhans cells have been used to stimulate primary mixed lymphocyte cultures.

L428 cells function as accessory cells for mitogen-induced, human T-cell proliferative responses

Purified human peripheral blood T-cells depleted of Ia-bearing cells and adherent cells do not proliferate in response to concanavalin A. The addition of 1% radiated L428 tumor cells reconstituted the proliferative response of the T-cells to a level comparable to that achieved with unfractionated MNL [19] (Fig. 2). When greater numbers of L428 tumor cells were added, the proliferative response was higher than that of the MNL. The L428 cells were approximately 30 times more potent than allogeneic adherent cells in reconstituting the response. The response of the T-cells plus the L428 cells followed the same time course and the response to various doses of concanavalin A was similar to the responses of MNL or T-cells plus allogeneic adherent cells. The increased proliferative response in the presence of the L428 cells as compared to that of the allogeneic adherent cells was not due to suppression of the cultures containing adherent cells by prostaglandins; the addition of indomethacin to cultures containing adherent cells did not result in increased stimulation. Although monoclonal anti-Ia antibody totally blocked allogeneic stimulation, the mitogen-induced proliferative responses of the MNL or the T-cells plus L428 cells were unaffected by concentrations of anti-Ia antibody that saturated the Ia receptors on the L428 cells. This raises the possibility that, although an Ia-positive cell may be required as an accessory cell for mitogen-induced T-cell proliferative responses, direct interaction with the Ia molecule may not be necessary. Furthermore, neither supernatants from the L428 cell cultures nor human IL 1 could replace the accessory cells in generating a significant concanavalin A induced T-cell proliferative response.

The accessory cell function of the L428 cells also permitted study of the mitogen-induced proliferative response of purified T-cells from patients with Hodgkin's disease [19]. T-cells from patients were purified until they had no evidence of monocytes and were functionally unable to respond to mitogens. The L428 cells were then added to the patient T-cells and the proliferative response was compared to the proliferative response of normal donor T-cells plus L428 cells. In this system, evaluation of T-cell proliferation was independent of any suppressive effects of patient monocytes. As expected, patient MNL proliferation in the presence of concanavalin A was

Table I. Proliferative response to concanavalin A[a]

	Normal controls	Poor prognosis patients	p value
Peripheral blood Mononuclear leukocytes	91,000± 17,000	44,000± 18,000	0.002
T-Cells + 1×10^3 L 428	57,000± 12,000	36,000± 13,000	0.04
T-Cells + 1×10^4 L 428	209,000± 40,000	126,000± 55,000	0.009

[a] Mean ^{3}H-thymidine incorporation ± SEM.

suppressed in the entire population, primarily due to the suppression in patients with massive mediastinal disease, or with Stage IIIB or IV disease (poor prognosis group) (Table I). T-cells from patients with Stage I, II, or IIIA (good prognosis group) proliferated normally in the presence of the L428 tumor cells and concanavalin A. This suggests that the T-cells of these patients, as examined by this assay, can function normally. The T-cells from patients with poor prognosis disease show impaired mitogenic responses in the presence of the accessory cell (Table I). This impairment of mitogen-induced proliferation, compared to age and sex-matched normal controls, was seen when various numbers of accessory cells were utilized, at all doses of concanavalin A, and regardless of the duration of the culture. The magnitude of the reduction in T-cell proliferation in the presence of the L428 accessory cells was comparable to that observed when mononuclear leukocytes from these patients were stimulated with concanavalin A. Although a small number of patients have been studied an inherent T-cell defect is suggested in patients with advanced Hodgkin's disease.

L428 cells present soluble antigen to T-cells

L428 cells are capable of presenting soluble antigen to T-cells in a genetically restricted fashion [20]. T-cell lines were established from normal donors previously immunized with tetanus toxoid. The T-cells utilized were incapable of tetanus toxoid-induced proliferation unless antigen presenting cells were added to the cultures. The L428 cells expressed HLA-DR 5. T-cells from the two normal HLA-DR 5 donors demonstrated significant proliferative responses when cultured with tetanus toxoid and L428 cells. No proliferative response was observed when the L428 cells were used as antigen-presenting cells for T-cell lines of other DR types. The tetanus toxoid dose response curves were similar, regardless of whether autologous mononuclear leukocytes or L428 cells were used as antigen-presenting cells. T-cell proliferation induced by soluble antigen was also blocked by anti-Ia antibody.

Origin of Reed-Sternberg cells

Functionally, Hodgkin's disease cells can be classified as antigen-presenting cells. However, the exact cell of origin remains undefined. Antigen-presenting cell function has been demonstrated classically in isolated monocyte preparations, yet the L428 cells differ from monocytes in that they lack monocyte cell surface markers, Fc and complement receptors, phagocytosis and strong staining for nonspecific esterase and acid phosphatase. Antigen-presenting cell function has also been described in Langerhans cells, but the

L428 cells lack Fc and complement receptors and do not stain with the OK T6 monoclonal antibody that binds to the Langerhans cell (unpublished data). L428 cells have all of the known characteristics of human dendritic cells which have been shown to be antigen-presenting cells [21]. However, because of the lack of a positive marker to define human dendritic cells, the relationship of the L428 cells to dendritic cells cannot be conclusively resolved.

Monoclonal antibody to Reed-Sternberg cells

A murine monoclonal antibody, termed HeFi-1, was produced following immunization with the L428 Hodgkin's disease tissue culture cell line [22]. HeFi-1 selectively stained only the Reed-Sternberg or Hodgkin's cells in 18/18 cases of Hodgkin's disease including the nodular sclerosis, mixed cellularity, and lymphocyte depleted histologic subtypes. HeFi-1 did not stain any cells in normal lung, brain, salivary gland, thyroid, gallbladder, pancreas, liver, testis, breast, endometrium, or kidney. However, rare large cells at the edge of the lymphoid follicles were stained in normal tonsil, colon, and hyperplastic thymus. The identity of these cells is unknown but they may represent precursors of the Reed-Sternberg cells. There was no staining of any cells in 14 cases of B-cell non-Hodgkin's lymphoma; however, the malignant cells in 3/11 cases of non-Hodgkin's lymphoma that appeared to express T-cell markers were also stained with HeFi-1. Whether these putative T-cell lymphomas are actually non-Hodgkin's lymphomas, or lymphocytes depleted Hodgkin's disease, remains to be determined. A similar pattern of staining has been reported with another monoclonal antibody to the L428 cells [23]. Modulation of the HeFi-1 cell surface antigen on the L428 cells was not observed. HeFi-1 specifically immunoprecipitated a cell surface protein of approximately 120,000 daltons from the L428 cell line. The HeFi-1 monoclonal antibody should prove useful not only in the diagnosis, staging, and potential therapy of Hodgkin's disease, but also in determining the Reed-Sternberg cell origin.

References

1. Kaplan HS (1980). Hodgkin's Disease. Cambridge, Mass.: Harvard University Press.
2. Twomey JJ and Rice L (1980). Impact of Hodgkin's disease upon the immune system. Semin Oncol 7:114–125.
3. Bobrove AM, Fuks Z, Strober S and Kaplan HS (1975). Quantitation of T and B lymphocytes and cellular immune function in Hodgkin's disease. Cancer 36:169–179.
4. Posner MR, Reinherz EL, Berard J et al. (1981). Lymphoid subpopulations of peripheral blood and spleen in untreated Hodgkin's disease. Cancer 48:1170–1176.

24

5. Goodwin JS, Messner RP and Peake GT (1977). Prostaglandin producing suppressor cells in Hodgkin's disease. N Engl J Med 297:963–968.
6. Twomey JJ, Laughter AH and Farrow S (1975). Hodgkin's disease: An immunodepleting and immunosuppressive disorder. J Clin Invest 56:467–475.
7. Engleman EG, Benike C and Hoppe RT (1979). Suppressor cells of the mixed lymphocyte reaction in patients with Hodgkin's disease. Transplant Proc 4:1827–1829.
8. Hellinger SM and Herzig GP (1978). Impaired cell-mediated immunity in Hodgkin's disease mediated by suppressor lymphocytes and monocytes. J Clin Invest 61:1620–1627.
9. Fuks Z, Strober S and Kaplan HS (1976). Interaction between serum factors and T-lymphocytes in Hodgkin's disease: Use as a diagnostic test. N Engl J Med 295:1273–1278.
10. Fuks Z, Strober S and King DP (1976). Reversal of cell surface abnormalities of T-lymphocytes in Hodgkin's disease after *in vitro* incubation in fetal sera. J Immunol 117:1331–1335.
11. Deshazo RD, Ewel C, Londono S et al. (1981). Evidence for the involvement of monocyte-derived toxic oxygen metabolites in the lymphocyte dysfunction of Hodgkin's disease. Clin Exp Immunol 46:313–320.
12. Fisher RI and Bostick-Bruton F (1982). Depressed T-cell proliferative responses in Hodgkin's disease: Role of monocyte-mediated suppression via prostaglandins and hydrogen peroxide. J Immunol 129:1770–1774.
13. Fisher RI, Vanhaelen C and Bostick F (1981). Increased sensitivity to normal adherent suppressor cells in advanced Hodgkin's disease. Blood 57:830–835.
14. Vanhaelen CPJ and Fisher RI (1981).Increased sensitivity of lymphocytes from patients with Hodgkin's disease to concanavalin A-induced suppressor cells. J Immunol 127:1216–1220.
15. Fisher RI (1982). Implications of persistent T-cell abnormalities for the etiology of Hodgkin's disease. Cancer Treat Rep 66:681–688.
16. Schaadt N, Diehl V, Stein H et al. (1980). Two neoplastic cell lines with unique features derived from Hodgkin's disease. Int J Cancer 26:723–731.
17. Diehl V, Kirchner HH, Burrichter H et al. (1982). Characteristics of Hodgkin derived cell lines. Cancer Treat Rep 66:615–632.
18. Fisher RI, Bostick-Bruton F, Sauder DN et al. (1983). Neoplastic cells obtained from Hodgkin's disease are potent stimulators of human primary mixed lymphocyte cultures. J Immunol 130:2666–2670.
19. Fisher RI, Bates SE, Bostick-Bruton F et al (1984). Neoplastic cells obtained from Hodgkin's disease function as accessory cells for mitogen-induced human T-cell proliferative responses. J Immunol 132:2672–2677.
20. Fisher RI, Diehl V and Volkman DJ (1984). Hodgkin's disease is a tumor of antigen-presenting cells. Proc Amer Assoc Cancer Res 25:193.
21. Van Voorhis WC, Hair LS, Steinman RN and Kaplan G (1982). Human dendritic cells. Enrichment and characterization from peripheral blood. J Exp Med 155:1172–1187.
22. Hecht TT, Longo DL, Coggman J et al. (1984). Production and characterization of a monoclonal antibody that selectively binds Reed-Sternberg cells. J Immunol (in press).
23. Schwab U, Stein H, Gerdes J et al. (1982). Production of a monoclonal antibody specific for Hodgkin's and Sternberg-Reed cells of Hodgkin's disease and a subset of normal lymphoid cells. Nature 299:65–67.

4. Immunologic phenotypes of non-Hodgkin's lymphomas: Correlation with morphology and function

E. S. JAFFE, O. J. COSSMAN, L. M. NECKERS, R. M. BRAZIEL
and C. R. SIMRELL
*Laboratory of Pathology, National Cancer Institute, Bethesda,
Maryland, USA*

The non-Hodgkin's lymphomas (NHL) represent multiple diseases with diverse morphologic and clinical expressions. Morphologic classification schemes such as that proposed by Rappaport have been shown to be useful in predicting the clinical course [1]. However, in some instances distinctive morphologic entities may be very closely related clinically and/or biologically, whereas other diseases that share morphologic similarities may be clinically and biologically quite distinct (Table I). The application of mod-

Table I. Non-Hodgkin's lymphomas and related disorders

Summary of usual cell surface markers	
Small lymphocytic	usually B
with plasmacytoid features	B
Lymphocytic lymphoma,	B
intermediate differentiation	B
Follicular lymphomas	B
Diffuse, small cleaved cell	B
Diffuse mixed small and large cell	both B & T
Diffuse, large cell	usually B
Large cell, immunoblastic	75% T
	25% B
	Rare true histiocyte
Small non-cleaved cell	
Burkitt's	B
Non-Burkitt's	usually B
Lymphoblastic lymphomas	80% T + pre-T
	10% pre-B
	10% pre-pre-B
Mycosis fungoides/Sezary syndrome	T
Adult T cell leukemia/lymphoma	T

ern immunologic techniques and concepts has enabled us to develop a conceptual framework which we may use to decipher the morphologic diversity of these neoplasms [2]. This review will focus on the non-Hodgkin's lymphomas presenting primarily in adult life.

NHL are fascinating and instructive models when viewed as neoplasms of the immune system. The spectrum of B-cell lymphomas reflects the functional and anatomic heterogeneity of the normal humoral immune system. The neoplastic cells often retain the morphologic, functional, and migratory characteristics of their normal counterparts. Likewise, the functional heterogeneity of the T-cell system is reflected in its malignant expressions; malignant clonal expansions have been useful in the identification of normal cellular phenotypes not previously recognized.

In addition to immunologic phenotype, NHL can be classified according to their clinical grade. Most classification schemes and clinical protocols recognize two broad categories: favorable or low-grade and unfavorable or high-grade [3]. The low-grade lymphomas include the small lymphocytic malignancies and most follicular lymphomas in the Working Formulation [4]. Studies have contrasted the clinical behavior of these lesions, which, paradoxically, leads to a significant potential for cure and long-term survival for the high-grade lymphomas. In contrast, although the low-grade lymphomas have an indolent natural history, they are rarely, if ever, cured. In addition to the clinical differences between low-grade and high-grade lymphomas, the pathologic and experimental characteristics of these tumors can also be contrasted (Table II). These differences have prompted an analogy of the low-grade lymphomas as the benign tumors of the lymphoid system [15].

Table II. Pathologic and experimental characteristics of low grade and high grade malignant lymphomas

Low grade	High grade
1. Non-destructive growth pattern	1. Destructive growth pattern
2. Absence of cellular atypia	2. Presence of cellular atypia/anaplasia
3. Respect privileged sites	3. Invade privileged sites
4. Respond to regulatory influences	4. Autonomous
5. Fail to grow in culture	5. Immortalized in culture
6. Non-transplantable	6. Transplantable in immunodeficient host

Low-grade B-cell lymphomas

Well-differentiated or small lymphocytic malignancies (WDL)

The majority of these low grade lymphomas are monoclonal B-cell proliferations. The predominant surface immunoglobulin (sIg) is IgM with either κ or λ light chains [6]. IgD frequently coexists with IgM. The sIg is of low density, often difficult to detect, and the density of sIg in a given case is usually very homogenous. In some patients spontaneous differentiation toward plasma cells with concomitant immunosecretion may occur, i.e., Waldenstrom's macroglobulinemia [7]. Complement receptors are also present on the neoplastic cells with a predominance of receptors for C3d [8]. Morphologically, clinically, and immunologically, WDL and chronic lymphocytic leukemia (CLL) are closely related.

WDL appears to represent a block in B-cell differentiation. The non-neoplastic T-lymphocytes in some patients with CLL have defective helper-cell activity, which may be related to the differentiation blockade [9]. This helper-cell defect may also contribute to the hypogammaglobulinemia of CLL. In contrast to CLL, Waldenstrom's macro-globulinemia does not appear to be associated with a defect in helper cells. *In vitro* studies have shown that most cases of CLL and WDL tested are capable of proceeding to the state of abundant immunoglobulin secretion when stimulated by phorbol ester (TPA) in culture [10]. This indicates that these cells are arrested at a preterminal stage of B-cell differentiation, but retain the capacity to differentiate when appropriate signals are provided. The reason why these cells don't differentiate *in vivo* is not known.

Using monoclonal antibodies, typical CLL cells express a 65,000 dalton antigen (T65) normally found on T-cells identified with Leu 1, T101, and other similarly reactive antibodies [11, 12]. This antigen is rarely found on normal B-cells [13], and is never found on the cells of follicular lymphomas [14]. It is also not found on the cells of Waldenstrom's macroglobulinemia [12]. Some cases of CLL and WDL express the so-called common, acute lymphoblastic leukemia antigen, CALLA. CLL and WDL cells also react with monoclonal antibodies B1, BA1, and HLA-DE (Ia). We have recently determined that sIg, B1, and BA1, but not HLA-DR, are expressed in lower density in CLL-WDL than in IDL or follicular center cell lymphoma (FCC). The decreasing sequence of density of each of the first three markers proceeds as follows: FCC > IDL > WDL. Those same three markers are progressively lost as normal B-cells differentiate into plasma cells [15–18]. This suggests a sequential differentiation pathway for these three types of low grade B-cell lymphomas in man [14].

Lymphocytic lymphoma, intermediate differentiation (ML, INT)

Pathologically and immunologically ML, INT are intermediate between WDL and follocular lymphoma (FL) [19]. This too is a B-cell malignancy with abundant monoclonal sIg and avid C3 receptors. The cells have membrane-associated alkaline phosphatase activity, a feature also seen in lymphocytes of the primary follicle and lymphoid cuff [20].

The ratio of the number of cells bearing only C3d receptors to the total number of cells bearing complement receptors, for normal B-cells and the B-cells of FL, is approximately 0.3. However, for the cells of ML, INT and CLL/WDL this ratio is approximately 0.6 [8]. In this respect the cells of ML, INT resemble those of CLL/WDL.

Using monoclonal antibodies, the cells of ML, INT express T65 found on CLL cells as well as CALLA found on the cells of FL [14]. Thus, the cells of ML, INT have an intermediate antigenic phenotype. These cells also express B1, BA1, and BA2.

A higher proportion of cases of ML, INT synthesize λ sIg than other B-cell lymphomas, which usually express monoclonal κ. This feature also has been described for centrocytic lymphomas in the Kiel classification, which share many morphologic and phenotypic characteristics with ML, INT [21]. These lesions are probably closely related, if not identical.

Follicular (nodular) lymphomas (FL)

FL is the neoplastic equivalent of the lymphoid follicle [22]. The cells have B-cells features, regardless of cytologic subtype. The different cytologic subtypes also show identical surface markers [19]. Clinical and pathologic differences among subtypes appear to reflect kinetic differences of the various cell types. sIg is usually very abundant and the predominant immunoglobulin class is IgM. The C3 receptor is easily detected both in cell suspensions and in frozen tissue sections, and receptors for both C3b and C3d are present [8]. The cells are B1 and BA1 positive, and approximately 60% of cases express CALLA (with the J5 antibody) [14]. The neoplastic cells do not react with Leu 1 or T101, in contrast to WDL, CLL, and ML, INT [14].

Variable numbers of cytologically normal T-lymphocytes are present, and can be identified within, as well as between, the neoplastic follicles [19, 23]. The ratio of helper to suppressor T-cells, as identified by monoclonal antibodies, does not differ from that in normal lymph nodes [23, 24]. Although the T-cells are phenotypically normal, and do not appear to be a part of the neoplastic process, they may play a regulatory role vis-a-vis the neoplastic cells. Although the cells of FL usually do not spontaneously secrete Ig, they can be induced to secrete *in vitro* after removal of autologous T cells and replacement with allogenic T cells [24].

High-grade lymphomas

Diffuse aggressive lymphomas

Diffuse aggressive lymphomas include, in the Working Formulation, tumors of the mixed small and large cell as well as small non-cleaved (non-Burkitt) subtypes. They represent a morphologic end point for transformed cells of diverse origins. Clinically they are aggressive but, if a complete remission is obtained, it is likely to be sustained with a potential for long-term cure [25]. In keeping with the transformed or dedifferentiated nature of the neoplastic cells, they fail to demonstrate the homing patterns characteristic of low-grade B-cell or T-cell lymphomas, and have a destructive growth pattern.

Approximately 60% of these tumors have B-cell markers [26]. Cytologically, such tumors are often composed of the follicular center cell types described by Lukes and Collins: large cleaved, large non-cleaved, and small non-cleaved (Table III) [27, 28]. These tumors may occur as a manifestation of progression of a FL, or may apparently occur *de novo*. Cytologically and immunologically, such lesions cannot be distinguished. We have recently observed two patients with large-cell lymphoma who, having achieved a complete remission, relapsed at 5 and 9 years respectively with FL, mixed-cell type. This observation, plus the finding of coexistent FL at presentation in approximately 15% of patients with large-cell lymphomas, suggests that many, if not most, of these B-cell lesions are part of the spectrum of FL.

About 35% of diffuse lymphomas have mature T-cell markers and would be included in the broad category of peripheral T-cell lymphomas (PTL) (Table IV) [26–28]. Although morphologically heterogeneous, common histologic features include a polymorphous background, a prominent vascular component, and the presence of large cells with prominent nucleoli [29]. Although such features may suggest a diagnosis of Hodgkin's disease, the cytologic atypia of the smaller lymphoid cells, and the rarity of Reed-Sternberg-like cells, are features distinguishing these lesions from Hodgkin's disease. In another subtype composed predominantly of larger cells, an inflam-

Table III. Diffuse aggressive lymphomas

	Diagnoses in Working Formulation correlated with immunotype			
	B	*T*	*H*	*Null*
Mixed cell	1	10	—	1
Large cell	19	—	—	—
Immunoblastic	5	14	1	1
Small non-cleaved	6	1	—	—

matory background is usually not evident. The cells may have abundant pale cytoplasm, distinct cytoplasmic membranes, and highly convoluted or multi-lobated nuclei [30]. The nuclear chromatin is fine and evenly distributed, and nucleoli are small and inconspicuous. The pleomorphism of the process is amplified by the marked range in cell size.

When characterized by monoclonal antibodies, the cells of PTL are mature T-lymphocytes. They lack TdT and usually express either a helper or suppressor phenotype [28, 31]. However, these antigens are not clonal markers and should not be interpreted as such. For reasons not understood, the majority of PTL express the antigens identified by OKT4 and/or anti-Leu3a, indicative of the helper subtype. A characteristic and useful diagnostic feature is that the cells of PTL often express aberrant T-cell phenotypes [32]. For example, they may react with only one of several pan-T monoclonal antibodies. Thus, 3A1, an antibody that reacts with the vast majority of normal T cells, is negative in most cases of PTL.

The clinical presentation of PTL is usually one of generalized lymphadenopathy, often with hepatosplenomegaly. 'B' symptoms are frequent. In the National Cancer Institute (NCI) series, 80% of patients had Stage IV disease. Most frequent sites of extranodal disease included skin, liver, and bone marrow. Pulmonary involvement is also common. The natural history of the disease is acute or subacute, but in the NCI experience, those patients with T-cell markers had a similar complete remission rate to the forms of

Table IV. Classification of post-thymic T-cell malignancies

I.	T-cell chronic lymphocytic leukemia helper suppressor prolymphocytic
II.	Mycosis fungoides/Sezary syndrome
III.	Peripheral T-cell lymphomas Subtypes and/or related terms: Node-based T-cell lymphoma T-zone lymphoma AILD-like T-cell lymphoma Lymphoepitheloid cell (Lennert's) lymphoma Multilobated T-cell lymphoma
IV.	Adult T-cell leukemia/lymphoma (HTLV-associated disease)
V.	Angiocentric immunoproliferative lesions (Lymphomatoid granulomatosis) (Polymorphic reticulosis) Angiocentric lymphomas

aggressive combination chemotherapy used against diffuse aggressive B-cell lymphoma [28].

We have observed patients presenting with diffuse malignant lymphomas in which cell surface phenotyping indicated that mature T-cells were numerically predominant. However, further studies led us to believe that the T-cells were non-neoplastic and that they were admixed with a smaller population of monoclonal B-cells which represented the malignant population [33, 34]. We termed these cases *pseudo-peripheral T-cell lymphomas* [31].

This process was seen in six patients with established diagnoses of FL. They developed recurrent lymphadenopathy and a diffuse mixed lymphoid proliferation which effaced lymph node architecture after variable intervals (range, 1–14 years; median, 6 years). Lymph node biopsies were classified as malignant lymphoma, diffuse, mixed small and large cell (five cases) and diffuse, large cell (one case). T-cells numerically predominated (69%) and were phenotypically normal, with both helper and suppressor phenotypes (ratio, approximately 5:1). Monoclonal B-lymphocytes could be demonstrated by sIg staining in four of five cases, but such cells did not exceed 34% (mean, 25%). In one case, a monoclonal population was also identified by Southern blot analysis which demonstrated clonally rearranged, heavy and light chain immunoglobulin genes. Total B-cells in the remaining two cases were 11% and 10%. After conversion to this diffuse histology, the patients continued to follow an indolent clinical course. Thus, we postulated that the numerically predominant T-cells may represent a beneficial host response.

We have also observed *de novo* cases of pseudo-PTL, arising without an antecedent history of FL. Phenotypically, they are similar to those described above. However, there is insufficient experience with these lesions to comment on their clinical behavior.

Only rare cases of diffuse aggressive lymphomas (<5%) have histiocytic markers, i.e., diffuse reactivity for lysosomal enzymes, Fc and complement receptors in the absence of sIg, and phagocytic ability [2]. In our experience, less than 5% of cases fail to demonstrate any surface and/or cytoplasmic markers when carefully studied [28, 34]. Although such rare cases would be termed 'null', it is unlikely that they are derived from true 'null' cells but instead fail to demonstrate markers because of disordered differentiation.

Adult T-cell leukemia/lymphoma

This acute lymphoid malignancy has distinctive clinical, pathologic, and epidemiologic features and it should not be included in the broad category of diffuse aggressive lymphomas. It is associated with the unique human retrovirus HTLV, Type I. The presence of antibodies to HTLV-I coincides with a distinct clinico-pathologic syndrome characterized by generalized lymphadenopathy, hepatosplenomegaly, skin and peripheral blood involvement, and hypercalcemia. The disease is aggressive; the median survival is only 9 months. The disease was first described by Uchiyama et al. in southwestern Japan, where it is endemic [35]. Outside Japan, endemic foci of disease include the Caribbean basin and the southeastern United States. In both of these regions the disease is much more common in blacks [36, 37].

The most characteristic diagnostic feature is the presence of highly pleomorphic and lobated lymphoid cells in the peripheral blood [38, 39]. Also notable in our series was partially tartrate-resistant acid phosphatase activity in the neoplastic cells. The pathologic spectrum of the associated lymphomas is broad and encompasses several diffuse histologic subtypes in the Rappaport Classification, the Working Formulation, and the classification of the Japanese Lymphoma Study Group [38, 39]. However, differences in survival could not be correlated with differences in histologic subtype [39]. In two-thirds of patients with cutaneous involvement, epidermal infiltration resembling Pautrier microabscesses was observed. However, most cases can be readily distinguished from mycosis fungoides/Sezary syndrome on clinical and epidemiologic grounds.

The cells of ATL have a mature T-cell phenotype [39]. Although they react with OKT4/anti-Leu 3a, they function *in vitro* as suppressor cells [40, 41]. A characteristic feature is reactivity with anti-Tac, a monoclonal antibody directed against the T-cell growth factor receptor [41]. The hypercalcemia and osteolytic bone lesions frequently observed are probably secondary to a lymphokine produced by the malignant cells, either osteoclast activating factor (OAF) or an OAF-like substance [42].

Angiocentric immunoproliferative lesions (AIL) and angiocentric lymphomas

Angiocentric immunoproliferative lesions (AIL) are a related group of lymphoproliferative disorders for which several diagnostic terms have been employed: lymphomatoid granulomatosis, polymorphic reticulosis, and atypical lymphocytic vasculitis [43–46]. These lesions are all angiocentric and angiodestructive lymphoid proliferations comprised of an admixture of lymphocytes and other inflammatory cells. Despite the polymorphic character of the infiltrate, the lymphocytes may show some cytologic atypia, and approximately 30% of patients develop frank malignant lymphoma [47, 48]. Therefore, it has been argued that, in at least some patients, the disease may be neoplastic at the outset [49–51].

Although only a small number of cases has been studied phenotypically, in all cases examined by us, both AIL and angiocentric lymphomas, the cells have had mature T-cell characteristics. In addition, the neoplastic T-cells appear to retain the capacity to function. We have identified a factor in cell culture supernatants derived from angiocentric T-cell lesions which can augment the phagocytic activity of human macrophages (PIF) [52].

PIF activity was identified in 3/3 AIL and 2/2 angiocentric lymphomas arising in patients with a previous history of AIL. Fourteen non-angiocentric PTL were negative for PIF as were ten NHL of B-cell origin and two cases of Hodgkin's disease. PIF activity was also identified in one of two cases of T-cell lymphoblastic malignancies.

We hypothesize that such a phagocytosis-inducing factor may play a role in the pathogenesis of an erythrophagocytic syndrome seen in association with T-cell malignancies [49]. This syndrome is characterized by hepatosplenomegaly, fever, and pancytopenia. Pathologic examination reveals activation of normal histiocytes with marked erythrophagocytosis throughout the reticuloendothelial system, i.e., the splenic red pulp, bone marrow, hepatic, and lymph node sinuses. This syndrome appears with greater prevalence in angiocentric lymphoma than other B-cell or T-cell lymphomas. The detection of PIF activity in the culture supernatant of one case of T-acute lymphocytic leukemia (T-ALL) is also of interest, as a syndrome simulating malignant histiocytosis has been reported in patients with ALL. In most cases which have been appropriately analyzed, the neoplastic cells have been of the T-cell phenotype. A similar hemophagocytic syndrome has been described in association with exogenous or endogenous immunodeficiency and infections [53]. It is possible that in an immunodeficient state, elaboration of PIF might proceed unchecked by normal regulatory controls.

Conclusion

The application of modern immunologic techniques to NHL has resulted in improvements in classification and the recognition of distinctive clinicopathologic entities. Nearly all NHLs have markers of B or T lymphocytes. Particularly in the low-grade malignancies, the neoplastic cells retain the capacity for function. The low-grade B-cell lymphomas appear to be composed of cells arrested at different stages in the sequence of B-cell activation. PTLs are morphologically and functionally heterogeneous, but phenotypic analysis alone has not led to the identification of distinctive clinicopathologic syndromes. However, integration of phenotypic, functional, clinicopathologic, and virologic data does offer promise in the subclassification of these malignancies.

34

References

1. Rappaport H (1966). Tumors of the hematopoietic system. Atlas of tumor pathology. Section 3, fascicle 8. Washington, D.C.: Armed Forces Institute of Pathology.
2. Mann RB, Jaffe ES and Berard CW (1979). Malignant lymphomas: A conceptual understanding of morphologic diversity. Amer J Pathol 94:103–192.
3. Rosenberg SA (1979). Current concepts in cancer: Non-Hodgkin's Lymphoma – Selection of treatment on the basis of histologic type. N Engl J Med 301: 924–928.
4. Rosenberg SA, Berard CW, Brown BW et al. (1982). National Cancer Institute sponsored study of classification of non-Hodgkin's lymphomas: Summary and description of a Working Formulation for clinical usage. Cancer 49:2112–2135.
5. Jaffe ES (1983). Follicular lymphomas: Possibility that they are benign tumors of the lymphoid system. J Nat Cancer Inst 70:401–403.
6. Braylan RC, Jaffe ES, Burbach JV et al. (1976). Similarities of surface characteristics of neoplastic well differentiated lymphocytes from solid tissues and from peripheral blood. Cancer Res 36:1619–1625.
7. Pangalis GA, Nathwani BN and Rappaport H (1977). Malignant lymphoma, well differentiated lymphocytic. Its relationship with chronic lymphocytic leukemia and macroglobulinemia of Waldenstrom. Cancer 39:999–1000.
8. Cossman J and Jaffe ES (1981). Distribution of complement receptor subtypes in non-Hodgkin's lymphomas of B cell origin. Blood 58:20–26.
9. Fu SM, Chiorazzi N, Kunkel HG et al. (1978). Induction of *in vitro* differentiation and immunoglobulin synthesis of human leukemic B lymphocytes. J Exp Med 148:1570–1578.
10. Cossman J, Neckers LM, Braziel RM et al. (1984). *In vitro* enhancement of immunoglobulin gene expression in chronic lymphocytic leukemia. J Clin Invest 73:587–592.
11. Martin PJ, Hansen JA, Nowinski RC et al. (1980). A new human T cell differentiation antigen: Unexpected expression on chronic lymphocytic leukemia cells. Immunogenetics II:429–439.
12. Royston I, Majda JA, Baird SM et al. (1980). Human T cell antigens defined by monoclonal antigens: The 65,000 dalton antigen of T cells (T65) is also found on chronic lymphocytic leukemia cells bearing surface immunoglobulin. J Immunol 125:725–731.
13. Caligaris-Cappio F, Gobbi M, Bofil M and Janossy G (1982). Infrequent normal B lymphocytes express features of B-chronic lymphocytic leukemia. J Exp Med 155:623–628.
14. Cossman J, Neckers LM, Hsu SM et al. (1984). Low grade lymphomas: Expression of developmentally regulated B-cell antigens. Amer J Pathol 114:117–124.
15. Ferroni M, Viale G, Risso A and Pernis B (1976). A study of the immunoglobulin classes present on the membrane and in the cytoplasm of human tonsil plasma cells. Eur J Immunol 6:562–565.
16. Halper J, Fu SM, Wang CY et al. (1978). Patterns of expression of human 'Ia-like' antigens during the terminal stages of B-cell development. J Immunol 120:1480–1484.
17. Stashenko P, Nadler LM, Hardy R and Schlossman SF (1981). Expression of cell surface markers after human B lymphocyte activation. Proc Nat Acad Sci USA 78:3848–3852.
18. Abramson C, Kersey J and Le Bien T (1981). A monoclonal antibody (BA-1) reactive with cells of human B lymphocyte lineage. J Immunol 126:83–88.
19. Jaffe ES, Braylan RC, Nanba K et al. (1977). Functional markers: A new perspective on malignant lymphomas. Cancer Treat Rep 61:953–962.
20. Nanba K, Jaffe ES, Braylan RC et al. (1977). Alkaline phosphatase-positive malignant lymphomas. A subtype of B-cell lymphomas. Amer J Clin Pathol 68:535–542.
21. Swerdlow SH, Haveshaw JA, Murray LJ et al. (1983). Centrocytic lymphoma: A distinct clinicopathologic and immunologic entity. Amer J Pathol 113:181–197.

22. Jaffe ES, Shevach EM, Frank MM et al. (1974). Nodular lymphoma. Evidence for origin from follicular B-lymphocytes. N Engl J Med 290:813-819.
23. Harris NL and Bhan AK (1983). Distribution of T-cell subsets in follicular and diffuse lymphomas of B-cell type. Amer J Pathol 113:172-180.
24. Braziel RM, Neckers LM, Jaffe ES and Cossman J (1983). Follicular (nodular) B-cell lymphomas: Immunoregulation of immunoglobulin secretion. Blood 62(Suppl. 1):187a.
25. DeVita VT, Canellos OP, Chabner BA et al. (1975). Advanced diffuse histiocytic lymphoma, a potentially curable disease. Lancet 1:248-250.
26. Jaffe ES (1980). Non-Hodgkin's lymphomas as neoplasms of the immune system, pp 222-226. In: Berard CW, moderator. A multidisciplinary approach to non-Hodgkin's lymphomas. Ann Intern Med 94:218-235.
27. Jaffe ES, Strauchen JA and Berard CW (1982). Predictability of immunologic phenotype of morphologic criteria in diffuse aggressive non-Hodgkins's lymphomas. Amer J Clin Pathol 77:46-49.
28. Cossman J, Jaffe ES and Fisher RI. Immunologic phenotypes of diffuse aggressive non-Hodgkin's lymphomas: Correlation with clinical features. Cancer (in press).
29. Waldron JA, Leech JE, Glick AD et al. (1977). Malignant lymphoma of peripheral T-lymphocyte origin. Cancer 40:1604-1617.
30. Pinkus GS, Said JW and Hargreaves H (1979). Malignant lymphoma, T-cell type. A distinct morphologic variant with large multilobulated nuclei, with a report of four cases. Amer J Clin Pathol 72:540-550.
31. Jaffe ES, Cossman J and Fisher RI (1981). Immunologic, pathologic and clinical analysis of peripheral T-cell lymphomas. Blood 58(Suppl. 1):551.
32. Doggett RS, Wood GS, Horning S et al. (1984). The immunologic characterization of 95 nodal and extranodal diffuse large cell lymphomas in 89 patients. Amer J Pathol 115:245-252.
33. Jaffe ES, Longo DL, Cossman J et al. (1984). Diffuse B-cell lymphomas with T-cell predominance in patients with follicular lymphomas or "pseudo T-cell lymphomas". Lab Invest 50:27-28a.
34. Arnold A, Cossman J, Bakhshi A et al. (1983). Immunoglobulin gene rearrangements as unique clonal markers in human lymphoid neoplasma. N Engl J Med 309:1593-1599.
35. Uchiyama T, Yodoi j, Sagawa K et al. (1977). Adult T-cell leukemia: Clinical and hematologic features of 16 cases. Blood 50:481-492.
36. Catovsky O, Greaves MF, Rose M et al. (1982). Adult T-cell lymphoma-leukemia in blacks from the West Indies. Lancet I:639-643.
37. Blayney DW, Jaffe ES, Blattner Wa et al. (1983). The human T-cell leukemia/lymphoma virus (HTLV) associated with American adult T-cell leukemia/lymphoma (ATL). Blood 62:401-405.
38. Hanaoka M, Sasaki M, Matsumoto H et al. (1979). Adult T-cell leukemia: Histological classification and characteristics. Acta Pathol Jap 19(5):727-738.
39. Jaffe ES, Blattner WA, Blayney DW et al. (1984). The pathologic spectrum of HTLV-associated leukemia/lymphoma in the United States. Amer J Surg Pathol 8:263-275.
40. Uchiyama T, Sagawak, Takatsuki K and Uchino H (1978). Effect of adult T-cell leukemia cells pokeweed mitogen-induced B-cell differentiation. Clin Immunol Immunopathol 10:24-34.
41. Waldmann TA (1984). Function and phenotype of virus-associated neoplastic cells, pp. 553-554. In: Broder S, moderator. T-cell lymphoproliferative syndrome associated with human T-cell leukemia/lymphoma virus. Ann Intern Med 100:543-557.
42. Grossman B, Schecter GP, Horton JE et al. (1981). Hypercalcemia associated with T-cell lymphoma-leukemia. Amer J Clin Pathol 75:149-155.
43. Kassel SH, Echevarria RA and Guzzo FF (1969). Midline malignant reticulosis (so-called lethal midline granuloma). Cancer 23:920-935.

44. Liebow AA, Carrington CB and Friedman RJ (1972). Lymphomatoid granulomatosis. Hum Pathol 3:457–558.
45. De Remee RA, Weiland LH and McDonald TJ (1978). Polymorphic reticulosis, lymphomatoid granulomatosis: Two diseases or one? Mayo Clin Proc 53:634–640.
46. Saldana MJ, Patchefsky AS, Israel H et al. (1977). Pulmonary angitis and granulomatosis. The relationship between histological features, organ involvement and response to treatment. Hum Pathol 8:391–409.
47. Katzenstein A, Carrington CB and Liebow AA (1979). Lymphomatoid granulomatosis: A clinicopathologic study of 152 cases. Cancer 43:360–373.
48. Fauci AS, Haynes BF, Costa J et al. (1982). Lymphomatoid granulomatosis, prospective clinical and therapeutic experience over ten years. N Engl J Med 306:68–74.
49. Jaffe ES, Costa JC, Fauci A et al. (1983). Malignant lymphoma and erythrophagocytosis simulating malignant histiocytosis. Amer J Med 75:741–748.
50. Colby TV and Carrington CB (1982). Pulmonary lymphomas simulating lymphomatoid granulomatosis. Amer J Surg Pathol 6:19–32.
51. Jaffe ES. The pathologic and clinical spectrum of post-thymic T-cell malignancies. Cancer Invest. (in press).
52. Simrell CR, Crabtree GR, Cossman J et al. (1982). Stimulation of phagocytosis by a T-cell lymphoma derived lymphokine. In: Vitetta E (Ed.). B and T-Cell Tumors, 24:247–252. UCLA Symposia in Molecular and Cellular Biology. New York: Academic Press.
53. Risdall RJ, McKenna RW, Nesbit ME et al. (1979). Virus associated hemophagocytic syndrome, a benign histiocytic proliferation distinct from malignant histiocytosis. Cancer 44:993–1002.

5. Non-Hodgkin's lymphoma with multilobated nuclei is not a distinct pathologic entity

Ph. M. KLUIN[1], S. C. J. VAN DER PUTTE[1],
H. J. SCHUURMAN[2], L. H. P. M. RADEMAKERS[1], S. POPPEMA[3]
and J. A. M. VAN UNNIK[1]
[1] *Institute of Pathology and* [2] *Division of Immunopathology,*
University Hospital, Utrecht; and [3] *Institute of Pathology, University*
Hospital Groningen, the Netherlands

T-cell non-Hodgkin's lymphoma (NHL) of large multilobated cell type was originally described by Pinkus et al. in 1979 [1]. The 4 cases mainly presented in extranodal sites and were associated with a favorable clinical course. Consecutively T-lymphocyte derived tumors with multilobated cells have been reported to occur in lymph nodes [2–5] and in the skin [6, 7]. A separate entity may comprise human T-cell leukemia virus (HTLV) related adult T-cell leukemia/lymphoma in which multilobated cells are frequent [2, 8], especially in the pleiomorphic subtype. Clinical studies reveal a poor survival [9].

More recently multilobated lymphoma of B-lymphocyte lineage has been described [10–14]. Van der Putte [14] has demonstrated that B-multilobated cells may be related to follicle centre cells (FCC). Moreover, we reported 3 cases of malignant lymphoma of the bone which contained large multilobated cells and appeared to be of B-lymphocyte lineage [15]. In the present study the spectrum of lymphoid and non-lymphoid malignancies which contain multilobated cells is further outlined.

Materials and methods

NHL with multilobated nuclei as found in haematoxylin & eosin paraffin sections were selected from the files of the Institute of Pathology, Utrecht. Only cases which could be characterized by immunocytochemical tests on frozen tissue sections, paraffin sections or in cell suspension, by enzyme histochemistry and by electron microscopy were included. Some cases were sent for consultation. Part of the investigation was done in the Institute of Pathology of the University of Groningen. It focused on NHL, diffuse large cleaved (Lukes-Collins classification) or diffuse (anaplastic) centrocytic (Kiel classification).

Multilobated cells were defined by the presence of at least 3 round nuclear

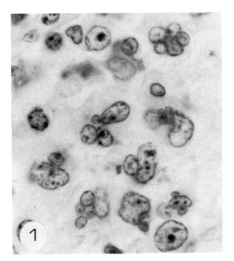

Figure 1. Cutaneous T-cell lymphoma with large multilobated cells.

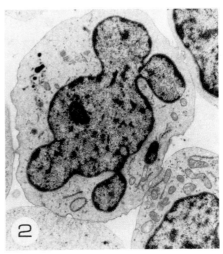

Figure 2. Blastic transformation in atypical Sezary's syndrome. Note the formation of peripheral lobules with an intact central area of the nucleus.

lobes or lobules that are interconnected by stalks, either to each other or to a central solid part of the nucleus. Cells with extensively cleaved or bilobated nuclei were excluded.

Results

Multilobated cells in T-NHL and normal T-cell dependent lymphoid tissues

After the original description by Pinkus et al. [1] we observed two patients with localized cutaneous lymphoma of the shoulder which contained large multilobated cells (Fig. 1). Most lymphoid cells showed reactivity with Leu-1, OKT3 and Leu-3a/OKT4 monoclonal antibodies. Both tumors showed very slow progression and periods of spontaneous regression, absence of dissemination and complete response to low dose radiotherapy (2500 rad).

One non-Caribbean and non-Japanese patient with atypical Sezary's syndrome presented with erythrodermia and leukocyte counts of $9800/mm^3$ with 50% small Sezary's cells. Lymph nodes with blastic transformation became involved after 9 months. A sudden terminal phase started with the appearance of blast cells with a distinct multilobation (Fig. 2). They were reactive with Leu-1 and OKT3 but weakly reactive with Leu-3a. Serum antibodies against HTLV antigens were not detectable. The patient died 2

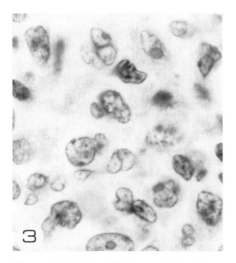

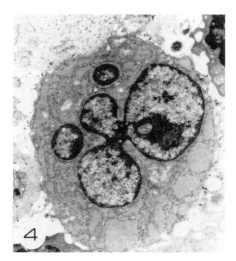

Figure 3. Follicular NHL, centroblastic/centrocytic with bi- and multilobated cells.

Figure 4. Follicular NHL centroblastic/centrocytic. Note the complete nuclear distortion. The cytoplasm shows plasmacytic differentiation with dilated cisternae of the RER.

years after the onset of disease. No HTLV related cases of adult T-cell leukemia/lymphoma were identified in the present series.

As a putative normal counterpart of T-multilobated lymphomatous cells we could demonstrate the presence of multilobated lymphoid cells within the normal thymus, especially in the cortico-medullary junction [7].

Multilobated cells in B-NHL and benign lymph nodes

First indications that B-NHL might contain multilobated cells were presented by Palutke et al. [10]. Recently we found multilobated cells (Fig. 3) in 21 cases of 42 follicular and diffuse FCC tumors. In 7 cases they were frequent. They were both inside and outside lymphomatous follicles. Ultrastructural analysis of 4 cases revealed 3 variants within a continuous spectrum: 1) large blast cells identical to centroblasts except for a slight nuclear lobation; 2) intermediate sized cells with a cytoplasmic structure of centrocytes with a more pronounced lobation; and 3) similar cells with plasmacytic organization of the cytoplasm (Fig. 4). Their existence was confirmed by the presence of monotypic cytoplasmic immunoglobulin in 3 of 4 cases. A remarkable feature was the absence of demonstrable surface immunoglobulin in all but one cases, tested both by immunocytochemistry on frozen tissue sections and by the sensitive direct antiglobulin rosetting reaction [16].

In a separate study, 14 cases of primary large cleaved or anaplastic cen-

40

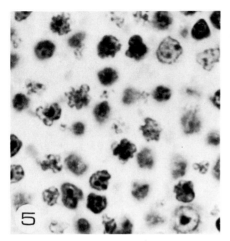

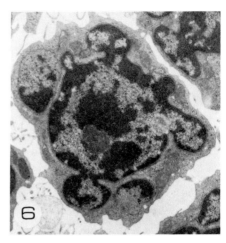

Figure 5. Small multilobated cells of the case which was diagnosed as B-CLL by clinical criteria (see text).

Figure 6. Same case as Figure 5. Note the peripheral lobation of the nucleus.

trocytic NHL were analyzed. Most tumors presented in extranodal sites, especially the nasopharynx. Strikingly, 4 of 14 cases contained almost only multilobated cells, while they were numerous in 3 others. Monotypic surface immunoglobulin was found in all but one of the tumors. No consistent immunologic phenotype could be demonstrated, using a panel of monoclonal antibodies: all cases were B 1 positive but two were negative for BA-1 and two others were negative for Vil-A_1. This anti-CALLA monoclonal antibody stained normal follicle centres in a 3-step immunoperoxidase assay as has been reported also by Stein [17].

Three cases of primary malignant lymphoma of the bone within the maxilla containing multilobated cells have been described recently [15]. These tumors met the criteria of primary reticulum cell sarcoma of the bone [18, 19]. Two cases were analyzed by immunohistology and possessed monotypic surface immunoglobulin and were B 1 positive. Some cells of one tumor contained also monotypic cytoplasmic immunoglobulin. An FCC origin was suggested by electron microscopy in the third case.

Recently we observed that primary B-cell lymphoma of the skin occasionally may contain multilobated cells and cannot be distinguished from cutaneous T-cell lymphoma by histologic criteria.

Forty reactive lymph nodes with non-specific inflammation and follicular hyperplasia were investigated [14]. In 11 cases multilobated cells were found in the follicle centres. They were numerous in 5 cases. Ultrastructurally the cytoplasm showed a centrocytic or plasmacytic differentiation; it contained cytoplasmic immunoglobulin of polytypic origin in the latter variant. These findings strengthened the concept of a FCC origin of large multilobated cells.

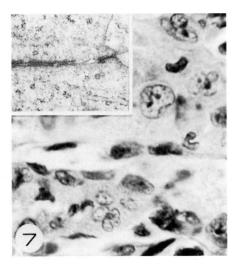 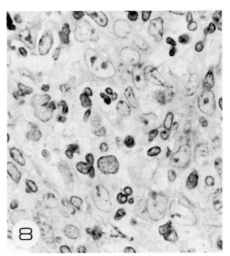

Figure 7. Multilobated cells in metastatic carcinoma (unknown primary). Inset: Desmo-
some in this tumor.

Figure 8. Multilobated cells in lymph node
involvement by myelomonocytic leukemia,
mimicking NHL.

A remarkable multilobation of small lymphoid cells was observed in one
case. The patient, aged 43 years, presented with mild lymphadenopathy,
splenomegaly and leukocyte counts of 140,000/mm^3. An involved lymph
node showed a diffuse infiltrate of small lymphocytes with almost round
nuclei and scarce so called prolymphocytes and paraimmunoblasts. However, groups of small cells with multilobated nuclei were apparent, in particular in imprints, glycolmethacrylate sections and by electron microscopy
(Figs. 5, 6). The first consideration of T-CLL was set aside by the (weak)
expression of surface IgM-IgD-λ; 50% of the leukemic cells formed spontaneous rosettes with mouse erythrocytes. Tissue lymphocytes showed ATP-
ase reactivity, faint staining for acid phosphatase and no staining for alkaline phosphatase and 5-nucleotidase. Leukemic and lymph node cells were
reactive with Leu-1 as observed in B-CLL.

Other tumors/leukemias with multilobated cells

An axillary lymph node with metastatic undifferentiated carcinoma of
unknown primary origin contained very irregular and sometimes clearly
multilobated nuclei (Fig. 7). Absence of all leukocyte markers and the presence of desmosomes confirmed the epithelial character.

Large round, beanshaped, bi- and multilobated nuclei are characteristic in
myelomonocytic leukemia. Therefore, leukemic infiltration into lymph
nodes mimicks NHL, especially diffuse types of FCC tumors (Fig. 8). How-

ever, Giemsa and naphtol-ASD-chloroacetate-esterase stainings may nicely demonstrate the myeloid origin of the tumor cells.

Discussion

In the present study was demonstrated that malignant lymphoma with multilobated cells is not uncommon, once this peculiar cell type has been recognized. Although most reports concern T-NHL [1–7], we demonstrated that B-NHL with multilobated cells may be much more frequent. In about 50% of NHL of FCC origin multilobated cells were found; they were frequent in about 17%. In selected cases of diffuse large cleaved lymphoma they were even more frequent (50%) and 30% of the tumors contained almost exclusively multilobated cells. In view of the vast majority of B-NHL over T-NHL in western countries, and especially the high frequency of FCC tumors, our data are likely to be applicable to other western countries.

The study on reactive lymph nodes and FCC tumors indicated a spectrum of centroblasts, centrocytes, plasmacytoid cells and multilobated cells with identical cytoplasmic differentiation. Therefore, multilobation may be considered as a variant of follicle centre cells.

The presence of multilobated cells in the case clinically diagnosed as B-CLL is difficult to explain since it cannot be related to the FCC reaction. However, B-CLL may be more heterogeneous than thought previously [20]. Lennert has suggested the possibility of B_1 and B_2 types of CLL, the post FCC (B_2) type showing more irregular nuclei than the B_1 type [21]. Possibly, the present case is related to the intermediate lymphocytic lymphoma (ILL) described by Berard which is of follicle mantle zone origin [22].

Necrosis was found in some cases of diffuse large cell NHL. This association may be of interest because Neftel has suggested that nuclear lobation could be induced by fever [23]. However, we found no consistent relation between nuclear lobation and fever or tissue necrosis. Artificial lobation may be caused by bad formalin fixation or subsequent histotechnical procedures. In our cases this was excluded as multilobation was found irrespective of the fixatives and embedding reagents used and also in cytologic imprints and in electron microscopy.

In conclusion we demonstrated that the presence of multilobated nuclei in benign or malignant lymphoid tissues does not imply a T-lymphocyte origin as may be suggested by the initial reports on T-NHL and on multilobated thymocytes. Multilobated B-cells originate in the normal FCC reaction and are also frequent in FCC tumors, especially in NHL of large cleaved subtype with localization in extranodal sites, such as the nasopharynx. The incidental finding of carcinoma and myelomonocytic leukemia with multilobated cells again stresses the importance of additional immunologic, enzymocytochemical and ultrastructural tests in these cases.

Acknowledgements

The authors thank Mrs. W. T. M. van Blokland and Mr. J. G. N. Geertzema for technical assistance. Dr R. L. H. Bolhuis, Daniel den Hoedt Hospital, Rotterdam and dr F. J. E. M. Blomjous, St Antonius hospital, Nieuwegein, kindly donated Vil-A$_1$ antibody and tissue sections, respectively.

References

1. Pinkus GS, Said JW and Hargreaves H (1979). Malignant lymphoma, T-cell type. A distinct morphological variant with large multilobated nuclei with a report of 4 cases. Amer J Clin Pathol 72:540–550.
2. Kikuchi M, Mitsui T, Matsui N et al. (1979). T-cell malignancies in adults: Histopathological studies of lymph nodes in 110 patients. Jap J Clin Oncol 9 (suppl):407–422.
3. Leong ASY, Dale BM, Lien SH et al. (1981). Node-based T-cell lymphoma. The clinical, immunological and morphological spectrum. Pathology 13:79–95.
4. Pallesen G, Madsen M and Hastrup J (1981). Large-cell T-lymphoma with hypersegmented nuclei. Scand J Hematol 26:72–79.
5. van der Putte SCJ, Toonstra J, van Prooyen HC et al. (1984). Sezary's syndrome with early immunoblastic transformation. Arch Dermatol Res 276:17–26.
6. van der Putte SCJ, Toonstra J, de Weger RA and van Unnik JAM (1982). Cutaneous T-cell lymphoma, multilobated type. Histopathology 6:35–54.
7. van der Putte SCJ, Schuurman H-J and Toonstra J (1982). Cutaneous T-cell lymphoma, multilobated type. expressing membrane differentiation antigens of precursor T-lymphocytes. Brit J Dermatol 107:293–300.
8. Hanaoka M (1982). Disease entity of adult T-cell leukemia: Cytological aspects and geographic pathology. Hanaoka M, Takutsuki K and Shimoyama M (Eds.). In: GANN Monogr Cancer Res 28:1–12. New-York: Plenum Press.
9. Kikuchi M, Mitsui T, Eimato T at al. (1982). Biopsy of adult T-cell leukemia. Hanaoka M, Takutsuki K and Shimoyama M (Eds.). In: GANN Monogr Cancer Res 28:37–50. New-York: Plenum Press.
10. Palutke M, Schnitzer B, Mirchandi I et al. (1980). T- and B-cell lymphomas look alike. Amer J Clin Pathol 74:360–361.
11. Weinberg DS and Pinkus GS (1981). Non-Hodgkin's lymphoma of large multilobated cell type. Amer J Clin Pathol 76:190–196.
12. Pileri S, Brandi G, Rivano MT et al. (1982). Report of a case of non-Hodgin's lymphoma of large multilobated cell type with B-cell origin. Tumori 68:543–548.
13. Cerezo L (1983). B-cell multilobated lymphoma. Cancer 52:2277–2280.
14. van der Putte SCJ, Schuurman H-J, Rademakers LHPM et al. Malignant lymphoma of follicle centre cells with marked nuclear lovation. Virch Arch (in press).
15. Kluin PhM, Slootweg PJ, Schuurman H-J et al. Primary B-cell malignant lymphoma of the maxilla with a sarcomatous pattern and multilobated nuclei. Cancer (in press).
16. Haegert DG, Hurd C and Coombs RRA (1978). Comparison of the direct anti-globulin rosetting reaction with direct immunofluorescence in the detection of surface membrane immunoglobulin on human peripheral blood lymphocytes. Immunology 34:533–538.
17. Stein H, Gerdes J and Mason DY (1982). The normal and malignant germinal centre. Clinics in Hematol 11:531–559.
18. Parker F and Jackson H (1939). Primary reticulum cell sarcoma of bone. Surg Gynecol Obstet 68:45–53.

19. Dosoretz DE, Raymond AK, Murphy GF et al. (1982). Primary lymphoma of bone. The relationship of morphologic diversity to clinical behavior. Cancer 50:1009–1014.
20. Catavsky D, Cherchi M, Brooks D et al. (1981). Heterogeneity of B-cell leukemias demonstrated by the monoclonal antibody FMC 7. Blood 58:406–408.
21. Lennert K (1981). Histopathology of Non-Hodgkin's Lymphomas. Berlin, Heidelberg, New-York: Springer-Verlag.
22. Berard CW, Jaffe ES. Braylan RC et al. (1978). Immunological aspects and pathology of the malignant lymphomas. Cancer 42:911–921.
23. Neftel KA, Stahel R and Müller O (1982). Letter to the editor. N Engl J Med 307:377.

6. Burkitt's lymphoma:
Multiparametric analysis of 55 cell lines
with special reference to morphometry

P. FELMAN, P. A. BRYON, O. GENTILHOMME, J. P. MAGAUD,
A. M. MANEL, B. COIFFIER and G. LENOIR
*Laboratoire Central d'Hématologie B, Centre Hospitalier Lyon-Sud,
Pierre-Bénite, France*

The term 'Burkitt's lymphoma' (BL) connotes a specific morphologic appearance which has been well described[1]. However, the boundaries of this entity from other related B-cell lymphomas, especially the small non-cleaved or undifferentiated non-Burkitt lymphomas, remain a matter of debate[2-4]. Morphologic differences between the two types of small non-cleaved lymphoma, Burkitt and non-Burkitt, as defined by the 'Working Formulation for Clinical Use'[5], are diversely appreciated by different investigators and even by the same investigator, upon repeated examinations[6]. Furthermore, the apparently specific translocation [8, 14] (q 24; q 32) has been found in non-Burkitt's types, large non-cleaved and immunoblastic lymphomas[7-9], suggesting the possibility of a polymorphous expression of Burkitt's lymphomas.

Beside morphologic, chromosomal and viral characteristics, the ability of Burkitt's cells to grow in long-term cultures represents an unusual feature, which may be considered as another typical characteristic of this lymphoma. Cell lines established from Burkitt's tumors constitute an attractive model for the study of the morphologic phenotype and its relationship with other characteristics. We have extensively investigated 55 BL cell lines and compared our results with data reported in the literature. Statistical determinations are based on variance analyses and the Chi square test.

Phenotypic expression of Burkitt's lymphoma cell lines

Morphology

BL cell lines have been widely studied for twenty years, but their morphologic expression has been quite poorly investigated, being chiefly examined by inverted microscope. Nilsson[10] and others[11, 12] considered the BL cells 'to retain their basic morphology when established as BL cell lines, with the exception of a slight increase in volume'. Profound diversity between different cell lines was found occasionally, but no morphologic heterogeneity in size and shape was noted within each cell line. However, in 1966, some unusual features were described about RAJI line cells including relatively large size, abundant basophilic cytoplasm and marked nuclear irregularity [13]. Magrath et al., observing 16 lines on Romanovsky's stained cytologic preparations, found important differences between EB-pos and EB-neg cell lines, the former showing heterogeneity in size and shape, and a strikingly decreased nuclear to cytoplasmic ratio [14].

The first attempts to quantify cell size in BL lines were realized on cell suspensions by electronic mean cell volume determination [14, 15] and revealed an important increase in cell size thought to result from a greater volume of cytoplasm. Our morphometric analysis of 55 BL cell lines (Table I) largely differed from previous similar analyses. Our technical conditions were closely related to usual histologic diagnostic procedures: cell suspension pellets were embedded in epoxy resin, cut at 2 μm [16] and observed under immersion lens. We characterized nuclear features including size, shape and area dispersion with a Leitz semi-automatic 'ASM' image analyzer. The wide diversity of histologic pictures was striking (Fig. 1 a, b, c, d, e). Although some BL lines retained the usual aspect of BL, the majority showed more or less important variations, including frequently pronounced irregularity of nuclear shape, increase of size, and sometimes a marked heterogeneity of size and shape within the lines. Five main cytologic subtypes could be identified, in part by morphometrically determined nuclear sizes and shapes: small cell lines (31 cases) with non-cleaved (13 cases) or irregular (18 cases) subtypes and large cell lines (24 cases) with non-cleaved (5 cases), irregular (9 cases) or immunoblastic (10 cases) subtypes. This large spectrum of morphologic and morphometric aspects is illustrated in Figs. 2 and 3. The diagram representing the relationship between size and shape

Table I. General data on Burkitt's cell lines

Geographic origin	Chromosomic analysis			EBV status	
	No.[a]	t (8; 14)	t variant	No.[a]	Positive lines
East Africa	13	6	6	13	12
North Africa	12	8	4	12	12
Europa	25	17	8	28	11
Others	2	1	1	2	2
Total number	52	33	19	55	37

[a] number of lines tested

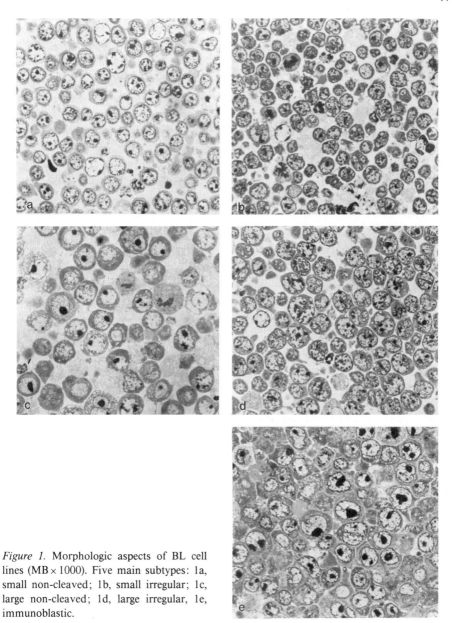

Figure 1. Morphologic aspects of BL cell lines (MB × 1000). Five main subtypes: 1a, small non-cleaved; 1b, small irregular; 1c, large non-cleaved; 1d, large irregular, 1e, immunoblastic.

permits the identification of the main cytologic subtypes of B-cell lymphomas [17]. Curves of nuclear size/shape distribution for the main subtypes underline the heterogeneity of morphologic expression of BL cell lines (Fig. 4).

Cytomorphometrical analysis performed on cytologic preparations, showed a simultaneous increase in nuclear area and cytoplasm, especially

48

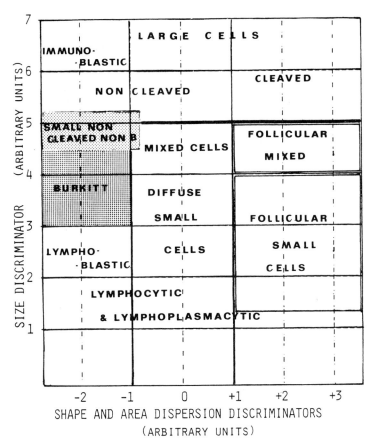

Figure 2. Pictorial representation of the relationship between size and shape for the main cytologic subtypes of B-cell lymphomas.

for the largest cells. Of note, a linear relationship exists between histomorphometric and cytomorphometric results, especially for the nuclear area (correlation test $r = 0.74$, $p < 0.001$).

Immunologic characteristics

BL cell lines are also heterogeneous according to immunoglobulin expression [10]. As have others before us, we identified three different immunoglobulin (Ig) phenotypes; a very immature phenotype, pre-B type, with only cytoplasmic heavy chain μ type, a mature phenotype sIg$^+$ cIg$^+$, and an intermediate sIg$^+$ cIg$^-$ phenotype. There was no agreement between Ig phenotype and morphologic subtypes, except the fact that 4 immunoblastic lines out of 9 showed pre-B phenotypes. Yet, the three groups differed according to morphometric determinations: the cμ^+ group was significantly

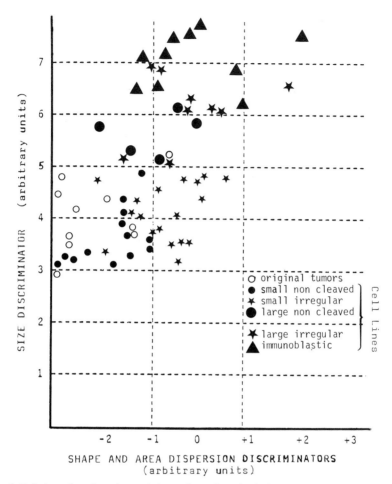

Figure 3. Relation of nuclear size and shape dispersion discriminators in 55 BL cell lines and ten related original tumors.

larger ($p<0.0001$ for mean nuclear area) and more heterogeneous ($p<0.025$ for area dispersion) than the 2 others, the most mature phenotype (sIg$^+$ cIg$^+$) was larger than the sIg$^+$ cIg$^-$ group ($p<0.05$). Furthermore, the cμ^+ group seemed restricted to African lines, with the exception of a Japanese line, and frequently associated with an immunoblastic appearance.

Most BL lines have been shown to express C_3, a BL specific antigen recognized by monoclonal antibody (mAB) 38; 13 and the common ALL antigen [10]. Few studies, however, have investigated several surface antigens expression as in ours [18]. Among the panel tested, four mAB were found to be interesting as regards morphologic characteristics: positivity for BL13, which recognizes B-cells from lymphoid follicles, and T 9, an antigen associated with transferrin receptors on proliferating cells, correlated with large-sized lines. On the other hand, positivity for J 5, recognizing CALL

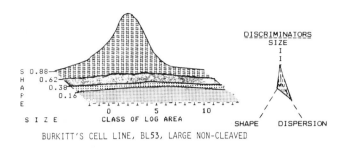

BURKITT'S CELL LINE, BL53, LARGE NON-CLEAVED

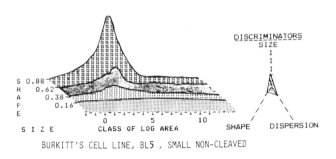

BURKITT'S CELL LINE, BL5 , SMALL NON-CLEAVED

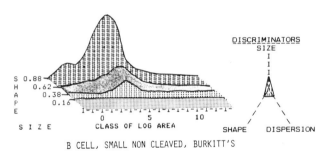

B CELL, SMALL NON CLEAVED, BURKITT'S

Figure 4. Size frequency distribution smoothed curves for 4 classes of shape in five cases of BL cell lines, and in one case of typical BL. On the right: size, shape and dispersion discriminator values.

antigen, and BA 1, more or less pan B marker, was significantly associated with small-sized lines.

Transforming factors

The transforming role of EBV has already been pinpointed [14], EB-pos lines being larger, less uniform in size and shape than EB-neg ones; our study confirms this difference for all morphometric parameters, size ($p < 0.001$), shape ($p < 0.05$), dispersion ($p < 0.01$). Moreover, increased nu-

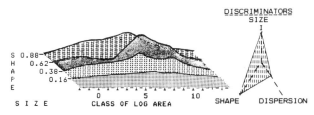

BURKITT'S CELL LINE, RAJI, LARGE IMMUNOBLASTIC

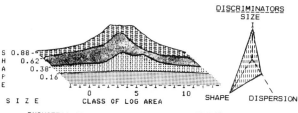

BURKITT'S CELL LINE, BL3 , LARGE IRREGULAR

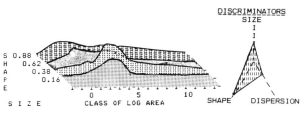

BURKITT'S CELL LINE, BL38, SMALL IRREGULAR

clear size seems to be related to geographical origin, African lines being significantly the largest cell lines ($p < 0.0001$). On the other hand, and contrary to findings of Magrath et al. [14], African lines remained the largest when compared with other EB-pos lines ($p < 0.001$). This feature may be explained in different ways, but it may be reasonably postulated that the influence of EBV on the behavior of BL cells in culture parallels the importance of infection. The fact that many of EB-pos Caucasian lines are derived from EB-neg biopsies, which implies an 'EBNA conversion' from a few EB-pos cells, is concordant with that hypothesis.

Cell kinetics may theoretically exert an influence on the increase in nuclear size; however, growth kinetics evaluated by doubling times did not seem to be significantly different between EB-pos and EB-neg lines [14]. In our study, the simultaneous determination of cell cycle was not performed, but the fact that T 9 positivity was associated with large cells is consistent with more intense growth kinetics.

Chromosomal abnormalities could partially account for phenotypic variability. There was no correlation between type of translocation and morphologic or immunologic characteristics. Moreover, in the 32 available caryotypes, we did not find an additional chromosomal aberration possibly related with morphology (Berger unpublished) [19, 20], especially for the unexpected immunoblastic pre-B lines, as recently proposed for ALL [21]. Hyperploidy may theoretically account for an increase in nuclear size; in most cases, increase in size was not associated with hyperploidy except for the largest line among the rare large cell EB-neg Caucasian lines.

Cell origin of BL

Differences in clinical presentation and relation with EBV between African and American BL as well as differences in corresponding BL lines led some authors to postulate a different cellular origin for BL according to geographic origin [14, 22]. Various racial or environmental factors could be involved. Our study confirms striking differences between lines from high endemic area (East Africa) and lines from low endemic areas (Europe, North

Table II. Influence of geographic factors

	East Africa	North Africa	Europe	*p* value
EBV + [a]	12/13	8/8	10/25	<0.005[c]
EBV − [a]	1	0	15	
t 2–8/2–8–9[a]	2/11	2/8	1/24	ns
8–14	6	6	15	
8–22	3	0	6	
cμ + [b]	6/13	0	0	<0.01[c]
sIg+ cIg− [b]	2	3/12	9/25	
sIg+ cIg+ [b]	5	9	16	
Small[b]	2/13	6/12	21/27	<0.0001[d]
Large[b]	5	3	5	
Immunoblastic[b]	6	3	1	

[a] Results expressed in number of patients.
[b] Results expressed in number of lines.
[c] X^2 test.
[d] Variance analysis.

Africa), as regards histologic appearance, EBV relation and immunologic phenotype (Table II). However, African lines present both the least and the most mature phenotypes and therefore encompass a broader spectrum of B-cell differentiation stages than do lines from other countries. This is not consistent with a more mature stage of differentiation for African Burkitt's lymphoma target cells [14].

Our observations would suggest a follicle center cell origin of BL. Twenty lines out of 54 tested, comprising both the least ($C\mu^+$) and the most mature lines, were positive for BL 13; the positivity of this marker strongly supports a peripheral origin of BL.

Two main patterns of reactivity with monoclonal antibodies were observed and related to geographic origin: BL 13 and T 9 were frequently expressed by African lines and among these nearly always by pre-B lines, whereas CALLA and BA 1 were expressed by Caucasian and North African lines, which, however, differed in terms of EBV relation. In addition, T 9 positivity was often expressed on Caucasian lines and nearly always on North African lines. Whether this association is related to a different cellular origin for African and non-African BL or reflects the incidence of other factors cannot be determined from our study. Many of the antigens tested could be characteristic of functional status (e.g. the transferrin receptor recognized by the OKT 9 mAB) rather than maturation stage; besides, surface antigen expression has been shown to vary in the same line at different times and from line to line in the same patient. On the other hand, we could not find a specific pattern related to the site of origin of the lines (primitive tumor, bone marrow, or fluids).

Burkitt's lymphoma entity: A reevaluation?

The possibility that the heterogeneity of BL cell lines may reflect some heterogeneity *in vivo* must be considered, particularly in view of the distinction between the two subtypes, Burkitt's and non-Burkitt's, of the small non-cleaved lymphomas. As far as we know, no comparison has yet been made between morphologic aspects of BL cell lines and the corresponding original Burkitt's tumors. We could review and measure histologic slides of ten original tumors only. The heterogeneity of this group according to size and shape was slight, except for one tumor which exhibited large and very irregular nuclei (morphometric data are represented in Fig. 3). At this point, it must be underlined that many typical BL have nuclear sizes smaller than those of macrophages, approximately between classes 4 and 5. Simultaneously, cytologic preparations from 18 original tumors were reviewed and classified into typical and atypical BL, the latter differing by a greater heterogeneity in size, and, in a variable percentage of cells, by a delicate chro-

54

matin pattern, irregular nuclei or sometimes large nucleoli. Lines derived from these two groups showed no differences concerning the number of large cell lines or the mean nuclear shape, and even some atypical BL showed typical BL appearance when established as lines. Neither did we find any difference as regards type of translocation, EBNA status, immunoglobulin profile or mAB expression. Moreover cell tumor or cell line morphology could be different in the same patient depending upon site of origin, typical in one, atypical in another.

As African BL represents the morphologic standard of reference for typical BL, we were interested by the morphometric analysis of some African Burkitt's tumors, previously reviewed by an international expert. In fact, the 7 tumors examined (not related with the cell lines studied), showed the same heterogeneity as non-endemic area tumors, with two cases mapped in the zone of small non-cleaved non-Burkitt's lymphoma.

The heterogeneity of African BL morphologic expression, and the fact that typical and atypical BL cannot be recognized on the basis of their derived cell lines lead us to question the validity of the distinction between Burkitt's and the so-called small non-cleaved non-Burkitt's lymphoma.

Acknowledgements

Chromosomal analysis was performed in part by J. Fraisse (Saint-Etienne) and IARC. We wish to thank M. Vuillaume for maintenance of cell lines and C. Bonnardel for providing African Burkitt's tumors.

References

1. Berard CW, O'Conor GT, Thomas LB (1969). Histopathological definition of Burkitt's tumor. Bulletin of WHO 40:601–607.
2. Grogan TM, Warnke RA, Kaplan HS (1982). A comparative study of Burkitt's and non-Burkitt's 'undifferentiated' malignant lymphoma. Cancer 49:1817–1828.
3. Miliauskas JR, Berard KW, Young RC et al. (1982). Undifferentiated non-Hodgkin's lymphomas (Burkitt's and non-Burkitt's types). The relevance of making this histologic distinction. Cancer 50:2115–2127.
4. Levine AM, Pavlova Z, Pockros AW et al. (1983). Small non cleaved follicular center cell (FCC) lymphoma: Burkitt and non-Burkitt variants in the United States. Cancer 52:1073–1079.
5. The Non-Hodgkin's Lymphoma Pathologic Classification Project. (1982). National Cancer Institute sponsored study of classifications of non-Hodgkin's lymphomas: Summary and description of a working formulation for clinical usage. Cancer 49:2112–2135.
6. Wilson JF, Jenkin RDT, Anderson JR et al. (1984). Studies on the pathology of non-Hodgkin's lymphoma of childhood. Cancer 53:1695-1704.
7. Bloomfield CD, Arthur DC, Frizzera G et al. (1983). Non-random chromosome abnormalities in Lymphoma. Cancer Res 43:2975–2984.

8. Yunis JJ, Oken MM, Kaplan ME et al. (1982). Distinctive chromosomal abnormalities in histologic subtypes of non-Hodgkin's lymphomas. N Engl J Med 307:1231–1236.
9. Sigaux F, Berger R, Bernheim A et al. (1984). Malignant lymphomas with band 8 q 24 chromosome abnormality: A morphologic continuum extending from Burkitt's to immunoblastic lymphoma. Brit J Haematol (in press).
10. Nilsson K and Klein G (1982). Phenotypic and cytogenetic characteristics of human B-lymphoïd cell lines and their relevance for the etiology of Burkitt's lymphoma. Adv in Cancer Res 37:319–379.
11. Minowada J, Klein G, Clifford P et al. (1967). Studies of Burkitt's lymphoma cells. Cancer 20:1430–1437.
12. Epstein MA and Barr YM (1965). Characteristics and mode of growth of a tissue culture strain (EB1) of human lymphoblasts from Burkitt's lymphoma J Nat Cancer Inst 34:231–238.
13. Epstein MA, Achong BG, Barr YM et al. (1966). Morphological and virological investigations on cultured Burkitt tumor lymphoblasts (strain RAJI) J Nat Cancer Inst 37:547–551.
14. Magrath IT, Pizzo PA, Whang-Reng J et al. (1980). Characterization of lymphoma – Derived cell lines: Comparison of cell lines positive and negative for Epstein-Barr virus nuclear antigen. 1; Physical, cytogenetic and growth characteristics. J Nat Cancer Inst, 63(3):465–474.
15. Nadkarni JS, Nadkarni JJ, Clifford P et al. (1969). Characteristics of new cell lines derived from Burkitt's lymphomas. Cancer 23:63–78.
16. Bryon PA (1976). Inclusion en époxy des biopsies médullaires pour le diagnostic hématologique. Pathol Biol 24:75.
17. Bryon PA, Felman P, French M and Coiffier B (1982). Méthodes quantitatives en hématologie 1. Histologie. Acta Hématol 45–53, Masson Paris.
18. Cohen JHM, Magoud JP, Lenoir GM et al. Immunologic phenotype of Burkitt's lymphoma cell lines according to geographic origin, Epstein-Barr virus status and type of chromosomal translocation (Submitted for publication).
19. Bernheim A, Berger R and Lenoir G (1981). Cytogenetic studies on African Burkitt's lymphoma cell lines: t(8; 14), t(2; 8) and t(8; 22) translocations. Cancer Genet and Cytogenet 3:307–315.
20. Bernheim A, Berger R and Lenoir G (1983). Cytogenetics studies on Burkitt's lymphoma cell lines. Cancer Genet Cytogenet 8:223–229.
21. Abromowitch M, Williams DL, Melvin SL and Stass S. (1984). Evidence for clonal evolution in pre-B cell leukemia. Brit J. Haematol 56:409–416.
22. Wright DH (1982). The identification and classification of non Hodgkin's lymphoma: A review. Diagn Histopathol, 5:73–111.

7. Regulation of T-cell colony formation in the absence of added growth factors, in patients with T-cell malignancies

V. GEORGOULIAS, M. ALLOUCHE and C. JASMIN

Unité d'Oncogénèse Appliquée, Hôpital Paul Brousse, Villejuif, France

T-cell colony growth in semi-solid media from normal T colony-forming cells (T-CFC) requires stimulation by phytohemagglutinin (PHA) [1–3], antigens [4], or T-cell growth factor (TCGF) and PHA [5–8]. TCGF, normally secreted by activated helper T-lymphocytes [9–12], allows continuous growth of normal PHA-stimulated [9–12] and neoplastic human T-cells [12–15]. Recent studies showed that TCGF can also be produced by fresh leukemic T-cells [14, 16] and human malignant T-cell lines after activation with PHA or phorbol diesters [17–19]. Some of these T-cell lines, although initially TCGF-dependent, can become TCGF-independent [13]. These data suggest that TCGF and probably other growth factors released by leukemic cells can play a role in the proliferation of these cells *in vitro*, and perhaps *in vivo*.

Therefore, we studied the mechanisms of proliferation of T-CFC from patients with T-cell acute lymphoblastic leukemia (T-ALL) and T-cell non-Hodgkin's lymphomas (T-NHL). We also investigated their capacity to generate colonies in the absence of added growth factors or mitogenic stimulation.

Materials and methods

Patients

Heparinized peripheral blood was obtained from 8 normal subjects, 15 patients with solid tumors, 5 with multiple myeloma, 5 chronic myelogenous, 5 acute non-lymphoid, 7 non-T non-B acute lymphoblastic leukemias and 22 patients with T-cell malignancies (17 with T-ALL and 5 with T-NHL). Fifteen patients were studied at initial presentation; 7 were studied while in relapse.

Cell preparation

Methods for obtaining different cell fractions have been described in detail elsewhere [20]. Briefly, peripheral blood mononuclear cells (MNC) were obtained by gradient density centrifugation (d = 1077). They were further separated into E-enriched (E+) and E-depleted (E−) cell fractions on the basis of 2-aminoethyl-isotio-uronium hydrobromide (AET)-treated sheep red blood cell (SRBC) rosette formation, followed by a second gradient density centrifugation.

Residual E^+ lymphocytes in the E^- cell fraction were eliminated by complement-mediated cytotoxicity with OKT3 monoclonal antibody (E^-OKT3$^-$ cells; 20). Both MNC and E^-OKT3$^-$ cells were depleted by plastic adherence as previously described [20]. Non-adherent cells were recovered by centrifugation of the cell suspension (MNCA$^-$ and E^-OKT3$^-$A$^-$ cells). Adherent cells (A$^+$) were obtained after vigorous washing of the plate. In some experiments, E^+ lymphocytes and A$^+$ cells were irradiated with 2500 and 7500 rad, respectively, using a ^{137}cesium source.

T-cell colony assay

$5-10 \times 10^5$ viable cells/ml from different cell fractions were seeded in 0.8% methylcellulose in culture medium supplemented with 20% fetal calf serum (FCS) and L-glutamine (2 mM) [20]. One-tenth ml of the cell preparation was seeded per well in 96 flat-bottomed well microtest plates.

E^-OKT3$^-$, and MNCA$^-$ or E^-OKT3$^-$A$^-$ cells (5×10^5/ml) were also co-cultured with autologous irradiated E^+ and adherent cells either in methylcellulose (one layer) or separately in an agar-methylcellulose double-layer, where the irradiated accessory cells were included in the agar (0.6%, v/v) underlayer. Controls consisted of seeding cell-containing methyl-cellulose on the top of cell-free agar underlayers. Triplicate cultures were incubated for 5–7 days at 37 °C in 5% CO$_2$ in air. Aggregates containing more than 50 cells were counted as colonies.

Preparation of conditioned media

10^6 MNC/ml were incubated for 2–7 days in growth medium supplemented with 10% FCS, and 2 mM L-glutamine. Supernatants were recovered, centrifugated, filtered through 0.45 μ and 0.22 μ Millipore filters and stored at 4 °C until use. The same procedure was used to obtain conditioned media (LCMA$^+$) from patients' adherent cells.

Media conditioned by PHA (1 % PHA-M)-stimulated patients' MNC were prepared as described above. All conditioned media were was tested for TCGF activity using a TCGF-dependent human T-cell line. Cell proliferation induced by different conditioned media was determined by tritiated thymidine (^{3}HTdR) incorporation [21]. Conditioned media were also tested for Interleukin 1 (IL1) activity by measuring their capacity to induce cell proliferation of CH3/J mouse thymocytes stimulated by concanavalin A [22].

Self-renewal capacity

Primary colonies were picked individually, pooled, dissociated and washed with cold growth medium (MEM); $5 \times 10^4 - 10^5$ viable cells/ml were replated in methylcellulose as for primary colony growth.

Blast and colony cell characterization

Fresh leukemic cells were phenotyped by indirect immunofluorescence using OKT-series (OKT3, T4, T6, T8, T10), cALLA (J5), anti-Ia (I1), and B1 monoclonal antibodies followed by F (ab')$_2$ fluoresceinated-goat anti-mouse immunoglobulin; they were also tested for AET-SRBC rosette formation [20].

Colonies of the same morphology and size were picked individually, pooled and washed. Cells were tested for AET-SRBC rosette formation and for the predominant markers detected on fresh leukemic cells. In control experiments, non-specific fluorescence was always less than 5 %. Slides were also prepared for morphologic examination, myeloperoxidase, PAS and acid phosphatase staining.

Results

Spontaneous colony formation

When $5 - 10 \times 10^5$ MNC/ml from patients with T-cell malignancies were seeded in methylcellulose in the absence of added growth factors or mitogenic stimulation, spontaneous colonies were obtained in samples from 18 of 22 patients (82 %) (Table I). Conversely, no spontaneous colony formation could be obtained from MNC of normal subjects or patients with non T-cell leukemias.

Spontaneous colony formation could also be obtained from E$^-$ OKT3$^-$

(in 9 out of 15 patients) and/or E^+ (in 4 out of 11 patients) cell fractions (Table I).

Colony characterization

Pooled MNC-derived colonies were composed mainly of lymphoblastoid cells. No macrophage or granulocytic cells were observed. Cytochemical

Table I. Clinical, hematologic and immunologic characteristics of patients with T-cell malignancies

Patient	% of blasts in P.B.	Blast phenotype[a]	Spontaneous colonies/10^5 cells[b]		
			MNC	$E^-OKT_3^-$	E^+
1	0 (R)[c]	$E^+T_3^+T_8^+$	29 ± 11	ND^d	ND
2	62 (R)	$E^+T_4^+T_6^+T_8^+$	106 ± 17	ND	ND
3	0 (R)	$E^+T_3^+T_8^+$	318 ± 12	ND	ND
4	61 (R)	E^+	284 ± 24	0	0
5	85 (P)	$E^+T_3^+$	0	0	ND
6	5 (R)	$T_6^+T_4^+T_8^+$	3 ± 2	0	800 ± 3
7	48 (R)	$E^+T_3^+T_8^+$	0	ND	ND
8	0 (P)	$E^+T_4^+T_6^+T_{10}^+$	34 ± 6	576 ± 83	960 ± 93
9	0 (P)	$E^+T_6^+$	36 ± 11	144 ± 24	ND
10	0 (R)	T_3^+	42 ± 6	380 ± 29	901 ± 82
11	98 (P)[e]	$E^+T_3^+T_4^+T_6^+T_8^+$	0	840 ± 59	102 ± 12
12	85 (P)	$T_9^+T_{10}^+$	676 ± 83	250 ± 23	0
13	47 (P)	T_8^+	486 ± 29	166 ± 27	0
14	0 (P)	$E^+T_3^+T_8^+$	198 ± 11	ND	ND
15	0 (R)	E^+	20 ± 2	ND	ND
16	0 (P)	$T_6^+T_{10}^+$	1373 ± 102	476 ± 82	0
17	68 (P)	T_3^+	47 ± 5	0	0
18	80 (R)	$T_{10}^+RFB1^+$[f]	238 ± 19	144 ± 19	0
19	0 (R)		182 ± 29	ND	ND
20	98 (P)	$RFB1^+$	16 ± 2	0	ND
21	90 (P)[g]	$E^+T_3^+T_{10}^+$	537 ± 49	240 ± 23	0
22	59 (P)	T_{10}^+	439 ± 12	0	0

[a] Based on expression of the antigen by more than 50% of the blast cells

[b] $5-10\times10^5$ cells from different cells fractions were seeded in methylcellulose in growth medium supplemented with 20% FCS and L-glutamine in the absence of added growth factors or mitogenic stimulation. Results are expressed as the mean number of colonies $\pm SD/10^5$ cells from triplicate wells

[c] R = studies at relapse; P = studied at presentation

[d] not determined

[e] percentage of blast cells in the malignant pleural effusion

[f] RFB1 is a monoclonal antibody recognizing myeloid precurors, both mature and immature T but not B cells (a gift from Dr G. Janossy, London, UK)

[g] cultures were performed from bone marrow cells where 90% of them were leukemic blasts

Table II. Phenotypic characterization of pooled spontaneous colonies obtained from unfractionated MNC and E^-OKT3 cells of patients with T-cell malignancies

Case	Predominant blast phenotype	MNC-derived colonies						E^-OKT3$^-$-derived colonies					
		E	OKT3	OKT4	OKT6	OKT8	OKT10	E	OKT3	OKT4	OKT6	OKT8	OKT10
8	$E^+T4^+T6^+T10^+$	42	23	23	75	15	65	76	42	30	68	ND	60
9	E^+T6^+	93	28	ND	77	47	56			not tested			
10	$T3^+$	65	28	ND	77	ND	87	58	5	ND	28	ND	65
11	$E^+T3^+T4^+T6^+T8^+$	No colony growth						68	12	69	53	49	56
12	$T9^+T10^+$	10	42	0	42	11	20	73	26	ND	64	14	ND
13	$T8^+$	85	86	88	71	48	53	41	27	65	78	65	ND
16	$T6^+T10^+$	32	30	10	80	ND	42			not tested			

Colonies were picked individually, pooled, washed, and stained either by indirect immunofluorescence using OKT-series monoclonal antibodies and FITC-goat antimouse immunoglobulin or tested for SRBC-rosette formation as described in 'Materials and methods'. Results are expressed as percentage of positive cells

ND: Not determined

staining showed that colony cells were myeloperoxidase-and PAS-negative. They displayed a spotlike acid phosphatase positivity over the Golgi apparatus.

In 6 patients, detailed phenotypic study of colonies did not reveal OKM1$^+$, J5$^+$, B1$^+$ or sIg$^+$ colony cells. Conversely, 13–86% and 10–93% of them where OKT3$^+$ and E$^+$, respectively. High reactivity with OKT6 (75–80% in 5 out of 7 patients) and OKT10 (56–87% in 4 out of 7 patients) monoclonal antibodies was also noted (Table II).

Pooled spontaneous colonies derived from the E$^-$OKT3$^-$ cell fraction also expressed, in all but one case, at least one specific T-cell marker. In 4 out of 5 patients, more than 60% of the colony cells were E$^+$, whereas only 5–42% of them were OKT3$^+$ (Table II). Moreover, in 4 out of 5 patients, 53–78% of the colony cells were OKT6$^+$, whereas in 3 patients more than 50% of the cells displayed the OKT10 antigen. The predominant phenotype of spontaneous colony cells (both MNC and E$^-$OKT3$^-$-derived) was quite similar to that observed on fresh leukemic cells.

Self-renewal capacity

Pooled primary spontaneous colony cells were replated in methylcellulose in the absence of added growth factors in order to determine their self-renewal capacity. Secondary spontaneous colonies could be obtained from both MNC- and E$^-$OKT3$^-$-derived primary colonies and were composed of E$^+$ cells (more than 40%; Table III). Spontaneous primary colonies could be transferred in methylcellulose without added growth factors up to 3 times.

Table III. Self-renewal capacity of primary MNC– and E$^-$OKT3$^-$-derived spontaneous T-cell colonies

| Patients | MNC-derived | | E$^-$OKT3$^-$-derived | |
	Primary	Secondary	Primary	Secondary
4	284±22	22±0.4 (48%)	–	–
6	3±2	5±5 (64%)	–	–
8	38±6	4±1 (ND)	576±83	12±2 (46%)
9	36±11	10±1 (41%)	144±24	5±2 (56%)
12	676±83	12±3 (38%)	250±23	9±3 (44%)
13	486±29	21±2 (42%)	166±27	18±4 (49%)

Pooled primary colonies from either unfractionated MNC or E$^-$OKT3$^-$ cell fraction were dissociated, washed and viable cells were replated in methylcellulose in the absence of added growth factors. Cultures were incubated as primary colonies. Results are expressed as the mean ±SD/10^5 and 10^4 seeded cells for (primary and secondary colony growth respectively), of triplicate wells. Percentages of SRBC-forming colony cells are presented in parentheses

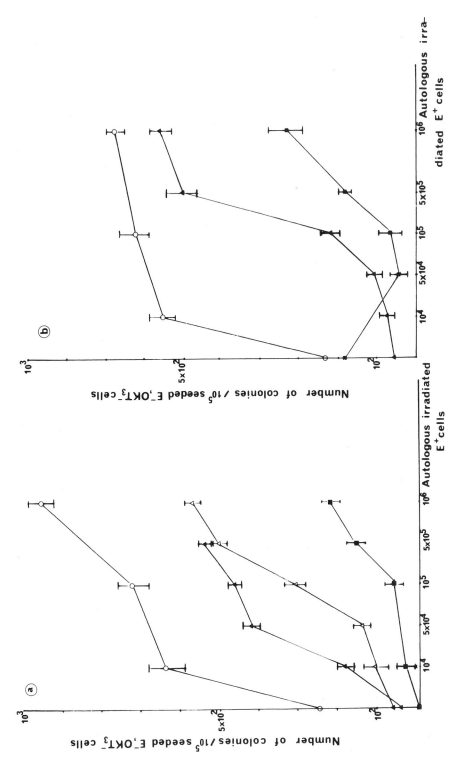

Figure 1. Effect of autologous irradiated E+ cells on spontaneous T-cell colony formation from patients' E−OKT3− cells seeded either in one (methyl-cellulose; a) or two layers (agar/methylcellulose; b) co-culture assays. Each symbol represents the same patient in the different culture assays.

Cellular cooperations regulate spontaneous colony growth

Table I also shows that, in 8 patients (No. 4, 12, 13, 16–18, 21, and 22), more spontaneous colonies were obtained from unfractionated MNC than from E⁻OKT3⁻ or E⁺ cell fractions. No spontaneous colony growth could be generated from purified E⁺ cells. Conversely, in 4 patients (8–11) more spontaneous colonies were obtained from E⁻OKT3⁻ cells than from MNC. Moreover, in 3 patients (6, 8 and 10) a significantly higher spontaneous plating efficiency was generated from purified E⁺ cells than from E⁻OKT3⁻ cells or MNC.

Table IV. Effect of adherent cells on colony formation from T-CFC of T-ALL patients

Patient	Spontaneous		Semi-purified IL2	
	MNC	MNCA⁻	MNC	MNCA⁻
12	676 ± 83	240 ± 17	ND	ND
13	486 ± 29	202 ± 19	476 ± 24	208 ± 24
18	238 ± 19	8 ± 1	258 ± 14	12 ± 3
21	537 ± 49	284 ± 22	612 ± 39	312 ± 28
22	439 ± 12	4 ± 1	503 ± 21	4 ± 2

MNC and adherent-depleted MNC (MNCA⁻) were seeded in methylcellulose either in the absence of added growth factors (spontaneous) or in the presence of 0.1 U/ml of semi-purified IL2 without PHA stimulation. Cultures were incubated as described in 'Materials and methods'. Resultats are expressed as the mean colony number $\pm SD/5 \times 10^4$ cells from triplicate wells

Table V. Effect of autologous adherent cells on spontaneous T-cell colony formation from patients' T-CFC

Number of irradiated adherent cells/ml	Co-culture in one layer	Co-culture in double layer
0	0	2 ± 1
10^4	25 ± 3	4 ± 1
10^5	165 ± 14	3 ± 2
10^6	670 ± 29	5 ± 3

Increasing numbers of irradiated (7000 rads) adherent cells were co-cultured with autologous MNCA⁻ from Patient No. 22 either in methylcellulose (one layer) or in the agar/methylcellulose double layer in the absence of added growth factors or PHA stimulation as described in 'Materials and methods'. Results are expressed as the mean number $\pm SD$ of colonies/5×10^4 cells from triplicate wells

E⁺ cells can enhance the spontaneous colony formation from some immature T-CFC

In 4 patients (12, 13, 16, 18) with immature blast cells (E⁻ OKT3⁻) where less colonies were obtained fromd E⁻ OKT3⁻ cells, autologous irradiated E⁺ cells enhanced, in a dose-dependent manner, colony formation from blast-enriched cell fraction either in a methylcellulose monolayer (Fig. 1A) or in an agar/methylcellulose double layer co-culture (Fig. 1B). Conversely, normal (allogeneic) irradiated E⁺ cells could not modify the plating efficiency from patients' E⁻ OKT3⁻ cells in either culture system.

Effects of adherent cells on spontaneous T-cell colony formation

In 5 patients, adherent cell depletion of MNC by plastic adherence resulted in decreased spontaneous colony growth. In 2, colony formation was completely abrogated (Table IV). Conversely, in 2 patients where spontaneous colony growth was observed from the E⁻ OKT3⁻ cell fraction (250 and 144 colonies/5×10^4 cells respectively), depletion of adherent cells did not modify the plating efficiency (248 and 127 colonies/5×10^4 cells respectively). Autologous irradiated A⁺ cells co-cultured with MNCA⁻ cells restored

Table VI. Endogenous production of TCGF and T-cell colony promoting activity (T-CPA) by patients' MNC

	TCGF activity (U/ml)		T-CPA (Colonies/5×10^4 normal E⁺ cells)	
Source of LCM	2-day	7-day	2-day	7-day
Normal MNC	0	0	0	0
Patient 1	ND	1.0	ND	70±12
8	ND	0	ND	0
10	0	ND	524±42	ND
11	0	0	264±19	278±25
12	0.3	0	294±23	48±7
13	0	0	145±12	14±3
17	0	0	248±29	14±2
18	0	0	244±19	258±27
20	0	0	374±25	60±8
22	0	0	608±39	18±3

TCGF activity was tested in a TCGF-dependent human T-cell line by ³HTDR incorporation as described in 'Patients and methods'. T-CPA was tested by seeding 5×10^5 normal peripheral blood E⁺ lymphocytes/ml in methylcellulose in the presence of 10% (v/v) of media conditioned by patients' unstimulated MNC for 2 and 7 days. Cultures were incubated as described in 'Materials and methods' and aggregates containing more than 50 cells were counted as colonies. Results are expressed as the mean number of colonies ±SD of 3 separate cultures.

colony formation, in a dose-independent manner, only in the single layer assay (Table V).

Endogeneous release of growth factors by patients' MNC

The spontaneous T-cell colony growth suggests an endogenous release of T-cell growth factor(s) by patients' MNC. Two out of 11 media conditioned (LCM) by unstimulated patients' MNC contained TCGF activity (Table VI), whereas IL1 activity was detected in 1 out of 8 LCM. Moreover, 2-day LCM from all patients were able to induce colony formation from normal E^+ clonogenic cells (Table VI), although 8 out of 9 LCM did not contain detectable amounts of IL2 activity. Generally minor T-cell colony promoting activity (T-CPA) was detected in some 7-day TCGF-free LCM (Table VI). Media conditioned by normal unstimulated MNC for 2 and 7 days did not display T-CPA.

Discussion

Peripheral blood clonogenic cells from patients with T-ALL and T-NHL can generate colonies in the absence of added growth factors and mitogenic stimulation. These colonies were of T-cell origin as demonstrated by their cytochemical and immunologic characterization. This phenomenon appears to be restricted to T-cell malignancies; MNC from non T-cell leukemic patients as well as normal subjects failed to exhibit spontaneous colony growth. The phenotype of pooled colonies obtained from both unfractionated MNC and E^- OKT3$^-$ cells varied from patient to patient. However, detailed phenotypic studies of colony cells suggest that colonies were mainly composed of immature cells (as assessed by the high proportion of OKT6$^+$ and OKT10$^+$ cells and the low frequency of OKT3$^+$ and/or E^+ cells [20] with a phenotype similar to that observed on original blasts.

Colonies obtained from E^- OKT3$^-$ cells were composed of E^+ and OKT3$^+$ cells (40–75 % and 20–45 % respectively), suggesting that, at least in some patients, immature T-CFC can also differentiate *in vitro* without added growth factors. Therefore, spontaneous colonies were not artifactual aggregates but true colonies derived from clonogenic cells which had the capacity to proliferate and differentiate *in vitro*. Self-renewal capacity of spontaneously proliferating T-CFC clearly demonstrates their stem-cell properties. Results from earlier studies indicated that T-CFC from T-cell malignancy patients, which proliferate *in vitro* in the presence of TCGF and PHA, did not display self-renewal capacity [20], in contrast to normal T-CFC [23].

In some patients, the number of colonies obtained from E⁻OKT3⁻ or/and E⁺ cells was lower than that obtained from unfractionated MNC. A minimum of 2×10^4/ml of MNC should be seeded to obtain spontaneous colony growth (data not shown). These observations suggest that cellular interactions regulate spontaneous colony growth. Co-culture experiments revealed that autologous, but not allogenic, E⁺ and adherent cells enhance spontaneous colony formation from E⁻OKT3⁻ and MNCA⁻ cells respectively, in a dose-dependent manner. Colony-enhancing activity of E⁺ cells was also demonstrated in the double layer culture assay, suggesting that this activity is mediated by diffusible factors. Conversely, adherent cells could restore colony formation from MNCA⁻ cells only in the single layer assay. Therefore, the colony-promoting activity of A⁺ cells could be due either to cell-to-cell contact or to short-range, non-diffusible soluble mediators. Patients' A⁺ cells seem to cooperate mainly with E⁺ cells, since colony growth from E⁻OKT3⁻ cell fraction could not be abrogated by adherent cell-depletion. Short-range mediators secreted by A⁺ cells might trigger autologous E⁺ cells to release other growth factors inducing the proliferation of immature T-CFC.

Spontaneous colony growth from T-CFC of patients with T-cell malignancies suggests that endogeneously released growth factors can induce the *in vitro* proliferation of some clonogenic T-cells. However, detectable amounts of constitutively released TCGF could be detected in LCM from only 2 of 11 patients. Unstimulated MNC from patients might release amounts of TCGF which are undetectable with the biological assay (less than 0.01 μ/ml), or consumed during the culture period. However, the frequent occurence of spontaneous colony growth indicate that other growth factors could be involved. All 2-day LCM induced T-cell colony formation from normal E⁺ lymphocytes in the absence of added TCGF or PHA. We suggest that this T-cell colony-promoting activity (T-CPA) is distinct from TCGF or IL1, since it was detected in TCGF and IL1-free conditioned media. The fact that T-CPA was lower in 7-day than in 2-day may indicate either its consumption by leukemic cells in culture or the presence of non-specific inhibitory factors.

In a previous study we indicated that T-CPA can be produced by blast-enriched cell fractions [24]. Therefore, our results suggest that *in vitro* proliferation of clonogenic T-cells from patients with T-cell malignancies is a multi-step process, involving adherent cells, presumably 'mature' E⁺ lymphocytes and leukemic cells.

Acknowledgements

We wish to thank Dr. F. Triebel for performing IL2 dosages and Mrs Martine Grosbois for secretarial help.

68

This work was supported by grants from the Association de la Recherche contre le Cancer ARC.

References

1. Rosenszajn L, Shohan D and Kalechman I (1975). Clonal proliferation of PHA-stimulated human lymphocytes in soft agar cultures. Immunology 29:1941–2055.
2. Glaësson MH, Rodger HB, Johnson GR et al. (1977). Colony formation by human lymphocytes in agar medium. Clin Exp Immunol 28:526–534.
3. Gerassi E and Sachs L (1976). Regulation of the induction of colonies *in vitro* by normal lymphocytes. Proc Nat Acad Sci USA 73:4546–4548.
4. Kornbluth J, Gorski A and Dupont B (1979). Alloantigen-activated lymphocyte colony formation in semi-solid agar. Transplant Proc 11:1978–1981.
5. Shen J, Wilson F, Shifrine M and Gershwin ME (1979). Selective growth of human T-lymphocytes in single phase semi-solid culture. J Immunol 119:1299–1305.
6. Triebel F, Robinson WA, Hayward AR and Coube de Laforest P (1981). Existence of a pool of T-lymphocyte colony forming cells (T-CFC) in human bone marrow and their place in the differentiation of the T-lymphocyte lineage. Blood 58:911–915.
7. Moreau JF and Miller RG (1983). Growth at limiting dilution of human T-cell depleted peripheral blood leukocytes. J Immunol 130:1139–1145.
8. Georgoulias V, Marion S, Consolini R and Jasmin C. Characterization of normal peripheral blood T- and B-cell colony forming cells: Growth factor(s) and accessory cell requirements for their *in vitro* proliferation (submitted for publication).
9. Ruscetti FN, Morgan DA and Gallo RA (1977). Functional and morphological characteristics of human thymus derived lymphocytes continuously growing *in vitro*. J Immunol 119:131–138.
10. Watson J (1979). Continuous proliferation of murine antigen specific helper T-lymphocytes in cultures. J Exp Med 150:1510–1516.
11. Mier JW and Gallo RC (1980). Purification and some properties of human T-cell growth factor from phytohemagglutinin-stimulated lymphocyte conditioned media. Proc Nat Acad Sci USA 77:6134–6138.
12. Ruscetti FN, Gallo RC (1981). Human T-lymphocyte growth factor: Regulation of growth and function of T-lymphocytes. Blood 57:379–394.
13. Poiezs BJ, Ruscetti FN, Mier JW et al (1980). T-cell lines from human T-lymphocytic neoplasias by direct response to T-cell growth factor. Proc Nat Acad Sci USA 77:6815–6819.
14. Gillis S, Mertelsmann R and Moore MAS (1981). T-cell growth factor (Interleukin 2) control of T-lymphocyte proliferation: Possible involvement in leukemogenesis. Transplant Proc 13:1884–1890.
15. Gootenberg JE, Ruscetti FW, Mier JW et al. (1981). Human cutaneous T-cell lymphoma and leukemia cell lines produce and respond to T-cell growth factors. J Exp Med 154:1403–1418.
16. Venuta S, Mertelsmann R, Wetle K et al. (1983). Production and regulation of Interleukin 2 in human lymphoblastic leukemias studied with T-cell monoclonal antibodies. Blood 61:781–787.
17. Solbach W, Barth S, Röllinghoff M and Nagner H (1981). Lymphocyte regulatory molecules in human leukemic cells and cell lines. Evidence for malignant proliferation of T-cells producing IL2 in Sezary syndrome. In: W. Knapp (ED.). Leukemia Markers, pp. 335–340. Academic Press.
18. Friedman SM, Tompson G, Halper JP and Knowles DH (1982). OT-CLL: A human T-cell

chronic lymphocytic leukemia line that produces IL2 in high titer. J Immunol 128:935–939.

19. Vyth-Dreese FA, Van Der Reijden HJ and De Vries JE (1982). Phorbol Ester-mediated induction and augmentation of mitogenesis and Interleukin 2 production in human T-cell lymphoproliferative diseases. Blood 60:1437–1446.

20. Georgoulias V, Auclair H and Jasmin C (1984). Heterogeneity of peripheral blood T-cell colony forming cells (T-CFC) of patients with T-cell malignancies. Leuk Res (in press).

21. Bertoglio J, Boisson N, Bonnet MC et al. (1982). First French workshop on standardization of human IL2: Joint report. Lymphokine Res 1:121–132.

22. Stosic-Grujicic S and Simic MM (1982). Modulation of interleukin 1 production by activated macrophages: *In vitro* action of hydrocortisone, colchicine and cytochalasin B. Cell Immunol 69:235–243.

23. Wu AM (1983). Regulation of self-renewal of human T-lymphocyte colony forming units (TL-CFUs). J Cell Physiol 117:101–108.

24. Georgoulias V, Triebel F, Kosmatopoulos C et al. T-cell colony growth in patients with T-cell malignancies: Growth factor(s) requirements for *in vitro* proliferation of peripheral blood T colony-forming cells (T-CFC). (Submitted for publication).

II. Cytogenetics

1. Banded chromosome abnormalities in non-Hodgkin's lymphoma. Correlations with morphology, immunologic phenotype and clinical course

C. D. BLOOMFIELD, D. C. ARTHUR, E. G. LEVINE,
G. FRIZZERA, K. J. GAJL-PECZALSKA, T. W. LEBIEN,
D. D. HURD and B. A. PETERSON
*Section of Medical Oncology, Department of Medicine and the
Departments of Laboratory Medicine and Pathology and Pediatrics,
University of Minnesota Health Sciences Center, Minneapolis,
Minnesota, U.S.A.*

Limited data are available regarding chromosomal abnormalities in malignant lymphoma, other than Burkitt's. The few reported studies of banded chromosomes have generally been based on small series (less than 50 cases) and have often included many incomplete karyotypes. Bone marrow, blood or effusions have frequently been studied rather than lymph nodes or other primary tumor masses, and relatively few patients have been studied at diagnosis. Moreover, for a given lymph node, chromosome findings have rarely been correlated with histology and immunologic phenotype. Since July 1978, we have been prospectively studying chromosomal abnormalities in lymph nodes from patients with lymphoma and correlating them with histology, immunologic phenotype and clinical findings [1, 2]. In this manuscript we briefly review our findings in the first 115 patients.

Materials and methods

Chromosomes from involved lymph nodes or other tumor masses from 115 patients (ages 8–85 years; median 55) with non-Hodgkin's malignant lymphoma were studied. In 73 patients, neoplastic tissue was analyzed at diagnosis prior to any treatment; in 42 patients, tissue was first studied at relapse. In all instances, the tumor was simultaneously studied for histology, immunologic markers, and G-banded chromosomes. Histologic classification was done using the International Working Formulation for Clinical Usage [3].

Immunologic phenotyping was based on study of both single cell suspensions and tissue frozen sections in all cases [4]. All cases were studied for surface (SIg) and cytoplasmic (CIg) immunoglobulin, and receptors for complement (C'), Fc, and unsensitized sheep erythrocytes (E). Seventy-nine

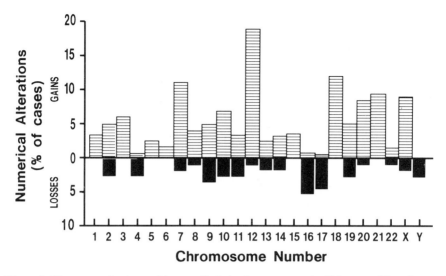

Figure 1. Histogram of gains and losses of whole chromosomes in 115 cases of lymphoma. A given patient may have more than one chromosome gained or lost.

cases were also studied with a panel of monoclonal antibodies including BA-1, BA-2 and BA-3 [5].

For cytogenic studies, a portion of the same tumor mass biopsied for histology and immunologic phenotyping was obtained directly from the surgical pathology laboratory and processed within one hour of biopsy. Metaphase chromosomes were harvested from direct preparations and unstimulated or methotrexate-synchronized short-term (24- and 48-hour) cultures using described methods [2]. G-banding was done using the Wright's technique of Sanchez et al. [6]. Photographs of metaphases were taken on high-contrast S0115 film, and multiple karyotypes were constructed in each case.

Chromosomes have been designated according to the ISCN (1978, 1981), and the karyotypes are expressed as recommended under this system [7, 8]. Chromosome abnormalities were designated as clonal if two or more metaphase cells had identical structural anomalies or extra chromosomes or if three or more metaphase cells had identical missing chromosomes.

Results

Clonal chromosome abnormalities were identified in 110 of the 115 patients. Two clones were identified in 12%. Most clones had multiple abnormalities. Abnormal karyotypes included gains of one or more whole chromosomes (without apparent structural abnormalities) in 58% of patients and losses of one or more whole chromosomes in 27% (Fig. 1). Chromo-

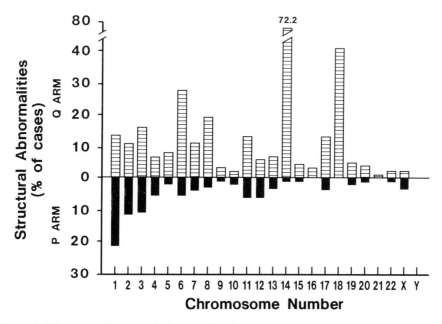

Figure 2. Histogram of structural abnormalities involving each chromosome in 115 cases of lymphoma. Structural rearrangements including translocations, deletions, duplications etc, are displayed for each chromosome arm.

somes most commonly gained were 12 (19% of patients), 18 (12%) and 7 (11%). Chromosomes most frequently lost were 16 (5%) and 17 (4%). Structural abnormalities were more frequent than numerical alterations, occurring in all except 12 patients. All chromosomes were affected, but with considerable variation in frequency. The chromosome long (q) arms were involved in 90% of patients and the short (p) arms in 50% (Fig. 2). The chromosome regions (by arm) most frequently rearranged were 14q (72% of patients), 18q (41%), 6q (28%), 1p (21%), 8q (19%), 3q (16%), 1q, 11q and 17q (14% each), 2p, 2q and 7q (11% each) and 3p (10%).

Structural abnormalities most frequently were translocations. Eighty-four different translocations were identified in 86 patients. Seven recurring translocations were identified: t(14; 18)(q32; q21) (in 35 patients), t(8; 14) (q24; q32) (in 10 patients) and t(3; 14)(p21; q32), t(5; 14)(q23; q32), t(8; 14)(q22; q32), t(11; 14)(q23; q32), t(14; 19)(q32; q13) in two each. Other common types of structural abnormalities included deletions, duplications and isochromosomes. Chromosomes regions most commonly rearranged were 14q32 (67% of patients), 18q21 (31%), 6q21 (15%), 8q24 (13%), 11q21–25 (11%) and 1p36 (10%).

A number of features of the karyotype differed significantly ($p < 0.009$) among histologic groups. These included the frequency of normal metaphase cells, the modal number of the abnormal clone, and the frequency of certain specific chromosome abnormalities (Table I). In histologic groups B, F and I, most cases had 20% or more normal metaphases and in groups G and J most cases had no normal cells. Interestingly, the modal number steadily increased as the follicular lymphomas included more large cells (a modal number of 47 in group B, 48 in group C and 49 in group D). The modal number was the same in large cell lymphomas whether they were nodular or diffuse (groups D and G).

No chromosome region or specific chromosome abnormality was restricted to a single histology, but several were frequent in only one or two groups. These included an extra 7 in follicular center cell tumors with large cells (groups C, D and G), an extra 8 in the follicular lymphomas, mixed small cleaved and large cell (C), t(8; 14)(q24; q32) in large and small noncleaved malignant lymphoma (G and J), 13p13 in C, 17q21–25 in D, and t(14; 18)(q32; q21) in follicular lymphomas (B-D) and diffuse large (follicu-

Table I. Karotype findings which differed significantly among histologies[a]

	International Working Formulation Groups									
	A[b]	B	C	D	F	G	H	I	J	
No. cases	19	28	8	9	13	23	4	3	5	
				Median value						*p* value
% Normal cells	18	22	7	15	20	0	12	45	0	.002
Modal number	46	47	48	49	47	49	48	46	46	<.001
			Frequency (%) of specific abnormality in each histology							
Chromosome or region altered										
6q21	21	29	25	22	23	39	75	0	20	.0085
+7	0	4	25	33	0	30	0	0	0	.0071
+8	0	4	38	11	0	0	0	0	0	.0018
8q	16	14	25	0	0	30	25	0	100	.0003
8q24	16	0	0	0	0	30	0	0	100	.0000
t(8;14) (q24;q32)	5	0	0	0	0	22	0	0	80	.0000
13p13	0	0	38	0	0	4	0	0	0	.0002
14q32	42	89	100	67	46	74	0	33	100	.0001
17q21-25	0	0	0	44	8	9	0	0	0	.0007
18q	16	68	63	44	15	52	0	0	20	.0013
18q21	5	64	63	44	0	26	0	0	20	.0000
t(14;18) (q32;q21)	0	61	63	44	0	26	0	0	20	.0000

[a] Only abnormalities with a *p* value <.009 are listed. This conservative *p* value has been chosen because of the large number of possibilities tested

[b] A-ML, small lymphocytic; B-ML, follicular, predominantly small cleaved; C-ML, follicular, mixed, small cleaved and large cell; D-ML, follicular, predominantly large cell; F-ML, diffuse, mixed small and large cell; G-ML, diffuse, large cell; H-ML, diffuse large cell immunoblastic; I-ML, lymphoblastic; J-ML, small non-cleaved

lar center) cell lymphoma (G). Rearrangements of specific chromosome regions, but not specific abnormalities, were occasionally found in 100% of a given histologic group.

Most (98) of the lymphomas in our series were B-cell. When the results of cytogenetic analysis were compared among broad immunologic groups (B, T, C', null) only abnormalities involving 18q differed significantly among the groups, occurring in all three cases of C' lymphoma, 44% of B lymphomas, but no T lymphomas ($p = 0.003$). Since most cases studied were B-cell (98), a detailed analysis of the distribution of chromosome abnormalities among lymphomas expressing different heavy and light chains was possible. No highly significant differences (all p values >0.03) in distribution were found. However, when the B-cell lymphomas were classified according to expression of the antigens identified by the monoclonal antibodies BA-1, BA-2 and BA-3, the distribution of certain chromosome abnormalities varied significantly (Table II). Most interesting was the frequent absence of BA-1 expression in lymphomas with chromosome rearrangements involving 5q and 6q.

Among the 73 patients studied at diagnosis prior to treatment, various aspects of the karyotype were studied relative to response to treatment, duration of first remission and survival. Median follow-up of the surviving patients in this group is 32 months (minimum of nine months). Sixty-five percent of patients achieved a complete remission. No significant correlations with cytogenetic findings were identified. However, duration of first remission was significantly shorter in patients demonstrating an abnormality of 1p (median 12 months vs. >48 months, $p = 0.01$). The length of survival varied significantly according to a number of aspects of karyotype

Table II. Chromosome abnormalities which differed significantly among B-cell monoclonal groups

	Expression of BA-1, BA-2, BA-3							BA-1 [a]		
	+ − −	− − −	+ + −	− + −	+ + +	+ − +		+	−	
No. cases	28	5	13	5	6	4	*p* value	51	12	*p* value
	% Chromosome abnormalities in each immunologic group									
1p abnl	4	40	46	20	0	50	.0085			
5q abnl	0	60	0	40	0	0	.0000	0	42	.0000
6q15	0	0	0	40	17	0	.0036			
6q21	18	60	8	60	0	0	.0157	12	50	.0086
+7	7	0	8	60	0	0	.0065			
16q abnl	0	0	0	0	0	50	.0000			

[a] Two additional cases were studied for BA-1 which were not studied for BA-2 and BA-3

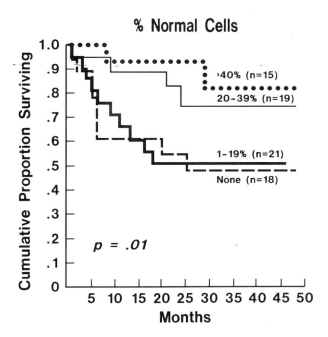

Figure 3. Survival of 73 patients with lymphoma according to the frequency of normal metaphases identified cytogenetically in a neoplastic lymph node studied pretreatment.

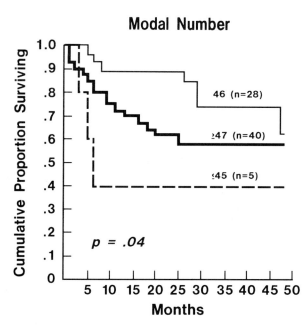

Figure 4. Survival of 73 patients with lymphoma according to the modal number of the primary clonal chromosome abnormality identified in a pretreatment neoplastic lymph node.

analysis. In particular, patients whose lymphomas had more than 20% normal metaphases survived significantly longer than those with fewer than 20% normal cells (Fig. 3). Similarly, patients with lymphomas whose clonal chromosome abnormality had a modal number of 46 survived longer than those with a modal number of ≥ 47 or ≤ 45 (Fig. 4). In addition, survival was worse in patients whose lymphoma had an extra 18 (median 7 months vs. >48 months, $p = 0.02$). Too few patients have been studied to determine if these various features of karyotype are independent risk factors.

Discussion

In this large study of G-banded chromosomes in lymphoma, clonal chromosome abnormalities have been found in 110 of 115 cases. Multiple recurring abnormalities were noted, some of which were associated with specific histologies or immunologic phenotypes. Certain aspects of cytogenetic analysis also seemed to correlate with patient survival. However, analysis is complicated by the multiple abnormalities found in most patients and the relatively small numbers of patients with each recurring abnormality studied. The clinical relevance of cytogenetic analysis for diagnosis, classification and prognosis in lymphoma obviously requires further study.

The biologic significance of these recurring clonal chromosome abnormalities is also unknown. However, it is of interest that 79% of patients had numerical or structural rearrangements that involve chromosomes or chromosome regions to which oncogenes have been mapped [9]. Detailed study of the role of oncogenes in lymphoma would appear to be a profitable endeavor.

Acknowledgements

Supported in part by the Coleman Leukemia Research Fund. Dr. Levine is a Fellow and Dr. LeBien a Scholar of the Leukemia Society of America.

References

1. Bloomfield CD, Arthur DC, Frizzera G et al. (1982). Chromosomal abnormalities in non-Hodgkin's malignant lymphoma. In: Vitetta E (Ed.). B and T Cell Tumors: Biological and Clinical Aspects, UCLA Symposia on Molecular and Cellular Biology, Vol. 24, pp.227–231. New York: Academic Press.
2. Bloomfield CD, Arthur DC, Frizzera G et al. (1983). Nonrandom chromosome abnormalities in lymphoma. Cancer Res 43:2975–2984.
3. Non-Hodgkin's Lymphoma Pathologic Classification Project (1982). National Cancer Insti-

tute-sponsored study of classifications of non-Hodgkin's lymphoma: Summary and description of a working formulation for clinical usage. Cancer 49:2112–2135.

4. Gajl-Peczalska KJ, Bloomfield CD, Frizzera G et al. (1982). Diversity of phenotypes of non-Hodgkin's malignant lymphoma. In: Vitetta E (Ed.). B and T Cell Tumors: Biological and Clinical Aspects, UCLA Symposia on Molecular and Cellular Biology, Vol. 24, pp. 63–67. New York: Academic Press.

5. Bloomfield CD, Gajl-Peczalska KJ, Frizzera G and LeBien TW. The clinical utility of cell surface markers in malignant lymphoma. In: Ford RJ, Fuller LM, Hagemeister FB (Eds.). New Perspectives in Human Lymphoma. New York: Raven Press (in press).

6. Sanchez O, Escobar JJ and Yunis JJ (1973). A simple G-banding technique. Lancet 2:269.

7. ISCN (1978). An international system for human cytogenetic nomenclature. Cytogenet Cell Genet 21:309–404.

8. ISCN (1981). An international system for human cytogenetic nomenclature in high-resolution banding. Cytogenet Cell Genet 31:1–23.

9. Bloomfield CD, Arthur DC, Levine EG et al. Chromosome abnormalities in malignant lymphoma. Biologic and clinical correlations. In: Modern Trends in Human Leukemia VI, Haematology and Blood Transfusion (in press).

2. Chromosomal aberrations in leukemic low-grade malignant B-cell lymphoproliferative neoplasias

G. GAHRTON, G. JULIUSSON, K. H. ROBERT, K. FRIBERG
and L. ZECH
*Division of Clinical Hematology and Oncology, Department of
Medicine, Huddinge Hospital and Karolinska Institute, and Institute
of Medical Cell Genetics, Medical Nobel Institute, Karolinska
Institute, Stockholm, Sweden*

The low-grade malignant B-cell lymphoproliferative disorders with leu-kemic cells in the peripheral blood (LMBLL) are practically all included in what is usually called chronic lymphocytic leukemia (CLL). When it became obvious that CLL was a heterogenous disease, it was subdivided in several groups, e.g. according to the Kiel classification [1]. New entities such as immunocytoma, prolymphocytic leukemia, and centrocytic lymphoma, were separated from CLL. Our original aim was to investigate the 'classical' CLL for possible presence of specific chromosomal aberrations. The study includes patients within the new subgroups, but only those who presented with a leukemic picture, i.e. a blood lymphocyte count of at least $5 \times 10^9/l$.

For a long time, CLL was considered not to be characterized by any spe-cific chromosomal abnormality [2]. This was in contrast to other hemato-poietic neoplasias, such as chronic myelocytic leukemia and the acute leu-kemias. It has become obvious that the reason chromosomal aberrations were not found was that CLL is characterized by the presence of mature lymphocytes with a low spontaneous mitotic index, and furthermore, the mitogens used to stimulate mitosis of lymphocytes were usually T-cell stimulators, such as phytohemagglutinin (PHA), while CLL in most cases is a B-cell malignancy [3].

The discovery of mitogens that primarily stimulated B-cells, so-called polyclonal B-cell activators (PBA) [4], opened new possibilities to study CLL B-lymphocytes. It was shown that PBA could induce DNA synthe-sis [5], mitosis [6], and immunoglobulin synthesis [7] in these cells. The immunoglobulins that could be detected intracellularly upon stimulation with PBA were monoclonal and of the same class as those present on the surface on lymphocytes before stimulation [7]. Thus, it was obvious that CLL leukemic cells were stimulated by PBA. In the cytogenetic studies, the most important finding was that PBA induced cell division, a prerequisite for such investigations [6]. We could then show that B-CLL leukemic cells had chromosomal aberrations, the most important of which was an extra chromosome 12 [8, 9]. The present work reports the clinical and prognostic importance of chromosomal abnormalities in LMBLL ('classical' CLL) [10, 11].

Materials and methods

Patients

Fifty-five patients with LMBLL were investigated as reported in [10] and [11]. According to Rai [12], 10 patients were in Stage 0, 20 in Stage I, 9 in Stage II, 8 in Stage III, and 8 patients in Stage IV. According to Binet [13], 27 patients were in Stage A, 10 in Stage B and 8 in Stage C. At diagnosis, all patients had blood lymphocyte counts of $\geq 5 \times 10^9/l$. The cell-surface immunoglobulin phenotype was μk in 6 cases, $\mu d k$ in 22, γk in 6, $\mu \lambda$ in 4, $\mu d \lambda$ in 12, while in 3 patients the fluorescence was too weak to make proper phenotype identification. Since the observation time was too short to analyze survival of the patients, the time from established disease to indication for treatment was analyzed. The guidelines for treatment were those of the Swedish Lymphoma Study Group [14], i.e., progressive disease with clear B-symptoms (fever, night sweats or weight loss not due to other causes), progressive disabling lymphadenopathy, progressive anemia or thrombocytopenia (hemoglobin level $< 100 \, g/l$ or platelet counts below $100 \times 10^9/l$).

Subclassification according to the Kiel classification [1] was based on the cytologic and morphologic pictures as well as immunocytochemistry of specimens obtained from lymph nodes, spleen, bone marrow, and peripheral blood.

Cell culture and mitogen stimulation

Cells for mitogen stimulation were obtained from lymph nodes, spleens, bone marrow, and peripheral blood. Lymphocytes were isolated by floatation on a Ficoll-Isopaque gradient [15]. The cells were then activated by Epstein-Barr virus (EBV), lipopolysaccharide from *Escherichia coli* (LPS), and tetradecanoylphorbolacetate (TPA) [6, 7, 11]. EBV stimulation was performed by incubation of the cells with 1 ml of the supernatant from the B95-8 cell line/10^7 cells for 1 h at 37 °C. LPS from *E. coli* was used at a final concentration of 100 μg/ml for stimulation of cells cultured at a concentration of 2×10^6 ml in Eagle's medium containing 10% heat-inactivated human AB serum. The cultures were harvested after an incubation for 4 days. During the last 90 minutes of culture, the cells were exposed to colchicine and hypotonic treatment with a 0.56% solution of potassium chloride for 5 minutes. Cells were fixed in methanol/acetic acid (3:1) for 40 minutes, centrifuged, suspended in fixative dropped onto slides and air dried. Cells were stained by the Q-banding technique [16]. Metaphases of good quality for chromosomal analysis were photographed in a fluorescence microscope. All metaphases were analyzed by conventional karyotyping. A clonal chromosomal abnormality was defined according to the International System for Human Cytogenetic Nomenclature (ISCN) [17] as follows: 1) gain of a specific chromosome in at least 2 cells; 2) loss of a specific chromosome in at least 3 cells; 3) identical structural aberrations in at least 2 cells. Patients were considered to have a normal karyotype if a normal karyotype was found in at least 12 cells, and if there was no evidence of a clonal aberration.

Results

Of the 55 patients, 43 had a sufficient number of metaphases for evaluation of chromosomal abnormalities. Of these, 32 patients had chromosomal aberrations. Sixteen patients had an extra chromosome 12, either as the only aberration (6 patients), or together with various other aberrations (10 patients). One patient had a partial duplication of chromosome 12 (the segment q13–q22). Fifteen patients had clonal chromosomal aberrations which did not involve duplications of chromosome 12. The aberrations were of different kinds. Six patients had a 14q+ marker chromosome, 4 patients had deletions on chromosome 11, 2 with the same breakpoint at q22, and 4 patients had deletions of chromosome 6 with different breakpoints. Two patients had a del(3) (p13) aberration. Seven patients had a complex karyotype with 3 or more clonal aberrations, while 15 patients had only one single aberration. Eleven patients had no apparent chromosomal aberrations in more than 12 metaphases studied.

According to the Kiel classification, the patients could be subgrouped in CLL 'proper' (CLL-Kiel) ($n = 22$), immunocytoma (IC) ($n = 29$), prolymphocytic leukemia (PLL) ($n = 2$), and centrocytic lymphoma ($n = 1$). One patient could not be subclassified. The chromosomal pattern could be evaluated in 17 patients with CLL-Kiel and 22 patients with IC, and in the 4 patients with other classifications. Clonal aberrations were found in 12 CLL-Kiel patients, 16 IC patients, and in all the other patients. With or without other aberrations, +12 were seen in 6 CLL patients, 10 IC patients and in the patient that was not subclassified. Thus, there was no clear difference in the frequency of the +12 abnormality between patients with CLL-Kiel or immunocytoma. Other aberrations were also seen in about the same frequency in these two groups, 6 in CLL-Kiel and 6 in IC. Of partic-

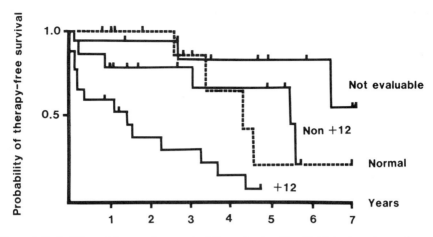

Figure 1. Probability of therapy-free survival for patients with: (1) Not adequate numbers of evaluable metaphases; (2) Normal chromosomal pattern; (3) Chromosomal abnormalities other than +12; (4) +12 with or without other abnormalities.

ular interest was that in both PLL patients a del(3)(p13) abnormality was found [18].

Patients with a complex karyotype, i.e. with 3 or more clonal aberrations, had the most aggressive disease. Both therapy-free survival and survival were significantly worse in this patient group than in patients with a normal karyotype or in those with only one or two clonal aberrations.

Patients with the +12 abnormality also had a poorer prognosis than patients with a normal karyotype (Fig. 1). As judged from the therapy-free survival, this was irrespective of whether +12 was the only abnormality or there were other changes in addition to the +12 abnormality. Thus, +12 as a single abnormality appeared to imply a less favorable prognosis than other single abnormalities [11].

Discussion

Although LMBLL is a heterogeneous disorder as judged from the cytomorphologic pattern and cytochemistry, the most specific chromosomal aberration, an extra chromosome 12, was found in most subgroups of LMBLL. This is in agreement with several reports by us [8–11] and others [19–21] that an extra chromosome 12 is the most common chromosomal abnormality in 'classical' CLL. The frequency of this aberration in the two main groups, CLL-Kiel and immunocytoma, was about the same, i.e. 6 of 17 (35%) in CLL-Kiel, and 10 of 22 (45%) in IC [11]. From the pathogenetic point of view, it is therefore possible that LBMLL with a +12 abnormality is a more distinct entity than a cytologically defined subgroup with various chromosomal abnormalities. This point is further strengthened by the prognostic implication of carrying a +12 abnormality. Those patients who had this aberration had a significantly poorer prognosis than patients who either had no abnormality, were not evaluable because of too few metaphases, or had chromosomal abnormalities other than +12 (Fig. 1). Also, there was the same poor prognosis in patients with +12 as a single aberration as in patients with +12 together with aberrations. Furthermore, patients with +12 as a single abnormality had a poorer prognosis than patients with other single abnormalities [11].

In many patients the +12 abnormality was present only in a minor fraction of the metaphases investigated. The nature of the normal metaphases is not clear, they could be normal B-cells. It is possible that such normal cells were more easily stimulated by PBA, and thus despite the dominating leukemic cell population a comparatively large fraction of normal metaphases were seen. They could also be normal T-cells, but this is less likely since EBV and LPS are specific B-cell stimulators. Appearance of +12 during progression of the disease cannot be excluded, which would imply that +12 is not involved in initiating the disease, but is a marker of progression.

One patient, previously described by us [22], had a partial duplication of chromosome 12, which indicates that the duplicated segment on q13-q22 may carry the important genes for disease development. It is of particular interest to note that the k-ras oncogene is located on chromosome 12, and some reports indicate that it may be located on the long arm [23]. Thus, it is possible that the duplication of this segment results in an equivalently increased gene dose, which leads to leukemic transformation. Alternatively, the oncogene may be activated by other mechanisms such as chromatid exchange as in the patient reported by us (above). Chromosomal translocations have been implicated in activation of oncogenes [24]. It is of interest to note that a fraction of patients with CLL have been shown to have an elevated amount of the enzyme serinehydroxymethyl transferase [25] in their lymphocytes. This enzyme is encoded on the long arm of chromosome 12 [26].

The importance of other chromosomal aberrations in LMBLL is less clear; they were of various kinds. The 14q+ marker chromosome seen in a number of other lymphoproliferative disorders [27] may have etiologic or pathogenetic importance. Other aberrations also seen in lymphoproliferative disorders were deletions on chromosome 6 and deletions on chromosome 11. One interesting finding was that two patients with prolymphocytic leukemia had the same abnormality on chromosome 3, a deletion, del(3)(p13) [18]. The number of chromosomal abnormalities other than +12 were many, while the number of patients with each of them was small. It was therefore not possible to analyze their prognostic implication. How-

86

ever, if several clonal abnormalities were present at the same time the prognosis was poor. This was true both regarding therapy-free survival and survival [11].

Acknowledgements

This work was supported by grants from the Swedish Cancer Society and the Karolinska Institute's Research Funds.

References

1. Lennert K. (1978). Malignant lymphomas other than Hodgkin's disease. Handbuch der speziellen patologischen Anatomie und Histologie. Band 1, Teil 3 B. Berlin, Heidelberg, New York: Springer-Verlag.
2. Mitelman F and Levan G (1978). Clustering of aberrations to specific chromosomes in human neoplasms. III. Incidence and geographic distribution of chromosome aberrations in 856 cases. Hereditas 89:207–232.
3. Rundles RW and Moore JO (1978). Chronic lymphocytic leukemia. Cancer 42:941–945.
4. Möller G (ed.) (1975). Subpopulation of B lymphocytes. Transplant Rev 24:1-236.
5. Robèrt KH, Möller E, Gahrton G et al. (1978). B-cell activation of peripheral blood lymphocytes from patients with chronic lymphatic leukaemia. Clin Exp Immunol 33:302–308.
6. Gahrton G, Zech L, Robèrt K-H and Bird AG (1979). Mitogenic stimulation of leukemia cells by Epstein-Barr virus. N Engl J Med 301:438–439.
7. Robèrt K-H (1979). Induction of monoclonal antibody synthesis in malignant human B-cells by polyclonal B-cell activators. Immunol Rev 48:123–143.
8. Gahrton G, Robèrt K-H, Friberg K et al. (1980). Extra chromosome 12 in chronic lymphocytic leukemia. Lancet 1:146–147.
9. Gahrton G, Robèrt K-H, Friberg K et al. (1980). Nonrandom chromosomal aberrations in chronic lymphocytic leukemia revealed by polyclonal B-cell-mitogen stimulation. Blood 56:640–647.
10. Robèrt K-H, Gahrton G, Friberg K et al. (1982). Extra chromosome 12 and prognosis in chronic lymphocytic leukaemia. Scand J Haematol 28:163–168.
11. Juliusson G, Robèrt K-H, Öst Å et al. (1984). Prognostic information from cytogenetic analysis in chronic B-lymphocytic leukemia and leukemic immunocytoma. Blood (in press).
12. Rai KR, Sawitsky A, Cronkite EP et al. (1975). Clinical staging of chronic lymphocytic leukemia. Blood 46:219–234.
13. Binet JL, Auquier A, Dighiero G et al. (1981). A new prognostic classification of chronic lymphocytic leukemia derived from multivariate survival analysis. Cancer 48:196–206.
14. Ideström K, Kimby E, Björkholm M et al. (1982). Treatment of chronic lymphocytic leukaemia and well-differentiated lymphocytic lymphoma with continuous low- or intermittent high-dose prednimustine versus chlorambucil/prednisolone. Eur J Cancer Clin Oncol 18:1117–1123.
15. Bøyum A (1968). Separation of leukocytes from blood and bone marrow. Scand J Clin Lab Invest Suppl 97, 21:31–50.

16. Caspersson T, Lomakka G and Zech L (1971). The 24 fluorescence patterns of the human metaphase chromosome — distinguishing characters and variability. Hereditas 67:89–102.
17. ISCN (1981). Report of the standing committee on human cytogenetic nomenclature. Cancer Genet Cytogenet 31:5–32.
18. Juliusson G, Robèrt K-H, Öst Å et al. (1984). Del (3) (p13) in B-prolymphocytic leukemia — a new nonrandom chromosomal aberration possibly correlated to the c-ras oncogene. (In preparation).
19. Morita M, Minowada J and Sandberg AA (1981). Chromosomes and causation of human cancer and leukemia. XLV. Chromosome patterns in stimulated lymphocytes of chronic lymphocytic leukemia. Cancer Genet Cytogenet 3:293–306.
20. Vahdati M, Graafland H and Emberger JM (1983). Karyotype analysis of B-lymphocytes transformed by Epstein-Barr virus in 21 patients with B-cell chronic lymphocytic leukemia. Hum Genet 63:327–331.
21. Han T, Ozer H, Sadamori N et al. (1984). Prognostic importance of cytogenetic abnormalities in patients with chronic lymphocytic leukemia. N Engl J Med 310:288–292.
22. Gahrton G, Robèrt K-H, Friberg K et al. (1982). Cytogenetic mapping of the duplicated segment of chromosome 12 in lymphoproliferative disorders. Nature 297:513–514.
23. Jhanwar SC, Neel BG, Hayward WS and Chaganti RSK (1983). Localization of c-ras oncogene family of human germ-like chromosomes. Proc Nat Acad Sci USA 80:4794–4797.
24. Klein G (1981). The role of gene dosage and genetic transpositions in carcinogenesis. Nature 294:313–318.
25. Bertino JR, Silber R, Freeman M et al. (1963). Studies on normal and leukemic leukocytes. IV. Tetrohydrofolate-dependent enzyme systems and dihydrofolic reductase. J Clin Invest 42:1899–1907.
26. Gerald PS and Grzeschik KH (1984). Report of the committee on the genetic constitution of chromosomes 10, 11 and 12. Cytogenet Cell Genet 37:103–126.
27. Mitelman F (1983). Catalogue of chromosome aberrations in cancer. Cytogenet Cell Genet 36:1–516.

3. Chromosome abnormalities in Burkitt lymphoma and Burkitt-type acute lymphoblastic leukemia

A. DE LA CHAPELLE
Department of Medical Genetics, University of Helsinki,
Helsinki, Finland

Specific association of non-random chromosomal rearrangements with distinct malignancies is now widely recognized. At the Sixth Human Gene Mapping Workshop in 1981, the best known associations of this type were assembled for publication as a committee report [1]. A greatly enlarged compilation of similar data has appeared as a result of the Seventh Human Gene Mapping Workshop held in 1983 [2]. As many as 54 recurrent associations between a break point and a neoplastic disorder were recorded. The number of disorders involved was 30. During the last year, several new associations of this type have been found. It is becoming increasingly clear that many of these are specifically related to the rearrangement, transcriptional activation, or amplification of cellular oncogenes located close to the breakpoints.

The breakpoints involved in recurrent structural chromosome abnormalities associated with Burkitt's lymphoma (BL) are close to the cellular myc oncogene on the one hand, and genes for immunoglobulins on the other. Molecular studies have shown structural rearrangements in these genes that alter their functions. Such events may play a key role in the mechanisms leading to malignant transformation of B-lymphocytes. It is believed that this may serve as a model for a better understanding of the mechanisms that lead to malignancy in other systems as well. For this reason the current interest in chromosome abnormalities associated with BL goes well beyond the scope of BL itself.

The observation of an abnormally long chromosome 14 in Burkitt cells by Manolov and Manolova [3] and the realization by Zech et al. [4] that the additional piece emanated from 8q, the (8; 14)(q24; q32) translocation are the early landmarks in BL cytogenetics. These discoveries as well as the more recent flood of information on variant translocations and other cytogenetic abnormalities have been expertly reviewed [5]. Key references can also be found in [1] and [2]. Hypotheses regarding the molecular consequences of these translocations were presented by Klein [6]. The molecular findings that largely confirm these hypotheses were recently reviewed [7–10]. In this paper, a critical analysis is given of chromosome abnormalities reported to occur in BL, considered together with acute lymphoblastic leukemia of Burkitt type as an entity.

Materials and methods

In the search for quantitative data on the types and frequency of cytogenetic abnormalities in BL, case reports and very small series must be omitted to avoid biased evaluations. The present review is based mainly on 5 reports presenting data on consecutive series, two on African [4, 11], and three exclusively or predominantly on non-African patients [12–14].

The terminology of the ISCN [15] is used throughout, and should be consulted for definitions of terms such as ploidy, modal number, stem-line, side-line, etc. Only clonal abnormalities found in relevant affected tissue were considered. The study of neoplastic cells in general, including BL, is seriously hampered by small numbers of mitoses and poor chromosomal morphology; both problems are clearly reflected in the reviewed reports. Therefore, some of the abnormalities were not found in the number of cells that is required for the abnormality to be designated as clonal. Moreover, designations such as 1q−, 6p−, 13q+, 14q+, etc. imply that a structural abnormality is present but its further delineation is not possible from the material at hand. In assessing the reports covered in this reveiw, the definitions of a clone established by the Second International Workshop on Chromosomes in Leukemia [16] were used with one modification. A typical abnormality, such as the t(8; 14) was considered clonal even when observed in only one cell if the same abnormality was observed in the same patient on other occasions, in other tissues, or in an established cell line derived from the patient. Finally, in the compilation of structural abnormalities by chromosome arm, incompletely defined rearrangements, such as 2p− or 18p+ were included if clonal, but assembled data on specific breakpoints mostly involved precisely defined abnormalities.

Results

General characteristics of the material

Relevant data are shown in Table I. The vast majority of the patients were studied at diagnosis. Of the non-African patients 72% had not received chemotherapy before the study. The corresponding figure was 86% for African patients.

Table I. Some parameters characterizing the patients included in the study and the stage at which the cytogenetic study was performed

	African[a]	Non-African
No. of patients	24	58
Median age, years	8	19
Male/female ratio	1.8	2.6
Studied at diagnosis	83%	100%
Studied at relapse	17%	0%
Studied prior to chemotherapy	86%	72%

[a] Data derived from a proportion of the patients only

Modal chromosome number

The dominating modal number is 46 (Fig. 1). Since all but two patients had structural or numerical abnormalities, the most typical stem-line in a BL tumor is pseudodiploid, i.e., has 46 chromosomes and one or several structural abnormalities. Side-lines are frequent; these have not been considered in the determination of modal number. The most common modal number other than 46 is 47. Other modal numbers were in the near-diploid range (43–53 chromosomes). No abnormalities of ploidy were seen.

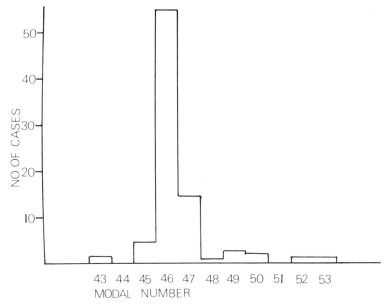

Figure 1. Modal number of chromosomes in direct preparations of involved tissue from 24 African and 58 non-African patients studied.

The typical translocations

The most common translocation, t(8; 14)(q24; q32) occurred in 71% of the non-African and 58% of the African patients (Table II). If two patients in whom the translocation was suspected but not confirmed are included, the figure for African patients is 67%. Thus over two-thirds of all patients have this translocation. Regarding the variant translocations, both occurred in non-African patients but not in African patients. Their absence in African patients should probably not be inferred from these data, however. First, both studies on African patients were performed before the existence of these translocations was well known. Second, the t(8; 22) is a minor translocation that might therefore have been overlooked. While the t(2; 8) could hardly be overlooked in banded preparations of reasonable quality, two of the patients in one series [11] who did not have the t(8; 14) had cells with 2p— and other markers which might have represented the t(2; 8). Third, the variant translocations have been found in *in vitro* cell lines from African patients [17]. It may be conclude that the the best estimate of the frequencies of the variant translocations are approximately 5% for t(2; 8) and approximately 10% for t(8; 22).

The question as to how many of the approximately 15% of the patients in whom none of the three typical translocations could be demonstrated might have had one if optimally studied, is harder to answer. Several facts hint that translocations may have remained undetected. First, the number of cells studied was often small. Second, the karyotypes without a typical translocation were often quite complicated. Third, in one patient, the t(8; 14) was not found in preparations of tumor tissue but occurred in an established cell line so that it probably had escaped detection in the tumor preparations. For the above reasons the total 85% frequency of the three typical translocations must be an underestimate. The significance of an entirely normal karyotype (in 2 patients), or of a cytogenetically normal clone (in 22% of the patients) alongside the abnormal ones in unclear.

Table II. Frequency of the three typical translocations involving band 8q24 and sites known to contain the three immunoglobulin loci

	African (N = 24)	Non-African (N = 58)
t(8;14) (q24;q32)	58 (67?)	71
t(2;8) (p11;q24)	0	5
t(8;22) (q24;q11)	0	9
None of the above	42 (33?)	15

Figures include three-way translocations (cf. text); question mark refers to two patients in whom the translocation was suspected but not confirmed

Three-way translocations

As is the case of the Philadelphia chromosome in chronic myeloid leukemia, translocations affecting two typical breakpoints may occasionally involve a third chromosome as well. In this series, four patients with such translocations were noted i.e. t(1; 8; 14)(q23; q24; q32), t(2; 8; 14)(p11 or 12; q24; q32), t(3; 8; 14)(q14; q24; q32) and t(8; 12; 14)(q24; p11; q32). The detailed structure of the resulting derivative chromosomes was not always apparent, however! Molecular methods are needed to clarify the effect the involvement of a third chromosome may have on the resulting gene rearrangements.

Recurrent structural rearrangements not involving known immunoglobulin loci

As shown in Table III, rearrangements in the middle and distal part of the long arm of chromosome 1 occur quite frequently in BL (19 cases). It is well known that rearrangements affecting this region are frequent in many malignancies, including myeloid and lymphoid leukemias and many solid tumors [18]. It will be of interest to see whether these rearrangements involve the ski oncogene, as of yet unknown oncogenes, or any of the numerous other genes that have been localized to this region. The hypothesis that rearrangements in 1q might be a requirement for tumor progression rather than induction of the transformed or malignant state is not supported by the present data. The question could perhaps be more adequately answered if tumors from untreated patients could be studied longitudinally during progression of the disease in the absence of treatment.

Table III. Recurrent structural rearrangements not involving known immunoglobulin loci

Rearrangement	No. of cases	Oncogene in region
dup;del;inv;t;(1) (q21-qter)	19	sk
13q$^+$	6	none
rob(13q22q)	2	none
del(2) (q)	2	none
t(1;6) (q21–23;q26–qter)	2	sk,myb
del(6) (q);6q$-$	3	
17p$+$	2	erb A1
i(17q)	2	

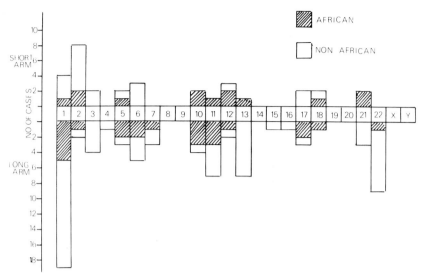

Figure 2. Frequency of clonal structural rearrangements by chromosome arm. 8q (with 72 entries) and 14q (with 62 entries) are not shown.

Other structural rearrangements

Seventy-two percent of the patients had at least one other abnormality in addition to the typical translocations listed in Table II. If the smaller number of African relative to non-African cases is kept in mind, there is no clearcut difference between these groups as shown in Fig. 2. The overall distribution is clearly non-random. Apart from 8q and the 2p, 14q and 22q arms carrying immunoglobulin loci, the most frequent sites of rearrangement are in 1q, 11q and 13q. As stated above, the 13q+ marker chromosome could not be analyzed in detail, so it may or may not represent one entity or one breakpoint. In the case of 11q, however, 6 of the 7 breakpoints were in the fairly narrow region in the proximal part of the long arm, 11q11–q14. None of these 6 abnormalities occurred more than once, however. While abnormalities of 11q are common in acute myeloid leukemia, they predominantly affect the distal half of the chromosome (Fourth International Workshop on Chromosomes in Leukemia [19]). In non-Burkitt, non-Hodgkin lymphoma, breakpoints in 11q have been observed but not with high frequency [20]. In future work special attention should probably be given to 11q1.

The total absence of structural rearrangements in chromosomes 19, 20, X and Y and the fact that the large chromosome 4 and chromosomes 15 and 16 have only one rearrangement each may be due to the relatively small series.

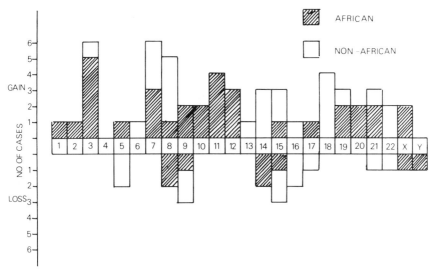

Figure 3. Frequency of clonal gains and losses of structurally normal chromosomes.

Gains and losses of structurally normal chromosomes

The chromosomes most often gained were Nos 3 and 7 (6 cases each) followed by Nos 8 (5 cases), 11 and 18 (4 cases). Since the modal number only very rarely is below 46, it follows that few chromosomes are lost (Fig. 3).

The frequent occurrence of +7 and relatively frequent observation of +3 has been reported in non-Burkitt lymphoma [20, 21]. An isochromosome of the long arm of chromosome 7, i(7q) is also common in some series of non-Burkitt lymphomas [22], but appears to be rare in BL, occurring only once in this series. Noteworthy is the absence of numerical aberration of chromosome 4 which had only one structural aberration. Finally, trisomy 12, a dominant aberration in chronic lymphocytic leukemia [23], is not common in BL.

The monoclonal nature of BL

The concept that BL is a monoclonal proliferation would be supported if the same cytogenetic abnormality could be found in BL tumors from different sites from the same patient on the same occasion. Only 5 patients could be evaluated for this feature. In 2 of these, the karyotypes were identical. In 3, differences occurred, but they could readily be caused by a combination of random loss and clonal evolution, since the same specific structural rearrangements were found. In no instance could the karyotypes be classified as being significantly different. On the basis of this limited material one may tentatively conclude that different tumors arise from a common ancestor cell. The alternative explanation, that independent tumors arise as different clones with identical karyotypes appears less likely but cannot be ignored.

The effect of treatment

All patients studied serially or only in relapse had received prior chemotherapy. In addition, several patients in whom the tissue studied was obtained at or soon after diagnosis, had already received some chemotherapy. In an attempt to study the effect of treatment on karyotype, the results from all suitable treated patients (N = 21) were compared with all those not treated (N = 53) for a number of parameters (Table IV). The frequency of single abnormalities was greater in untreated patients than in treated patients, respectively 64% and 36%. The reverse was seen with multiple abnormalities, the corresponding figures beings respectively, 19% and 81%. These differences are not statistically significant, possibly because of small sample sizes.

The occurrence of structural abnormalities involving 1q and 13q showed a similar, albeit weaker effect. Figures for the two most common numerical abnormalities, +3 and +7 were too small to allow conclusions, but no trend of a similar effect was noted here. There are a number of possible explanations for the trend toward more structural abnormalities following therapy. Chemotherpay may induce structural chromosome rearrangements in BL cells, and these altered cells may continue to proliferate in a clonal fashion. Alternatively, however, chemotherapy may select clones with multiple abnormalities. It should be noted that in most treated cases more time

Table IV. Comparison of clonal cytogenetic abnormalities in patients treated and untreated with chemotherapy at the time of sampling

Abnormality	Untreated N = 53		Treated N = 21	
	No.	%	No.	%
None or single	19	36	4	19
More than one	34	64	17	81
Structurally abnormal 1q	12	23	7	33
13q+	4	8	3	14
+3	5	9	1	5
+7	3	6	1	5

None of the differences are statistically significant

had elapsed, sometimes months or years, between diagnosis and sampling than in untreated cases. Thus an untestable third hypothesis must be that the observed alterations are due to spontaneous clonal evolution.

Established cell lines

Much of the spectacular progress in molecular studies on BL is due to work performed on cell lines established from BL tissue. It is therefore of particular interest to examine to what extent karyotypes of *in vitro* BL cell lines are representative of the *in vivo* situation. It seems well established that many cell lines retain the typical translocations listed in Table II [24]. The cell lines Daudi, Ramos, BL2, LY47, LY67 and others are much-studied examples of this [3, 4, 25]. It also seems clear that, analogous to *in vitro* lines from other sources, additional abnormalities, both structural and numerical, arise in BL lines during prolonged growth *in vitro* [3, 4, 26]. These phenomena are not the object of the present review.

Discussion

Typical translocations occurring with high frequency (85 % in BL tissue studied directly after sampling *in vivo*), result in the juxtaposition of the cellular oncogene myc with immunoglobulin genes. Molecular studies during the past 3 years have already gone a long way in clarifying exactly where the genes break and join, and have shown alterations in their structure and function. These studies in BL have led the way to an emerging broader understanding of the genetic mechanisms associated with and probably responsible for at least one step in the induction of the malignant state in mammalian cells.

Cytogenetic studies are now being widely used in the evaluation of patients with lymphoma, most of whom have a cytogenetic abnormality. Unfortunately, non-random recurring chromosomal abnormalities are not specifically and uniquely associated with any histologic or immunologic subclasses of malignant non-Hodgkin lymphoma [20]. The typical translocations associated with BL described in this paper may come closest to showing such specificity since they occur in over 85 % of Burkitt tumors. However, since t(8; 14) occurs in other lymphoid malignancies as well [14], they are not diagnostic of BL. In one of the series reviewed here, one of the typical translocations with a break point in 8q24 occurred in 14 of 16 BL patients, but was not found in any of 134 patients belonging to other subgroups of non-Hodgkin lymphoma or ALL that were studied by banding during the same period [14]. How rarely or often they actually occur in other neoplasias needs to be further studied. The picture emerging from the present review is that other structural aberrations found in BL together with or in the absence of the typical translocations, may not offer particular landmarks for diagnostic purposes. This certainly appears to hold for numerical aberrations which are few and mostly involve chromosomes observed in abnormal dosage in other malignancies as well.

Acknowledgements

Aided by grants from the Sigrid Jusélius Foundation, the Academy of Finland, the Foundation Baltzar W.A. von Platen and the Folkhalsan Institute of Genetics.

References

1. Berger R, Bernheim A and de la Chapelle A (1982). Chromosome rearrangements in acquired malignant diseases. Cytogenet Cell Genet 32:205-207.
2. de la Chapelle A and Berger R (1984). Report of the committee on chromosome rearrangements in neoplasia and on fragile sites. Cytogenet Cell Genet 37:274-311.
3. Manolov G and Manolova Y (1972). Marker band in one chromosome 14 from Burkitt lymphomas. Nature 237:33-34.
4. Zech L, Haglund U, Nilsson K and Klein G (1976). Characteristic chromosomal abnormalities in biopsies and lymphoid cell lines from patients with Burkitt and non-Burkitt lymphomas. Int J Cancer 17:47-56.
5. Zech L (1983). Chromosome abnormalities in malignant diseases of the lymphatic system, pp. 269-295. In: Molander DW (Ed.). Diseases of the Lymphatic System. New York: Springer-Verlag.
6. Klein G (1981). The role of gene dosage and genetic transpositions in carcinogenesis. Nature 294:313-318.
7. Perry RP (1983). Consequences of *myc* invasion of immunoglobulin loci: Facts and speculation. Cell 33:647-649.
8. Nowell P. Dalla-Favera R, Finan J et al. (1983). Chromosome translocations, immunoglobulin genes, and neoplasia, pp. 165-182. In: Rowley JD and Ultmann JE (Eds.). Chromosomes and Cancer. New York: Academic Press.
9. Cory S. C-*myc* oncogene activation by chromosome translocation in mouse and man. In: Andersson LC, Ekblom P, Gahmberg CG and Klein G (Eds.). Gene Expression During Normal and Malignant Differentiation. Academic Press (in press).
10. Klein G. Oncogene activation by chromosomal translocations. In: Andersson LC, Ekblom P, Gahmberg CG and Klein G (Eds). Gene Expression During Normal and Malignant Differentiation. Academic Press (in press).
11. Bigger RJ, Lee EC, Nkrumah Fk and Whang-Peng J (1981). Direct cytogenetic studies by needle aspiration of Burkitt's lymphoma in Ghana West Africa. J Nat Cancer Inst 67:769-776.
12. Douglass EC, Magrath IT, Lee EC and Whang-Peng J (1980). Cytogenetic studies in non-African Burkitt lymphoma. Blood 55:148-155.

13. Berger R and Bernheim A (1982). Cytogenetic studies on Burkitt's lymphoma-leukemia. Cancer Genet Cytogenet 7:231–244.
14. Knuutila S, Elonen E, Heinonen K et al. (1984). Chromosome abnormalities in 16 Finnish patients with Burkitt's lymphoma or L3 acute lymphocytic leukemia. Cancer Genet Cytogenet 13:139–151.
15. ISCN (1978). Birth Defects Original Article Series, Vol. 14, No. 8. New York: The National Foundation.
16. Second International Workshop on Chromosomes in Leukemia (1980). General Report. Cancer Genet Cytogenet 2:93–96.
17. Lenoir GM, Preud'homme JL, Bernheim A and Berger R (1982). Correlation between immunoglobulin light chain expression and variant translocation in Burkitt's lymphoma. Nature 298:474–476.
18. Brito-Babapulle V and Atkin NB (1981). Break points in chromosome no. 1 abnormalities of 218 human neoplasms. Cancer Genet Cytogenet 4:215–225.
19. Fourth International Workshop on Chromosomes in Leukemia (1984). Cancer Genet Cytogenet 11:249–360.
20. Bloomfield CD, Arthur DC, Frizzer G et al. (1983). Nonrandom chromosome abnormalities in lymphoma. Cancer Res 43:2975–2984.
21. Yunis JJ, Oken MM, Kaplan ME et al. (1982). Distinctive chromosomal abnormalities in histologic subtypes of non-Hodgkin's lymphoma. N Engl J Med 307:1231–1236.
22. Mitelman F (1983). Catalogue of chromosome aberrations in cancer. Cytogenet Cell Genet 36:1–516.
23. Gahrton G, Robert K-H. Friberg K et al. (1980). Nonrandon chromosomal aberrations in chronic lymphocytic leukemia revealed by polyclonal B-cell-mitogen stimulation. Blood 56:640–647.
24. Douglass EC, Magrath IT, Lee EC and Whang-Peng J (1980). Serial cytogenetic studies of nonendemic Burkitt's lymphoma cell lines. J Nat Cancer Inst 65:891–895.
25. de la Chapelle A, Lenoir G, Boué J et al. (1983). Lambda Ig constant region genes are translocated to chromosome 8 in Burkitt's lymphoma with t(8;22). Nucl Acids Res 11:1133–1142.
26. Zhang S, Zech L and Klein G (1982). High-resolution analysis of chromosome markers in Burkitt lymphoma cell Lines. Int J Cancer 29:153–157.

4. DNA content and proliferation in non-Hodgkin's lymphoma: Flow cytofluorometric DNA analysis in relation to the Kiel classification

B. CHRISTENSSON[1], B. TRIBUKAIT[2] and P. BIBERFELD[1]

[1]Department of Pathology, Karolinska Hospital, and [2]Department of Radiobiology, Karolinska Institute, Stockholm, Sweden

The Rappaport classification is widely used for diagnosis and treatment of non-Hodgkin's lymphomas (NHL) [1–3]. However, it has become increasingly inconsistent with the rapidly changing concepts of the functional diversity of the immune system. Attempts have, therefore, been made to incorporate immunologic concepts into the morphologic classification of NHL [4, 5]. The clinical applicability of these newer classifications as well as their capacity to identify biologically distinct tumor groups is currently under study.

It is generally accepted that the transformation of small lymphoid cells to large blastlike cells is associated with metabolic and proliferative activity. Large cell lymphomas are considered to be highly proliferative and are associated with rapid tumor growth and poor prognosis. This assumption is the general basis for the histologic differentiation between HGM and LGM in the Kiel classification. Malignancy grading between the CB/CC and CB as well as between IC and IB is dependent on the frequency of cells with blastlike morphology. The validity of the histologic division into HGM and LGM is dependent on the accuracy with which the frequency of large presumably proliferative cells can be detected.

Some previous reports have shown the usefulness of quantitative methods for determination of cell proliferative activity in lymphomas, both by thymidine incorporation [6–9] and by DNA FCF [10–16]. In addition, DNA-FCF studies give information about the DNA content of the tumor cells. In contrast to most other solid malignancies, the majority of non-Hodgkin's lymphomas have only minor deviations in the DNA content compared to normal diploid cells [12–14]. This has also been confirmed by cytogenetic studies showing only low numbers of extrachromosomes in the majority of non-Hodgkin's lymphomas and lymphatic leukemias [17–21 and Bloomfield et al., this vol.]. In the present report the proliferative activity and DNA content of 208 cases of NHL and lymphatic leukemias was related to the Kiel classification and these variables were used as biological probes for estimating the accuracy of the histologic malignancy grading.

Materials and methods

Patients

Including both children and adults, 208 patients with non-Hodgkin's lymphoma or lymphatic leukemia were studied. Over 90 % of the patients were analyzed prior to treatment and in 50 cases more than one biopsy was analyzed.

Preparation of tissue specimens

Unfixed biopsy material was obtained and divided into three parts, one part fixed in formol sublimate fixation (B5) [22] for conventional histology and immunoperoxidase (PAP) staining. Another part was quick-frozen in streaming carbon dioxide and stored at $-70\,°C$ until cryosectioning for immunofluorescence (IFL) and marker studies. From the third part a suspension of viable cells was obtained by mincing the tissue and passing it through a wire mesh. The cell suspension was used for immunologic studies and DNA determinations by FCF. Cells for FCF analysis were pelleted and suspended in $-20\,°C$ absolute ethanol.

Histologic diagnosis was based on slides stained with haematoxylin-eosin, PAS, Giemsa and Lendrum stains. In cases where bone marrow or peripheral blood was used for FCF analysis, the representativity of the material was analyzed by immunophenotyping and/or morphology of Giemsa stained smears or cytospin preparations. The diagnosis was further substantiated whenever possible on histologic specimens from the same patient. Slides were classified according to the Kiel classification [11, 23].

The low grade malignancy (LGM) group included the MLL, CLL, PLL, HCL, mycosis fungoides (MF), Sezarys syndrome (Sez), IC, CC, CB/CC follicular (CB/CC FOLL) and the CB/CC follicular and diffuse (CB/CC F & D) groups whereas the high grade malignancy (HGM) group contained the CB F & D, lymphoblastic undifferentiated (LBU), lymphoblastic Burkitt type (LBBL), IB and ALL.

Immunophenotype analysis

Suspended lymphoma cells from tumor or bone marrow biopsies or peripheral blood were analysed for the presence of receptors for sheep erythrocytes and complement factor 3 using erythrocyte indicator techniques [24]. The indirect IFL technique [24] was used to study the expression of Ig heavy and light chain isotypes and/or antigens reactive with the monoclonal antibodies OKT-3, 4, 8, Na1/34, J5 and OKIa. Additional immunohisto-chemical analysis was in certain cases performed on cryostat sections using the same panel of reagents [24, 25]. A lymphoma was considered monoclonally Ig positive when the K/L ratio was above 3.5 or below 0.5 and the number of light chain positive cells was above 22%. These criteria excluded all normal and reactive lymph nodes and PBL tested.

Flow-cytofluorometry (FCF)

Ethanol fixed suspended cells were enzyme digested (RNAse, pepsin) and ethidium bromide stained [26]. The DNA content of the G0/G1 peak was expressed as the ratio between the channel number for the G0/G1 peak of the lymphoma and for the lymphocyte standard, rendering a DNA content of 1 to diploid and 2 to tetraploid tumors. Tumors with a DNA content between 0.95 and 1.05 were designated as 'neardiploid'. Tumors in this range without discernable extra peaks could not with certainty be considered as aneuploid. An aneuploid population with tetraploid DNA content was defined by a peak exceeding the G2/M peak found in normal cells by 3 S.D. The mean value for the G2/M peak of normal controls was subtracted from the tetraploid G1 peak when calculating the proportion of cells in the aneuploid G0/G1 peak. In these cases, also a G2/M peak in the octaploid region was found. The proportions of cells in G0/G1, S and G2/M phases were calculated using a simplified method described by Baisch et al. [27]. A good agreement was found between the proportion of S-phase cells calculated in this way and labelling index in non-Hodgkin's lymphomas (unpublished data).

Statistical analysis

Differences in the S-phase frequency distributions and DNA content distribution in different groups were calculated by the Kruskal-Wallis test. Differences in the frequency of aneuploid lymphomas in different groups were calculated by Fisher's exact test or by Chi-square analysis whenever appropriate. Stepwise discriminant analysis was performed according to the method of Wilks [28] after log transformation of the S-phase and DNA content values. Correlation computations were made by the Spearman rank correlation method.

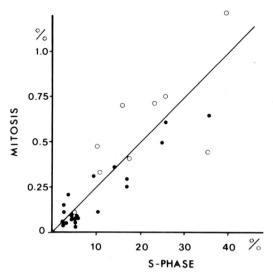

Figure 1. Correlation of the frequency of mitotic figures in histologic sections to the S-phase frequency in lymphomas and reactive lymphnodes (r = 0.86, p<0.001). Filled circles are "near diploid' and open circles are aneuploid cases.

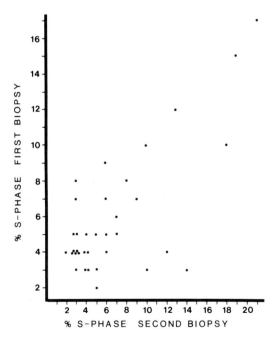

Figure 2. Correlation of the frequency of S-phase cells in multiple biopsies from different sites at diagnosis (r = 0.73, p<0.01).

Results

Cell sample representativity

The representativity with regard to tumor cells in the cell suspensions obtained from lymphoma specimens was demonstrated in several ways. The mitotic frequency in tissue sections correlated well with the S-phase frequency in 29 biopsies. (r = 0.86, $p < 0.001$) (Fig. 1). In aneuploid B-lymphomas, the frequency of monoclonal light chain restricted cells correlated well with the frequency of aneuploid cells (r = 0.81, $p < 0.001$, data not shown).

In 40 cases, two biopsies taken from different anatomic sites at diagnosis were analyzed. A good correlation in S-phase frequency was found between biopsies (Fig. 2, r = 0.73, $p < 0.01$). Moreover, in 10 cases both diagnostic and relapse biopsies were analyzed. Also in these cases, a good correlation between the S-phase frequencies was found (r = 0.83, $p < 0.01$, data not shown). Furthermore, none of the post-treatment biopsies showed DNA content values significantly different from those taken at diagnosis.

DNA analysis in relation to morphology

Of 208 patients analyzed, 146 (70%) had lymphomas with 'neardiploid' DNA content. The mean S-phase frequency was 8.3% in the whole population, 7.3% in the 'neardiploid', and 12.8% in the aneuploid group.

Table I gives the frequency of aneuploid tumors and the mean values of the frequency of cells in S-phase for 'neardiploid' and aneuploid tumors, respectively, in relation to the groups of the Kiel classification and also the mean S-phase frequency of the non-neoplastic control lymph nodes. The frequency of the different immunophenotypes is also listed.

A statistically significant difference between the S-phase frequency distributions of LGM (mean = 5.4%) and HGM (mean = 15.5%) was found both for tumors with 'neardiploid' (LGM mean = 5.0%, HGM mean = 14.1%, $p < 0.001$) and aneuploid (LGM mean = 6.5%, HGM mean = 18.8%, $p < 0.01$) DNA content. A significant difference in the S-phase frequency distribution was also found between the CB/CC F & D and CB groups, both for lymphomas with 'neardiploid' ($p < 0.001$) and aneuploid ($p < 0.01$) DNA content.

A mean S-phase frequency below 7% was found in all LGM lymphoma groups. However, the CB/CC F & D had a more heterogeneous S-phase frequency distribution than the other LGM lymphomas (Fig. 3).

The HGM lymphomas had clearly higher mean S-phase frequencies and wider ranges. Moreover, the S-phase distributions for the HGM lymphomas

Table I. Flow cytofluorometric analysis of DNA content and S-phase fractions

Diagnosis	No. of cases	Biopsy site					DNA		Mean S-phase %		Immunophenotype			
		LN	Spl	BL	BM	Other	Near dipl	aneuploid	Near dipl	aneuploid	B	T	N B/T	Not tested or inconclusive
Non-neopl. lymph nodes	30	30					30		5.5					
ML lymphocyt (MLL)	9	7	2				8	2	4.6	3.5	6	3		
CLL	22	9	2	8	3		19	3	4.4	4.1	19	3		
PLL	4			3	1		3	1	6	5	3	1		
HCL	7		4	2	1		7	0	3.6		5		2	
MF	2	1				1	1	1	4.5	7.6		1		1
Sézary (Sez)	4	1		3			1	3	6.9	8		4		
Immunocytoma (IC)	37	30	4		1	2	31	6	4.8	6.5	34		1	2
Centrocytic (CC)	10	9	1				6	4	5.4	5.9	10			
CB/CC F	16	14	2				13	3	5.4	4.9	16			
CB/CC F+D	37	34	1			2	20	17	5.9	7.9	35	1		1
CB F+D	16	16					12	4	16.4	28.5	13	1	2	
LB Burkitt	4	2		1	1		3	1	35.0	22.2	4			
LB Undiff	9	8				1	5	4	14.1	12.2		1	6	2
IB	8	8					2	6	12.8	19.5	6	1		
ALL	23	1		10	12		16	7	8.7	12.8	1	1	21[a]	
Total	208	140	16	27	19	6	146	62			152	17	33	6

[a] 14 cALLA+, 1 cALLA− Ia+

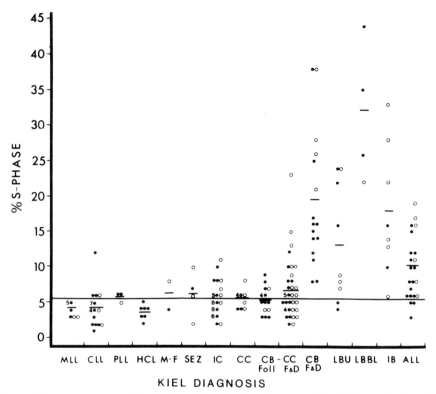

Figure 3. S-phase frequency distribution of the morphologic types of the Kiel classification. The line at the 5.5% level indicates the mean S-phase frequency of the controls. Filled circles are 'near diploid' and open circles are aneuploid cases.

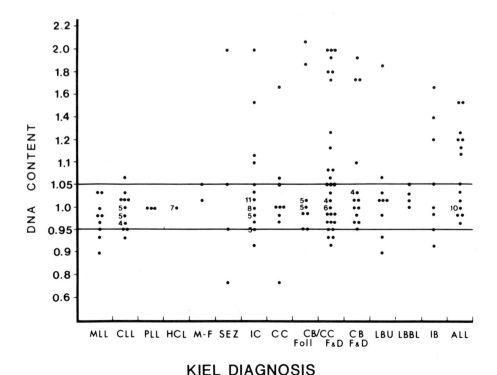

Figure 4. DNA content distribution in relation to the morphologic types of the Kiel classification.

and the CB/CC F & D lymphomas showed a considerable overlap (Fig. 3). The difference in S-phase frequency distribution between the aneuploid HGM lymphomas (mean = 18.8%) and the 'neardiploid' ones (mean = 14.1%) was not statistically significant.

Fig. 4 shows the DNA content distribution in relation to morphology. A weak but significant difference was found in the DNA content distribution between the LGM (mean = 1.07) and the HGM (mean = 1.11) groups ($p < 0.05$) although the frequency of aneuploid NHL did not differ significantly in the LGM (27%) and HGM (37%) groups. The CB/CC F & D (46%) and IB (75%) had the highest frequencies of aneuploid tumors in the LGM and HGM groups, respectively.

Although most aneuploid tumors were found in the hyper- or hypodiploid ranges, FC derived lymphomas occasionally had DNA contents in the tetraploid range. In fact all but three of the tumors with DNA contents over 1.6 were FC derived (Fig. 5).

The frequency of aneuploid tumors was markedly higher in the CB/CC F & D (46%), as compared to the CB/CC FOLL (19%) group. However, the proliferative activity was quite similar in both groups.

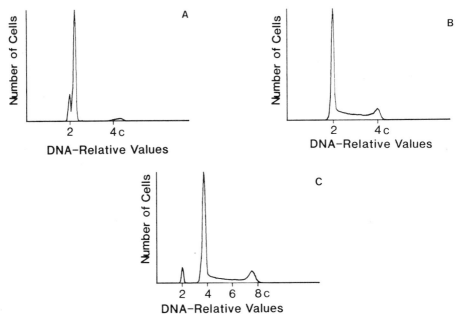

Figure 5. DNA histograms for: A) An IC lymphoma of lymphoplasmocytic type, positive for IgG, kappa. The DNA content of the G0/G1 peak was 1.10; 90% of the cells were in the aneuploid population with 5.2% of the cells in S-phase. B) A IgM, kappa positive CB diffuse lymphoma with a 'near diploid' DNA content and 38.4% of the cells in S-phase. C) A CB diffuse lymphoma positive for IgM, IgD and lambda. The DNA content of the G0/G1 peak was 1.7; 95% of the cells were in the aneuploid population with 28.3% of the cells in S-phase.

DNA analysis in relation to immunology

No significant differences in S-phase frequency distributions were found between C3d receptor positive and negative lymphomas or between lymphomas with different heavy and light chain isotypes. Neither did B and T lymphomas show any significant differences in the S-phase frequency distributions.

The frequency of aneuploid lymphomas was similar (30%) in the B-, T- and non-B/T lymphoma groups. The frequency of lymphomas expressing various light and heavy chain isotype combinations were not significantly different in 'neardiploid' and aneuploid tumors.

Stepwise discriminant analysis

To further analyze the relative importance of S-phase and DNA content for the malignancy grading of different types of NHL stepwise discriminant analysis was used. The S-phase frequency but not the DNA content variable was found to be significantly discriminating between the HGM and LGM groups (Wilk's lambda = 0.62).

Using this discriminant model for classification 94% of the LGM lymphomas were allocated to the low proliferative group by their S-phase frequency values. In contrast only 62% of the HGM cases were classified to the high proliferative group whether the 38% of the HG lymphomas, allocated to the low proliferative group by their S-phase frequency values, have a better clinical prognosis than the other is currently under investigation.

We also tried to differentiate between lymphocytic-IC (Group 1), FC derived (Group 2) and lymphoblastic/immunoblastic (Group 3) lymphomas by discriminant analysis using S-phase frequency and DNA content as discriminating variables. In this discriminant model, in addition to the S-phase frequency, the DNA content had a weak but significantly discriminating capacity (Wilk's lambda = 0.73 and 0.93, respectively). The S-phase frequency was the most important variable, especially for Groups 1 and 3 whereas the DNA content was more important for Group 2 than for Groups 1 and 3.

Discussion

The establishment of a new lymphoma classification requires that its capacity to more efficiently divide lymphomas into clinically and biologically relevant groups can be shown. We have previously analyzed the predictive capacity of the Kiel classification with respect to survival and its relation to the immunophenotype of NHL [24, 29]. In the present report the Kiel classification was studied in relation to the proliferative activity and DNA content of NHL as measured by FCF analysis. These variables were also used as biological probes to estimate the accuracy of the histologic malignancy grading.

Obviously the representativity with regard to tumor cell composition of the cell suspensions for the tumor samples is of major importance in flow analysis. In the present study this was evidenced by the good correlation of the frequency of mitotic figures in tissue sections to the S-phase frequency in cell suspensions and also by the good correlation of the observed frequency of monoclonal Ig positive to the frequency of aneuploid cells in aneuploid B-lymphomas. Furthermore, good concordance was found for the S-phase frequencies in multiple biopsies from different sites of the same patient, indicating the homogenous proliferative activity in tumor irrespective of site.

The limitations for the detection of an abnormal DNA content as a marker for aneuploidy in FCF-analysis depend upon instrumentation, cell preparation and staining [30]. Although the methods used for cell fixation, enzyme digestion and ethidium bromide staining gave a low coefficient of variation ($2.87\% + -0.53$) other factors may also determine the sensitivity of the method. The possibility to detect small variations in the DNA content also depends on the relative number of admixed non neoplastic cells in the tumor sample. Based on these considerations, we determined a 'neardiploid' DNA content range (0.95–1.05) within which we could not with certainty identify cell populations with abnormal DNA content.

Assuming that all chromosomes had equal amounts of DNA, this range would equate a range of chromosome numbers from 43 to 49 and would thus indicate that a loss or gain of approximately 3 chromosomes would be needed to detect a DNA content abnormality under the conditions used in the present study. This estimate of the numerical chromosome abnormality required to detect distinct differences in the DNA histograms is in accordance with the findings in other correlative cytogenetic and FCF-DNA analyses [17, 21].

Based on our definition of aneuploidy (<0.95 or >1.05), the overall frequency of aneuploid NHL was 30% (LGM 27%, HGM 37%). These figures are in agreement with the frequency of aneuploid NHL with more than 5% deviation in the modal chromosome number from the normal [46] number as determined by cytogenetic methods [18 and Bloomfield et al., this vol.]. However, our frequencies of aneuploid NHL are lower than those reported by Diamond et al. [12, 13], Barlogie et al. [14] and Shackney et al. [31]. This disparity is probably mostly related to differences in the criteria used for the definition of aneuploidy. Different classifications, variations in patient selection as well as differences in cell preparation and staining might also interfere with these results.

The presence of aneuploidy has been implicated as a prognostic factor in human cancer [32] and to be related to biological subtypes of ALL [33]. In the present study, as expected, high frequencies of aneuploid tumors were found in the HGM (IB 75%) but also in the LGM (CB/CC F & D 46%) group. Interestingly with few exceptions NHL with DNA content in the tetraploid range were FC derived. In accordance with our findings of a high DNA content in FC derived lymphomas Yunis et al. [18] reported high numerical chromosomal abnormalities in these lymphomas. Also Kvaløy et al. [9] observed a high DNA content in FC derived lymphomas.

The lack of any significant correlation between the proliferative activity and DNA content in NHL of the same histologic type indicates that quantitative DNA content abnormalities in NHL may not necessarily be associated with rapid tumor growth. This is in line with suggestions that specific chromosomal abberrations, like the translocation of the c-onc gene in Burkitt's lymphoma, may be more important than net changes in DNA content for the induction of uncontrolled proliferation and the development of neoplasia in NHL and lymphatic leukemias [34–36].

Our finding of a highly significant difference in the S-phase frequency distribution of the HGM and LGM groups indicates that, in general, there is a correlation between the proliferation rate of the tumor and its morphological and clinical behavior. However, the wider S-phase frequency distribution found in the CB/CC F & D as compared to the IC, lymphocytic and the other LGM FC derived lymphomas, indicated a greater heterogeneity in the FC derived NHL. A few cases in the other LGM groups were found which had increased S-phase frequencies indicating some proliferative heterogeneity also within these groups. These tumors may belong to a group with intermediate prognosis.

Also the HGM lymphomas had a considerable proportion of low proliferating cases. These findings have prompted clinical studies on the possible use of ploidy and proliferation as additional prognostic markers independent of morphology.

The mean S-phase frequencies of the LGM and HGM groups of the Kiel classification in this study were quite similar to those reported in other FCF-DNA studies [10–14] and comparable to those obtained with labeling index methods [7, 8, 37]. However, the use of different histologic classifications prevented a closer comparison.

The S-phase frequency in the individual case has to be interpreted in relation to the frequency of neoplastic cells, as indicated by light chain restriction or aneuploidy. Especially in FC derived lymphomas an admixture of low proliferative T cells may bias the estimation of tumor cell proliferation. This has been evidenced in cases where non-neoplastic T cells and tumor cells have been analyzed separately after separation by immunologic methods or centrifugal elutriation (unpublished data).

The stepwise discriminant analysis confirmed our impression that the S-phase variable was a strong discriminator between the HGM and LGM groups. The high concordance rate (94%) between low proliferation and low malignancy grading morphologically indicates a good accuracy of the Kiel classification in the distinction between low and high proliferating lymphomas. Thus only 6% of the high proliferating lymphomas were classified as of low grade malignancy.

However, the proliferative heterogeneity found also within distinct morphologic types of the HGM group indicates that in large cell lymphomas the proliferative capacity of the large cells may not be easily recognized morphologically. The possibility to use S-phase analysis in addition to morphology as an independent marker of the biological behavior of the tumor may be of prognostic importance and is currently under study.

Discriminant analysis of the three morphologically separable groups lymphocytic/IC, FC derived and lympho/immunoblastic lymphomas showed that in addition to S-phase frequency DNA content was a significant, albeit weaker discriminator. In this model DNA content mostly influenced the group of FC derived lymphomas, supporting our previous observations that a fraction of these lymphomas have a characteristically high DNA content.

Our finding that the Kiel classification identifies lymphomas with high proliferative activity is in accordance with our previous findings [29] that this classification have a good capacity to predict clinical prognosis. However, our findings of a proliferative heterogeneity, especially within the HGM group, indicate that S-phase determination by flow cytofluorometry may provide an additional prognostic marker independent of morphology and immunology.

Acknowledgements

This work was supported by grants from the Swedish Cancer Society. The foundations of the Karolinska Institute, Stockholm Cancer Society, Robert Lundbergs Foundation and the Royal Academy of Sciences, Stockholm.

The skillful technical assistance of Marianne Ekman, Margareta Andersson, Inga-Lill Linder and Britta Randers is gratefully acknowledged.

References

1. Fisher RI, Hubbard SM, DeVita VT et al. (1981). Factors predicting long-term survival in diffuse mixed, histiocytic, or undifferentiated lymphoma. Blood 58:45-51.

2. Rosenberg SA (1979). Non-Hodgkin's lymphoma — Selection of treatment on the basis of histologic type. Engl J Med 301:924–928.
3. Kim H, Zelman RJ, Fox MA et al. (1982). Pathology panel for lymphoma clinical studies: A comprehensive analysis of cases accumulated since its inception. J Nat Cancer Inst 68:43–67.
4. Lennert K (1978). Malignant lymphomas other than Hodgkin's disease. In: Handbuch der speziellen pathologischen Anatomie und Histologie, Berlin, Heidelberg, I Band, Teil 3B. New York: Springer-Verlag.
5. Lukes RJ, Taylor CR, Chir B et al (1978). A morphological and immunological surface marker study of 299 cases of non-Hodgkin lymphomas and related leukemias. Amer J Pathol 90:461–485.
6. Silvestrini R, Piazza R, Riccardi A and Rilke F (1977). Correlation of cell kinetic findings with morphology of non-Hodgkin's malignant lymphomas. J Nat Cancer Inst 58:499–504.
7. Costa A, Bonadonna G, Villa E et al. (1981). Labeling index as a prognostic marker in non-Hodgkin's lymphoma. J Nat Cancer Inst 66:1–5.
8. Lang W, Kienzle B and Diehl V (1980). Proliferation kinetics of malignant non-Hodgkin's lymphomas related to histopathology of lymph node biopsies. Virchows Arch A Path Anat Histol 389:397–407.
9. Kvalöy S, Godal T, Marton PF et al (1981). Spontaneous (H-3)-Thymidine uptake in histological subgroups of human B-cell lymphomas. Scand J Haematol 26:221–234.
10. Scarffe JH and Crowther D (1981). The pre-treatment proliferative activity of non-Hodgkin's lymphoma cells. Europ J Cancer 17:99–108.
11. Diamond LW and Braylan RC (1980). Flow analysis of DNA content and cell size in non-Hodgkin's lymphoma. Cancer Res 40:703–712.
12. Diamond LW, Braylan RC, Bearman RM et al (1980). The determination of cellular content in neoplastic and non-neoplastic lymphoid populations by flow cytofluorometry. Flow Cytometry IV:478–482.
13. Diamond LW, Nathwani BN and Rappaport H (1982). Flow cytometry in the diagnosis and classification of malignant lymphoma and leukemia. Cancer 50:1122–1135.
14. Barlogie B, Latreille J, Freireich EJ et al. (1980). Characterisation of hematologic malignancies by flow cytometry. Blood cells 6:719–744.
15. Braylan RC, Fowlkes BJ, Jaffe ES et al. (1978). Cell volumes and DNA distributions of normal and neoplastic cells. Cancer 41:201–209.
16. Kruth HS, Braylan RC, Benson NA and Nourse VA (1981). Simultaneous analysis of DNA and cell surface immunoglogulin in human B-cell lymphomas by flow cytometry. Cancer Res 41:4895–4899.
17. Barlogie B, Hittelman W, Spitzer G et al. (1977). Correlation of DNA distribution abnormalities with cytogenetic findings in human adult leukemia and lymphoma. Cancer Res 37:4400–4407.
18. Yunis J, Oken M, Kaplan ME et al. (1982). Distinctive chromosomal abnormalities in histologic subtypes of non-Hodgkin's lymphoma. N Engl J Med 307:1231–1236.
19. Bloomfield CD, Rowley JD, Goldman AI et al (1983). Chromosomal abnormalities and their clinical significance in acute lymphoblastic leukemia. Cancer Res 43:868–873.
20. Morita M, Minowada J and Sandberg AA (1981). Chromosomes and causation of human cancer and leukemia. XLV. Chromosome patterns in stimulated lymphocytes of chronic lymphocytic leukemia. Cancer Genet Cytogenet 3:293–306.
21. Bunn Jr PA, Whang-Peng J, Carney DN et al. (1980). DNA content analysis by flow cytofluorometry and cytogenetic analysis in mycosis fungoides and Sezary syndrome. J Clin Invest 65:1440–1448.
22. Mason DY and Biberfeld P (1980). Technical aspects of lymphoma immunohistology. J Histochem Cytochem 28:731–745.

23. Gerard-Marchant R, Hamlin I, Lennert K et al. (1974). Classification of non-Hodgkin's lymphomas. Lancet II:406–408.

24. Christensson B, Lindemalm C, Johansson B et al. (1983). Correlation of immunophenotype to morphology in unfavourable non-Hodgkin's lymphoma. Acta Path Microbiol Immunol Scand sect A 91:425–433.

25. Porwit- Ksiazek A, Christensson B., Lindemalm C et al (1983). Characterisation of malignant and non-neoplastic cell phenotypes in highly malignant non-Hodgkin lymphomas. Int J Cancer 32:667–674.

26. Tribukait B (1984). Flow cytometry in surgical pathology and cytology of tumors from the genito- urinary tract. In: Koss G, Coleman DV (Eds.). Adv. Clin Cytol Vol. 2:163–198.

27. Baisch H, Göhde W and Linden WA (1975). Analysis of PCP-data to determine the fraction of cells in various phases of the cell cycle. Radiat Environ Biophys 12:31–39.

28. Klecka WR (1981). Discriminant Analysis. In: SPSS second edition, pp. 434–467. New York: McGraw-Hill.

29. Lindemalm C, Christensson B, Johansson B et al. (1983). A clinico-pathological and immunological study of unfavourable non-Hodgkin lymphomas: Comparison of the Rappaport and Kiel classifications. Acta Path Microbiol Immunol Scand sect A 91:435–443.

30. Taylor IW and Milthorpe BK (1980). An evaluation of DNA fluorochromes, staining techniques, and analysis for flow cytometry. I. Unperturbed cell populations. J Histochem Cytochem 28:1224–1232.

31. Shackney SE, Skramstad KS, Cunningham RE et al. (1980). Dual parameter flow cytometry studies in human lymphomas. J Clin Invest 66:1281–1294.

32. Barlogie B, Raber M, Schumann J et al. (1983). Flow cytometry in clinical research. Cancer Res 43:3982–3997.

33. Look AT, Melvin SL, Williams DL et al (1982). Aneuploidy and percentage of S-phase cells determined by flow cytometry correlate with cell phenotype in childhood leukemia. Blood 60:959–963.

34. Neel BG, Jhanwar SC, Chaganti RS and Hayward WS (1982). Two human c-onc genes are located on the long arm of chromosome 8. Proc Nat Acad Sci USA 79:7842–7846.

35. Taub R, Kirsch I, Morton C et al (1982). Translocation of the C-myc gene into the immunoglobulin heavy chain locus in human Burkitt lymphoma and murine plasmacytoma cells. Proc Nat Acad Sci USA 79:7837–7841.

36. Dalla-Favera R, Bregni M, Erikson J et al. (1982). Human C-MYC ONC gene is located on the region of chromosome 8 that is translocated in Burkitt lymphoma cells. Proc Nat Acad Sci USA 79:7824–7827.

37. Hansen H, Koziner B and Clarkson B (1981). Marker and kinetic studies in the non-Hodgkin's lymphomas. Amer J Med 71:107–123.

5. Oncogenes in human neoplasms

G. M. COOPER
Dana Farber Cancer Institute and Department of Pathology, Harvard Medical School, Boston, MA 02115, USA

The biologic activity of tumor DNA, detected by transfection of NIH 3T3 mouse cells, has led to the identification of transforming genes which are activated in a variety of human and animal neoplasms. The DNA of many tumors efficiently induces transformation of NIH 3T3 cells. In contrast, the DNA of normal cells lacks efficient transforming activity, even the normal DNA of the same individual animals or patients whose tumor DNA induces transformation. These findings imply that the development of many neoplasms involves dominant genetic alterations leading to activation of transforming genes, which are then detectable by their biologic activity in this gene transfer assay.

Application of this approach to naturally occurring tumors led to identification of activated transforming genes in chicken B-cell lymphomas [1], a human bladder carcinoma cell line [2, 3], and carcinogen-induced rodent carcinomas and neuroblastomas [3]. Subsequently, activated transforming genes have been detected in many different types of neoplasms (carcinomas, sarcomas, neuroblastomas, melanomas, lymphomas and leukemias) of human, rodent and avian origin. Some of the transforming genes identified by this approach are related to the ras genes of Harvey and Kirsten sarcoma viruses, whereas others are unrelated to described retroviral transforming genes.

Distribution of activated genes in neoplasms

Three ras genes have been identified as biologically active transforming genes in neoplasm DNA: ras^H, ras^K and ras^N [4–8]. These genes have been detected in many different types of neoplasms including carcinomas, sarcomas, melanomas, neuroblastomas, lymphomas, and leukemias of myeloid and lymphoid origin.

Ras genes seem to contribute to the development of neoplasms arising from many types of differentiated cells. This is consistent with the fact that they are expressed in the normal vertebrate cells which have been examined. Yeast also contain functional ras genes, suggesting that these genes play a fundamental role in cell proliferation which is highly conserved in evolution; however, ras genes function as active transforming genes in only a small fraction (approximately 10–20%) of individual neoplasms. Thus, ras activation apparently is not necessary for the development of neoplasms, although it occurs in many types of tumors. Data from recent studies suggest that ras activation may occur late in tumor progression. For example, Albino et al. [9] reported detection of an activated ras^N gene in only one out of five metastases of one melanoma patient. This discovery suggests that ras activation may impart a selective advantage to a clone of neoplastic cells, but is not essential for formation of a primary neoplasm or even its metastatic derivatives.

Other transforming genes detected by transfection have been activated in neoplasms of specific cell types. For example, Burkitt's lymphoma-1 (Blym-1) has been detected as an activated transforming gene in surface immunoglobulin-positive B-cell lymphomas of chicken, mouse or human origin [1, 10, 11]. However, distinct transforming genes are activated in T-cell neoplasms, and in B-cell neoplasms representing other stages of B-lymphocyte differentiation [10, 12]. Activation of these transforming genes appears specific to the neoplasms representing discrete stages of B- and T-lymphocyte differentiation, and occurs in the majority (80–100%) of individual neoplasms of the appropriate cell type [10]. The spectrum of activation of these genes in neoplasms thus suggests that they play a more reproducible role than the ras genes in the development of specific tumor types.

Ras gene activation and function

All ras genes closely encode proteins of approximately 21,000 daltons, called p21. Experimental manipulations of the normal human ras^H gene have shown that over-expression of the normal gene product induces cell transformation [13]. However, activation of ras genes in human tumors is commonly a consequence of structural, rather than regulatory, mutations [14–22]. The mutations in tumors which have been analyzed alter either codon 12 or codon 61. At either of these positions, substitution of multiple different amino acids is sufficient to endow p21 with transforming activity. In addition, most activating mutations appear to induce alterations in the p21 conformation, which are detectable by abnormal electrophoretic mobilities [16, 19, 22]. These observations suggest that substitution of abnormal amino acids at these critical loci may inactivate a regulatory domain of p21, thus resulting in abnormal p21 function *in vivo*.

Studies of viral ras proteins have indicated that they are localized to the inner face of the plasma membrane [23, 24] and modified by acylation [25]. The only established biochemical activity common to all viral ras-transforming proteins is guanine nucleotide binding [23, 26].

To clarify the biochemical basis of the transforming activity of mutant p21 in human tumors, we compared the biochemical properties of p21 encoded by normal and activated human ras genes. These experiments indicated that both normal and transforming human p21 were localized to the plasma membrane, and were modified to similar extent by post-translational acylation [27]. Neither normal nor activated p21 wee glycosylated or phosphorylated [16, 27]. Thus, the subcellular localization and post-translational processing of human p21 are not altered by ras gene activation.

Because guanine nucleotide binding represented the only known biochemical activity of p21, we investigated the possibility that mutational activation altered the affinity or specificity of p21 for nucleotides. However, the GTP binding affinities of both normal and activated human p21 were indistinguishable (K_D of 1–2×10^{-8} M), and both the normal and activated proteins were specific for GTP and GDP binding [27]. Thus mutational activation of p21 does not directly affect its nucleotide-binding properties.

To determine the physiology of ras proteins, we identified other cellular proteins with which p21 might interact [28]. Immunoprecipitation of extracts of human carcinoma cell lines with anti-p21 monoclonal antibodies revealed a second protein of approximately 90,000 daltons. This coprecipitated protein was identified as the transferrin receptor by three criteria: 1) comigration in both reducing and non-reducing gels; 2) immunologic reactivity with monoclonal antibody raised against transferrin receptor; and 3) identity of partial proteolysis maps of the 90,000 dalton co-precipitated protein and transferrin receptor. Co-precipitation of transferrin receptor, detected with three different ras monoclonal antibodies, was dependent on the presence of ras proteins in cell extracts. This complex was dissociated by the addition of transferrin to cell extracts, suggesting that transferrin binding induces a change in conformation of the receptor, leading to dissociation of ras proteins.

Transferrin is an iron-binding protein required for the growth of most cells in culture. Expression of transferrin receptor is closely correlated with cell proliferation. Furthermore, monoclonal antibodies against transferrin receptor inhibit cell growth, in some cases even if iron is supplied in an alternate form. Transferrin and its receptor thus appear to play a fundamental role in the growth of many differentiated cell types. This interaction between ras proteins and transferrin receptor suggests p21 may function with this cell surface receptor in regulation of cell growth, perhaps by transducing growth signals mediated by transferrin binding. The role of p21 in this respect may be analogous to other membrane guanine nucleotide binding proteins, such as the adenyl cyclase G-proteins and transducin [29].

Blym transforming genes

The Blym-1 transforming gene was first identified in DNA of chicken B-cell lymphomas [1], and was isolated as a molecular clone by sib-selection [30]. The cloned chicken Blym-1 gene was unusually small (only about 600 nucleotides), and the nucleotide sequence indicated that it encoded a small protein of 65 amino acids [30]. Comparison of the predicted chicken Blym-1 amino acid sequence to sequences of known cellular proteins revealed partial homology (36%) between the chicken Blym-1 protein and the amino-terminal region of transferrin family proteins [30]. This homology was concentrated in regions which were conserved between different members of the transferrin family, suggesting a common ancestry for chicken Blym-1 and a region of the transferrins as well as a possible functional relationship.

Blot hybridization analysis indicated that the chicken Blym-1 gene was a member of a small family of related genes, which were present in human as well as chicken DNA. We therefore investigated the possibility that the transforming gene detected by transfection of Burkitt's lymphoma DNA might be a member of the human gene family homologous to chicken Blym-1. A genomic library of DNA from a Burkitt's lymphoma was screened using chicken Blym-1 probe. A biologically active human transforming gene, designated human Blym-1, was isolated [11]. This human homolog of chicken Blym-1 represents the transforming gene detected by transfection of all six Burkitt's lymphoma DNA studied.

Restriction mapping and nucleotide sequencing indicate that human Blym-1, like chicken Blym-1, is quite small (approximately 700 nucleotides) [11, Diamond et al., personal communication]. The sequence of human Blym-1 also predicts a small protein (58 amino acids) consisting of two exons, and rich in lysine and arginine. Alignment of the human and chicken Blym-1 amino acid sequences indicates 33% amino acid identities. The human and chicken Blym-1 proteins therefore are related ($p < 0.005$), but the significant divergence occurring between the two sequences suggests the chicken and human genes may represent distant members of the Blym family.

The human Blym-1 sequence also displays significant homology (20%) to the amino-terminal region of transferrins. Amino acids which are conserved between the chicken and human Blym-1 genes also tend to be conserved between different members of the transferrin family. It is unlikely that this homology to transferrin shared by both chicken and human Blym-1 genes, developed by chance. Instead, this homology probably reflects some functional property of the Blym transforming proteins. In view of the molecular interaction between ras proteins and transferrin receptor, these findings raise the hypothesis that the Blym transforming genes may also affect cell proliferation via a pathway related to transferrin and its surface receptor.

Oncogene activation and pathogenesis of neoplasms

The development of neoplasms *in vivo* clearly involves progressive preneoplastic and neoplastic stages rather than a single-step conversion of a normal cell to a fully neoplastic cell. Therefore, the transforming genes detected by transfection of tumor DNA represents only one event in neoplasm development. In fact, many neoplasms involve activation of at least two distinct oncogenes, suggesting that different oncogenes may function at different stages of neoplasm development.

In chicken B-cell lymphomas, the Blym-1 gene is detected by the transfection assay [1]. However, a different gene (myc) is activated in the same tumors by adjacent integration of viral DNA [31]. Blym-1 and myc are unrelated to each other, and are not closely linked in cellular DNA [32]. Thus, their co-activation in these neoplasms represents two distinct events. Since both genes are activated in the vast majority (90%) of individual lymphomas, both appear to play important roles in the disease process.

Human myc and Blym-1 genes are also both activated in Burkitt's lymphomas. In this disease, human myc is translocated from chromosome 8 to an immunoglobulin locus [33, 34]. In the same tumors, human Blym-1, located on chromosome 1 [35], is detected as an active transforming gene in the transfection assay [11]. Thus, the same two oncogenes are involved in B-cell lymphomas of both chicken and man. The activation of both myc and Blym genes in Burkitt's lymphoma in two different species strongly supports the causal role of these genes in the disease process.

Outgrowth of pre-neoplastic transformed lymphoid follicles is the first stage in development of B-cell lymphoma in the chicken [36]. Approximately 10–100 hyper-proliferative lesions out of approximately 10^5 lymphocyte follicles are observed in the bursa. These pre-neoplastic follicles retain the organization of normal lymphoid follicles, and the majority appear to regress under normal physiologic controls which mediate regression of the bursa. However, a small fraction (< 5%) of these pre-neoplastic follicles may progress to clonal neoplasms [36].

Activation of both myc and Blym-1 has occurred in the earliest detectable clonal bursal neoplasms [32]. Since the disease process is initiated by infection with a virus that activates myc, it may be speculated that activation of myc is directly responsible for pre-neoplastic follicle proliferation, but is insufficient to induce the full neoplastic phenotype. Activation of Blym within some pre-neoplastic lymphocytes would then represent a second event responsible for progression to neoplasia. Data from studies of the biologic effects of an activated myc gene on bursal lymphocytes support this hypothesis (Neiman et al., personal communication). Activated myc was introduced into bursal lymphocytes through infection with the retrovirus HB1, which contains a myc gene recovered by recombination from chicken DNA [37]. Infected lymphocytes were then transplanted to chicken embryos pretreated with cyclophosphamide to ablate their endogenous bursal lymphocyte population. Histologic examination of the bursas of these transplanted embryos indicated that the HB1 myc gene acutely induced formation of pre-neoplastic follicles. DNA from these pre-neoplastic follicles did not induce transformation of NIH 3T3 cells, indicating that Blym-1 was not activated. These results indicate that myc alone can induce the initial pre-neoplastic stage of lymphomagenesis, and suggest that activation of Blym-1 is associated with further progression to neoplasia.

In addition to myc and Blym-1 activation in B-cell lymphomas, pairs of transforming genes are similarly implicated in several other types of neoplasms. Mouse plasmacytomas involve activation of myc by chromosomal translocation [38, 39], as well as activation of a distinct transforming gene detected by transfection [40]. Abelson virus-induced mouse pre-B-cell lymphomas involve the viral abl gene as well as a distinct and unlinked NIH 3T3 transforming gene [40]. Murine leukemia virus-induced T-cell lymphomas and mouse mammary tumor virus-induced carcinomas involve activation of genes by virus integration (MLVI and MMTVint) [41–43], and of unrelated transforming genes detected by transfection [12, 44]. The activation of two distinct transforming genes in neoplasms thus appears to be a common occurrence. By analogy to the myc and Blym-1 combination, these genes may function at distinct stages of tumor development.

References

1. Cooper GM and Neiman PE (1980). Transforming genes of neoplasms induced by avian lymphoid leukosis viruses. Nature 287:656–658.
2. Krontiris TG and Cooper GM (1981). Transforming activity of human tumor DNAs. Proc Nat Acad Sci USA 78:1181–1184.
3. Shih C, Padhy LC, Murray M and Weinberg RA (1981). Transforming genes of carcinomas and neuroblastomas introduced into mouse fibroblasts. Nature 290:261–264.
4. Der CJ, Krontiris TG and Cooper GM (1982). Transforming genes of human bladder and lung carcinoma cell lines are homologous to the ras genes of Harvey and Kirsten sarcoma viruses. Proc Nat Acad Sci USA 79:3637–3640.
5. Parada LF, Tabin CJ, Shih C and Weinberg RA (1982). Human EJ bladder carcinoma oncogene is homologue of Harvey sarcoma virus ras gene. Nature 297:474–478.
6. Santos E, Tronick SR, Aaronson SA et al. (1982). T24 human bladder carcinoma oncogene

is an activated form of the normal human homologue of BALB — and Harvey — msv transforming genes. Nature 298:343–347.

7. Hall A, Marshall CJ, Spurr NK and Weiss RA (1983). Identification of transforming gene in two human sarcoma cell lines as a new member of the ras gene family located on chromosome 1. Nature 303:396–400.

8. Shimizu K, Goldfarb M, Perucho M and Wigler M (1983). Isolation and preliminary characterization of the transforming gene of a human neuroblastoma cell line. Proc Nat Acad Sci USA 80:383–387.

9. Albino AP, LeStrange R, Oliff AI et al. (1984). Transforming ras genes from human melanoma: A manifestation of tumour heterogeneity? Nature 308:69–72.

10. Lane M-A, Sainten A and Cooper GM (1982). Stage-specific transforming genes of human and mouse B- and T-lymphocyte neoplasms. Cell 28:873–880.

11. Diamond AD, Cooper GM, Ritz J and Lane MA (1983). Identification and molecular cloning of the human blym transforming gene activated in Burkitt's lymphomas. Nature 305:112–116.

12. Lane M-A, Sainten A, Doherty KM and Cooper GM (1984). Isolation and characterization of a stage-specific transforming gene, Thym-1, from T-cell lymphomas. Proc Nat Acad Sci USA 81:2227–2231.

13. Chang EH, Furth ME, Scolnick EM and Lowy DR (1982). Tumorigenic transformation of mammalian cells induced by a normal human gene homologous to the oncogene of Harvey murine sarcoma virus. Nature 297:497–483.

14. Capon DJ, Chen EY, Levinson AD et al. (1983). Complete nucleotide sequences of the T_{24} human bladder carcinoma oncogene and its normal homologue. Nature 302:33–37.

15. Capon DJ, Seeburg PH, McGrath JP et al. (1983). Activation of ki-ras[2] gene in human colon and lung carcinomas by two different point mutations. Nature 304:507–513.

16. Der CJ and Cooper GM (1983). Altered gene products are associated with activation of cellular ras[k] genes in human lung and colon carcinomas. Cell 32:201–208.

17. Reddy EP, Reynolds RK, Santos E and Barbacid M (1982). A point mutation is responsible for the acquisition of transforming properties by the T24 human bladder carcinoma oncogene. Nature 300:149–152.

18. Shimizu K, Birnbaum D, Ruley MA et al. (1983). Structure of the ki-ras gene of the human lung carcinoma cell line Calu-1. Nature 304:497–500.

19. Tabin CJ, Bradley SM, Bargmann CI et al. (1982). Mechanism of activation of a human oncogene. Nature 300:143–149.

20. Taparowsky E, Suard Y, Fasano O et al. (1982). Activation of the T24 bladder carcinoma transforming gene is linked to a single amino acid change. Nature 300:762–765.

21. Taparowsky E, Shimizu K, Goldfarb M and Wigler M (1983). Structure and activation of the human n-ras gene. Cell 34:581–586.

22. Yuasa Y, Srivastava SK, Dunn CY et al. (1983). Acquisition of transforming properties by alternative point mutations within c-ras/n-ras human proto-oncogene. Nature 303:775–779.

23. Furth ME, Davis LJ, Fleurdelys B and Scolnick EM (1982). Monoclonal antibodies to the p21 products of the transforming gene of Harvey murine sarcoma virus and of the cellular ras gene family. J Viral 43:294–304.

24. Willingham MC, Pastan I, Shih TY and Scolnick EM (1980). Localization of the src gene product of the Harvey strain of msv to plasma membrane of transformed cells by electron microscopic immunocytochemistry. Cell 19:1005–1014.

25. Sefton BM, Trowbridge IS, Cooper JA and Scolnick EM (1982). The transforming proteins of Rous sarcoma virus, Harvey sarcoma virus and Abelson virus contain tightly bound lipid. Cell 31:465–474.

26. Scolnick EM, Papageorge AG and Shih TY (1979). Guanine nucleotide-binding activity as an assay for src protein of ras-derived murine sarcoma viruses. Proc Nat Acad Sci USA

76:5355–5359.

27. Finkel T, Der CJ and Cooper GM (1984). Activation of ras genes in human tumors does not affect localization, modification, or nucleotide binding properties of p21. Cell 37:151–158.

28. Finkel T and Cooper GM (1984). Detection of a molecular complex between ras proteins and transferrin receptor. Cell 36:1115–1121.

29. Gilman AG (1984). G proteins and dual control of adenylate cyclase. Cell 36:577–579.

30. Goubin G, Goldman DS, Luce J et al. (1983). Molecular cloning and nucleotide sequence of a transforming gene detected by transfection of chicken B-cell lymphoma DNA. Nature 302:114–119.

31. Hayward WS, Neel BG and Astrin SM (1981). Activation of a cellular oncogene by promoter insertion in ALV-induced lymphoid leukosis. Nature 290:475–480.

32. Cooper GM and Neiman PE (1981). Two distinct candidate transforming genes of lymphoid leukosis virus-induced neoplasms. Nature 292:857–858.

33. Dalla-Favera R, Bregni M, Erikson J et al. (1982). Human c-*myc* onc gene is located on the region of chromosome 8 that is translocated in Burkitt lymphoma cells. Proc Nat Acad Sci USA 79:7824–7827.

34. Taub R, Kirsch I, Morton C et al. (1982). Translocation of the c-*myc* gene into the immunoglobin heavy chain locus in human Burkitt lymphoma and murine plasmacytoma cells. Proc Nat Acad Sci Usa 79:7837-7841.

35. Morton CC, Taub R, Diamon A et al. (1984). Mapping of the human *Blym-1* transforming gene activated in Burkitt lymphomas to chromosome 1. Science 223:173–175.

36. Neiman PE, Jordan L, Weiss RA and Payne LN (1980). Malignant lymphoma of the bursa of Fabricus. Analysis of early transformation. Cold Spring Harbor Conf on Cell Proliferation 7:519–528.

37. Bister K, Jansen HW, Graf T et al. (1983). Genome structure of HBI, a variant of acute leukemia virus MC29 with unique oncogenic properties. J Virol 46:337–356.

38. Shen-Ong GLC, Keath EJ, Piccoli SP and Cole MD (1982). Novel myc oncogene RNA from abortive immunoglobin-gene recombination in mouse plasmacytomas. Cell 31:443–452.

39. Crews S, Barth R, Hood L et al. (1982). Mouse c-myc oncogene is located on chromosome 15 and translocated to chromosome 12 in plasmacytomas. Science 218:1319–1321.

40. Lane M-A, Neary D and Cooper GM (1982). Activation of a cellular transforming gene in tumours induced by Abelson murine leukaemia virus. Nature 300:659–661.

41. Tsichlis PN, Strauss PG and Hu LF (1983). A common region for proviral DNA integration in Mo MuLV-induced rat thymic lymphomas. Nature 302:445–449.

42. Nusse R and Varmus HE (1982). Many tumors induced by the mouse mammary tumor virus contain a provirus integrated in the same region of the host genome. Cell 31:99–109.

43. Peters G, Brookes S, Smith R and Dickson C (1983). Tumorigenesis by mouse mammary tumor virus: Evidence for a common region for provirus integration in mammary tumors. Cell 33:369–377.

44. Lane M-A, Sainten A and Cooper GM (1981). Activation of related transforming genes in mouse and human mammary carcinomas. Proc Nat Acad Sci USA 78:5185–5189.

6. Stage specific transforming genes in lymphoid neoplasms

M. A. LANE [1,2], H. A. F. STEPHENS [1,2], M. B. TOBIN [1]
and K. DOHERTY [1]
1 Laboratory of Molecular Immunobiology, Dana Farber Cancer Institute, and 2 Department of Pathology, Harvard Medical School, Boston, Massachusetts, USA

Identification of activated cellular transforming genes in a variety of neoplasms has been greatly facilitated by the use of the NIH 3T3 transfection assay. A unique property of the NIH 3T3 cells is that they have the ability to undergo transformation following integration of dominantly acting genes, possibly because they have already progressed some way down the path toward overt malignancy. These cells have the ability to be transformed by a variety of transforming genes and therefore may represent a multi potential cell capable of responding to many different growth stimulatory signals.

Utilizing the transfection assay, members of the ras ras^H, ras^K, ras^N family have been found to be activated in 10–20% of of all neoplasms assayed. Because ras genes are transcribed in all cells at all stages of differentiation, it is likely that these genes may be 'at risk' to an activating event in all cells at some statistically low level. This finding may or may not imply a mechanism of protection for ras genes which prevents them from being activated in all tumors. Following exposure to chemical carcinogens however, ras gene activation in particular cell systems seems to increase but it is not yet clear from analysis of these systems whether the carcinogens utilized interact specifically with the genes encoding ras proteins [1].

Stage specific transforming genes, in contrast to ras genes, appear to be activated quite discretely in cells of a particular lineage, representative of a particular stage of differentiation. The lymphoid system, in which cell lineages and differentiative pathways have been best characterized has provided the most useful system for analysis of stage specific transforming genes. As we previously reported, a common gene is activated in multiple isolates of pre-B-tumors of both humans and mice [2]. This gene differs both from the gene found to be activated in multiple intermediate B-cell neoplasms and from that activated in mature B-neoplasms. The first of the B-lineage stage specific transforming genes to be isolated and characterized, Blym1 was initially identified in chicken bursal lymphomas. Cloning and sequencing of this gene indicated that it encoded a small protein of 8 KD which shared homology with the amino terminal domains of transferrin family molecules [3]. Chicken Blym1 was utilized as a probe to isolate human Blym1 from Burkitt's lymphomas and it was determined that human Blym1 gene also shared homology with the transferrins. Blym1, the gene activated in a variety of intermediate B-cell tumors, is therefore, well conserved evolutionarily, and is expressed in multiple tumor isolates from several different species including humans, but differs by restriction endonuclease inactivation patterns from genes activated in pre-B or mature B-tumors. Blym1 activation has not been detected in tumors of other cell lineages or B cell tumors at different stages of differentiation and therefore unlike ras genes represents a uniquely stage and lineage specific gene [4].

Within the T-lymphoid lineage two different stage specific genes have been found to be activated in neoplasms of rodent and human species. Isolated from a BALB/c T lymphoma, Tlym1 is representative of the gene activated in multiple isolates of pre-T and intermediate T-tumors. Tlym1 differs from the gene activated mature T neoplasms as the two genes have differing patterns of susceptibility to restriction endonuclease inactivation.

Tlym1 was isolated by sib selection and transfection of a transforming gene — enriched λ Charon 30 library containing cell DNA inserts in the 8 kb range. A single phage was isolated containing cell DNA inserts in the 8 kb range. A single phage was isolated containing a cellular insert of 8.7 kb which was biologically active. To facilitate further mapping a 4.7 kb Hind-Bam fragment containing an EcoR1 site was subcloned into PBR322. This fragment which contains the transforming region of the gene was chosen because digestion with EcoR1 was previously shown to inactivate the transforming activity of Tlym1 [2, 5].

Hybridization of a flanking sequence probe to BALB/c liver DNA and to S49 tumor DNA indicated that activation of this gene did not occur as a result of gross rearrangements or deletions in cell DNA. Hybridization of coding sequence probe to human DNA under conditions of slightly relaxed stringency indicated that this sequence was conserved between mouse and human species [5].

Hybridization of the 4.7 kb fragment containing the transforming region to lymphoid cellular RNA detected major message species of 0.6, 0.7 and 1.6 kb in both T- and B-cells and in addition, a message of 1.8 kb in RNA from a T-suppressor clone. These message sizes were of interest to us because of a report by Peter Rigby and his colleagues concerning their isolation of cDNA clones by subtractive RNA hybridization from SV40 transformed cells. One group of genes referred to as Set 1 genes shared extensive sequence homology with MHC 1 genes from the TL/QA region. Set 1 genes used as probes detected messenger RNA of 0.6, 0.7 and 1.6 kb, and appeared to possess a novel repeat element having a structure similar to a transposon, as it was flanked by direct repeat sequences [6].

Because of the similarity of RNA messenger sizes identified by both Tlym1 and Set 1 genes, and because Tlym1 had been isolated from a thymic lymphoma it was of interest to determine whether Tlym1 did encode a gene within the MHC I region and it was of particular interest to determine whether our gene encoded an altered TL or QA product.

Tlym1 was found to hybridize to pMHC1 [7] described by Seidman and coworkers as a probe crossreactive with most MHC I region genes; to 64-c, reported by Rigby's group to contain exons four, five and six of the Set 1 gene; and to 64-E which contained their Set 1 sequence [6]. The results of these experiments indicate that Tlym1 shares homology with Class 1 MHC genes.

As Tlym1 contained a ClaI site, some further analysis was possible based upon the report by Steinmetz et al. [8] defining thirteen clusters containing 36 genes within the BALB/c MHC I region. From their reported analysis of ClaI sites within the gene clusters, we have been able to rule out all but nine genes mapping to four clusters. Clusters one and six map to QA regions, while clusters three and five map to TL regions as determined by these authors. If the genes contained in the thirteen clusters constitute all of the genes encoded within the MHC I region then this retrospective analysis further localizes Tlym1 to the QA/TL region of the MHC I complex, provided the cosmid clusters contain all of the MHC region genes.

An antisera crossreactive with all MHC I products was used to immunoprecipitate Tlym1 protein products from ^{35}S labeled cell extracts and supernates. This antisera precipitated a 44 kd protein from the supernates of multiple Tlym1 transformants which was not present in supernates from untransformed NIH 3T3 cells, NIH 3T3 cells transformed by ras genes or NIH 3T3 cells transformed by a mouse Blym1 gene. These findings further confirm that Tlym1, is an MHC I product and demonstrates that this gene encodes a secreted protein product. Use of Tlym1 transformant supernates in a soft agar colony growth factor assay indicated that these supernates had the ability to stimulate NIH 3T3 cells to form large numbers of colonies while control supernates from normal NIH 3T3 cells stimulated very few cells to produce colonies after 14 days culture.

Genes in the TL/QA region encode cell surface expressed proteins in the range of 40–45 thousand daltons, which have been found to be associated with beta-2 microglobulin. TL antigens are expressed in a highly stage specific manner and have been found only on thymus cells. TL negative strains in which thymic leukemias develop often express a novel TL on their surface. At present, the biological role of the TL antigens is unclear.

QA1 antigens have been detected on approximately two thirds of all Thyl+ cells and are found on one class of helper T-cells as well as a feedback suppressor cell. QA2 is also found on a majority of Thyl+ cells and is expressed on some but not all T-cell leukemias. Proliferation to the mitogens ConA and PhA can be blocked if T-cells are pretreated with antiserum directed against the QA2 antigen. QA3 is also expressed predominantly on Th-1 positive cells and behaves as does QA2 in mitogen studies.

The antigens QA4 and QA5 have a different tissue distribution and appear not to be present on thymic cells. These antigens are present on Ig-cells from spleen and lymph nodes and are additionally expressed on B-cell blasts following lipopolysaccharide stimulation [9].

At the nucleic acid level, the sequences encoding TL and QA do not exhibit extensive polymorphism and in some cases share homology of 80% or more, while the genes encoding H-2 seem to be more extensively polymorphic. For these reasons it will be of use to distinguish TL products from QA products utilizing specific serologic reagents.

In summary, Tlym1 is the first of the cellular transforming genes found to encode a secreted protein product and it appears that this gene shares substantial homology to genes encoded within the TL/QA region of the major histocompatibility complex. It is therefore attractive to speculate that this gene functions in T-cell lymphomas by producing a secreted product which may associate with the T-cell receptor to provide an autologous growth stimulus. When this gene is integrated into NIH 3T3 cells the secreted protein product may function with a somewhat lower affinity by associating with other receptors involved with the initiation of proliferation.

Acknowledgements

The authors thank J. Seidman, Dept. of Genetics, Harvard Medical School for pMHCI and for MHCI Crossreactive Antisera; P. W. J. Rigby Imperial College, London, for 64-C and 64-E. The authors also wish to thank L. Hood and S. Hunt, California Institute of Technology, H. Cantor and G. Freeman, Dana-Farber Cancer Institute, and T. Boyse and F. W. Shen, Sloan-Kettering Memorial Laboratory, for useful and productive discussions. This work was supported by CA33108. M. A. Lane is a Scholar of the Leukemia Society of America.

References

1. Cooper GM and Lane MA (1984). Cellular transforming genes and oncogenesis. Biochem Biophys Acta (in press).
2. Lane MA, Sainten A and Cooper GM (1982). Stage-specific transforming genes of human and mouse B- and T-lymphocyte neoplasma. Cell 28:873–880.
3. Goubin G, Goldman DS, Luce J et al. (1983). Molecular cloning and nucleotide sequence of a transforming gene detected by transfection of chicken B-cell lymphoma DNA. Nature 302:114–119.

4. Diamond A, Cooper GM, Ritz J and Lane MA (1983). Identification and molecular cloning of the human Blym transforming gene activated in Burkitt's lymphomas. Nature 305:112–116.

5. Lane MA, Sainten A, Doherty KM and Cooper GM (1984). Isolation and characterization of a stage specific transforming gene, Tlym-I, from T-cell lymphomas. Proc Nat Acad Sci USA 81:2227–2231.

6. Brickell PM, Latchman DS, Murphy D et al. (1983). Activation of a Qa/TLa class I major histocompatibility antigen gene is a general feature of oncogenesis in the mouse. Nature 306:756–760.

7. Evans GA, Margulies DH, Camerini–Otero RD et al. (1982). Structure and expression of a major histocompatibility antigen gene H-2L^d. Proc Nat Acad Sci USA 79:1994–1998.

8. Steinmetz M, Winoto A, Minard K and Hood L (1981). Clusters of genes encoding mouse transplantation antigens. Cell 28:489–498.

9. Flaherty L (1980). TLA-region antigens. In: The Role of the Major Histocompatibility Complex in Immunology, p 33. New York: Garland STPM Press.

III. Biochemical markers

1. DNA synthetic and degradative pathways in malignant lymphomas

A. V. HOFFBRAND[1] and A. D. HO[2]

[1] *Department of Haematology, Royal Free Hospital and School of Medicine, Hampstead, London, UK and*
[2] *Medizinische Universitäts-Poliklinik, Heidelberg, FRG*

This review concerns those enzyme reactions which have proved valuable in diagnosis or treatment of lymphomas. Of particular value is the measurement of a number of enzymes involved in purine or pyrimidine synthesis or degradation, e.g., terminal deoxynucleotidyl transferase (TdT) and the purine enzymes, adenosine deaminase (ADA), purine nucleoside phosphorylase (PNP) and 5′nucleotidase (5′NT), thymidine phosphorylase and thymidine kinase (TK). During development, lymphoid populations show remarkable changes in the concentrations of these enzymes and the neoplasms derived from them show a 'frozen' biochemical profile similar to the corresponding normal cell of origin. The explanation of these changes in enzyme concentration may be partly related to the change from proliferation dominance in early cells to differentiation and functional development in later cells. It may also provide a mechanism for selection of clones destined to develop or die. Recent interest in the relation of cell proliferation to membrane protein phosphorylation has led to studies in our and other laboratories of protein phosphorylation in normal and malignant lymphoid tissues. This topic is dealt with at the end of this review. Relevant recent reviews in these areas include those by van Laarhoven and de Bruyn [1] and van de Griend and colleagues [2].

Terminal deoxynucleotidyl transferase (TdT)

This enzyme catalyses the polymerisation of single stranded DNA onto a free 3-OH′ end of an oligo- or poly-deoxynucleotide primer without template direction. The preferred substrate is deoxyguanosine triphosphate (dGTP). The enzyme can be measured biochemically or tested for by indirect immunofluorescence, immunoperoxidase, alkaline phosphatase-antialkaline phosphatase (APAP) or avidin-biotin complex (ABC) techniques [3]. The latter techniques have the advantage that single cell analysis can be carried out and double or triple markers detected on each cell. A recent study in non-Hodgkin's lymphomas (NHL) showed excellent concordance between the biochemical and immunologic methods, but concluded the ABC method was preferable in lymphoma diagnosis. The function of the enzyme is unknown although it has been proposed to play a role in generation of diversity in lymphoid precursors in the bone marrow or thymic cortex, the only two normal tissues that contain it [4, 5]. It is expressed at the stage of T- and B-lymphoid development when gene rearrangement is occurring and it is possible that at this stage it is active in altering the DNA base sequence. Alternatively, Ma et al. [6] suggested that it may have a role in polymerizing excess, unbalanced deoxyribonucleoside triphosphates (dNTP) in early thymic cortical cells which have little ability to degrade dNTP but have ability to degrade active kinases which phosphorylate salvaged nucleotides. This may help to prevent toxicity to the key enzyme in DNA synthesis, ribonucleotide reductase. Unlike the replicative DNA polymerase, TdT activity is unrelated to the cell cycle [7]. Therefore, detection of its presence in leukemia or lymphoma cells does not depend on their proliferative status. No specific inhibitor of TdT has yet been found, and an inborn lack of TdT has not been described in humans.

TdT is usually present in common and null, non-B, non-T, acute lymphoblastic leukemia (c-ALL and null-ALL), pre-B-ALL and Thy-ALL blast cells and also in the cells of patients with chronic granulocytic leukemia in lymphoid blast transformation. Only one type of lymphoma shows TdT activity, histologically, the lymphoblastic lymphoma which on immunological testing has been invariably shown to be of T-cell type. This tumor overlaps in children with Thy-ALL, and is thought to arise in early cortical thymocytes or in prothymocytes. A recent study showed the cells of 25 such patients to be positive, whereas the cells of 117 patients with NHL of other types were negative, except in one case of large cell immunoblastic lymphoma which was positive by the enzyme assay only [3]. TdT is not detectable in identifiable B-cell tumors (SIg$^+$), mature T-cell tumors (T-CLL, T-PLL, Sezary's syndrome and mycosis fungoides) and in Hodgkin's disease.

An advantage of TdT detection in lymphoma (and leukemia) diagnosis is that cells outside the marrow (or thymus) which show the presence of TdT are invariably malignant. Thus, detection of a single TdT positive cell in the cerebrospinal fluid, a pleural aspirate, or a lymph node or testicular biopsy section demonstrates the presence of tumor. Moreover, cells doubly positive for nuclear TdT and T-cell surface antigens are abnormal even in the bone marrow providing an extremely sensitive method of detecting residual Thy-ALL cells.

Purine metabolic enzyme (ADA, PNP, 5'NT)

Normal tissues

Particular interest in these enzymes arose when congenital deficiency of adenosine deaminase (ADA) was recognized as a cause of severe combined immune deficiency with failure of both T- and B-cell development. ADA catalyses the conversion of deoxyadenosine and adenosine to deoxyinosine and inosine respectively. High concentrations of ADA are now known to occur in early cortical thymocytes and the levels fall as the T-cells mature [8]. B-cells, other haemopoietic cells and other tissues have lower levels of ADA. In contrast, PNP and 5'NT concentrations rise as T-cells mature in the thymus, 5'NT concentrations ultimately being higher in T_8 than in T_4 lymphocytes [8, 9]. Mature B-cells, however, have higher 5'NT levels than T-cells. The dependence of early thymocytes (and the lymphomas and leukemias derived from them) on ADA to degrade deoxyadenosine, normally salvaged from plasma, makes them exquisitely sensitive to ADA deficiency (or inhibition by deoxycoformycin). Toxicity is thought to result from accumulation of dATP which in proliferating cells inhibits ribonucleotide reductase, lowers the cell concentrations of the other 3 dNTP and so switches off DNA synthesis. In non-proliferating cells, postulated mechanisms include inhibition of S-adenosyl homocysteine hydrolase (SAHH) with accumulation of S-adenosyl homocysteine (SAH) which inhibits S-adenosyl methionine (SAM) mediated reactions [10], depletion of ATP with possible reduction in protein phosphorylation [11], and interference by adenosine with synthesis or metabolism of RNA [12] and in particular of polyadenylated RNA leading to G0-G1 interface arrest [13–15]. Although SAHH activity is higher in B- than T-cells, it has been difficult to show an exact correlation in resting or proliferating cells between cell toxicity and the degree of inhibition of SAHH, e.g. by deoxyadenosine when ADA is inhibited by deoxycoformycin (dCF) or EHNA.

The overall differences between early T-cells and more mature T-cells or early or late B- or myeloid-cells in the balance between purine and pyrimidine synthesis or degradation appears to be due to increased activities in early T-cells of synthetic enzymes e.g. deoxyadenosine, deoxyguanosine and deoxycytidine kinases and deoxyadenosine mono- and di-phosphate kinases, with lower activities of degradative enzymes e.g. ecto-ATPase, 5'nucleotidase, thymidine phosphorylase and endonucleotidases [16]. On the other hand, the endogenous production of deoxyadenosine has been shown to be greater in B- than T-lymphoblasts [17]. The susceptibility of T-cells to deoxyadenosine toxicity is also explained in terms of the variation between lymphoid populations in the degree of functional separation of DNA precursors into synthetic and degradative compartments. Using thymine nucleotides as a model and established tumor cell lines, early T-cells have been shown to have a tight multi-enzyme complex for channelling thymine nucleotides derived from salvage or de novo synthesis into DNA. They have little degradative ability [18].

The explanation for the changes in purine enzymes of developing T-cells has been postulated to allow for clonal selection of those T-cells which recognize self, interact with thymic epithelial cells and are rescued from self-destruction by cell-cell enzyme transfer or enzyme induction preventing the build-up of dATP and other metabolites dependent on ADA for degradation [6]. External nucleosides may selectively kill or impair function of one or other lymphoid population. The recent observation by Cohen et al. [19] that deoxyadenosine selectively impairs human T-cell suppressor (compared with helper) function, even though proliferative responses of T_8^+ and T_8^- populations are equally affected, suggests suppressor function has a different proliferative need. Moreover, deoxyguanosine has been shown to selectively impair suppressor compared to helper function in mice.

The differences in synthesis and degradation of deoxynucleotides between T- and B-cells makes T-cells susceptible to deoxyribonucleoside toxicity, particularly when they are immature and have greater synthetic or less degradative ability. Thus, it has been shown that when ADA activity is blocked by deoxycoformycin, deoxyadenosine is toxic to T-cell lines at concentrations which leave B and myeloid lines intact.

Lymphomas

ADA can be detected biochemically, antigenically or by the immunoperoxidase technique. High ADA levels are a feature of Thy-ALL and immature T-cell lymphomas. On the other hand, these tumors show low levels of PNP and 5′NT. In individual cases, however, a high level of ADA is not diagnostic since high levels may also occur in B lymphoma cells. The changes in enzymes seen as normal T-cells mature can be partly reproduced by treating T leukemic/lymphoma cells (Molt 4) with the inducing agent phorbol ester [20]. Changes in ADA levels occur during B- as well as T-cells development. Immunohistochemical staining shows positive nuclear staining in normal small cleaved lymphocytes (centrocytic cells) and weak nuclear or cytoplasmic stain in large lymphoid cells. Similarly, centrocytic lymphomas show strongly positive staining, while centroblastic tumours show weaker staining and immunoblastic tumors are negative [21]. The levels of all three enzymes, ADA, PNP and 5′NT are lower in B-CLL cells than in normal adult peripheral blood B lymphocytes and more closely resemble those of cord blood lymphocytes [22, 23]. In diffuse, well-differentiated lymphoma and CLL, the pattern of all the three purine enzymes differs from that in immunocytoma. This variant of CLL with intracytoplasmic Ig shows significantly higher 5'NT levels than the usual form [22].

In more mature T-cell tumors (e.g. Sezary's syndrome and mycosis fungoides) the pattern of purine enzymes resembles that of mature T-lymphocytes with higher PNP and 5'NT levels and lower ADA levels. This pattern is also reproduced in chronic Tγ-lymphocytosis cells but these cells have been found to have a higher ADA activity and a higher ADA/PNP ratio than in chronic T-cell malignant disease [2].

Deoxycoformycin.

This ADA inhibitor has proved effective in obtaining a remission in patients with Thy-ALL resistant to other therapy. In our own experience, patients with acute leukemia of non-thymic phenotypes have been resistant [24]. The drug has been less widely used in T-cell lymphoma but in isolated cases, e.g. of mycosis fungoides, has proved effective in achieving temporary remission [25]. In some cases, relapsing blast cells after dCF therapy have shown an altered expression of surface antigens compared to the original blast cells, suggesting adenosine or deoxyadenosine accumulation may affect synthesis of particular proteins. Surprisingly, dCF has also proved effective therapy against some B-cell tumors, including B-cell NHL, CLL (which has a low ADA level), hairy cell leukemia and occasional cases of common-ALL [25, 26]. Major toxic effects have included acute tubular necrosis with renal failure and central nervous system damage. Other side-effects have been iritis, nausea and vomiting, hemolysis and biochemical evidence of liver damage.

The possibility of using dCF alone or in combination with deoxyadenosine (AdR) *in vitro* for selectively depleting marrow of T-cell tumor cells prior to autologous bone marrow transplantation has been explored. Combinations of dCF (10^{-6} M) and AdR (10^{-5} M) are toxic to Thy-ALL (lymphoma lines) but fail to inhibit the growth of normal marrow myeloid progenitors. A similar selective effect has been shown by viability testing, ^{3}H-thymidine uptake and T-cell colony assays. However, in order to achieve >95% toxicity to T-cells, 72-hour incubation was needed [27]. More recently, a shorter time interval (18 hours) was shown necessary to kill clonogenic T-cells while leaving the viability of myeloid colony forming cells intact (Russell, Bellingham and Hoffbrand, unpublished).

PNP deficiency leads to selective T-cell depletion with normal B-cell immunity, even though PNP levels are similar in T- and B-cells. Deoxyguanosine kinase activity is greater in T- than B-cells and excess deoxyguanosine leads to excessive accumulation of dGTP in T-cells only, which is thought to inhibit ribonucleotide reductase.

A PNP inhibitor, 8-aminoguanosine, has also been studied in combination with deoxyguanosine. Some synergism against T-cell tumors has been found without toxicity to early myeloid cells [28]. However, 8-aminoguanosine has been found to reduce toxicity of deoxyguanosine to mature T-cells, suggesting that deoxyguanosine toxicity in these cells is not due to dGTP accumulation but probably to degradation of GdR by PNP to metabolites which inhibit purine synthesis. B-cell proliferation is inhibited by deoxyguanosine by a pathway dependent on PNP activity, suggested to be via degradation of deoxyguanosine to guanosine, which after salvage is phosphorylated to GMP and so to GTP [29].

2-Chloradeoxyadenosine (CdA)

A structural analogue of deoxyadenosine that is not degraded by ADA is selectively toxic at nanomolar concentrations to human T-lymphoblastoid cell lines, particularly those with high ratios of deoxycytidine kinase to deoxynucleotidase [30]. In these cells, it was 1000-fold more active than deoxyadenosine plus deoxycoformycin. It also inhibits at nM concentrations the growth of some c-ALL lines but not of normal bone marrow cells or colony-forming myeloid progenitors. Unlike most purine and pyrimidine antagonists, CdA inhibits resting normal peripheral blood T-cells and also inhibits slowly dividing T-cells in patients with mycosis fungoides. In replicating cells, the compound is incorporated into DNA and this is a potential mechanism of toxicity. The toxicity in resting cells takes longer (at least 2 days) and the mechanism for this is uncertain. CdA is phosphorylated and enters the cell nucleotide pool where it may interfere with ATP mediated reactions. CdA and other deoxyadenosine analogues obviously have therapeutic potential in the treatment of slowly dividing T-cell tumors resistant to existing cycle-specific agents.

Other enzymes

Thymidine phosphorylase

This enzyme removes the sugar deoxyribose from thymidine. It is concerned in the degradation and possible recycling of thymine. Among normal hemopoietic cells, the level is higher in B-cells and myeloid cells than in T-cells, a pattern that is reproduced in leukemic/lymphoma cell lines [7]. Although there is a wide variation within each phenotypic cell type, the mean levels were lower in immature compared with more mature T-cell tumors or normal T-lymphocytes which in turn are substantially lower than in mature B-cells.

Thymidine kinase

The concentration of this enzyme involved with salvage of thymidine is known to be raised in proliferating compared to resting cells. Among lymphomas, this has also been found [31]. The fetal isoenzyme TK_1 closely parallels changes in DNA synthesis whereas TK_2 remains constant throughout the cell cycle. The relative proportion of TK_1 to TK_2 isoenzymes is increased, in rapidly growing lymphoma and in CLL in patients with pleomorphic immature cells in the peripheral blood at a late stage of the disease compared with the TK_2 isoenzyme which is present in patients with more typical morphology and benign course.

Lactate dehydrogenase (LDH)

The LDH isoenzyme pattern changes as T-cells mature [2]. Thymocytes show an approximately equal proportion of heart (H) to muscle (M) type isoenzyme, whereas in mature T-lymphocytes, the heart type dominates. This change in pattern is reflected in T-cell tumors, patients with Thy-ALL showing a thymocyte-like pattern, whereas those with chronic T-cell malignancies showed a pattern more closely resembling that of mature T-cells.

Tyrosine phosphorylation

The roles of protein kinases that phosphorylate cell proteins on tyrosine residues in cell proliferation is currently under intense investigation since some growth factors (epidermal growth factor, platelet-derived growth factor) have been shown to stimulate tyrosine phosphorylation in their receptors. It is not yet known whether T-cell growth factor (IL2) acts by a similar mechanism. In relation to the current review, it has been suggested that the block in G0-G1 interface caused by deoxyadenosine stimulated lymphocytes may be due to inhibition of phosphorylation of a membrane or intracellular protein due to interference with ATP metabolism. Blast-like proliferation induced by lectin treatment of T-lymphocytes is correlated with activation of a tyrosine protein kinase (TPK). Lymphoma lines have been shown to contain an active TPK [32]. We have found that the enzyme activity for an artificial substrate is highest in resting lymphocytes and CLL cells than in lectin-stimulated lymphocytes, proliferating leukemia or lymphoma lines [33]. Moreover, the kinase activity falls within the first few hours when lymphocytes are stimulated into cycle by phytohemagglutinin. The exact proteins phosphorylated on the membranes and in the cytosol of normal and leukemic lymphoid cells are currently being studied but it is already apparent that myeloid cells and myeloid leukemia cell lines show

138

substantially less tyrosine phosphorylation of proteins than lymphoid cells at an equivalent stage of development.

References

1. Van Laarhoven JPR and de Bruyn CHMM (1983). Purine metabolism in relation to leukemia and lymphoid cell differentiation. Leuk Res 7:451–480.
2. Van de Griend RJ, van der Reijden HJ, Bolhuis RLH et al. (1983). Enzyme analysis of lymphoproliferative diseases: A useful addition to cell surface phenotyping. Blood 62:669–676.
3. Braziel RM, Keneklis T, Donlon JA et al. (1983). Terminal deoxynucleotidyl transferase in non-Hodgkin's lymphoma. Amer J Clin Pathol 80:655–659.
4. Baltimore D (1974). Is terminal deoxynucleotidyl transferase a somatic mutagen in lymphocytes? Nature 248:409–411.
5. Bollum FJ (1979). Terminal deoxynucleotidyl transferase as a hematopoietic cell marker. Blood 54:1203–1215.
6. Ma DDF, Sylwestrowicz T, Janossy G and Hoffbrand AV (1983). The role of purine metabolic enzymes and terminal deoxynucleotidyl transferase in intrathymic T-cell differentiation. Immunol Today 4:65–68.
7. Srivastava BIS and Minowada J (1983). Terminal transferase immunofluorescence, enzyme markers and immunological profile of human leukemia – lymphoma cell lines representing different levels of differentiation. Leuk Res 7:331–338.
8. Ma DDF, Sylwestrowicz TA, Granger S et al. (1982). Distribution of terminal deoxynucleotide transferase, purine degradative and synthetic enzymes in sub-populations of human thymocytes. J Immunol 129:1430–1435.
9. Massaia M, Ma DDF, Sylwestrowicz N et al. (1982). Enzymes of purine metabolism in human peripheral lymphocyte subpopulations. Clin Exp Immunol 50:148–154.
10. Hershfield MS (1979). Apparent suicide inactivation of human lymphoblast S-adenosylhomocysteine hydrolase by 2'-deoxyadenosine and adenine arabinoside: A basis for direct toxic effects of analogs of adenosine. J Biol Chem 254:22–25.
11. Siaw MFE, Mitchell BS, Koller CA et al. (1980). ATP depletion as a consequence of adenosine deaminase inhibition in man. Proc Nat Acad Sci USA 77:6157.
12. Matsumoto SS, Yu J and Yu AL (1983). Inhibition of RNA synthesis by deoxyadenosine plus deoxycoformycin in resting lymphocytes. J Immunol 131:2762–2766.
13. Fox RM, Kefford RF, Tripp EH and Taylor IW (1981). GI-phase arrest of cultured human leukemic T-cells induced by deoxyadenosine. Cancer Res 41:5141.
14. Kefford RF, Fox RM, McCairns E et al. (1983). Terminal incorporation of 2'-deoxyadenosine into polyadenylate segments of polyadenylated RNA in GI-phase-arrested human T-lymphoblasts. Cancer Res 43:2252.
15. Redelman D, Bluestein HG, Cohen AH et al. (1984). Deoxyadenosine (AdR) inhibition of newly activated lymphocytes: Blockade at the GO-GI interface. J Immunol 132:2030–2038.
16. Carson DA, Kaye J and Wasson DB (1981). The potential importance of soluble deoxynucleotidase activity in mediating deoxyadenosine toxicity in human lymphoblasts. J Immunol 126:348–353.
17. Iizasa T, Kubota M and Carson DA (1983). Differential production of deoxyadenosine by human T and B lymphoblasts. J Immunol 131:1776–1779.
18. Taheri MR, Wickremasinghe RG and Hoffbrand AV (1982). Functional compartmentalisation of DNA precursors in human leukaemoblastoid cell lines. Brit J Haematol 52:401–410.

19. Cohen AH, Bluestein HG and Redelman D (1984). Deoxyadenosine modulates human suppressor T-cell function and B-cell differentiation stimulated by staphylococcus aureus protein A. J Immunol 132:1761–1766.
20. Ho AD, Ma DDF, Price G and Hoffbrand AV (1983). Effect of thymosin and phorbol ester on purine metabolic enzymes and cell surface phenotype in a malignant T-cell line (Molt-3). Leuk Res 7:779–786.
21. Chechik BE, Schrader WP, Perets A and Fernandes B (1984). Immunohistochemical localization of adenosine deaminase in human benign extrathymic lymphoid tissues and B-cell lymphomas. Cancer 53:70–78.
22. Ho AD, Dörken B, Ma DDF et al. (1984). Purine degradative enzymes and immunological phenotypes in chronic B-lymphocytic leukemia: Identification of leukemic immunocytoma as a separate entiti. (Submitted).
23. van Laarhoven JPRM, de Gast GC, Spierenburg TTh and DeBruyn CHMM (1983). Enzymological studies in chronic lymphocytic leukemia. Leuk Res 7:261–267.
24. Prentice HG, Smyth JF, Ganeshaguru K et al. (1980). Remission induction with adenosine deaminase inhibitor 2'-deoxycoformycin in Thy-lymphoblastic leukaemia. Lancet 2:170–172.
25. Spiers ASD, Ruckdeschel JC and Horton J (1984). Effectiveness of pentostatin (2'-deoxycoformycin) in refractory lymphoid neoplasms. Scand J Haematol 32:130–134.
26. Spiers ASD and Parekh SI (1984). Complete remission in hairy cell leukaemia achieved with Pentostatin. Lancet i:1080–1081.
27. Lee N, Russell N, Ganeshaguru K et al. (1984). Mechanisms of deoxyadenosine toxicity in human lymphoid cells *in vitro*: Relevance to the therapeutic use of inhibitors of adenosine deaminase. Brit J Haematol 56:108–120.
28. de Fouw NJ, Ma DDF, Michalevicz R et al. (1984). Differential cytotoxicity of deoxyguanosine and 8-aminoguanosine for human leukaemic cell lines and normal bone marrow progenitor cells. Haematol Oncol 2 (in press).
29. Spaapen LJM, Rijkers GT, Staal GEJ et al. (1984). The effect of deoxyguanosine on human lymphocyte function. II. Analysis of the interference with B lymphocyte differentiation *in vitro*. J Immunol 132:2318–2323.
30. Carson DA, Wasson DB, Taetle R and Yu A (1983). Specific toxicity of 2-chlorodeoxyadenosine toward resting and proliferating human lymphocytes. Blood 62:737–743.
31. Ellims PH, Van Der Weyden MB and Medley G (1981). Thymidine kinase isoenzymes in human malignant lymphoma. Cancer Res 41:691–695.
32. Gacon G, Piau J-P, Blaineau C et al. (1983). Tyrosine phosphorylation in human T lymphoma cells. Biochem Biophys Res Comm 118:843–850.
33. Piga A, Taheri MR, Yaxley JC et al. (1984). Higher tyrosine protein kinase activity in resting than in proliferating normal or leukaemic blood cells. (Submitted).

2. Enzymes involved in adenosine metabolism in normal or leukemic lymphocytes

J.C. MANI, J.C. BONNAFOUS, G. CLOFENT, J. FAVERO,
A. GARTNER and J. DORNAND
*Laboratoire de Biochimie des Membranes, ER CNRS 228, Ecole
Nationale Supérieure de Chimie, Montpellier, France*

Normal lymphocytes have very low levels of *de novo* purine biosynthesis. These cells are highly dependent on the purine salvage pathway and the uptake of extracellular purines, mainly adenosine. The discovery that several immunodeficiencies are linked to deficiencies of some enzymes involved in adenosine metabolism has focused attention on relationships between this metabolism and lymphocyte differentiation and function.

An arrest of B- or T-lymphocytes in an early stage of differentiation might explain some immunodeficiencies and some properties of leukemic lymphocytes. Recently, several enzymes involved in adenosine metabolism were found useful to characterize several leukemias.

Enzymes of adenosine metabolism

Several years ago, we showed the presence on lymphocyte plasma membranes of an ecto-ATPase activated by either Ca^{2+} or Mg^{2+} ions [1]. The physiologic role of this enzyme is poorly understood, but it appears to be involved in a chain of nucleotide-degrading enzymes leading to adenosine:

$$ATP \xrightarrow{\text{ecto-ATPase}} ADP \xrightarrow{\text{ecto-ADPase}} AMP \xrightarrow{\text{ecto-5'N}} Adenosine$$

The presence of ecto-ADPase and ecto-5'nucleotidase (ecto-5'N) on lymphocyte membranes was demonstrated by Gillian et al. [2]. These enzymes are coupled to the uptake of adenosine by lymphocytes [3], increasing the pool of purines in these cells.

Another mechanism allows lymphocytes to overcome their low *de novo* purine biosynthesis, namely the purine salvage pathway in which nucleotides resulting from nucleic acid catabolism are metabolized as follows:

$$
\begin{array}{c}
\text{Ado} \quad \overset{\text{AK}}{\underset{5'\text{N}}{}} \quad \text{AMP} \ \rightleftarrows \ \text{ADP} \ \rightleftarrows \ \text{ATP} \\
\end{array}
$$

Ado   **AK**   AMP ⇄ ADP ⇄ ATP
   5′N

↓ADA   AMP-DA

   5′N

Ino   IMP ⇄ GMP ⇄ GDP ⇄ GTP

     HGPRT
  PNP

    HX → Uric
           acid

dIno ← dIMP ⇄ dGMP ⇄ dGDP ⇄ dGTP

↑ADA   AMP-DA
    dAK

dAdo   dAMP ⇄ dADP ⇄ dATP
  5′N

The major enzymes of this metabolism are adenosine deaminase (ADA), purine nucleoside phosphorylase (PNP), 5′nucleotidase (5′N), hypoxanthine-guanine phosphoribosyl transferase (HGPRT), AMP deaminase (AMP-DA) and the purine kinases.

Adenosine metabolism enzymes and lymphocyte maturation

Adenosine and adenosine deaminase appear to play a crucial role in lymphocyte maturation [4]. In humans, adenosine can induce lymphocyte ma-

Table I. Nucleotide-degrading ecto-enzymes in mouse and human lymphocyte populations (nmol/h/mg)

Cell population	ecto-ATPase	ecto-ADPase	ecto-5′N
Mouse unseparated thymocytes	360	170	30
Mouse PNA+ immature thymocytes	180	65	30
Mouse PNA− mature thymocytes	680	190	280
Mouse unseparated splenocytes	1350	350	300
Mouse SBA− T splenocytes	1320	n.d.	370
Mouse SBA+ B splenocytes	1200	n.d.	280
Mouse lympho node lymphocytes	1450	n.d.	100
Mouse bone marrow lymphocytes	n.d.	n.d.	200
Human unseparated thymocytes	660	n.d.	50
Human PNA+ immature thymocytes	n.d.	n.d.	50
Human PNA− mature thymocytes	n.d.	n.d.	204
Human PBL	1650	n.d.	245
Human tonsil lymphocytes	1650	n.d.	225

turation [5]. Adenosine deaminase deficiency leads to severe combined immunodeficiency (SCID) characterized by the lack of mature B and T lymphocytes [6]. On the other hand, some enzymes, like ecto-5'N, display different activities in mature or immature lymphocytes.

We measured most of adenosine metabolism enzymes in several lymphocyte populations in order to correlate their activities with the maturation level of the cells. Table I shows the activities of the ecto-enzymes involved in sequential nucleotide hydrolysis, both in human and mouse lymphocyte populations. These activities appear higher in blood and peripheral lymphoid organ lymphocytes than in thymocytes. When thymocytes are fractionated by peanut agglutinin, the immunocompetent PNA⁻ subpopulation behaves as mature peripheral cells with high ecto-enzyme values, while immature PNA⁺ thymocytes display very low activities. A striking difference between mature and immature cells is in ecto-5'N activity which is correlated both with adenosine transport into lymphocytes [7] and with the activation of adenylate cyclase through adenosine receptors [8]. The relationship between ecto-5'N and adenosine-induced adenylate cyclase stimulation appears correlated with the involvement of cyclic AMP in the maturation of lymphocyte by adenosine.

Ecto-5'N deficiency was observed in peripheral blood lymphocytes from patients with X-linked congenital agammaglobulinemia. This disease is characterized by the absence of mature B-cells and low serum immunoglobulin levels [9]. It was also observed in hypogammaglobulinemia [10] and

Table II. Purine salvage pathway enzymes in mouse thymocyte and splenocyte subpopulations (nmol/h/mg)

Enzyme specific activity	Thymocytes			Splenocytes			
	Unseparated	PNA⁺	PNA⁻	unseparated	SBA⁺	SBA⁻	
Adenosine kinase	140	120	132	61	n.d.	n.d.	
Deoxyadenosine kinase	32	40	27	21	n.d.	n.d.	
dAMP kinase	540	n.d.	n.d.	990	n.d.	n.d.	
Cytosolic 5'N with 5'AMP	38	33	20	45	32	57	
with 5'IMP	50	45	40	60	51	75	
with 5'dAMP	104	120	90	120	144	70	
S-adenosyl-homocysteine hydrolase: −hydrolysis	56	56	55	70	n.d.	n.d.	
− synthesis	134	122	134	127	n.d.	n.d.	
Purine nucleoside phosphorylase	520	460	600	1200	n.d.	n.d.	
Adenosine deaminase	28000	29400	8000	2700	2400	3500	
AMP-deaminase	30	20	270	880	750	700	

infectious mononucleosis [11]. It is unclear if ecto-5′N deficiency in immunodeficient patients is a cause or a consequence of cell immaturity. Substances which induce thymocyte maturation, such as thymosin f5 [12] or interleukine [13], increase ecto-5′N in immature cells. Substances which inhibit ecto-5′N activity, such as concanavalin A, *Lens culinaris* agglutinin, Zn^{2+}, Ni^{2+} or Hg^{2+}, display mitogenic properties.

Enzyme activities of the purine salvage pathway are reported for mouse lymphocytes (Table II). Few or no differences were observed for kinases, cytosolic 5′nucleotidase, S-adenosyl-homocysteine hydrolase or purine nucleoside phosphorylase. Two enzymes, adenosine deaminase and AMP-deaminase, presented widely different activities in mature and immature thymocytes. Their activities were also determined in human lymphocytes (Table III). An inverse relationship occurs for ecto-5′N and ADA activities as a function of maturation level [14]. The ratio ecto-5′N/ADA can be used as maturation marker, instead of TdT (Terminal deoxynucleotidyl transferase) level. Low ecto-5′N/ADA ratios correspond to high TdT levels and immature cells whereas high ratios correspond to low TdT levels and mature cells [15].

Adenosine deaminase catalyses the irreversible hydrolytic deamination of adenosine to inosine, and of deoxyadenosine to deoxyinosine. Inherited deficiency of adenosine deaminase results in the fatal infantile syndrome of SCID [6]. The correlation of ADA deficiency with SCID the first association made between an enzyme deficiency and a disease of specific immunity. It represented the first evidence that an intact purine salvage pathway was essential to maintain normal immune function. Deoxyadenosine and adenosine concentrations are increased in patients with SCID. Deoxyadenosine is cytotoxic and causes a selective accumulation of the corresponding deoxyribonucleoside triphosphate (dATP). Recent data show that different lymphoid cells display very different sensitivity to this nucleoside cytotoxicity. It appears that the most important factor regulating this cytotoxicity is whether cells can degrade accumulated d-ATP [16]. As reported by Edwards et al. [17], we found that thymocytes strongly accumulate d-ATP when incubated with ADA inhibitors and 20 μM deoxyadeno-

Table III. Adenosine deaminase and AMP-deaminase activities (nmol/h/mg) in human lymphocyte populations

Lymphocyte populations	AMP-DA	ADA
PNA⁺ immature thymocytes	n.d.	25800
PNA⁻ mature thymocytes	n.d.	13200
Tonsil lymphocytes	600	6000
Peripheral blood lymphocytes	670	4200

sine [18], while splenocytes accumulate only small amounts of this nucleotide under the same conditions. Since these cell populations have similar activities for purine salvage pathway enzymes (kinases, cytosolic nucleotidase) except for AMP-DA, d-ATP might not be able to accumulate in splenocytes because of high AMP-DA levels in these cells. This hypothesis could also explain why PNA$^+$ thymocytes are more sensitive to the toxic effects of deoxyadenosine than PNA$^-$ thymocytes [19], although both populations display the same deoxyadenosine kinase activities in the presence of ADA inhibitors [20].

Other correlations have been found between deficiency in purine metabolism enzymes and specific diseases. A deficiency of purine nucleoside phosphorylase, which catalyses the readily reversible conversion of inosine, deoxyinosine, guanosine and deoxyguanosine to their respective bases, has been described in patients with T-cell deficiency and normal B-cell function [21]. Again, as for ADA deficiency and SCID, the enzyme deficiency is not simply a marker for immunodeficiency disease, but a cause of it.

Adenosine metabolism enzymes in lymphoblastoid cell lines

Enzymes which displayed different activities among lymphocyte populations were assayed in several lymphoblastoid cell lines. Depending on their origin and the presence of certain surface markers, these cell lines can be classified as B, T or null lymphoblasts. Several authors have tried to assess the stage of maturation of such cell lines [22].

As in normal lymphocytes, the differences between the activities of purine metabolism enzymes appear more related to the maturation stage of the cells than to their T, B or null character (Table IV). Lymphoblasts of T-ALL origin, known as immature cells (high TdT level), behave like immature lymphocytes with low ecto-5'N, low AMP-DA and high ADA activities. Normal B-cell lines from both ALL patients and normal individuals possess mature cell character (low TdT level) and behave like normal PBL for ADA (low), ecto-5'N and AMP-DA (high) activities.

The very low ecto-5'N activity in T-ALL lymphoblasts is due to the absence of enzyme molecules on the cell surface [23] and not to changes in kinetic parameters [13] or to the presence of an inhibitor as suggested by Sun et al. [24]. The decrease of ecto-5'N activity by lymphoblast cell supernatants reported by these authors is not caused by an inhibitor, but is an artefact due to an incorrect enzyme assay [25]. The absence of ecto-5'N on T-ALL lymphoblasts was supported by immunofluorescent experiments [23].

Table IV. Adenosine metabolism enzymes (nmol/h/mg) and TdT level of human lymphoblastoid cell lines

Cells	T/B character	Origin	ecto-ATPase	ecto-5'N	ADA	ecto-5'N/ADA $\times 10^c$	AMP-DA	TdT level (H: high; L: low)
Normal PBL	T-B	Normal blood	1650	245	4200	65	670	L
Ichikawa	T	T-ALL[a]	325	10	12000	0.8	n.d.	H
CEM	T	T-ALL	405	22	9000	2.4	37	H
RPMI 8402	T	T-ALL	n.d.	40	15000	2.7	n.d.	H
1301	T	T-ALL	n.d.	27	10800	2.5	23	H
H-SB2	T	T-ALL	225	0	21600	0	40	H
MOLT-3	T	T-ALL	n.d.	0	48000	0	40	H
MOLT-4	T	T-ALL	390	11	44000	0.2	20	H
JM	T	T-ALL	n.d.	35	14400	2.4	n.d.	H
JURKAT	T	T-ALL	n.d.	50	12000	4.2.	n.d.	H
REH	Null	Null-ALL	580	41	12600	3.2	n.d.	H
NALM-16	Null	Null-ALL	n.d.	14	18000	0.8	n.d.	H
K-562	Null	CML-BC[b]	820	74	2400	31	n.d.	L
CCRF-SB	B	T-ALL	2100	110	2100	52	180	L
RAJI	B	Burkitt	n.d.	130	4200	31	n.d.	L
EBV-lymphoblasts[c] (4 cell lines)	B	Normal B cells	2000	180	3750	45	160	L

[a] T-cell acute lymphocytic leukemia

[b] Chronic myeloid leukemia, blast crisis

[c] Epstein-Barr virus-transformed normal B-cells

Adenosine metabolism enzymes in leukemic patients

An arrest of B- or T-lymphocytes in an early stage of differentiation might explain some properties of leukemic lymphocytes. The B-cell origin of several lymphoid proliferations, such as chronic lymphocytic leukemia (CLL) and most lymphoblastic lymphomas, is well documented [26]. The proliferating monoclonal B-cells may either be arrested at a given stage of differentiation or conversely correspond to a clone of B-lymphocytes that pursues uninterrupted maturation up to plasmocytes. The first pattern corresponds to CLL lymphoblasts and most B-type lymphomas (e.g. Burkitt's lymphoma).

Neoplastic diseases featured by proliferating T-cells, e.g. Sezary syndroma and a few T-CLL, are less common than B-cell malignancies. Lymphoblasts from 70% of ALL patients are characterized by the absence of B or T-cell markers; 25–30% of ALL patients have T-lymphoblasts (T-ALL). Very few patients display acute leukemia with B-cell markers (B-ALL) and most of these B-ALL cases may in fact correspond to lymphomas with a leukemic presentation [26]. ALL lymphoblasts present characteristics of immature lymphocytes; T-ALL cells look like thymocytes rather than peripheral T-cells.

Adenosine metabolism enzymes were useful for the characterization of several leukemias. Table V displays activities observed in a few patients. From these and many other data [27], it appears that T-ALL and B-ALL have low ecto-5'N and PNP, but ADA levels are high in B-ALL and low in T-ALL. Null-ALL displays ecto-5'N levels higher than control PBL, normal PNP and ADA values. T-CLL has normal and B-CLL has low ecto-5'N activities. Ecto-5'N was also low in Sezary syndrome. Myeloid leukemia can be characterized by its ecto-5'N activity: low for acute myeloid leukemia

Table V. Adenosine metabolism enzymes in PBL lymphocytes from normal or leukemic patients

Cell origin	Enzyme activities (nmol/h/mg or nmol/h/10^6 cells [x])			
	Ecto-ATPase	Ecto-5'N	ADA	AMP-DA
Normal PBL	1650/77 [x]	245/10 [x]	4200	670
Pre-B ALL	n.d.	10	600	105
Pre-B prolymphocytic leukemia	n.d.	15	300	340
Pre-B hairy cell leukemia	n.d.	15	15	280
T-ALL (10 cases)	n.d.	1.1 [x]	n.d.	n.d.
B-CLL	n.d.	20	1200	150
B-CLL (8 cases)	13 [x]	0.4 [x]	n.d.	n.d.

(AML) and chronic myeloid leukemia (CML) in chronic phase or myeloid blast crisis (CML-MBC), above normal for CML in lymphoid blast crisis (CML–LBC) [28].

References

1. Dornand J, Mani JC, Mousseron-Canet M and Pau B (1974). Propriétés d'une ATPase Ca^{++} ou Mg^{++} dépendante des membranes plasmiques de lymphocytes. Effet de la concanavaline A sur les ATPases membranaires. Biochimie 56:1425–1432.
2. Gillian PS, Tarulata S, Webster ADB and Peters TJ (1982). Studies on the kinetic properties and subcellular localization of adenine nucleotide phosphatases in peripheral blood lymphocytes from control subjects and patients with common variable primary hypogammaglobulinaemia. Clin Exp Immunol 49:393–400.
3. Dornand J, Bonnafous JC and Mani JC (1979). Role of adenosine transport in lymphocyte stimulation. In: Kaplan JG (Ed.). Molecular Basis of Immune Cell Function, pp. 426–428. Amsterdam: Elsevier.
4. Shore A, Dosch HM and Gelfand EW (1981). Role of adenosine deaminase in the early stages of precursor T cell maturation. Clin Exp Immunol 44:152–155.
5. Astaldi A, Leupers CJN and Schellekens PTA (1981). Adenosine induces immunological maturation of thymocytes. Immunobiology 159:93.
6. Hirschhorn S, Bajaj S, Borkowsky W et al. (1979). Differential inhibition of adenosine deaminase deficient peripheral blood lymphocytes and lymphoid cell lines by deoxyadenosine and adenosine. Cell Immunol 42:418–423.
7. Dornand J, Bonnafous JC, Gavach C and Mani JC (1979). 5'Nucleotidase-facilitated adenosine transport by mouse lymphocytes. Biochimie 61:973–978.
8. Bonnafous JC, Dornand J and Mani JC (1980). 5'Nucleotidase-adenylate cyclase relationships in mouse thymocytes: A reevaluation of the effects of concanavalin A on cyclic AMP levels. Febs Lett 110:30–34.
9. Thompson LF, Boss GR, Spielgelberg HL et al. (1979). Ecto-5'nucleotidase activity in T- and B-lymphocytes from normal subjects and patients with congenital X-linked agammaglobulinemia. J Immunol 123:2475–2478.
10. Johnson SM, Asherson GL, Watts RNE et al. (1977). Lymphocyte purine 5'nucleotidase deficiency in primary hypogammaglobulinemia. Lancet 1:168–170.
11. Quagliata F, Faig D, Conklyn M and Silber R (1974). Studies on the lymphocyte 5'nucleotidase in chronic lymphocytic leukaemia, infectious mononucleosis, normal subpopulations and PHA stimulated cells. Cancer Res 34:3197–3202.
12. Ho AD, Ma DF, Price G and Hoffbrand VA (1983). Effect of thymosin and phorbol ester on purine metabolic enzymes and cell surface phenotype in a malignant T-cell line (Molt-3). Leuk Res 7:779–786.
13. Dornand J, Gartner A, Bonnafous JC et al. (1984). Ecto-5'nucleotidase and lymphocyte differentiation. In: Kreutzberg GW and Zimmermann H (Eds). Proceedings of the International Erwin Riesch Symposium on Ecto-Enzymes. (In press).
14. Dornand J, Bonnafous JC, Favero J and Mani JC (1982). Ecto-5'nucleotidase and adenosine deaminase activities of lymphoid cells. Biochem Med 28:144–156.
15. Dornand J, Bonnafous JC, Favero J and Mani JC (1982). Inverse relationships of 5'nucleotidase and adenosine deaminase activities among human lymphoid cells. In: Serrou B, Rosenfeld C and Daniels J (Eds.) Current Concepts in Human Immunology and Cancer Immunomodulation, pp. 395–401. Amsterdam: Elsevier.
16. Sylwastrowicz T, Piga A, Murphy P et al. (1982). The effect of deoxycoformycin and

deoxyadenosine on deoxyribonucleotide concentrations in leukemic cells. Brit J Haematol 51:623–630.

17. Edwards NL, Mitchell BS, Fox IH and Mond JJ (1982). Plasma membrane 5'nucleotidase and dATP accumulation in murine lymphocytes. J Clin Chem Clin Biochem 20:365.

18. Dornand J, Barbanel AM, Bonnafous JC et al. (1984). AMP-deaminase and cytosolic 5'nucleotidase involvement in lymphocyte maturation. In: Peeters H (Ed.). Protides of the Biological Fluids, pp. 663–666. London: Pergamon Press.

19. Sidi Y, Umiel T, Trainin N et al. (1982). Differences in the activity of adenosine deaminase and of purine nucleoside phosphorylase and in the sensitivity to deoxypurine between subpopulations of mouse thymocytes. Thymus 4:147–154.

20. Ma DF, Sylwestrowicz TA, Granger S et al. (1982). Distribution of terminal deoxynucleotidyl transferase and purine degradative and synthetic enzymes in subpopulations of human thymocytes. J Immunol 129:1430–1435.

21. Carson DA, Lakow E, Wasson DB and Katamani N (1981). Lymphocyte dysfunction caused by deficiencies in purine metabolism. Immunol Today 234–238.

22. Minowada J (1978). Markers of human leukemia-lymphoma cell lines reflect hematopoietic cell differentiation. In: Serrou B and Rosenfeld C (Eds.). Human Lymphocyte Differentiation: Its Application to Cancer, pp. 337–344. Amsterdam: Elsevier.

23. Dornand J, Bonnafous JC, Favero J et al. (1984). An immunofluorescent technique for the determination of cell surface 5'nucleotidase. In: Rosenfeld C, Serrou B and Viallet P (Eds). Fluorescent Techniques and Membrane Markers in Cancer and Immunology. (In press).

24. Sun AS, Holland JM, Lin K and Ohnuma T (1983). Implications of a 5'nucleotidase inhibitor in human leukemic cells for cellular aging and cancer. Biochim Biophys Acta 762:577–584.

25. Dornand J, Bonnafous JC, Favero J et al. (1984). The proposed 5'nucleotidase inhibitor in human cells is an artefact. Biochim Biophys Acta (in press).

26. Cooper MD and Seligmann M (1977). B- and T-lymphocytes in immunodeficiency and lymphoproliferative diseases. In: Loor F and Roelants GE (Eds.). B- and T-Cells in Immune Recognition, pp. 377–405, London: J Wiley and Sons.

27. Mani JC, Bonnafous JC, Favero J and Dornand J (1983). Purine metabolism enzymes in lymphocytes. Clin Immunol Newsletter 4:53–58.

28. Koya M, Kanoh T, Sawada H et al. (1981). Adenosinedeaminase and ecto-5'nucleotidase activities in various leukemias with special reference to blast crisis: Significance of ecto-5'nucleotidase in lymphoid blast crisis of chronic myeloid leukemia. Blood 58:1107–1111.

3. Purine metabolism in normal and pathologic lymphoid cell differentiation

H. J. SCHUURMAN[1], J. P. R. M. VAN LAARHOVEN[3] and
G. C. DE GAST[2]
*Division of [1] Immunopathology and [2] Immunohematology, University
Hospital, Utrecht, the Netherlands, and [3] Department of Human
Genetics, University Hospital St. Radboud, Nijmegen, the Netherlands*

Intact purine metabolism is pivotal for proper functioning of (lymphoid) cells. During the generation of immunocompetent lymphocytes of T- or B-cell lineage, and during subsequent differentiation into effector cells, cell divisions occur which require DNA synthesis. Studies of the causal relationship between deficiency of certain purine nucleotide metabolizing enzymes and deficiencies in immune function, revealed several privileged pathways in purine metabolism (Fig. 1). These pathways are different for T- and B-cells in different stages of maturation, and are related to purine enzyme activities [1, 2]. Assessment of purine nucleotide metabolizing enzymes in lymphoreticular malignancies [3, 4] showed enzyme activities that could be related to normal lymphoid cell differentiation. In addition, the purine enzyme make-up of lymphoid cells may be applied in malignant cell typing and permits estimation of the effectiveness of enzyme-directed chemotherapy. This survey focuses on these different aspects.

Purine metabolism in normal lymphoid cell differentiation

Purine enzyme make-up [5–7].

This has been best documented for lymphocytes of the T-cell lineage: T-lymphocytes in different stages of maturation differ in enzyme make-up (Table I). Interpretation of these data must take into account biophysical cell properties, such as cell size and density, which underly the isolation of different subpopulations. Differences in enzyme activities may only reflect these biophysical properties. This phenomenon is eliminated if enzyme activity ratios are considered: in general, the ADA/PNP enzyme activity ratio decreases during the maturation of lymphocytes from cortical thymocytes, to more mature (medullary) cells, to immunocompetent peripheral blood T-lymphocytes (Table I). This ratio is therefore a useful marker for

Table I. Activities of some enzymes involved in purine metabolism in normal human lymphocyte subpopulations [a]

| | T cell lineage [b] | | | | | |
| | thymocytes | | peripheral blood cells | | | blood non-T lympho-cytes [b] |
	small immature	medium-sized more mature	T	T_γ	$T-T_\gamma$	
ADA	730	970	100	130	100	130
PNP	40	83	160	100	150	440
ADA/PNP	21	13	0.62	1.3	0.7	0.3
ecto-5'NT	0.35	2.0	8.6	4.3	7.0	13
dCK	0.08	0.18	0.05			
ecto-5'NT/dCK	4.4	12	190			
AK			4.8	2.7	4.6	13
ecto-5'NT/AK			1.4	1.6	1.5	1.0
AdKin	85	170	220	400	200	780
HGPRT			5.7	5.1	5.0	11
APRT			11	6.1	11	11
AMPD			160	93	140	360

| | T cell lineage [c] | | | | | |
| | thymocytes | | | peripheral blood cells | | blood B-cells [c] |
	prothym	cortical	medullary	T	T8	T4	
ADA	480	300	130	54	45	74	26
PNP	85	27	120	130	75	99	92
ADA/PNP	5.6	11	1.1	0.31	0.60	0.75	0.28
ecto-5'NT	8.3	4.1	25	30	33	9.7	38
dCK	1.2	0.50	0.31	0.30	0.1	0.3	1.5
ecto-5'NT/dCK	6.9	8.2	81	100	330	32	25
AK	4.8	1.4	3.1	3.2	0.3	0.3	0.5
ecto-5'NT/AK	1.7	2.9	8.1	9.4	110	32	76
TK	9.0	2.2	1.5				
TdT	23	22	2.7	<0.3			

[a] Values in nmol/10^6 cells.hr, for TdT in pmol/10^8 cells.hr
[b] Data from ref 5, 10: thymocyte separation by cell-size or cell-density
[c] Data from ref 3, 6, 7: thymocyte separation by cell-density in combination with surface marker expression

153

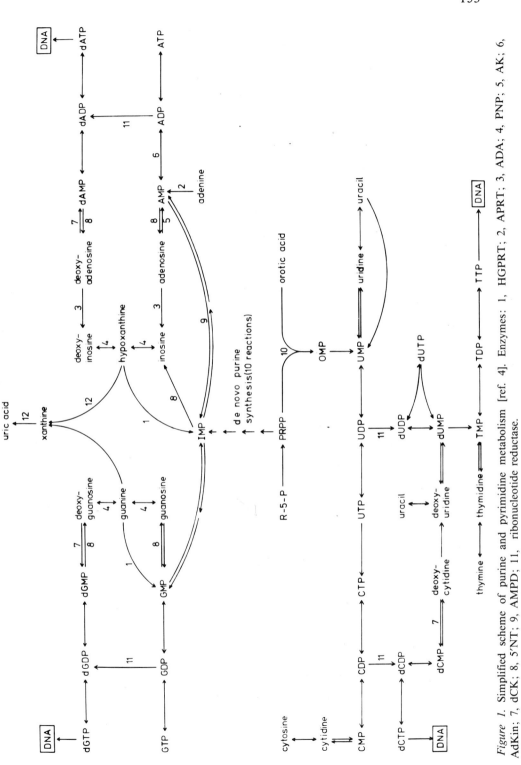

Figure 1. Simplified scheme of purine and pyrimidine metabolism [ref. 4]. Enzymes: 1, HGPRT; 2, APRT; 3, ADA; 4, PNP; 5, AK; 6, AdKin; 7, dCK; 8, 5'NT; 9, AMPD; 11, ribonucleotide reductase.

T-cells in different stages of maturation. However, the small 'prothymocyte' fraction of the thymus reveals a value below that of cortical thymocytes [6]. The ecto-5′NT/dCK enzyme activity ratio increases from immature to mature T-lymphocyte subpopulations.

In contrast to the T-cell lineage, there are almost no data on the purine enzyme make-up of B-lymphocytes at different stages of maturation. B-cells in peripheral blood, which form part of the recirculating B-cell pool (including B-cells in primary follicles and mantles of secondary follicles in lymphoid tissues and small B-lymphocytes in the bone marrow) have been characterized (Table I). Compared with T-cells, there is a high ecto-5′NT activity. Additional semiquantitave data have been obtained in enzyme histochemistry, in particular for 5′NT and ATPase. B-cells in germinal centres (centrocytes and centroblasts) are negative for these enzymes, whereas B-cells in the mantle zone and in primary follicles are positive [8]. This positivity was originally used to discriminate B-cells from T-lymphocytes (which are negative) in lymphoid tissue sections. Plasma cells are ATPase positive, but 5′NT negative.

Purine metabolic pathways (Fig. 1)

To illustrate privileged pathways in different lymphocyte subsets, the ecto-5′NT/dCK enzyme activity ratio can be used. The phosphorylation of purine (deoxy)nucleoside to (deoxy)ribonucleotide is positively influenced by nucleoside kinase activity (reaction 7 in Fig. 1), whereas 5′NT activity affects dephosphorylation (reaction 8). In immature thymocytes, (deoxy)nucleosides are more easily converted into (toxic) dNTP, such as dATP and dGTP, than in mature peripheral blood T-lymphocytes (Table I). In thymocytes, concentrations of (deoxy)nucleosides (for (deoxy)adenosine under conditions of blocked ADA activity) that inhibit the *in vitro* proliferative response and accumulate as intracellular dNTP are lower than in peripheral blood T-cells [9]. For thymocyte subpopulations, the 50% inhibitory dose is inversely correlated with the ecto-5′NT/dCK ratio [10]. Furthermore, freshly isolated thymocytes show larger dNTP pools than peripheral T-cells [11]. It should be noted, however, that the ecto-5′NT activity is assumed to reflect intracellular 5′NT activity. The characteristics of intracellular 5′NT apparently differ from those of ecto-5′NT [12]. Apart from phosphorylation, deoxyguanosine mediated intoxication of lymphocytes *in vitro* can follow PNP mediated conversion into guanine (reaction 4 in Fig. 1) and subsequent HGPRT mediated salvage into GMP (reaction 1). The occurrence of this pathway, in which there is no accumulation of dGTP but accumulation of intracellular GDP and GTP, has been described both for peripheral blood T-cells [13] and B-cells [14]. The high ecto-5′NT activity of B-cells (Table I) makes the intoxication by phosphorylation (conversion into dGTP) unlikely. The inhibition of cell function may be related to disturbance of the cAMP/cGMP balance which is known to interfere with cell function [15].

In mammalian cells, the only route of dNTP synthesis is the ribonucleotide reductase mediated conversion of nucleoside diphosphates into their deoxy analogs (reaction 11 in Fig. 1). dATP is a potent inhibitor of ribonucleotidase activity; dGTP inhibits reduction of GDP, CDP and UDP, but not of ADP. The composition of the intracellular dNTP pool is of utmost importance in cell proliferation. It has been reported [11] that the dCTP pool is the smallest dNTP pool in S-phase thymocytes: this pool regulates cellular DNA synthesis.

Physiologic significance

The purine metabolism in immature thymocytes is unfavorable for cell function, due to the formation of toxic dNTP. This phenomenon has led to speculations on the relation between purine metabolism and generation of immunocompetence. In the thymus cortex this is under control of the epithelial cell microenvironment. Only those thymocytes which are in close contact with the supporting thymic stromal are believed to escape dNTP mediated suicide [16]. Similarly, the presence of TdT in immature lymphocytes such as cortical thymocytes may have physiologic significance. This enzyme acts as a DNA polymerase that catalyses the coupling of dNTP to a free 3′OH of DNA. By altering the base composition of DNA in this way, TdT may function in the generation of immunologic diversity [17] or participate in somatic mutations after gene rearrangements [18].

Purine metabolism in pathologic lymphoid cell differentiation

Purine enzyme make-up [3, 4, 19–22]

This has been best documented for blood and bone marrow samples from patients with leukemia (Table II). The data presented confirm other studies [23, 24].

At first, the purine enzyme make-up can be applied as marker for subtypes of lymphoid malignancies. In this aspect, T-ALL is distinguished from other forms of ALL by a high ADA activity. Similarly, preB-ALL reveals a high 5′NT activity. High activities of AdKin are found in nonT-nonB-ALL, especially in leukemic cells that express the cALL marker [21]. For CLL, T-CLL cells have a higher activity of ADA, PNP and even more pronounced, 5′NT than B-CLL cells. Within the B-CLL group, cases without paraproteinemia have a higher activity of ADA and a lower activity of 5′NT than those with paraproteinemia [22].

Secondly, the purine enzyme make-up can be used to relate the status of pathologic lymphoid cells to normal lymphoid cell differentiation. In this relation, it should be emphasized that normal and pathologic cells can differ in their biophysical properties that influence absolute enzyme activities. This influence is eliminated when enzyme activity ratios are considered. For normal T-cell differentiation, changes in purine enzyme make-up are available (Table I): the high ADA/PNP enzyme activity ratio and low ecto-5′NT/dCK ratio of T-ALL cells resembles that of immature T-lymphocytes in the normal thymus cortex. T-CLL cells are more like mature peripheral blood T-cells in this aspect. The data on TdT form further evidence for these relationships. These similarities are in agreement with phenotype data of malignant cells [25]. For cells of the B-cell lineage this relation cannot be

Table II. Activities of some enzymes involved in purine metabolism in pathologic human lymphocyte populations [a]

| | | | | | | B-CLL | | |
| | | | | | | | paraproteinemia | |
	Control [b]	T-ALL	c-ALL	preB-ALL	B-ALL	total	without	with
ADA	130	1070	510	420	120	49	56	29
PNP	210	120	200	190	290	130	125	150
ADA/PNP	0.69	8.6	2.5	2.2	0.41	0.38	0.45	0.19
5′NT	18	1.0	28	78	0.50	3.8	1.2	12
ecto-5′NT	7.6	0.8	8.8		0.15	2.3	1.4	5.1
AK	7.9	6.3	5.1			17	17	20
ecto-5′NT/AK	1.0	0.13	1.7			0.13	0.084	0.26
AdKin	270	280	980	760	270	770	720	920
HGPRT	6.9	11	14	8.6		7.0	6.9	7.1
APRT	14	6.9	10			13	13	14
AMPD	270	150	250			190	180	230

	null-ALL [c]	c-ALL	T-ALL	T-CLL	B-CLL
ADA	320	380	390	71	26
PNP	68	106	62	78	36
ADA/PNP	4.7	1.7	6.3	0.9	0.7
5′NT	22	41	3.9	18	3.6
TdT	29	59	36	0.6	<0.3

[a] Values in nmol/10^6 cells.hr, for TdT in pmol/10^8 cells.hr
[b] Data from ref. [4, 21, 22]
[c] Data from ref. [3, 19, 20]

made, as normal B-lymphocytes at different stages of maturation have not been characterized for purine enzyme make-up. However, the purine enzyme make-up of pathologic cells may give some information on this aspect. Assuming an increase in maturation stage going from c-ALL → preB-ALL → B-ALL → B-CLL, there is a decrease in ADA/PNP activity mainly due to a decrease in ADA activity. If B-CLL cells in patients with paraproteinemia are more differentiated than in those without paraproteinemia, this decrease extends to the stage of mature B-cells. 5'NT activity increases start at the B-ALL stage to the level of normal blood B-lymphocytes at the B-CLL level, but at a very early stage (c-ALL and preB-ALL) there is a high 5'NT activity.

Enzyme-directed chemotherapy.

The effect of drugs which interfere with DNA synthesis of proliferating malignant lymphoid cells may depend on the purine enzyme make-up of the cells. For instance, agents such as 6-mercaptopurine and 8-azaguanine inhibit cell proliferation after conversion to toxic nucleotides. This conversion involves the salvage pathway mediated by HGPRT (reaction 1 in Fig. 1). Cells with a high activity of HGPRT and with a low net dephosphorylating capacity (which results in degradation of the nucleotide into nucleoside) are expected to be sensitive to these drugs. For leukemia this concerns T-ALL and B-ALL: due to the high 5'NT activity null-ALL and c-ALL are expected to be more resistant.

The pharmacologic manipulation of naturally occurring (deoxy)ribonucleotides has been the subject of many studies. Thymidine has been proposed as anti-cancer drug [26]; the conversion product after thymidine kinase mediated phosphorylation is dTTP (Fig. 1), which interferes with the composition of the dNTP pool. Depletion of the dCTP pool may occur similar to that in S-phase thymocytes [11], and this may inhibit DNA synthesis. Thymidine *in vitro* especially affects proliferating cells [27]. In agreement with the proposed mode of action, preliminary clinical applications have shown a reduction of peripheral blast counts in those leukemias characterized by a high thymidine kinase over phosphorylase enzyme activity ratio, i.e. the net capacity of the cell to convert thymidine into dTTP or into thymine. This was found in T-ALL: there was no clinical effect for B-lymphoma derived leukemic blasts with a low ratio [28]. The effect of thymidine appears to be only the arrest of cells in S-phase (compatible with data on normal thymocytes [11]); to obtain remission, combination therapy with S-phase reagents (such as cytosine arabinoside) has been proposed [26, 28].

The inhibition of ADA activity by agents such as deoxycoformycin has a profound effect on lymphoid cell function. The block in conversion of adenosine to inosine (reaction 3 in Fig. 1) results in increased levels of adenosine and its conversion products after phosphorylation such as (deoxy)ATP and cyclic AMP. A number of mechanisms have been proposed for the inhibition of cell proliferation [1, 2, 4]. These mechanisms include inhibition of pyrimidine nucleotide synthesis, adenosine mediated inhibition of PRPP formation and subsequent inhibition of *de novo* purine and pyrimidine synthesis, (deoxy)adenosine mediated inhibition of S-adenosyl-homocysteine hydrolase activity with subsequent blockade of (DNA) methylation reactions, dATP mediated allosteric inhibition of ribonucleotide reductase with subsequent blockade of dNTP formation, and interference by cAMP in blastogenesis and lymphoid effector cell function. In cultures of cells of T-ALL cell lines with low concentrations of deoxyadenosine and blocked ADA activity, there is an arrest of cells in G1-phase and accumulation of dATP: both phenomena could be inhibited by deoxycytidine addition [29]. This suggests a main role for ribonucleotide reductase in growth inhibition. The formation of dATP is largely dependent on the net capacity of the cell to phosphorylate (deoxy)adenosine, indicated above by the ecto-5'NT/dCK enzyme activity ratio. As a better estimate, a correlation between soluble 5'NT and deoxyadenosine toxicity has been found [30], and an even better correlation seems to exist with ecto-ATPase [31]. This dATP inactivating enzyme was absent from deoxyadenosine sensitive T-ALL and null-ALL cell lines, but was present on EB-virus transformed B-lymphocytes. These cells are resistant to deoxyadenosine intoxication at low concentrations, but are blocked in S-phase at high doses of deoxyadenosine. Under these conditions T-ALL cell lines are not arrested in G1-phase but are directly killed, which suggest that other mechanisms of cell inhibition may be operative, in addition to ribonucleotide reductase inhibition [29]. The mechanism of inhibition of DNA methylation seems of little importance [32, 33], but a perturbation in dATP/ATP balance due to dATP mediated activation of AMPD (resulting in lowered levels of ATP, reaction 9 in Fig. 1) may play a role [34].

Deoxycoformycin has been applied in treatment of acute lymphoblastic malignancies with variable success. The success of treatment was related to the capacity of the malignant cell to accumulate dATP during *in vitro* culture with deoxycoformycin and deoxyadenosine [35–37]. This conversion is particularly facilitated in T-ALL (related to the low 5'NT/dCK enzyme activity ratio, Table II). In agreement with the involvement of ribonucleotide reductase inhibition, the increase in dATP is associated with a decrease in other dNTP [26]. In addition, the success of treatment is influenced by the capacity of the cell to degrade the accumulated dATP during *in vitro* culture (possibly ecto-ATPase mediated, see above) [37].

Similar to deoxycoformycin treatment, therapy focusing on guanosine toxicity has been opened for investigation since inhibitors of PNP have become available. Under conditions of blocked PNP activity, accumulation of guanosine and its conversion products after phosphorylation such as cGMP and dGTP are expected. The disturbance of the cGMP/cAMP balance affects lymphocyte proliferation [15], and dGTP inhibits ribonucleotide reductase activity; depletion especially of dCTP is expected. For the PNP inhibitor 8-aminoguanine, a selective effect on T-lymphocyte growth but not B-lymphocyte growth has been shown, associated with accumulation of dGTP [38]. The finding of S-phase cells in a PNP-deficient child [39] suggest that treatment of lymphoid malignancies by PNP inhibition will result in S-phase arrest. It can be proposed to evaluate therapy by PNP inhibition, especially in T-lymphoblastic malignancies, similar to the recommendations for deoxycoformycin treatment [36]. Such treatment may be effective in combination with S-phase reagents.

References

1. Mitchell BS and Kelley WN (1980). Purinogenic immunodeficiency diseases: Clinical features and molecular mechanisms. Ann Intern Med 92:826–831.
2. Watts RWE (1983). Purine enzymes and immune function. Clin Biochem 16:48–53.
3. Hoffbrand AV, Ma DDF and Webster ADB (1982). Enzyme patterns in normal lymphocyte subpopulations, lymphoid leukaemias and immunodeficiency syndromes. Clin Haematol 11:719–741.
4. van Laarhoven JPRM and de Bruyn CHMM (1983). Purine metabolism in relation to leukemia and lymphoid cell differentiation. Leuk Res 7:451–480.
5. van Laarhoven JPRM, Spierenburg GTh, Collet H et al. (1984). Purine interconversion pathways in T, B, T_y and T-T_y-cells from human peripheral blood. Adv Exp Med Biol 165B:111–118.
6. Ma DDF, Sylwestrowicz TA, Granger S et al. (1982). Distribution of terminal deoxynucleotidyl transferase and purine degradative and synthetic enzymes in subpopulations of human thymocytes. J Immunol 129:1430–1435.
7. Massaia M, Ma DDF, Sylwestrowicz TA et al. (1982). Enzymes of purine metabolism in human peripheral lymphocyte subpopulations. Clin Exp Immunol 50:148–154.
8. Müller-Hermelink HK (1974). Characterization of the B-cell and T-cell regions of human lymphatic tissue through histochemical demonstration of ATPase and 5'nucleotidase activities. Virchow Arch B Cell Pathol 16:371–378.
9. Cohen A, Lee JWW, Dosch H-M and Gelfand EW (1980). The expression of deoxyguanosine toxicity in T-lymphocytes at different stages of maturation. J Immunol 125, 1578–1582.
10. Schuurman HJ, van Laarhoven JPRM, Broekhuizen R et al. (1983). Lymphocyte maturation in the human thymus. Relevance of purine nucleotide metabolism for intrathymic T-cell function. Scand J Immunol 18:539–549.
11. Cohen A, Barankiewicz J, Lederman HM and Gelfand EW (1983). Purine and pyrimidine metabolism in human T-lymphocytes. Regulation of deoxyribonucleotide metabolism. J Biol Chem 258:12334–12340.
12. Carson DA and Wasson BD (1982). Characterization of an adenosine 5'-triphosphate- and deoxyadenosine 5'-triphosphate-activated nucleotidase from human malignant lymphocytes. Cancer Res 42:4321–4324.

13. Spaapen LJM, Rijkers GT, Staal GEJ et al. (1984). The effect of deoxyguanosine on human lymphocyte function. I. Analysis of the the interference with lymphocyte proliferation *in vitro*. J Immunol 132:2311–2317.

14. Spaapen LJM, Rijkers GT, Staal GEJ et al. (1984). The effect of deoxyguanosine on human lymphocyte function. II. Analysis of the interference with B-lymphocyte differentiation *in vitro*. J Immunol 132:2318–2323.

15. Hadden JW and Coffey RG (1982). Cyclic nucleotides in mitogen-induced lymphocyte proliferation. Immunol Today 3:299–304.

16. Ma DDF, Sylwestrowicz T, Janossy G and Hoffbrand AV (1983). The role of purine metabolic enzymes and terminal deoxynucleotidyl transferase in intrathymic T-cell differentiation. Immunol Today 4:65–68.

17. Baltimore D (1974). Is terminal deoxynucleotidyl transferase a somatic mutagen in lymphocytes? Nature 248:409–411.

18. Gearhart PJ (1982). Generation of immunoglobulin variable gene diversity. Immunol Today 3:407–412.

19. Ganeshaguru K, Lee N, Llewellin P et al. (1981). Adenosine deaminase concentrations in leukemia and lymphoma: Relation to cell phenotypes. Leuk Res 5:215–222.

20. Ma DDF, Massaia M, Sylwestrowicz TA et al. (1983). Comparison of purine degradative enzymes and terminal deoxynucleotidyl transferase in T-cell leukemias and in normal thymic and post-thymic T-cells. Brit J Haematol 54:451–457.

21. van Laarhoven JPRM, Spierenburg GTh, Bakkeren JAJM et al (1983). Purine metabolism in childhood acute lymphoblastic leukemia: Biochemical markers for diagnosis and chemotherapy. Leuk Res 7:407–420.

22. van Laarhoven JPRM, de Gast GC, Spierenburg GTH and de Bruyn CHMM (1983). Enzymological studies in chronic lymphocytic leukemia. Leuk Res 7:261–267.

23. Blatt J, Bunn PA, Carney DD et al (1982). Purine pathway enzymes in the circulating malignant cells of patients with cutaneous T-cell lymphoma. Brit J Haematol 52:97–104.

24. Demeocq F, Viallard JL, Boumsell L et al. (1982). The correlation of adenosine deaminase and purine nucleoside phosphorylase activities in human lymphocytes subpopulations and in various lymphoid malignancies. Leuk Res 6:211–220.

25. Foon KA, Schroff RW and Gale RP (1982). Surface markers on leukemia and lymphoma cells: Recent advances. Blood 60:1–19.

26. Schornagel JH (1982). Studies on the reversal of methotrexate toxicity by thymidine and on the role of thymidine as an anti-cancer drug. Thesis, Utrecht.

27. Howell SB, Teatle R and Mendelsohn J (1980). Thymidine as a chemotherapeutic agent: Sensitivity of normal human marrow, peripheral blood T-cells, and acute nonlymphocytic leukemia. Blood 55:505–510.

28. Kufe DW, Beardsley P, Karp D et al. (1980). High dose thymidine infusions in patients with leukemia and lymphoma. Blood 55:580–589.

29. Fox RM, Kefford RF, Tripp EH and Taylor IW (1981). G1-phase arrest of cultured human leukemic T-cells induced by deoxyadenosine. Cancer Res 41:5141–5150.

30. Carson DA, Kaye J and Wasson DB (1981). The potential importance of soluble deoxynucleotidase activity in mediating deoxyadenosine toxicity in human lymphoblasts. J Immunol 126:348–352.

31. Fox RM, Piddington SK, Tripp EH and Tattersall MHN (1981). Ecto-adenosine triphosphate deficiency in cultured human T- and null-leukemic lymphocytes. J Clin Invest 68:544–552.

32. Kefford RF, Helmer MA and Fox RM (1982). S-adenosylhomocysteine hydrolase inhibition in deoxyadenosine-treated human T-lymphoblasts and resting peripheral blood lymphocytes. Cancer Res 42:3822–3827.

33. Russel NH, Prentice HG, Lee N et al. (1981). Studies on the biochemical sequelae of therapy

in Thy-1 acute lymphoblastic leukemia with the adenosine deaminase inhibitor 2'deoxyco-formycin. Brit J Haematol 49:1-9.

34. Bagnara AS and Hershfield MS (1982). Mechanism of deoxyadenosine-induced catabolism of adenine ribonucleotides in adenosine deaminase-inhibited human T-lymphoblastoid cells. Proc Nat Acad Sci USA 79:2673-2677.

35. Matsumoto SS, Yu AL, Bleeker et al. (1982). Biochemical correlates of the differential sensitivity of subtypes of human leukemia to deoxyadenosine and deoxycoformycin. Blood 60:1096-1102.

36. Prentice HG, Russell NH, Lee N et al. (1981). Therapeutic selectivity of and prediction of response to 2'deoxycoformycin in acute leukemia. Lancet 2:1250-1253.

37. Sylwestrowicz T, Piga A, Murphy P et al. (1982). The effects of deoxycoformycin and deoxyadenosine on deoxyribonucleotide concentrations in leukaemic cells. Brit J Haematol 51:623-630.

38. Kazmers IS, Mitchell BS, Dadonna PE et al. (1981). Inhibition of purine nucleoside phosphorylase by 8-aminoguanosine: Selective toxicity for T-lymphoblasts. Science 214:1137-1139.

39. Rijkers GT, Zegers BJM, Spaapen LJM et al. (1984). Mononuclear cells in S-phase in a patient with purine nucleoside phosphorylase deficiency. Adv Exp Med Biol 165B:171-174.

4. Purine degradative enzymes in the malignant cells of patients with B-cell leukemia

A. D. HO[1], B. DÖRKEN[1], W. HUNSTEIN[1] and
A. V. HOFFBRAND[2]
[1] *Medizinische Universitäts-Poliklinik, Heidelberg, FRG and*
[2] *Department of Haematology, Royal Free Hospital and School of Medicine, London, UK*

The purine degradative enzymes adenosine deaminase (ADA), purine nucleoside phosphorylase (PNP) and ecto-5'-nucleotidase (5-NT) seem to play an important role in the development of both T- and B-lymphocytes [1–4]. Inherited deficiencies of ADA and PNP are associated with various immune defects. Furthermore remarkable differences in enzyme activities of these purine enzymes and terminal deoxynucleotidyl transferase (TdT) have been reported among immunologic subclasses of acute lymphocytic leukemia (ALL) [5–8]. Studies of these enzymes in normal T-cell precursors have shown that different thymic subsets in different stages of maturation are characterized by specific enzyme patterns with a fall in TdT and ADA activities and a rise in PNP and 5'NT activities during T-cell maturation [9, 10]. Further investigations have shown that the enzyme patterns of malignant T-cells are comparable to the enzymatic make up of normal T-lymphocytes in defined stages of development [11, 12]. For example, the blasts of T-ALL have high levels of TdT and ADA activities but low levels of PNP and 5'NT, an enzyme pattern which corresponds to that of prothymocytes, their normal counterparts.

In B-cell derived malignancies, the significance of these enzymes remains to be established. The enzyme changes during normal B-cell maturation have not yet been defined. Nevertheless, circulating B-cells have up to 4 times higher 5'NT levels than do T-lymphocytes [13]. Cord blood B-cells are reported to have a much lower 5'NT activity than adult B-cells [14]. We have investigated the activities Tdt, ADA, PNP and 5'NT in the circulating malignant cells of 48 patients with different B-cell neoplasias and have correlated these data with clinical and phenotypical features.

Materials and methods

B-cell leukemias or lymphomas were classified according to the Kiel classification [15]. Diagnosis was established by morphology (histology or cytology), studies of surface membrane (SmIg) and cytoplasmic immunoglobulins (CIg) and analysis with monoclonal antibodies against B-cell differentiation antigens (B 1, HD-6, HD-28, HD-37, HD-39). There were 5 patients with common acute leukemia (cALL), which were clearly B committed as the blasts were B 1 positive, 14 patients with chronic B lymphocytic leukemia (B-CLL), 4 patients with prolymphocytic leukemia (PLL), 4 patients with centrocytic lymphomas (diagnosis in CC was established primarily by histologic and histoimmunologic examination of lymph node biopsy) and 21 patients with immunocytoma (IC), defined by the presence of CIg. The IC patients showed similar leukocyte counts and proportions of B neoplastic cells (usually >90%) in the peripheral blood to the patients with CLL.

Cells

Leukemic cells were obtained from the peripheral blood by Ficoll-Isopaque gradient centrifugation. Only cell suspensions with at least 75% monoclonal malignant B-cells as indicated by monoclonal SmIg or by expression of monoclonal differentiation antigens were used for enzyme analysis. Viability of the cells was always more than 95%, as revealed by trypan-blue (0.2%) dye exclusion test.

Immunologic markers

The reagents used were: monovalent rabbit antibodies conjugated with FITC against human μ, δ, γ and α heavy chains and against κ and λ light chains, polyvalent rabbit antibody against human Ig (G+A+M), conjugated with TRITC, all obtained from MEDAC (F.R. Germany). The monoclonal antibodies B1 and OKT 3 were obtained from Coulter Electronics (Hialeah, U.S.A.) and from Orthodiagnostics (Raritan, N.J., U.S.A.) respectively.

Surface immunoglobulins were detected by incubating 10^6 cells with the corresponding FITC conjugated rabbit antibody. After incubation for 30 min at room temperature, cells were washed and resuspended in phosphate buffered saline containing 0.2% sodium azide [10]. Cell surface antigens as defined by the appropriate monoclonal antibodies were detected utilizing FITC-conjugated goat anti-mouse Ig, as described [10].

Enzyme assays

TdT activity was assayed as described [10]. All purine enzyme assays except 5'NT were performed on cell extracts, the methods have been described in detail elsewhere [8]. Cells were suspended in the appropriate buffer and were disrupted by freezing in liquid nitrogen and thawing at 37 °C thrice. The disrupted cell suspension was centrifuged for 60 min at 30,000 rpm (60,000 g) at 4 °C in an ultracentrifuge.

ADA was measured in a mixture containing ^{3}H-adenosine (1 mM, 0.6 µCi) and 10 µl of cell extract (in 0.5 mM potassium phosphate buffer with 1 mM β-mercaptoethanol pH 7.4) in a final volume of 50 µl. ADA activity was expressed in Units/10^8 cells (1 Unit = 1 µmol substrate converted/hr).

PNP was assayed by incubating 10 µl cell extract and inosine (2 mM 0.1 µCi) in phosphate buffer (25 mM pH 7.4) in a total volume of 100 µl for 40 min at 37 °C PNP activity was expressed in Units/10^6 cells (1 Unit=1 nmol substrate converted/hr). The 5'NT assay was done on intact cells; 1×10^6 cells in 50 µl of saline-Tris buffer (0.04 M, pH 7.4) were incubated with equal volume of reaction mixture containing 2-^{3}H-adenosine monophosphate (0.1 mM, 0.4 µCi) and magnesium chloride (3 mM) for 15 min at 37 °C. 5'NT activity was expressed in Units/10^6 cells (1 Unit = 1 nmol substrate converted/hr).

Statistical analysis

Tests for statistical differences of the means were performed according to the Student t-test.

Results

The activities of the enzymes TdT, ADA, PNP, and 5'NT are summarized in Fig. 1 and 2. Malignant cells of cALL were characterized by high levels of TdT (mean $\pm$ SD = 29.4 $\pm$ 25.8 U/10^8 cells), ADA (mean = 53.2 $\pm$ 28.3 U/10^8 cells) and 5'NT (mean = 33.3 $\pm$ 2.6 U/10^6 cells) but moderate levels of PNP (mean = 127.7 $\pm$ 27.4 U/10^6 cells). The levels of TdT activity in all the other malignant B-cells were very low to not detectable (mean = 0.1 U/10^8 cells, range: <0.1 to 1.9 U/10^8 cells). Leukemic cells of B-CLL were characterized by low activities of ADA (mean $\pm$ SD = 2.2 $\pm$ 1.2 U/10^8 cells) PNP (mean = 68.9 $\pm$ 35.7 U/10^6 cells) and also of 5'NT (mean = 2.8 $\pm$ 2.2 U/10^6 cells). Circulating cells of PLL were shown to have also low levels of ADA (mean = 1.6 $\pm$ 1.1 U/10^8 cells), PNP (mean = 55.9 $\pm$ 36.0 U/10^6 cells) and 5'NT (mean = 1.4 $\pm$ 0.9 U/10^6 cells). In CC, ADA activity was again low (mean = 2.4 $\pm$ 2.2 U/10^6 cells), but PNP (mean = 84.6 $\pm$ 19.9 U/10^6 cells) and 5'NT (mean =

166

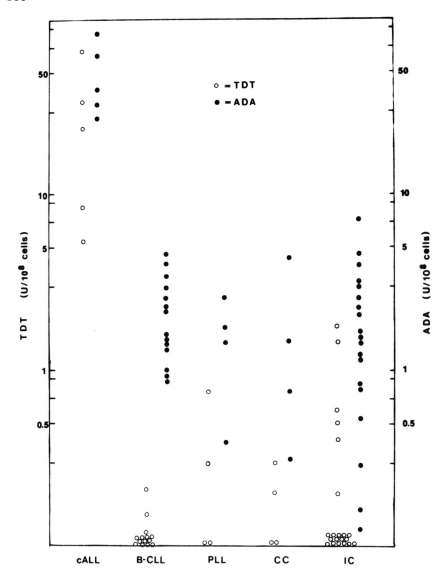

Figure 1. Enzyme activities of terminal deoxynucleotidyl transferase (TdT) and adenosine deaminase (ADA) in malignant cells of common acute lymphocytic leukemia (cALL), chronic B lymphocytic leukemia (B-CLL), prolymphocytic leukemia (PLL), centrocytic lymphoma (CC) and leukemic immunocytoma (IC). Each dot or circle represents the value of one patient. The enzyme activities are shown in logarithmic scale.

7.3 ± 8.5 U/10^6 cells) activities were moderately high. In malignant cells of IC, low activity of ADA (mean = 2.4 ± 2.3 U/10^8 cells) was again observed, but the activities of PNP (mean = 116.0 ± 59.1 U/10^6 cells) and 5′NT (mean) = 18.1 ± 14.2 U/10^6 cells) were relatively high. Thus the malignant cells of cALL have a very different enzyme pattern as compared to

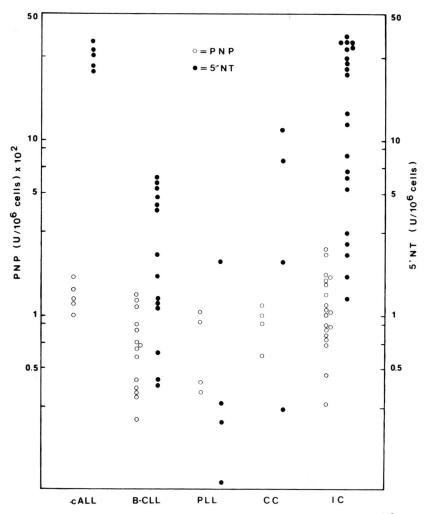

Figure 2. Enzyme activities of purine nucleoside phosphorylase (PNP) and ecto-5′-nucleotidase (5′NT) in malignant cells of cALL, B-CLL, PLL, CC and IC. Each dot or circle represents the value of one patient. The enzyme activities are given in logarithmic scale.

the other B neoplasms. Between B-CLL and IC, the differences in PNP ($p < 0.01$) and in 5′NT ($p < 0.001$) are significant. For PLL and CC, more data are yet required for statistical analysis.

Discussion

In this study we have demonstrated that different enzyme patterns occur in subsets of B-cell neoplasms. The blasts of cALL are shown to have distinctive high levels of TdT, ADT and 5′NT, as shown by other authors [8, 12].

In contrast, the malignant cells of B-CLL are characterized by very low levels of all the enzymes TdT, ADA, PNP and 5'NT. Though TdT and ADA activities are also invariably low in all the other malignant B cells investigated, differences in PNP and 5'NT could be found. Leukemic cells of IC have significantly higher levels of 5'NT ($p < 0.001$) and PNP ($p < 0.01$) than those of B-CLL. The malignant cells of CC seem to have intermediate values of PNP and 5'NT as compared to B-CLL and IC. However, no statistical analysis could be attempted in view of the small numbers.

In contrast to the well defined maturation pathway of the T-cells, the pathways of B-cell development seem to be very complex [16]. The phenotypes and purine enzyme patterns of the T-cell malignancies are relatively well defined in relation to the normal equivalent cell [11, 17, 18]. The complexity of B-cell types in non-Hodgkin's lymphomas has led to the suggestion that a large number of divergent pathways may exist within multiple compartments of B-cell development [19]. Up till now, the definition of maturation stages in B-cells has been based on Ig expression and on Ig secretory activity. Cells of CLL probably derive from early B-cells [15, 16, 20]. Upon primary antigen stimulation the normal virgin B-cell undergoes transformation into an immunoblast, which then gives rise to lymphoplasmacytoid cells and plasma cells. A further response to antigenic stimulation is the development of germinal centers. In the germinal center, centroblasts originate from the virgin lymphocytes and give rise to centrocytes and these ultimately to memory cells (not shown in figure). Memory cells can also be transformed directly to immunoblasts and lymphoplasmacytoid cells. Malignant cells of IC probably derive from memory cells and during the development of lymphoplasmacytoid cells [15].

Though the enzyme patterns of normal precursors in different stages of B-cell maturation are still yet to be defined, it is known that cord blood B-cells, which are considered to be immature, have a much lower 5'NT activity than adult B-cells [13, 21]. Referring to the similarity in 5'NT activity between cord blood cells and CLL, some authors even suggested that cord blood lymphocytes might be the normal counterparts of CLL [22]. In the later stages of B-cell development it seems that maturation is associated with an increase in 5'NT activities. Thus the enzyme pattern of the leukemic cells of IC seems also to show that they are more mature than the cells of CLL, supporting the above proposed pathway of B-cell maturation.

The present study has emphasized the value of purine enzyme studies in defining subsets of B-cell neoplasia. The enzymatic profile may be a useful supplement to immunologic phenotype in approaching the stages of maturation arrest represented by the leukemic population. Further studies of these enzymes in other non-Hodgkin's-lymphomas might be valuable for the understanding of B-maturation.

Acknowledgements

Supported in part by the Tumorzentrum Heidelberg/Mannheim, F.R. Germany.

References

1. Giblett ER, Anderson JE, Cohen F et al. (1972). Adenosine-deaminase deficiency in two patients with severely impaired cellular immunity. Lancet 2:1067–1069.
2. Giblett ER, Ammann AJ, Wara DW et al. (1975). Nucleoside-phosphorylase deficiency in a child with severely defective T-cell immunity and normal B-cell immunity. Lancet 1:1010–1013.
3. Johnson SM, North ME, Asherson GL et al. (1977). Lymphocyte purine 5'-nucleotidase deficiency in primary hypogammaglobulinaemia. Lancet 1:168–170.
4. Barton RW and Goldschneider I (1979). Nucleotide-metabolizing enzymes and lymphocyte differentiation. Mol Cell Biochem 28:135–147.
5. Coleman MS, Greenwood MF, Hutton JJ et al. (1978). Adenosine deaminase, terminal deoxynucleotidyl transferase (TdT) and surface markers in childhood acute leukemia. Blood 52:1125–1131.
6. Blatt J., Reaman GH, Levin N and Poplack DG (1980). Purine nucleoside phosphorylase activity in acute lymphoblastic leukemia. Blood 56:380–382.
7. Ganeshaguru K, Lee N, Llewellin P et al. (1981). Adenosine deaminase concentrations in leukaemia and lymphoma: A relation to cell phenotypes. Leuk Res 5:215–222.
8. Sylwestrowicz TA, Ma DDF, Murphy PP et al. (1982). 5'Nucleotidase, adenosine deaminase and purine nucleoside phosphorylase activities in acute leukaemia. Leuk Res 6:475–482.
9. Barton RW and Goldschneider I (1979). Nucleotide-metabolizing enzymes and lymphocyte differentiation. Mol Cell Biochem 28:135.
10. Ma DDF, Sylwestrowicz TA, Granger S et al. (1982). Distribution of terminal deoxynucleotidyl transferase and purine degradative and synthetic enzymes in subpopulations of human thymocytes. J Immunol 129:1430–1435.
11. Ma DDF, Massaia M, Sylwestrowicz TA et al. (1983). Comparison of purine degradative enzymes and terminal deoxynucleotidyl transferase in T-cell leukaemias and in normal thymic and post-thymic T-cells. Brit J Haematol 54:451–457.
12. Van Laarhoven JPRM, Spierenburg GT, Bakkeren JAJM et al. (1983). Purine metabolism in childhood acute lymphoblastic leukemia: Biochemical markers for diagnosis and chemotherapy. Leuk Res 7:407–420.
13. Massaia M, Ma DDF, Sylwestrowicz TA et al. (1982). Enzymes of purine metabolism in human peripheral lymphocyte subpopulations. Clin Exp Immunol 50:148–154.
14. Rowe M, de Gast CG, Platts-Mills TAE et al. (1979). 5'Nucleotidase of B- and T-lymphocytes isolated from human peripheral blood. Clin Exp Immunol 36:97–101.
15. Lennert K (Ed.) (1978). Malignant Lymphomas Other than Hodgkin's Disease. Berlin, Heidelberg, New York: Springer-Verlag.
16. Ezdinly EZ and Nanus DM (1983). B-lymphoproliferative disorders: A proposed unified pathogenetic pathway. Hematol Oncol 1:297–319.
17. Blatt J, Reaman G and Poplack D (1980). Biochemical markers in lymphoid malignancies. N Engl J Med 303:918–922.
18. Blatt J, Bunn PA, Carney DD et al. (1982). Purine pathway enzymes in the circulating malignant cells of patients with cutaneous T-cell lymphoma. Brit J Haematol 52:97–104.
19. Godal T and Funderud S (1982). Human B-cell neoplasms in relation to normal B-cell

differentiation and maturation processes. Adv Cancer Res 36:211–255.

20. Johnstone AP (1982). Chronic lymphocytic leukaemia and its relationship to normal B-lymphopoiesis. Immunol Today 3:343–348.

21. Rowe M, de Gast CG, Platts-Mills TAE et al. (1980). Lymphocyte 5′-Nucleotidase in primary hypogammaglobulinaemia and cord blood. Clin Exp Immunol 39:337–343.

22. Kramers MTC, Catovsky D, Cherchi M and Galton DAG (1977). 5′Nucleotidase in cord blood lymphocytes. Leuk Res. 1:279–281.

5. Lymphocyte uroporphyrinogen synthase activity as a diagnostic test in lymphoproliferative disorders — preliminary results

M. LAHAV [1, 2], O. EPSTEIN [1], N. SCHOENFELD [1], M. SHAKLAI [3] and A. ATSMON [1, 2]

[1] Laboratory of Biochemical Pharmacology, [2] Department of Internal Medicine B and [3] Hematology Unit, Beilinson Medical Center, Petah Tiqva and The Sackler Faculty of Medicine, Tel Aviv University, Ramat Aviv, Israel

Uroporphyrinogen synthase (EC 4.3.1.8) (UROS), an enzyme in the heme biosynthetic pathway, converts porphobilinogen to uroporphyrinogen. Lymphocyte UROS (L-UROS) is an inducible enzyme [1] and its activity is increased in erythroleukemia cells [2]. Recent observations [3, 4] showed the presence of circulating malignant lymphocytes in the blood of patients with lymphoproliferative diseases (LPD) without apparent peripheral involvement.

In a previous study we showed that patients with LPD have elevated erythrocyte UROS activity, and preliminary studies revealed that L-UROS is possibly an even more sensitive test for the presence of active LPD [5]. In this study, we determined the enzyme activity in lymphocytes of a larger group of patients with active LPD, of a healthy control group and of patients with various other diseases. Our data suggest that determination of L-UROS activity may serve as a valuable test for the diagnosis of LPD.

Materials and methods

L-UROS activity was determined in 70 patients with active LPD. The group included patients with chronic lymphocytic leukemia, Hodgkin's disease and various types of non-Hodgkin's lymphoma. The diagnosis was determined histologically according to the classification of Rappaport [6]. In 14 of the 70 patients L-UROS activity had been determined before treatment was started. The other patients had been treated for various periods.

A control group consisted of 70 healthy volunteers. The distribution of age and gender between the two groups did not differ statistically.

L-UROS activity was also measured in 15 patients suffering from various epithelial malignancies (cancer of colon, breast, gall bladder, ovary, pancreas, lung, rectum, stomach, kidney, tongue) thymoma as well as chronic and acute myeloid leukemia. L-UROS activity was determined in a group of

15 patients with various infectious diseases including infectious mononucleosis, hepatitis, influenza and various bacterial infections.

Lymphocytes were prepared from heparinized blood according to usual methods. The lymphocytes were suspended in 0.05 M tris buffer, pH 8.2, homogenized and kept frozen at $-20\,°C$ up to a maximum of seven days. The homogenate was thawed, sonicated, 20×0.4 sec., and UROS activity was measured by an adaptation of the method of Magnussen et al. [7]. Enzyme activity was expressed as pmoles of porphyrins/mg protein/hr (pmol porph/mg prot/h). Determinations were made in duplicate and each value shown is the average of the duplicates.

Statistical analysis was performed by a single classification analysis of variance followed by an aposteriori test (SS-STP) or by Student's t-test. Specificity of the L-UROS activity as a test for the diagnosis of LPD

$$\text{was calculated as: } \frac{\text{total patients with active disease}}{\text{true positive results}}$$

$$\text{and the sensitivity as: } \frac{\text{total patients without disease}}{\text{true negative results}}.$$

Results

L-UROS activity of all the patients and of the control group are shown in Fig. 1.

The mean value ± 1 SD of L-UROS activity of the healthy control group was 12.3 $\pm$ 2.6 pmol porph/mg prot/h. An L-UROS activity of 17.5 pmol porph/mg prot/h, which was the mean + 2 SD, was arbitrarily chosen as the upper limit of normal values.

The mean enzyme activity of LPD patients was significantly higher ($p < 0.001$) than that of the controls 43.6 $\pm$ 22 pmol porph/mg prot/h. We did not observe differences in mean L-UROS activity between various subgroups or different clinical stages of LPD, or between treated and untreated patients with active LPD.

As shown in the figure, all control values were below the arbitrary limit of normal. Only two out of the 70 LPD patients had an L-UROS activity below this limit.

The mean L-UROS activity of patients with non-lymphoid malignant diseases was 14.7 $\pm$ 4.9 pmol porph/mg prot/h. Among those patients with various infectious diseases, the mean was 13.5 $\pm$ 2.8 pmol porph/mg prot/h and none of the values in this latter group exceeded the upper limit of normal as defined above.

Based on these results, the specificity and sensitivity of the determination of L-UROS activity as a diagnostic test for LPD were both 97%.

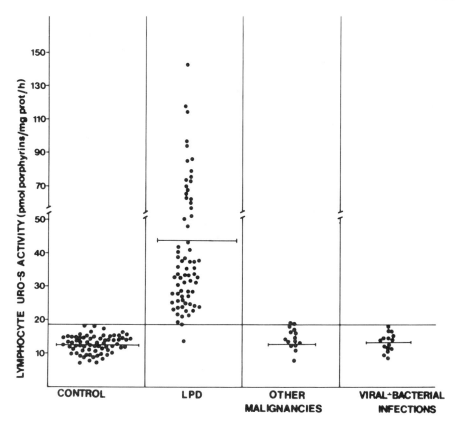

Figure 1. L-UROS activity of a control group, patients with LPD, patients with other malignancies and patients with infectious diseases. The line at 17.5 pmol porph/mg prot/h is the mean + 2 SD of the control group, the value chosen as the upper limit of normal.

Discussion

The determination of UROS activity in peripheral lymphocytes seems to be a simple highly sensitive and specific test for diagnosing LPD. This test had extremely high sensitivity and specificity, both 97%, in our patient material.

According to these results, determination of L-UROS activity may be very helpful in screening all patients with pyrexia of unknown origin, lymphadenopathy, etc. for the presence or absence of LPD. When a positive diagnosis cannot be made by cytologic examination of needle aspiration of nodules or tumors, an L-UROS determination may aid in the final evaluation of the patient. However, in spite of the high specificity and sensitivity of the test, histologically proven diagnosis of LPD is essential before treatment is initiated.

174

We do not know yet whether L-UROS is elevated in all the peripheral lymphocytes of patients with LPD, or whether only a small subset of circulating lymphocytes have very high UROS activity, thus raising the average activity. Preliminary investigations indicate the likelihood of the latter possibility. The biochemical mechanisms underlying the increased L-UROS activity in LPD are unknown and many biologic and biochemical problems remain to be solved.

References

1. Sassa S, Zalar GL and Kappas A (1978). Studies in porphyria. VII. Induction of uroporphyrinogen-I synthase and expression of the gene defect of acute intermittent porphyria in mitogen-stimulated human lymphocytes. J Clin Invest 61:499–508.
2. Sassa S (1976). Sequential induction of heme pathway enzymes during erythroid differentiation of mouse Friend leukemia virus-infected cells. J Exp Med 143:305–315.
3. Ault KA (1979). Detection of small numbers of monoclonal B-lymphocytes in the blood of patients with lymphoma. N Engl J Med 300:1401–1405.
4. Marikovsky Y, Resnitzky P and Reichman N (1978). Surface charge characteristics of peripheral blood lymphocytes in chronic lymphatic leukemia and malignant lymphoma. J Nat Cancer Inst 60:741–748.
5. Epstein O, Lahav M, Schoenfeld N et al. (1983). Erythrocyte uroporphyrinogen synthase activity as a possible diagnostic aid in the diagnosis of lymphoproliferative diseases. Cancer 52:828–832.
6. Rappaport H (1966). Tumors of the hematopoietic system. In: Atlas of Tumor Pathology, section 3, fascicle 8, pp. 97–161. Washington DC: Armed Forces Institute of Pathology.
7. Magnussen CR, Levine JB, Doherty JM et al. (1974). A red cell enzyme method for the diagnosis of acute intermittent porphyria. Blood 44:857–868.

6. Enzymatic and ultrastructural properties of the plasma membrane in human leukemias, in non-Hodgkin's lymphomas and in human lymphoblastoid cells

G. A. LOSA
Laboratory of Cellular Pathology, Ticino Institute of Pathology, Locarno, Switzerland

Ectoenzymes in lymphoblastic leukemias and in non-Hodgkin's lymphomas

We have showed that mononuclear cells of patients with primary immunodeficiency displayed a remarkable scattering of surface enzyme activities, whereas normal peripheral blood lymphocytes and non proliferating cells of patients with recurrent infections of the respiratory tract did not [1, 2]. Almost complete lack of correlations between ectoenzyme activities was also noted in immunodeficient cells, in contrast to a broad correlation level in control lymphocytes [1]. On this basis, an hypothesis was developed suggesting a dynamic rearrangements of integral and associated constituents of the plasma membrane in acute pathologic situations leading to a discrete enzyme expression. This view was strenghtened by an enzymatic analysis of blood and reticuloendothelial cell malignancies. Specific activity changes of the ectoenzymes were recorded in cells isolated from patients with acute lymphoblastic leukemia. Cellular immunologic phenotype was defined by conventional surface and cytochemical markers [3, 4]. The contribution of the surface enzyme analysis to the identification of differentiation stage and cell origin has been clearly documented by a recent report [5] showing that acute undifferentiated leukemia (AUL; Ia^+, $cALLA^-$) could be distinguished into three groups owing to the expression of the plasma membrane enzyme γ-glutamyltranspeptidase (Glupase) and the soluble terminal transferase (TdT). Thus, a leukemic population at a given stage of differentiation expresses a surface immunologic phenotype accompanied by biochemical characteristics of their plasma membrane.

In a current study to focus the relationship between enzymatic and immunologic surface properties, we observed multimodal distribution profiles of ectoenzyme activities in cells isolated from diffuse non-Hodgkin's lymphomas (NHL), characterized by an heterogenous immunologic phenotype (Fig. 1). It was therefore not surprising that the enzyme activities did not corre-

176

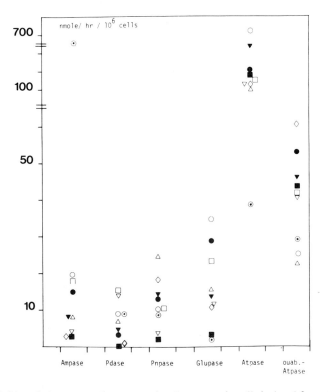

Figure 1. Activities of plasma membrane associated enzymes in cells isolated from diffuse NHL. Ampase: 5'-nucleotidase; Pdase: alkaline phosphodiesterase; Pnpase, alkaline phosphomonoesterase: Glupase, γ-glutamyltranspeptidase: Atpase, adenosine triphosphatase: ouab.-Atpase, ouabain dependent adenosine triphosphatase. The immunologic phenotype of these nine cases is tabulated hereunder.

| Case | Immunologic phenotype (% positive cells) | | |
	Leu 1	sIg	Anae
1○	37	41 (> k)	6
2●	34	39 (> λ)	24
3□	45	28 (> λ)	13
4△	33	34 > λ)	2
5▽	13	20 —	13
6▼	18	12 —	—
7■	21	7 (> k)	4
8◇	18	15 —	1
9⊙	0	4 —	1

late with each other, with the exception of the 5'-nucleotidase and the Glupase, as documented in Table I. In contrast, some cases of diffuse NHL with a homogenous cell population that predominantly expressed monoclonal surface immunoglobulins (μ, λ) showed a low level as well as a faint scattering of the various enzyme activities. Finally, a great deal of enzyme variations was also recorded in human lymphoblastoid cells [6].

These findings prompted us to examine whether changes in plasma membrane enzyme activities should be considered as a peculiar trait of the malignancy, or as a trait inherent to the high proliferative capacity of cells at a given stage of differentiation. To answer this question, we devised an ultrastructural and biochemical approach. The study included equilibrium density centrifugation with subsequent enzymatic analysis of isolated membranes combined to morphometric quantitation of intramembrane particles on freeze-fracture preparations of human lymphoblastoid cells. The immunologic phenotype of the three lymphoblastoid cell lines (Reh-6, Nalm-1, Raji), assessed by staining with monoclonal antibodies and polyclonal antiimmunoglobulin antisera, indicated a differentiation level progressing from the common-like type (Ia$^+$, cALLA$^+$, sIg$^-$) to an immature B stage (Ia$^+$, sIg$^+$).

Enzymatic and freeze fracture analysis of human lymphoblastoid cells

Due to different growth kinetics of the three lymphoblastoid cell lines, cells were harvested at the beginning of the plateau phase ($\sim 10^9$ cells), washed and homogenized in a tris-potassium-magnesium buffer solution (TKM)

Table I. Correlations between activities of plasma membrane-associated enzymes in NHL

		r_s	p value
5'-nucleotidase versus	γ-glutamyltranspeptidase	0.96	0.01
	alkaline phosphomonoesterase	0.32	ns
	alkaline phosphodiesterase	0.46	ns
	adenosine triphosphatase	0.36	ns
alkaline phosphodiesterase versus			
	γ-glutamyltranspeptidase	0.29	ns
	alkaline phosphomonoesterase	0.05	ns
	adenosine triphosphatase	0.29	ns
alkaline phosphomonoesterase versus			
	γ-glutamyltranspeptidase	0.36	ns
	adenosine triphosphatase	0.11	ns
adenosine triphosphatase versus			
	γ-glutamyltranspeptidase	0.43	ns

These correlations were calculated with enzymatic activities measured in cells from NHL
r_s = Spearman rank correlation coefficient

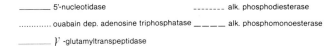

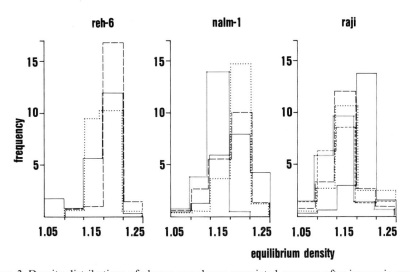

Figure 2. Density distributions of plasma membrane associated enzymes after isopycnic centrifugation of total homogenates from human lymphoblastoid cell lines.
Cell line Reh-6: Ia$^+$, cALLA$^+$, sIg$^-$, Leu 5$^-$; dCell line Nalm-1: Ia$^+$, cALLA$^+$, cIgM$^+$; Raji : Ia$^+$, cALLA$^-$, sIg$^+$; (Ia: immune associated antigen; cALLA: common acute lymphoblastic leukemia antigen; sIg: surface immunoglobulins; cIgM: cytoplasmic immunoglobulins of the class M).

containing 60% sucrose.[2] Homogenates were subjected to discontinuous sucrose gradient ultracentrifugation at 100,000 g for 12 hours. Membrane fractions were quantitatively collected, thoroughly washed and assayed for protein content as well as activities of several marker enzymes for the plasma membrane and subcellular organelles. Fig. 2 illustrates the data obtained

Table II. Morphometric analysis of protoplasmic and external faces of plasma membranes

	Particles density (Np/μm^2)	
Cell line	Plasma membrane PF	Plasma membrane EF
Reh 6	904.62 $\pm$ 516.92	255.38 $\pm$ 347.69
Nalm 1	1754.64 $\pm$ 752.64	337.53 $\pm$ 428.80
Raji	971.14 $\pm$ 498.12	340.12 $\pm$ 402.65

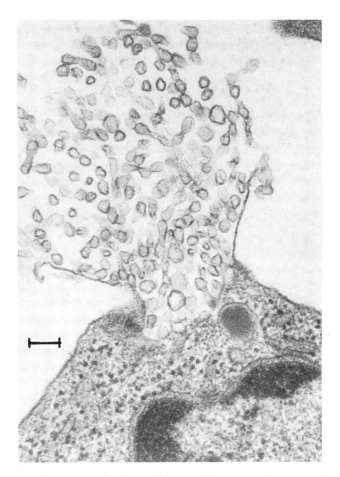

Figure 3. Electron microscopy view of membrane shedding from a leukemic cell. (72000× :⊢⊣ 138 nm).

from triplicate gradient experiments for each cell line. Cells of the Reh-6 line lacked or did not express a detectable activity of alkaline phosphodiesterase (PDAse) and Glupase. The Nalm-1 line, partially committed for the synthesis of cytoplasmic IgM, showed a Glupase activity but its distribution profile, as a function of density, remained distinct from that of the ouabain-dependent adenosine triphosphatase and other enzymes. In the membrane fractions of Raji cells, PDAse was detectable while all plasma membrane enzymes, except 5′-nucleotidase, displayed uniform activity profiles. The pronounced codistribution of different enzymes indicates that constituents associated to the external membrane leaflet are more homogeneously distributed in Raji cells than in less differentiated cells. The latter (Reh-6, Nalm-1), on the contrary, had membranes with zones of preferential enzyme location. The non-homogeneous distribution of constituents in plasma membrane of lymphoid cells has been already documented by others [7, 8, 9].

We also analyzed the behavior of the integral and transmembrane glycoproteins by recording the density (Np/μm^2) and the density distributions of the intramembrane particles as visualized on freeze fracture preparations.

The morphometric analysis [10] of both external and protoplasmic faces of the plasma membrane from the three cell lines revealed no significant differences in particle density (Table II) or in particle density distributions [11]. Ultrastructural data, therefore, seem to disagree with the enzymatic data. The asymmetric arrangement of membrane provides for a reasonable interpretation; integral constituents of the plasma membrane structure may be homogeneously distributed in mature and immature cells, constantly adapting to the dynamic processes of differentiation and proliferation. In contrast, the externally associated ectoconstituents that provide functional and cellular mechanisms may be progressively inserted into the membrane and distributed according to the developmental state.

Membrane rearrangement and membrane shedding

A variety of mechanisms may be proposed on the basis of enzyme activity variations, e.g. different rates of enzyme synthesis, posttranslational modification of enzyme proteins, modification of the phospholipid environment of the plasma membrane, and inactivation or activation through exogenous

Table III. Protein content and membrane 5'-nucleotidase activity in membrane vesicles and in cells isolated from patients with common lymphoblastic leukemia

c-ALL	Membrane vesicles (100000 g)		Intact cells 5'-nucleotidase nmole/hr/10^6 cells
	Protein $\mu g/ml$	5'-nucleotidase nmole/hr/mg	
1	1466	514.5	33.2
2	1500	762.2	—
3	377	0.0	52.7
4	775	190.5	—
5	922	38.1	44.5
6	637	0.0	—
7	390	99.2	—
8	604	0.0	—
9	375	0.0	—
10	500	4542.8	91.7
11	375	270.1	—
control	10-15	0.0	20.1 (mononuclear cells)

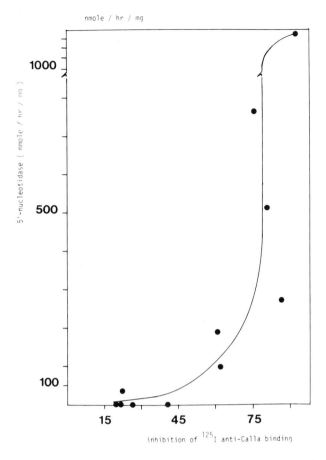

Figure 4. Relationship between 5′nucleotidase and cALLA antigen (% inhibition of ^{125}I anti-cALLA binding) in membrane vesicles isolated by ultracentrifugation of sera from patients with acute lymphoblastic leukemia (Ia+, cALLA+).

molecules (fibronectin, laminin, others?). The method by which proliferating cells adapt and indefinitely keep their plasma membrane in a particular stage of differentiation is unknown. A putative mechanism which deserves particular attention is the shedding of membrane fragments, largely documented in many cell types [12–14], which implies a continuous rearrangement of the plasma membrane. Fragment extrusion seems to involve specific portions of the plasma membrane of proliferating, pathologic lymphoid cells; gradient centrifugation showed plasma membrane associated enzymes generally do not codistribute along with membrane vesicles of the same density. Further evidence of membrane shedding was provided by the analysis of pellets recovered by high speed centrifugation (100,000 g/30 minutes) of sera from patients with acute lymphoblastic leukemia of the common type (Ia+, cALLA+). The pellets contained membrane vesicles as identified by electron microscopy and biochemical assays (Fig. 3, Table III). Biochemical heterogeneity characterized these fragments, as some pellets contained cALLA antigen as well as membrane 5′-nucleotidase activity, whereas others lacked both [15]. However, simultaneous expression of both antigens on membrane vesicles occurred in a sigmoidal way. The functional meaning of such a codistribution remains to be explored (Fig. 4).

The level of cALLA and of 5′-nucleotidase activity measured on the membrane pellets was unrelated to the level of both constituents on the intact cells isolated from the corresponding patient blood, as documented in Table III. In our opinion, these findings show that membrane shedding is a general and relevant phenomenon of proliferating cells, whereas the rate of shedding and the membrane composition are peculiar to each type of lymphoblastic leukemia.

Conclusions

Proliferating and pathologic cells are characterized by distinct activity levels of plasma membrane associated enzymes that are defined by the developmental state of the cell population. The progression of differentiation could be biochemically followed through the progressive appearance of ectoenzyme activities and through the increasing homogeneous distribution of these constituents on the outer surface of the plasma membrane, as evidenced by equilibrium density experiments.

To ensure the necessary antigenic make-up of the surface, proliferating cells extrude membrane fragments at specific rates from preferential domains of the plasma membrane. Experimental evidence is provided by membrane vesicles that bear cALLA antigen and 5′-nucleotidase activity, vesicles that are obtained by ultracentrifugation from sera of patients with common lymphoblastic leukemia and from culture media of human lymphoblastoid cell lines.

Acknowledgements

The collaboration of the members of the Laboratory of Cellular Pathology is gratefully acknowledged.

References

1. Losa G, Morell A and Barandun S (1982). Correlations between enzymatic and immunologic properties of human peripheral blood mononuclear cells. Amer J Path 107:191–201.

2. Maestroni G and Losa G (1984). Clinical and immunobiological effects of an orally administered bacterial extract. Int J Immunopharmacol 6:111–117.
3. Morell A, Carrel S, Von Fliedner V et al. (1983). Expression of immunological markers and of ectoenzyme activities on leukemic cells. Verh Dtsch Ges Path 67:517–521.
4. Losa G (1982). Enzymatic properties in pericellular membranes of leukemic cells. Adv Exp Med Biol 145:377–384.
5. Heumann D, Grob JP, Von Fliedner V and Losa G (1984). Activity of membrane associated γ-glutamyltranspeptidase in acute leukemia. Proc. Second International Conference on Malignant Lymphoma, Lugano: 103.
6. Losa G and Morell A (1980). Enzyme profiles in plasma membrane of human leukemic cell cultures. Eur J Cell Biol 22:535.
7. Resch K, Loracher A, Mähler B et al. (1978). Functional mosaicism of the lymphocyte plasma membrane. Biochim Biophys Acta 511:176–193.
8. Anderson L, Gahmberg C, Kimura A and Vigzell H(1978). Activated human T-lymphocytes display new surface glycoproteins. Proc Nat Acad Sc USA 75:3455–3458.
9. Sachs DH, Kiszkiss P and Kim KJ (1980). Release of Ia antigens by a cultured B-cell line. J Immunol 124:2130–2135.
10. Losa G and Weibel E (1983). Freeze fracture and enzymatic analysis of membrane vesicles in subcellular fractions of rat liver. Cell Molec Biol 29:129–137.
11. Conti A and Losa G (1984). Organizzazione biochimica ed ultrastrutturale delle membrane di cellule leucemiche umane coltivate *in vitro*. Boll Soc Tic Sc Nat LXXI.
12. Liepins A and Hillman A (1981). Shedding of tumor cell surface membranes. Cell Biol Int Rep 5:15–26.
13. De Broe M, Wieme R, Logghe G and Roels F (1977). Spontaneous shedding of plasma membrane fragments by human cells *in vivo* and *in vitro*. Clin Chim Acta 81:237–245.
14. Dainiak N Cohen C (1982). Surface membrane vesicles from mononuclear cells stimulate erythroid stem cells to proliferate in culture. Blood 60:583–594.
15. Carrel S, Buchegger F, Heumann D et al. (1984). Detection of the common acute leukemia antigen (cALLA) in the serum of leukemia patients. (Submitted for publication).

IV. Clinico-pathologic correlations

1. Prognostic significance of cytologic subdivision in nodular sclerosing Hodgkin's disease: An analysis of 1156 patients

K. A. MACLENNAN, M. H. BENNETT, A. TU, B. VAUGHAN
HUDSON, M. J. EASTERLING, C. VAUGHAN HUDSON AND
A. M. JELLIFFE
*British National Lymphoma Investigation, Department of Oncology,
The Middlesex Hospital Medical School, London, UK*

Nodular sclerosis is the most commonly recognized histopathologic subtype of Hodgkin's disease in many studies [1–5]. In the clinical trials of the British National Lymphoma Investigation (BNLI) [6], 75% of the cases have been classified as nodular sclerosis. Cellular nodules may have a wide variety of histologic appearances which may range from a predominance of lymphocytes to lymphocyte depletion with numerous Hodgkin's cells [7]. A clear need has emerged for further histopathologic subdivision within this group in order to provide additional prognostic information. Several reports on this theme have been published, but the numbers of cases examined in these studies have been rather small [8–13]. In two previous publications we described the prognostic significance of a cytologic subdivision of nodular sclerosing Hodgkin's disease in a group of laparotomized or Stage IV patients [14] and in a group of patients who had not undergone staging laparotomy [15]. We now present the combined results of our histologic analysis of 1156 cases of nodular sclerosing Hodgkin's disease included in which are patients from the previous two studies. The prognostic significance of this cytologic subdivision is discussed and the relationship to anatomic stage is reviewed.

Materials and methods

A total of 1194 cases have been reviewed, 1113 which had been previously classified as nodular sclerosis and a further 81 cases which have been added after reappraisal of other histologic subtypes of Hodgkin's disease. All patients had been entered into the clinical trials of the BNLI, at least three years prior to this study. Thirty-eight cases have been excluded either because the histopathologic material was unavailable for review or because information regarding clinical follow-up was inadequate. The remaining 1156 patients form the basis for this report. Of these, 856 either underwent

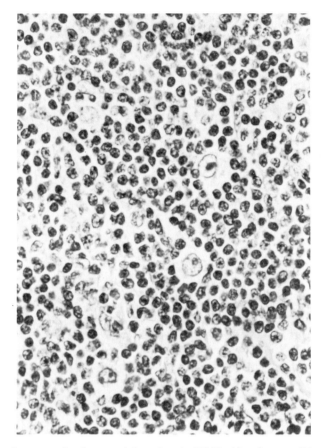

Figure 1. Lymphocyte predominant nodular sclerosis, NS(L). Abundant small lymphocytes and occasional typical lacunar cells. H & E × 450.

staging laparotomy or had evidence of visceral organ involvement (Stage IV disease).

All the pathologic material has been reviewed by at least one of the pathologist involved in this study (MHB, KAM and AT). The criteria used for subclassification were essentially similar to those applied in the Lukes and Butler classification [16, 17] for lymphocyte predominant, mixed cellularity and lymphocyte depleted Hodgkin's disease. Since these criteria were being applied to the cellular nodules of nodular sclerosis, nodule formation, lacunar cells and at least a minimal degree of intranodal collagen band formation were a prerequisite.

Lymphocyte predominant nodular sclerosis

This was subdivided into lymphocytic predominance (L) and lymphocytic and histiocytic predominance (L/H). Lacunar cells and classifical Reed-

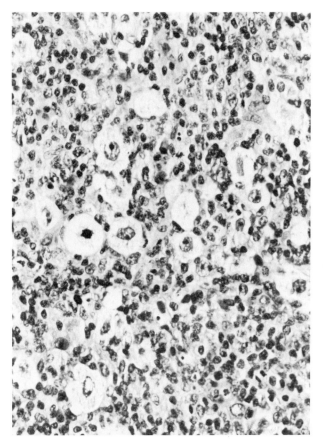

Figure 2. Mixed cellularity nodular sclerosis, NS (MC). Plentiful lacunar cells in a cellular background containing lymphocytes, histiocytes and plasma cells. H & E × 450.

Sternberg cells were scanty (Fig. 1). If areas of the lymph node showed more plentiful Hodgkin's cells within a lymphocytic or lymphocytic and histiocytic background, then this was interpreted as indicating progression to the mixed cellularity form of the disease and these cases were designated L-MC and L/H-MC. Some cases showed the cytologic features of the lymphocytic or lymphocytic/histiocytic forms of the disease, but, throughout the node, classical Reed-Sternberg and lacunar cells were rather too numerous. These cases were classified as having the mixed cellularity form of the disease of either a lymphocytic type (MC-L) or lymphocytic/histiocytic type (MC-L/H).

Mixed cellularity nodular sclerosis

This was the most commonly observed cytologic pattern and showed a

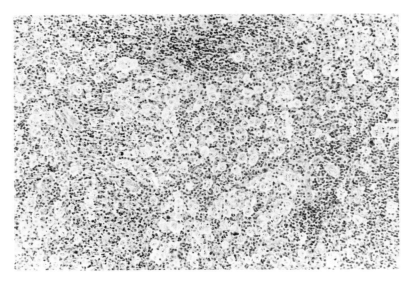

Figure 3. Mixed cellularity — Pleomorphic subtype of nodular sclerosis, NS (MC-Pleo). Numerous atypical and highly malignant appearing lacunar cells are present but there is no evidence of lymphocyte depletion. H & E × 125.

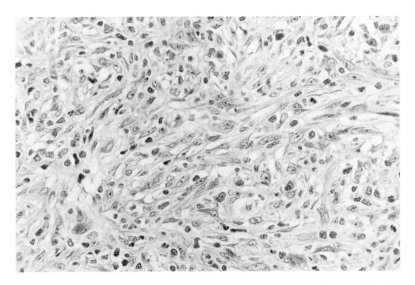

Figure 4. Fibro-histiocytic variant of lymphocyte depleted nodular sclerosis, NS (LDf). The centre of a cellular nodule showing depletion of lymphocytes and proliferating bland appearing fibroblasts and histiocytes. There is a relative paucity of Hodgkin's cells. H & E × 450.

varying mixture of lymphocytes, plasma cells, histiocytes and eosinophils as well as easily detectable lacunar and Reed-Sternberg cells (Fig. 2). A small proportion of cases in this group contained large areas with numerous pleomorphic and highly malignant appearing Hodgkin's cells, but without evi-

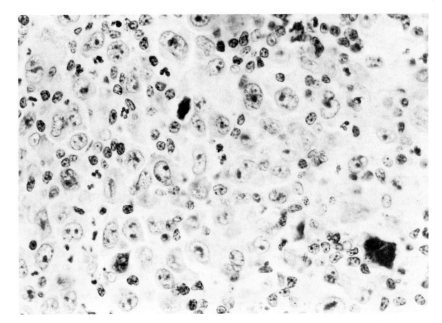

Figure 5. Reticular variant of lymphocyte depleted nodular, NS (LDr). A sheet of mononuclear Hodgkin's cells with marked depletion of lymphocytes. H & E × 450.

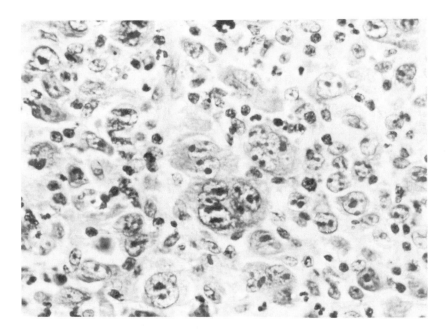

Figure 6. Pleomorphic variant of lymphocyte depleted nodular sclerosis, NS (LD pleo). Bizarre and anaplastic appearing Hodgkin's cells with depletion of lymphocytes. H & E × 600.

dence of lymphocyte depletion. These cases have been designated mixed cellularity-pleomorphic (MC-Pleo) (Fig. 3).

Lymphocyte depleted nodular sclerosis

This designation has only been used when the majority of the nodules show lymphocyte depletion. Three basic cytologic patterns were found. These were:

1) Fibrohistiocytic (LD-f) which is composed of relatively bland appearing fibroblasts and histiocytes, with few lacunar or Reed-Sternberg cells (Fig. 4). It is important only to apply these cytologic criteria to the cellular nodules and not to areas of developing sclerosis.

2) Reticular (LD-r) which is composed of sheets of relatively uniform, primitive mononuclear and lacunar cells (Fig. 5).

3) Pleomorphic (LD-pleo) which is characterized by the presence of bizarre and anaplastic giant cells in addition to the presence of lacunar and primitive mononuclear cells (Fig. 6).

The latter two forms of lymphocyte depletion are frequently associated with necrosis of the cellular nodules. Any combination of these three patterns may occur within the same lymph node.

In some lymph nodes only a proportion of the cellular nodules will show lymphocytic depletion. These areas are however very obvious, even with the scanning objective. We have described this cytologic pattern as mixed cellularity with progression to lymphocyte depletion (MC-LD). The occurrence of scanty, small and easily missed areas of lymphocyte depleted cytology do not appear to have prognostic significance and can be safely ignored [15].

Rarely, all the cellular nodules showed lymphocyte depletion, but, despite careful searching, no Reed-Sternberg cells could be found. These cases have been classified as a typical histiocytic Hodgkin's disease because the appearances of the cellular nodules were identical to those cases of lymphocyte depleted nodular sclerosis which did contain classical Reed-Sternberg cells.

After histologic classification the clinical details were examined and survival curves were calculated using the life table method. Statistical comparison of survival curves was carried out using the log rank test as described by Peto et al. [18].

Results

The total numbers in each of the twenty-three cytologic subtypes is shown in Table I. In order to reduce the complexity of this, and in the light of previous findings [14, 15], subtypes with essentially similar cytologic features have been combined to form four major groups (Table I):

1) Cases with a predominantly lymphocytic (L) or lymphocytic and histiocytic (L/H) background with or without focal mixed cellularity type cytology (L-MC, L/H-MC).

2) Mixed cellularity type cytologies (MC-L, MC-LH and MC); also included in this group are cases with areas of bland fibro-histiocytic lymphocyte depletion. This type was previously shown to have a good prognosis [15].

Table I. Histologic grade and cytologic subtype of nodular sclerosing Hodgkin's disease

Classification	No. of Patients (%)
GRADE I	828 (71.6)
LP L/H±MC	146 (12.6)
L	60
L/H	28
L-MC	42
L/H-MC	16
MC	682 (59.0)
MC (L)	86
MC (L/H)	38
MC	505
MC-LDF	53
GRADE II	328 (28.4)
MC+LDR or Pleo	252 (21.8)
MC-Pleo	78
MC-LDR	82
MC-LDP	16
MC-LDFR	39
MC-LDFPleo	13
MC-LDRPleo	12
MC-LDFRPleo	12
LD	76 (6.6)
LDF	14
LDR	19
LDPleo	5
LDFR	7
LDFPleo	4
LDRPleo	7
LDFRP	9
AH	11

194

HODGKIN'S DISEASE

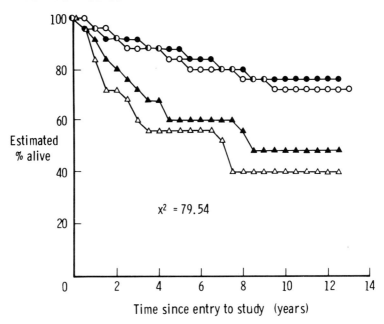

Figure 7. Actuarial survival of the four major groups of NS.
O: LP, L/H + or − MC; ●: MC; ▲: MC + LDr or pleo; △: LD.

3) Mixed cellularity type cytologies with extensive areas of lymphocyte depleted reticular or pleomorphic cytology (MC-Pleo and MC-LD except MC-LDF).

4) Predominantly lymphocyte depleted cytologies (LD).

The actuarial survivals for these four major cytologic groups are shown in Fig. 7. It can be seen that there is little difference in the survival of the L and L/H groups compared with that of the mixed cellularity subtypes. These two major groups have been amalgamated to form a group of low grade malignancy which we have termed Grade 1 NS. There is a slight prognostic advantage for the mixed cellularity group with lymphocyte depleted reticular or pleomorphic areas over the predominantly lymphocyte depleted cytologies. This is not of sufficient magnitude to be clinically useful and these two groups have been combined to form a higher grade malignant group termed Grade 2 NS. There is a very large difference in survival between these two grades (Fig. 8) and this difference is statistically significant ($p < 0.0001$).

In order to assess whether the difference in survival between the two histologic grades is due to a disproportionate representation of older pa-

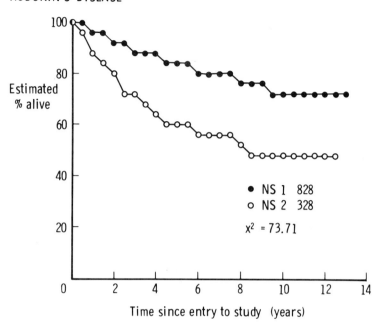

HODGKIN'S DISEASE

Figure 8. Actuarial survivals of Grade 1 and Grade 2 nodular sclerosis presenting at all stages.

tients, males or advanced stage in the Grade 2 group, we have assessed their relative frequency in each histologic grade (Table II). It is evident that the distributions of age, stage and sex are similar in the two grades and thus play little part in the difference in survival. Some factors such as systemic symptoms, an elevated ESR, anemia [19] and lymphocytopenia [20], are related to the intrinsic, and biologic aggressiveness of the disease. As might be expected, these are represented with a higher relative frequency in the cytologically more malignant Grade 2 group (Table II).

Table II. Distribution of prognostic variables by histologic grade

	Percent patients	
Variable	Grade I	Grade II
Age > 49 yrs	17.5	19.8
Males	63.5	57.0
Pathologic stages III-IV	53.8	61.1
B Symptoms	27.0	49.8
ESR ≥ 40 mm/hr	37.3	58.6
Anemia	30.3	52.0
Absolute lymphocyte count < 1500/mm³	33.9	47.4

196

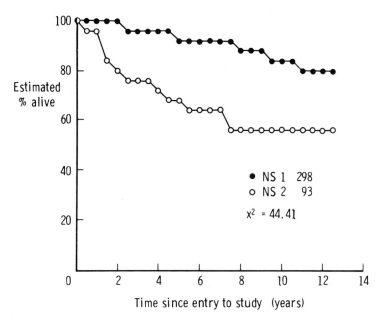

Figure 9. Actuarial survivals of Grade 1 and Grade 2 nodular sclerosis in patients presenting with pathologically staged I and II disease.

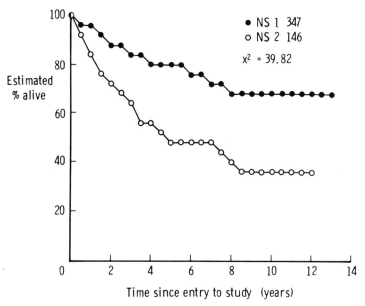

Figure 10. Actuarial survivals of Grade 1 and Grade 2 nodular sclerosis in patients presenting with pathologically staged III and IV disease.

The anatomic stage is regarded as an important factor in the prognostic assessment of patients with Hodgkin's disease. We have, therefore, examined a group of patients who had undergone staging laparotomy or had Stage IV disease, and compared the effect upon survival of histologic grade in cases presenting at a similar stage. The first group examined were those patients presenting with Stages I and II disease (Fig. 9). We found a very large difference in survival between the two histologic grades ($p < 0.001$). Analysis of patients with Stages III and IV disease (Fig. 10) also revealed a large difference in survival ($p < 0.0001$).

Discussion

One of the first histopathologic classifications of Hodgkin's disease to gain widespread acceptance was that of Jackson and Parker [21]. This classification, although providing a clear discrimination in prognosis between the paragranuloma, granuloma and sarcoma groups, was clinically of little help because the majority of cases were classified as Hodgkin's granuloma, which had an extremely variable survival [22]. Smetana and Cohen [23], in an analysis of cases from the AFIP recognized a sclerotic variant of Hodgkin's granuloma which had a superior survival to the group as a whole. Lukes and colleagues termed this nodular sclerosis [16, 24, 25], recognizing it distinctive natural history and mode of spread. Strum and Rappaport [26] emphasized the unique position of nodular sclerosis by convincingly demonstrating the consistency of this histologic pattern in sequential biopsies and by recognizing the progression of the cellular phase of the disease to the classical form in some cases. As pathologists became more familiar with the criteria for diagnosis of nodular sclerosis, not only did the relative frequency of this subtype rise but also the wide spectrum of cytologic appearances was recognized [7].

Several studies have attempted to histologically subdivide nodular sclerosing Hodgkin's disease into prognostically distinct groups [8–13]. Most of these studies subclassified nodular sclerosis into lymphocyte predominant, mixed cellularity and lymphocyte depleted types on the basis of the cellular background and the relative number of lacunar and Reed-Sternberg cells. Cross [8], on the other hand, subdivided nodular sclerosis into well and poorly differentiated forms by assessing the number of mature lymphocytes present and the degree of anaplasia of the 'reticulum cells'. In this histologic study of nodular sclerosis, we have used not only the cellular background and relative numbers of lacunar and Reed-Sternberg cells, but also have utilized the degree of cytologic atypia of the Hodgkin's cells as a basis for subdivision.

We present here a histologic review of 1156 patients with nodular sclerosing Hodgkin's disease, which we believe to be the largest published series. Our observations endorse the conclusions of other workers that subtypes with lymphocyte depleted cytology have a reduced survival when compared to those with lymphocyte predominant cytology. In addition we have shown that the mixed cellularity categories are divisible into two distinct prognostic groups, those with extensive areas of lymphocyte depleted or pleomorphic cytology being associated with a decreased survival. One interesting exception to this is mixed cellularity with areas of bland appearing, fibro-histiocytic lymphocyte depletion; this is not associated with a decreased survival. However, when the entire lymph node shows a fibro-histiocytic, lymphocyte depleted cytologic appearance, the survival is similar to the lymphocyte depleted group as a whole.

The difference in survival between the two histologic grades appears to be relatively independent of stage. The stage distribution between the two grades appears similar. In a group of patients in whom the anatomic extent of disease was accurately determined, either by staging laparotomy or by evidence of visceral organ involvement, the decreased survival of the Grade 2 histologic group, as compared to the Grade 1, is apparent in patients presenting with Stages I and II as well as in those presenting with Stages III and IV disease.

The presence of a reduced pretreatment hemoglobin or peripheral blood lymphocyte count, a raised ESR and the occurrence of systemic B symptoms, have been associated with a more aggressive natural history of Hodgkin's disease [4, 20, 21, 27, 28]. All these have been observed to have an increased relative frequency in the Grade 2 histologies, when compared to the Grade 1. We feel this may reflect the intrinsic malignant potential of this group.

In conclusion, we have been able to subdivide nodular sclerosis into two distinct prognostic grades on the basis of the cytologic appearances of the cellular nodules. Although other workers have been unable to show any prognostic relevance to histopathologic subtyping in Hodgkin's disease [29], we believe that the strict application of the cytologic criteria, originally proposed by Lukes and Butler [16, 25], to nodular sclerosis, will permit the recognition of a group of patients who have a poor prognosis. It also appears from this study that only easily recognized areas of pleomorphic or lymphocyte depleted cytology have prognostic relevance. This makes the subdivision of nodular sclerosing Hodgkin's disease, into favorable and poor prognostic groups, easy to perform without special training. The Grade 2 group constitutes approximately 30% of all cases of nodular sclerosis and these patients may require intensive therapy, even when it is confined to an early stage.

References

1. Kadin ME, Glatstein E and Dorfman RF (1971). Clinical-pathologic studies of 117 untreated patients subjected to laparotomy for the staging of Hodgkin's disease. Cancer 27:1277–1294.
2. Chelloul N, Burke J, Motteram R et al. (1972). HL-A antigens and Hodgkin's disease. Report on the histological analysis. In: Histocompatibility Testing. Copenhagen: Munkgaard.
3. Kirschener RH, Abt AB, O'Connell MJ et al. (1974). Vascular invasion and hematogenous dissemination of Hodgkin's disease. Cancer 34:1159–1162.
4. Kaplan HS (1980). Hodgkin's Disease. 2nd ed. Cambridge. Mass.: Harvard University Press.
5. Bergsagel DE, Alison RE, Beon HA et al. (1982). Results of treating Hodgkin's disease without a policy of staging laparotomy. Cancer Treat Rep 66:717–731.
6. Jelliffe AM and Vaughan Hudson G (1981). The evolution of the British National Lymphoma Investigation. Clin Radiol 32:483–490.
7. Noiman RS (1978). Current problems in the histopathological diagnosis and classification of Hodgkin's disease. Path Ann 13:289–328.
8. Cross RM (1968). A clinicopathologic study of nodular sclerosing Hodgkin's disease. J Clin Path 21:303–331.
9. Keller AR, Kaplan HS, Lukes RJ and Rappaport H (1968). Correlation of histopathology with other prognostic indicators in Hodgkin's disease. Cancer 22:437–499.
10. Patchevsky AS, Brodovsky H, Southard M et al. (1973). Hodgkin's disease. A clinical and pathological study of 235 cases. Cancer 32:150–161.
11. Cionini L, Argonini L, Biti GP and Bondi R (1978). Prognostic significance of histologic subdivision of Hodgkin's disease nodular sclerosis. Acta Radiologica (Oncology) 17:65–73.
12. Carbone A (1979). Histologic subclassification of nodular sclerosis Hodgkin's disease. Tumori 65:743–751.
13. Mann RB, Jaffee ES and Berard CW (1979). Malignant lymphomas, a conceptual understanding of morphologic diversity. Amer J Path 94:103–192.
14. Bennett MH, Tu A and Vaughan Hudson B (1981). Analysis of grade 1 Hodgkin's disease. Clin Radiol 32:491–498.
15. Bennett MH, MacLennan KA, Easterling MJ et al. (1983). The prognostic significance of cellular subtypes in nodular sclerosing Hodgkin's disease: An analysis of 271 non-laparotomised cases. Clin Radiol 34:497–501.
16. Lukes RJ and Butler JJ (1966). The pathology and nomenclature of Hodgkin's disease. Cancer Res 26:1063–1081.
17. Lukes RJ (1971). Criteria for involvement of lymph node, bone marrow, spleen and liver in Hodgkin's disease. Cancer Res 31:1755–1767.
18. Peto R, Pike MC, Armitage P et al. (1977). Design and analysis of randomized clinical trials requiring prolonged observation of each patient. II. Analysis and examples. Br J Cancer 35:1–39.
19. MacLennan KA, Vaughan Hudson B, Easterling MJ et al. (1983). The presentation haemoglobin level in 1103 patients with Hodgkin's disease. Clin Radiol 34:491–495.
20. MacLennan KA, Vaughan Hudson B, Jelliffe AM et al. (1981). The pretreatment peripheral blood lymphocyte count in 1100 patient with Hodgkin's disease: The prognostic significance and the relationship to the presence of systemic symptoms. Clin Oncol 7:333–339.
21. Jackson H Jr and Parker F Jr (1947). Hodgkin's Disease and Allied Disorders. New York: Oxford University Press.
22. Jelliffe AM and Thompson AD (1955). The prognosis in Hodgkin's disease. Brit J Cancer 9:21–36.

23. Smetana HF and Cohen BM (1956). Mortality in relation to histologic type in Hodgkin's disease. Blood 11:211–224.
24. Lukes RJ (1963). Relationship of histologic features to clinical stage in Hodgkin's disease. Amer J Roentgenol 90:944–955.
25. Lukes RJ, Butler JJ and Hickes EB (1966). Natural history of Hodgkin's disease as related to its pathologic picture. Cancer 19:317–344.
26. Strum SB and Rappaport H (1971). Interrelations of the histologic types of Hodgkin's disease. Arch Path 91:127–134.
27. Tubiana M, Attie E, Flamant R et al. (1971). Prognostic factors in 454 cases of Hodgkin's disease. Cancer Res 31:1801–1810.
28. Hoppe RT, Cox RS, Rosenberg SA and Kaplan HS (1982). Prognostic factors in pathologic Stage III Hodgkin's disease. Cancer Treat Rep 66:743–749.
29. Colby TV, Hoppe RT and Warnke RA (1982). Hodgkin's disease: A clinicopathologic study of 659 cases. Cancer 49:1848–1858.

2. Comparison of the Working Formulation of non-Hodgkin's lymphoma with the Rappaport, the Kiel, and the Lukes-Collins Classifications. Correlations and prognostic value

J. ERSBØLL, H. B. SCHULTZ, N. I. NISSEN, P. HOUGAARD and K. HOU-JENSEN
The Finsen Institute, and Statistical Research Unit, University of Copenhagen, Denmark

The Rappaport classification of non-Hodgkin's lymphoma [1] gained universal acceptance as a valuable basic diagnostic language for communication of therapeutic results among medical centers in the period 1968-75. Recognition that non-Hodgkin's lymphomas represent neoplasms of the lymphocytic immune system has resulted in new classifications based upon modern concepts of the T- and B-lymphocyte systems [2, 3]. Other newer classification schemes have challenged the terminology used by Rappaport [4–6], and the Rappaport system itself has been modified several times [7–9]. The existence and the use of many histologic classifications for the non-Hodgkin's lymphomas prompted the United States National Cancer Institute to sponsor a large international multi-institutional clinicopathologic study comparing six classifications. The results were published in 1982, and two important conclusions were reached [10]: 'First, each system is successful in separating a large group of patients into subgroups with a spectrum of prognoses varying from good to poor survival. Second, no system appears superior to any other in this respect'. Based on this study, the investigators reached consensus on a 'Working Formulation of non-Hodgkin's Lymphoma for Clinical Usage'.

Before an international classification can be generally accepted, its value should be confirmed independently in a number of large series. The purposes of this article are: 1) to evaluate the terminology of the Working Formulation in relation to three commonly used classifications—Rappaport, Kiel, Lukes-Collins—following the guidelines for translation of the NCI-sponsored study; and 2) to compare the prognostic value of the Working Formulation to that of the three established classifications. Our study is based on 658 consecutive patients with non-Hodgkin's lymphoma treated between 1970 and 1979 at the Finsen Institute in the Department of Internal Medicine.

Materials and methods

Criteria for inclusion in the study were reviewed and confirmed diagnosis of lymphoma, no previous therapy, as well as treatment and follow-up completed in our department. Six hundred and fifty-eight patients fulfilled these requirements.

Pathologic materials were reviewed by one pathologist (H.B.S.) without knowledge of the clinical history, and classified independently according to the Rappaport Classification [1], the Kiel Classification [2, 11], the Lukes-Collins Classification [3], and the Working Formulation [10]. Diagnoses were made on hematoxylin and eosin stained sections. Whenever possible, Giemsa, periodic acid-Schiff, reticulin, and methyl-green pyronin stained sections were also examined.

Medical records were reviewed and interpreted by one clinician (J.E.). All patients were staged according to the Ann Arbor system [12]. The department participates in the Cancer and Leukemia Group B, and all eligible patients with Stages III-IV disease were entered on six different CALGB studies. Combinations of cyclophosphamide, vincristine and prednisone were given in the period 1970-76. For unfavorable histologic subtypes doxorubicin was added in the period 1976-79, whereas patients with favorable

Table I. Translation guidelines as published in the NCI report [10]

Working Formulation	Rappaport	Kiel	Lukes-Collins
SL	DWDL	CLL, IC/1, IC/2	SL, PL
F-SC	NPDL	CB/CC	FCC-SC
F-M	NM	CB/CC	FCC-SC, FCC-LC
F-L	NH	CB/CC	FCC-LC, FCC-LNC
D-SC	DPDL	CC	FCC-SC
D-M	DM	CB/CC, IC/3	FCC-SC, LC, LNC
D-L	DH	CB/CC, CC, CB	FCC-LC, LNC
IB	DH	IB, T-zone	IBS (T-or B-cell type)
LB	LB	LB-conv, LB-NOS	T-convoluted
SNC	DU	LB-Burk, LB-NOS	FCC-SNC

Abbreviations: *Working Formulation:* F-(follicular), D-(diffuse), SL (small lymphocytic), SC (small cleaved cell), M (mixed small and large cell), L (large cell), IB (immunoblastic), LB (lymphoblastic), SNC (small noncleaved cell). *Rappaport classification:* D (diffuse), N (nodular), WDL (well differentiated lymphocytic), PDL (poorly differentiated lymphocytic), M (mixed lymphocytic-histiocytic) H (histiocytic), U (undifferentiated). *Kiel classification:* IC/1 (lymphoplasmacytic), IC/2 (lymphoplasmacytoid), IC/3 (lymphoplasmacytoid polymorphic), CB/CC (centroblastic/centrocytic), LB-conv (lymphoblastic, convoluted), LB-NOS (lymphoblastic unclassified), LB-Burk (LB, Burkitt's type). *Lukes-Collins classification:* PL (plasmacytoid lymphocytic), FCC (follicular center cell) LC (large cleaved cell), LNC (large noncleaved cell), SNC (small noncleaved cell, IBS (immunoblastic sarcoma), U-cell (undefined cell).

histologic subtypes received COP. For patients with Stage I-II, treatment consisted of extended field radiotherapy with or without combination chemotherapy as described [13]. Second line therapy varied.

All clinical and pathologic data were registered in a common form and computerized. The terms of the 10 major subtypes of the Working Formulation were compared one by one with the corresponding categories of the three other systems. The extent of accordance was assessed following the translation guidelines as indicated in the NCI-study (Table I shows the relations among terms of the 4 systems, and the abbreviations as used throughout this article).

Survival was measured from the date of diagnosis to the date of death or last date of follow-up: March 31, 1983. Survival curves were constructed using the Kaplan-Meier method [14] and compared with the logrank test [15]. The Cox proportional hazards model [16] was used to assess the relative effect of histologic subtype on prognosis after adjusting for the effect of age, sex, clinical stage and symptoms. For each classification, a standard histologic subtype with favorable prognosis was selected, to which all other subtypes were compared (Rappaport: NPDL; Kiel: CB/CC; Lukes-Collins: FCC-SC; Working Formulation: F-SC). The overall prognostic information of each system was also assessed with the Cox model by including two classifications simultaneously as covariates. The statistical significance of adding one classification to another was evaluated by a Chi-square test of change in maximized log-likelihood. A significance level ≥ 0.05 implies that no further information is provided, and that the two systems can be substituted for one another in terms of prognostic value.

Results

Six hundred and two patients could be classified according to the ten major subtypes of the Working Formulation. The distribution of diagnoses using all four systems is shown in Table II. Following the translation guidelines of the NCI-study (Table I) our results are commented upon to emphasize the similarities and discrepancies.

Interclassification comparisons and correlations

Follicular lymphomas.
Each of the four systems recognizes two principal types of architectural pattern, follicular or diffuse. In this comparative analysis we shall not distinguish between total and partial follicularity, since the Rappaport system makes no provision for such distinction. Within follicular lymphomas the

Table II. Distribution of diagnoses using four classifications

Working Formulation		Rappaport		Kiel		Lukes-Collins	
SL	(51)	DWDL	(40)	CLL	(26)	PL	(23)
		DPDL	(9)	IC/2	(16)	B-SL	(15)
		DM	(2)	IC/1	(7)	T-SL	(13)
				IC/3	(1)		
				CC	(1)		
F-SC	(93)	NPDL	(89)	CB/CC	(89)	FCC-SC	(91)
		NM	(4)	CC	(5)	FCC-LC	(2)
F-M	(34)	NM	(29)	CB/CC	(33)	FCC-LC	(34)
		NPDL	(5)	IC/3	(1)		
F-L	(23)	NH	(23)	CB	(20)	FCC-LNC	(20)
				CB/CC	(2)	FCC-LC	(1)
				IB	(1)	FCC-SNC	(1)
						B-IBS	(1)
D-SC	(32)	DPDL	(30)	CC	(16)	FCC-SC	(32)
		DWDL	(2)	CB/CC	(16)		
D-M	(50)	DM	(26)	CB/CC	(19)	FCC-LC	(37)
		DPDL	(22)	IC/3	(13)	LEL	(5)
		DH	(2)	CC	(9)	PL	(2)
				LEL	(5)	T-IBS	(2)
				IB	(1)	B-IBS	(3)
				T-zone	(1)	T-SL	(1)
				others	(2)	others	(1)
D-L	(76)	DH	(71)	IB	(35)	FCC-LNC	(55)
		DPDL	(3)	LB-NOS	(15)	FCC-LC	(12)
		DU	(2)	others	(10)	U-cell	(8)
				IC/3	(5)	others	(1)
				CC	(4)		
				CB	(4)		
				CB/CC	(3)		
IB	(146)	DH	(97)	IB	(100)	B-IBS	(98)
		DM	(43)	LEL	(24)	T-IBS	(24)
		DU	(4)	IC/3	(18)	LEL	(24)
		DPDL	(2)	T-zone	(4)		
LB	(66)	DPDL	(38)	LB-NOS	(40)	U-cell	(39)
		DU	(18)	LB-conv	(25)	T-conv	(25)
		DH	(10)	IB	(1)	IBS	(2)
SNC	(31)	DU	(25)	LB-Burk	(24)	FCC-SNC	(31)
		DH	(4)	LB-NOS	(4)		
		NH	(2)	CB	(2)		
				others	(1)		

number of cytologic subtypes ranges from one (Kiel system) to three (Rappaport and Lukes-Collins systems, the Working Formulation). Lymphomas categorized as follicular in the Working Formulation were in 98% to 100% of the cases also recognized as follicular in the three other systems. The extent of accordance for F-SC and F-M lymphomas was high, since 96% to 98%, and 85% to 100% of the cases respectively were correctly assigned into related terms of the reference systems. The F-L subtype was translated into related terms of the Rappaport and Lukes-Collins systems in 100% and 86% of the cases respectively. In contrast, our interpretation of the equivalent term to F-L in the Kiel system differed from the translation guidelines. According to the NCI-study, the F-L subtype is equivalent to CB/CC (with large centrocytes and a large number of centroblasts). Our F-L category corresponded to CB in 86% of the cases. Such interpretation is consistent with results of the Kiel Lymphoma Study Group [17] who divided the nodular histiocytic subtype of Rappaport (equivalent to F-L) into CB (63%) and CB/CC (22%). The criteria for separating a CB/CC lymphoma with a high content of centroblasts from a CB lymphoma are not well-defined, and the actual number of centroblasts is not the decisive factor. The existence of follicular centroblastic lymphomas has not been foreseen in the NCI-study.

Diffuse small cell lymphomas.
Each system makes provision for a lymphoma entity with histologic features indistinguishable from the tissue manifestations of chronic lymphocytic leukemia. This entity can be further subdivided depending upon the presence or absence of plasmacytoid lymphocytes. In the Working Formulation the subtypes is termed small lymphocytic. For SL lymphomas the extent of accordance varied between 78% (Rappaport system) and 100% (Lukes-Collins system). Cases with a higher number of mitotic figures were classified as DPDL lymphomas in the Rappaport system.

The Working Formulation introduces a lymphoma subtype termed diffuse small cleaved cell which represents the diffuse counterpart of the follicular lymphoma of corresponding cell type. The translation guidelines seem illogical, since the same diffuse lymphoma composed of predominantly small cleaved cells (centrocytes), and a few large noncleaved cells (centroblasts) will be translated into two different categories of the Working Formulation depending upon the use of the Kiel system (D-M) or the Lukes-Collins system (D-SC). Consequently, the Kiel system separated the D-SC subtype into CB/CC (50%) and CC (50%). For the other systems, 94% (Rappaport system) and 100% (Lukes-Collins system) of the cases were correctly translated.

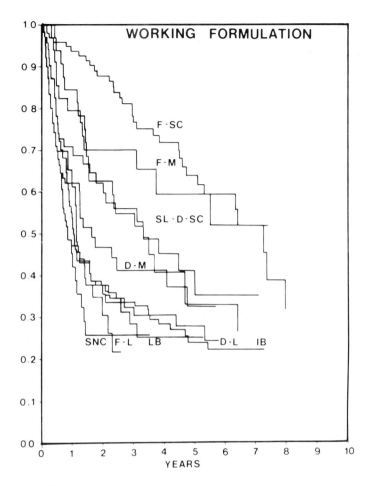

Figure 1. Survival according to the Working Formulation.

Diffuse large cell lymphomas.

Large cell lymphomas encompass the D-M, D-L, and IB subtypes of the Working Formulation. The cellular composition of these lymphomas is rarely monomorphic, and the borderlines among subtypes are not always well-defined. The many attempts of subdividing the diffuse histiocytic subtype of Rappaport into different morphologic subsets with or without different prognoses reflect the difficulties in classifying these lymphomas. Most inconcistencies between the translation guidelines and our classification results were observed in large cell lymphoma categories. Summarizing the results, the heterogeneous mixed cell subtype was translatable in 51% (Rappaport system), 65% (Kiel system), and 75% (Lukes-Collins system) of the cases. The D-L subtype was correctly translated in 13% (Kiel system), 89% (Lukes-Collins system), and 95% (Rappaport system) of the cases. The IB

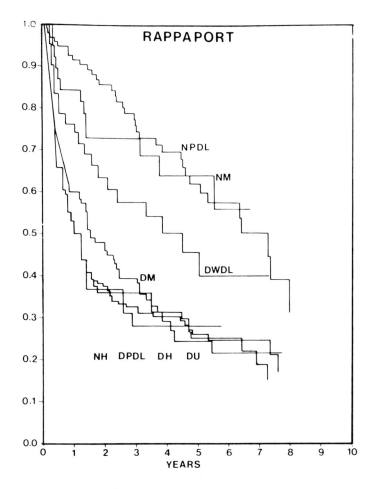

Figure 2. Survival according to the Rappaport classification.

subtype corresponded to related terms in 66% (Rappaport system), 88% (Kiel system), and 100% (Lukes-Collins system) of the cases. Our interpretation of the term 'immunoblastic' and its separation from 'centroblastic' accounts for the defective translation of the D-L subtype into related terms of the Kiel system. The criteria for classifying a lymphoma as CB have changed in the last decade. In the original Kiel series [2] the CB subtype was rare (0.5% of all lymphomas), in the current version of the Kiel system [11] it represents 5.5% of the population, and in the prospective study of the Kiel Group [17] the frequency has increased to 13%. Another example of different interpretation of the term 'immunoblastic' is given in one of the reports on the NCI-study [18]. The diffuse histiocytic subtype of Rappaport was subclassified by Lukes using the Lukes-Collins system, and by Lennert using the Kiel system. The term 'immunoblastic' was used by Lukes in 20%

208

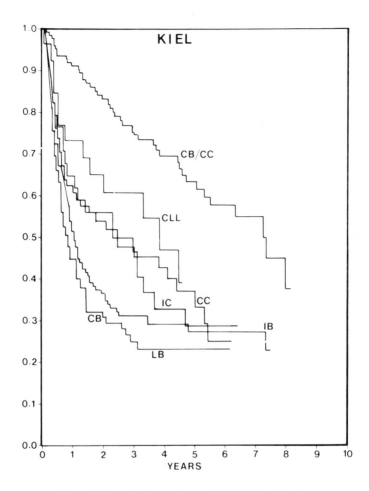

Figure 3. Survival according to the Kiel classification.

of the cases, and by Lennert in 40% of the cases. In the present study only the monomorphic subtype of CB was recognized as CB, the polymorphic subtype was in most cases categorized as IB or other subtypes of the high malignancy grouping.

Lymphoblastic and small noncleaved cell lymphomas.
The lymphoblastic lymphoma entity has equivalents in both the Rappaport and the Kiel systems, regardless of the subdivision into convoluted nuclei or non-convoluted nuclei subtypes. Our comparisons showed an almost 100% accordance between these two systems and the Working Formulation considering the LB subtype. In contrast, only the convoluted nuclei subtype of Lukes-Collins is included in the LB category. The NCI-report offers no directions for translating the nonconvoluted nuclei subtype into related

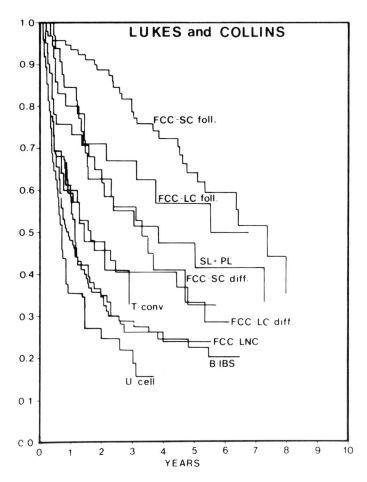

Figure 4. Survival according to the Lukes-Collins classification.

terms of the Lukes-Collins system. In our study the LB subtype was separated into convoluted cell type (38%) and undefined cell type (59%) using the Lukes-Collins system.

The small noncleaved cell type encompasses two entities, the Burkitt and non-Burkitt subtypes. The extent of accordance among systems was high since 81% (Rappaport), 90% (Kiel), and 100% (Lukes-Collins) of the cases were correctly assigned to related categories.

Prognostic significance of the Working Formulation

Survival curves for each system are shown in Fig. 1, 2, 3 and 4. In keeping with the results of the NCI-study, examination of the curves demonstrated

Table III. The prognostic significance of histologic subtype evaluated by Cox analysis [a]

Working Formulation	RR	p	Rappaport	RR	p	Kiel	RR	p	Lukes-Collins	RR	p
F-SC	1.00	–	NPDL	1.00	–	CB/CC	1.00	–	FCC-SC	1.00	–
F-M	1.43	0.27	NM	1.03	0.93	IC/1	106	0.92	B-SL	1.00	0.99
SL	1.61	0.07	DWDL	1.26	0.41	CLL	1.16	0.62	T-SL	1.39	0.37
D-SC	1.68	0.06	DPDL	2.85	0.0001	IC/2	1.65	0.14	PL	1.68	0.08
D-M	2.61	0.0002	DM	2.88	0.0001	CC	1.93	0.004	FCC-LC	1.85	0.02
D-L	3.28	0.0001	DU	3.22	0.0001	IC/3	2.36	0.0003	T-IBS	2.20	0.02
SNC	3.56	0.0001	DH	3.42	0.0001	T-zone	2.63	0.18	LEL	3.06	0.0001
IB	3.89	0.0001	NH	4.35	0.0001	LEL	2.83	0.0001	FCC-LNC	3.22	0.0001
F-L	4.22	0.0001				IB	3.00	0.0001	FCC-SNC	3.28	0.0001
LB	5.00	0.0001				LB-Burk	3.56	0.0001	B-IBS	3.52	0.0001
						CB	3.63	0.0001	U-cell	4.66	0.0001
						LB-NOS	3.74	0.0001	T-conv	5.20	0.0001
						LB-conv	4.76	0.0001			

[a] Age, sex, Ann Arbor Stage, and symptoms included in the Cox model

that each system was equal to any other in separating a population into subpopulations with prognoses ranging from a median survival of > 7 years to < 1 year. Table III shows the results of the Cox analyses for each of the systems after the adjustment for the prognostic effect of age, sex, clinical stage and symptoms at presentation. Besides the prognostic significance of histologic subtype, poor survival was associated with higher age, male sex, Stages II-IV disease and presence of B-symptoms when considering the total population. The results of the Cox analysis demonstrated that our intermediate malignancy grouping was prognostically heterogeneous, since the D-SC subtype had a relative risk and survival similar to those of the SL subtype (median survival 3.5 years), whereas the F-L and D-L subtypes had survivals not different from those of other subtypes of the high grade grouping (median survival 1.1 years). Another important result of the Cox analyses was that lymphomas belonging to related entities within the four classifications had relative risk values of the same magnitude.

Table IV provides an example of the Cox analyses including two schemes simultaneously. The relative risk values can be used for an analysis of the following issues: 1) the significance of plasmacytoid lymphocytes in SL lymphomas; 2) the significance of follicular architectural pattern in lymphomas that are cytologically identical; 3) the significance of the subdivision of large cell lymphomas into FCC types and non-FCC types; and 4) the overall

Table IV. Cox analysis including two schemes simultaneously. Working Formulation by Lukes-Collins

Working Formulation	F-SC	F-M	SL	D-SC	D-M	D-L	SNC	IB	F-L	LB
Lukes-Collins										
FCC-SC	1.00			1.82						
B-SL			1.18							
T-SL			1.73							
PL			2.14							
FCC-LC		1.52		2.85	3.16					
T-IBS								2.83		
LEL								3.97		
FCC-LNC					3.93				4.22	
FCC-SNC							4.01			
B-IBS								4.48		
U-cell					14.58					5.10
T-conv										6.29

The relative risk values have to be compared to the risk value of the combined subset FCC-SC/F-SC = 1. The Cox model includes age, sex, Ann Arbor Stage and symptoms. Subsets with less than 5 patients are omitted prognostic information of adding one scheme to another. Summarizing the results, the following conclusions were reached: 1) The presence or absence of plasmacytoid differentiation within SL lymphomas had no prognostic significance; 2) the presence of follicular pattern within the same cytologic subtypes (F-SC vs D-SC, F-M vs D-M, and F-L vs D-L) implied a favorable prognosis significantly superior to that of the diffuse counterpart, except for the F-L subtype in which the importance of pattern was wiped out by the importance of cell type; 3) no significant difference in prognosis was evident when comparing the FCC and non-FCC subtypes of large cell lymphomas; and 4) addition of each of the three established classifications to the Working Formulation in the Cox model provided no further prognostic information ($p \geq 0.05$).

Discussion

The terminologic analysis demonstrated that the Working Formulation is more similar to American systems than to the Kiel system. However, the conceptual differences between the Kiel classification and the Working Formulation are altogether of minor importance and at least some of them can be removed by small adjustments of the translation guidelines. The overall accordance between our classification results and the translation guidelines of the NCI study was high, since 75% (Kiel system), 82% (Rappaport system), and 89% (Lukes-Collins system) of our non-Hodgkin's lymphomas were correctly assigned to related categories of the Working Formulation.

The prognostic value of the Working Formulation was in our study equal to that of the three reference systems, and none of these was superior to any other in predicting prognosis. We find the Working Formulation useful with a terminology which is simple and easily understood, but do we really need it as a new classification? The modified Rappaport scheme is very similar to the Working Formulation, and it suffices to substitute the term 'nodular' with 'follicular', and to separate the diffuse 'histiocytic' subtype into 'large cell' and 'immunoblastic' subtypes, after which the two systems are identical for practical purpose.

Acknowledgements

The project was supported by grants from the Danish Cancer Society, the Danish Medical Research Counsil, and the Elna C. Nielsen Foundation. The authors thank Niels Keiding, Head of the Statistical Research Unit, University of Copenhagen for his advices and discussions. The assistance of Mr. Michael Davidsen is greatly appreciated.

References

1. Rappaport H (1966). Tumors of the hemopoietic system. In: Atlas of Tumor Pathology, Section 3, Fascicle 8. Washington DC: US Armed forces Institute of Pathology.
2. Lennert K, Mohri N, Stein H and Kaiserling E (1975). The histopathology of malignant lymphoma. Br J Haematol (suppl) 31:193–203.
3. Lukes RJ and Collins RD (1974). Immunologic characterization of human malignant lymphomas. Cancer 34:1488–1503.
4. Dorfman RF (1974). Classification of non-Hodgkin's lymphoma. Lancet 1:1295.
5. Bennett MH, Farrer-Brown G, Henry K and Jelliffe AM (1974). Classification of non-Hodgkin's lymphomas. Lancet 2:405–406.
6. Mathe G, Rappaport H, O'Conor GT and Torlani H (1976). Histological and cytological typing of neoplastic diseases of hemopoietic and lymphoid tissues. In: WHO International Histological Classification of Tumours, no 14. Geneva: World Health Organization.
7. Nathwani BN, Kim H and Rappaport H (1976). Malignant lymphoma lymphoblastic. Cancer 38:964–983.
8. Rappaport H 1977). Non-Hodgkin's lymphomas: Roundtable discussion of histopathologic classifications. Cancer Treat Rep 61:1037–1042.
9. Nathwani BN (1979). A critical analysis of the classifications of non-Hodgkin's lymphomas. Cancer 44:347–384.
10. The Non-Hodgkin's Lymphoma Pathologic Classification Project (1982). National Cancer Institute sponsored study of classification of non-Hodgkin's lymphomas: Summary and description of a working formulation for clinical usage. Cancer 49:2112–2135.
11. Lennert K and Mohri N (1978). Histopathology and diagnosis of non-Hodgkin's lymphomas. In: Malignant Lymphomas Other Than Hodgkin's Disease, pp. 111–469. New York: Springer Verlag.
12. Carbone PP, Kaplan HS, Musshoff K et al. (1971). Report on the Committee on Hodgkin's Disease Staging Classification. Cancer Res 31:1860–1861.
13. Nissen NI, Ersbøll J, Hansen HS et al. (1983). Randomized study of radiotherapy versus radiotherapy plus chemotherapy in stage I-II non-Hodgkin's lymphomas. Cancer 52:1–7.
14. Kaplan EL and Meier P (1958). Nonparametric estimation from incomplete observations. Amer J Stat Assoc J 53:457–481.
15. Peto R, Pike MC, Armitage P et al. (1977). Design and analysis of randomized clinical trials requiring prolonged observation of each patient. II. Analysis and examples. Br J Cancer 35:1–39.
16. Cox DR (1972). Regression models and life tables (with discussion). J Roy Statist Soc B 34:187–220.
17. Krüger G, Grisar T, Lennert K et al. (1981). Histopathological correlation of the Kiel with original Rappaport classification of malignant non-Hodgkin's lymphomas. Blut 43:167–181.
18. Hoppe RT (1982). A Working Formulation of Non-Hodgkin's Lymphomas for Clinical Usage: Clinicopathological and prognostic correlations. In: Rosenberg SA and Kaplan HS (Eds.). Malignant Lymphomas. Etiology, Immunology, Pathology, Treatment, pp. 469–483. New York: Academic Press.

3. Bone marrow and blood involvement by non-Hodgkin's lymphoma: Clinicopathologic features and prognostic significance in relationship to the Working Formulation

E. MORRA [1], M. LAZZARINO [1], E. ORLANDI [1],
D. INVERARDI [1], A. CASTELLO [2], A. COCI [2], U. MAGRINI [2]
and C. BERNASCONI [1]
[1] *Divisione di Ematologia, Ospedale Policlinico San Matteo and*
[2] *Istituto di Anatomia ed Istologia Patologica, Università di Pavia,
Pavia, Italy*

Bone marrow (BM) biopsy is a valuable staging procedure for patients with malignant non-Hodgkin's lymphomas (NHL). In cases presenting with nodal involvement, a positive bone marrow finding would allow diagnosis of Stage IV disease without the need for more aggressive procedures. Previous studies have evaluated the frequency and pattern of bone marrow involvement in the various pathologic subtypes of the NHL classified according to the Rappaport [1–5], Lukes and Collins [6, 7], and Kiel [8–11] schemes. Furthermore, the results of Bartl's study [10] applying the Kiel classification to BM biopsies, indicated the prognostic significance of BM disease in NHL. As concerns peripheral blood involvement by malignant lymphomas, the leukemic phase has been the subject of several studies, all based on the Rappaport [12–14], Lukes and Collins [7], WHO [15, 16] and Kiel systems [17].

To date, no studies have been reported on BM and blood disease in NHL, classified using the NCI sponsored New Working Formulation (NWF) of NHL [18]. The current study was therefore undertaken with the aim of assessing clinico-pathologic features and prognostic significance of BM and blood involvement in 137 consecutive cases of NHL, classified according to the NWF.

Materials and methods

One hundred and thirty-seven consecutive previously untreated adult patients with NHL, diagnosed at the Division of Hematology, Policlinico S. Matteo, Pavia, from January 1978 to March 1983 were classified using the Kiel system and reviewed according to the New Working Formulation. In the majority of patients (114 cases) the diagnosis was made by examination of lymph node biopsies. Single cases with primary extranodal involvement were diagnosed by biopsies from other sites: skin (6 cases), gastrointestinal tract (12 cases), orbital tissues (2 cases), bone marrow (2 cases), uterus (1 case). The patients ranged in age from 16 to 73 years. There were 79 males and 58 females. The median time of follow-up was 23 months (range 3–70+). The minimum follow-up period for surviving patients was 12 months. Patients with CLL, as well as cases with lymphoblastic lymphoma with blood and BM disease undistinguishable from acute lymphoblastic leukemia were excluded from this study. The extent of the disease was staged according to the Ann Arbor classification. All cases underwent unilateral BM biopsy and peripheral blood examination as part of their initial evaluation. The BM biopsies were obtained from the posterior superior iliac spine with Jamshidi needles, fixed, dehydrated and embebbed in plastic without decalcification. Sections were cut 2–3 μ thick and stained with Giemsa or Dominici for cytologic details, and Gomori's silver impregnation for reticulin fibres [19].

The adopted criteria for BM and blood involvement have been reported in prior studies [10, 17]. Four major patterns of lymphoma involvement were defined: 1) diffuse interstitial with minimal replacement of BM cells, 2) diffuse massive with extensive replacement of BM cells, 3) focal with paratrabecular location, and 4) focal non paratrabecular with nodular infiltrates randomly distributed in the central intertrabecular areas. The extent of BM disease was classified into three categories: < 30% replacement, 30–70%, and greater than 70% replacement of hematopoietic BM cells. Blood specimens were obtained at diagnosis and subsequently at each monthly visit. BM examination was usually repeated as part of restaging after treatment and in case of relapse or progressive disease. The initial treatment of the 55 patients classified by the NWF as having low grade malignant lymphoma (LGML), and of the 56 cases with intermediate grade malignant lymphoma (IGML) consisted of radiotherapy alone or radiotherapy followed by chemotherapy (chlorambucil or CVP) in most patients with Stages I and II. Patients with advanced disease (Stages III and IV) were treated with the CVP regimen. The 26 patients with high grade malignant lymphoma (HGML) were given intensive chemotherapy programs including vincristine, anthracyclines, cyclophosphamide, bleomycin and prednisone. The same regimens were used in cases of documented histologic progression towards high grade malignancy. Survival was measured from histologic diagnosis of lymphoma and from the onset of the leukemic phase. Survival curves were calculated according to Berkson and Gage [20] and compared by the generalized Wilcoxon technique of Gehan [21]. The corrected X^2 test was used for percentage differences.

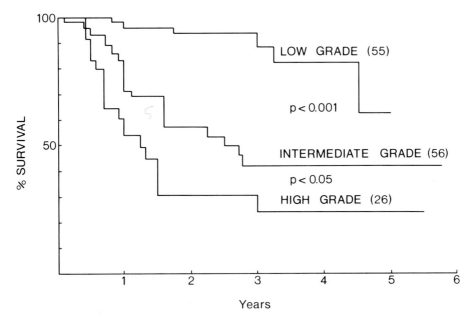

Figure 1. Actuarial survival of 137 patients with NHL grouped into the three major prognostic categories of the Working Formulation.

Results

Table I shows the classification of the 137 cases according to the Kiel system and the NWF of non-Hodgkin's lymphomas. Fig. 1 reports the actuarial survival curves of all cases grouped into the three major prognostic categories of the NWF.

The overall incidence of BM involvement at diagnosis was 38 % (52/137). The frequencies of BM disease in the three major NWF groups were the following: 51 % (28/55) for LGML, 32 % (18/56) for IGML, and 23 % (6/26) for HGML (Table II). As concerns the proliferation pattern, the paratrabecular location was characteristic of cases in which small cleaved cells predominated in the bone marrow. If we consider the prognostic significance of BM status at the time of diagnosis, the survival curves of LGML, IGML, and HGML were not significantly affected by the presence or absence of marrow disease (Fig. 2). Nevertheless, among the 52 patients with BM infiltration at diagnosis, a focal pattern of involvement and a low extent of marrow disease (< 30 % replacement) discriminated groups with better prognosis (Fig. 3). Fifty-three patients had two or more BM biopsies. Of 29 patients with BM disease at diagnosis who underwent repeat BM histology, the disappearance of marrow involvement at restaging after primary chemotherapy was obtained, independently of the degree of malignancy, in 13

Table I. Classification of 137 consecutive cases of NHL according to the Kiel system and the Working Formulation

Kiel		Working Formulation		Grade	
Lymphocytic	(13)	Small lymphocytic	(28)	LOW GRADE	(55)
Lymphoplasmacytic/lymphoplasmacytoid	(15)				
Cb/Cc (small), foll. ± diff.	(27)	Follicular, small cleaved cell	(20)		
		Follicular, mixed, small cleaved and large cell	(7)		
Cb/Cc (large), foll ± diff.	(2)	Follicular, large cell	(2)	INTERMEDIATE GRADE	(56)
Cc (small)	(9)	Diffuse, small cleaved cell	(9)		
Cb/Cc (small), diff.	(12)	Diffuse, mixed, small and large cell	(26)		
Lymphoplasmacytic/-cytoid, polymorphic	(14)				
Cc (large)	(2)	Diffuse, large cell	(19)		
Cb/Cc (large), diff.	(1)				
Cb	(16)				
Immunoblastic	(16)	Immunoblastic	(16)	HIGH GRADE	(26)
Lymphoblastic convoluted	(4)	Lymphoblastic convoluted	(4)		
Lymphoblastic unclassified	(6)	Lymphoblastic nonconcoluted	(6)		
Lymphoblastic, Burkitt	–	Small noncleaved cell	–		

Cb: centroblastic; Cc: centrocytic.

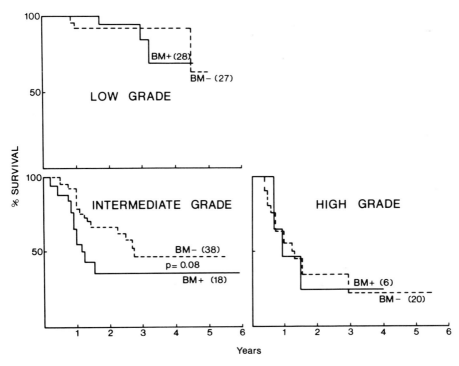

Figure 2. Actuarial survival of low grade, intermediate grade and high grade malignant lymphomas according to bone marrow involvement at diagnosis.

cases (45%). All these showed a low extent (<30%) of marrow disease at diagnosis whereas the median BM replacement at diagnosis was 60% (range 20–98%) in the remaining 16 patients. Nevertheless, survival was not significantly improved by the clearing of BM infiltration.

Peripheral blood involvement by lymphoma, detected by routine hematologic investigation, was found at diagnosis in 16% of all cases (22/137)

Table II. Incidence of BM and blood involvement in 137 patients with NHL grouped into the three major prognostic types of the WF

| | No. of cases | BM+ at diagnosis | Leukemic patients | | | Median time to leukemic conversion (mos) |
			Total No. of cases	Leukemic at presentation	Leukemic during course	
LGML	55	28	19	12	7	12
IGML	56	18	16	7	9	10
HGML	26	6	10	3	7	7
Total	137	52	45	22	23	

220

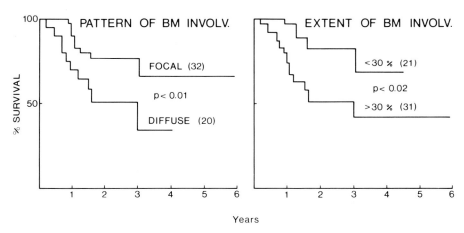

Figure 3. Actuarial survival according to the pattern and extent of BM involvement in 52 NHL with BM disease at diagnosis.

and in 42% (22/52) of patients with marrow disease at presentation (Table II). Additional 23 patients developed leukemic spread during their clinical course, after a median time from diagnosis of 10 months. Thirteen of them did not show BM infiltration at presentation, but all developed BM disease

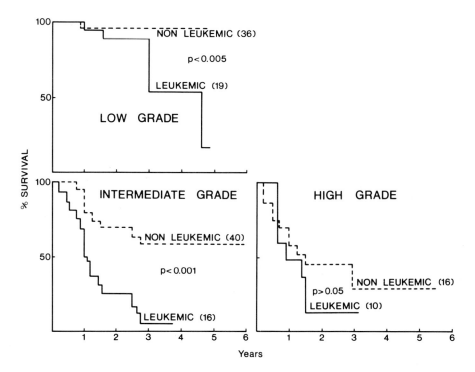

Figure 4. Actuarial survival of low grade, intermediate grade and high grade malignant lymphomas in relation to the occurrence of blood involvement.

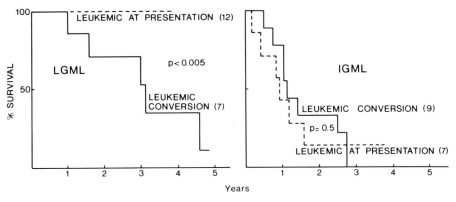

Figure 5. Actuarial survival of leukemic low grade and intermediate grade malignant lymphomas according to the time of blood involvement.

at the time of leukemic conversion. Therefore, the overall incidence of peripheral blood involvement by lymphoma was 33% (45/137). In 27 out of 35 patients (77%) who underwent trephine biopsy at the time of leukemic spread, the pattern of BM manifestations was predominantly diffuse. Comparison of the survival curves of all leukemic and non-leukemic cases shows that leukemic spread significantly affects prognosis of LGML and IGML (Fig. 4). On the other hand, the analysis of survival curves of leukemic patients in these two NWF groups according to the time of blood involvement (Fig. 5) showed that survival of LGML with subsequent leukemic progression was significantly shorter than that of patients who were leukemic at the time of diagnosis. In fact, a shift to a less differentiated lymph node histology was documented in five LGML patients with late leukemic spread. These patients exhibited a BM histology and a cytologic peripheral pattern mainly characterized by mature cells, even when nodal histology at that moment showed conversion to a less differentiated cell type. Once leukemic progression occurred, the median survival did not exceed 7 months. These cases of secondary leukemic conversion of LGML proved to be associated with less responsive disease, more extensive BM involvement in all cases and clinical features more typical of HGML: systemic symptoms (6/7), bulky disease (6/7), mediastinal masses (2/7). In contrast to LGML, in patients with IGML, either initial or subsequent blood involvement was associated with the same poor prognosis (Fig. 5). As regards HGML, the median survival of leukemic and non-leukemic cases did not differ statistically (Fig. 4).

Discussion

In this study on 137 consecutive patients with non-Hodgkin's lymphoma classified according to the NWF, the overall incidence of BM involvement at diagnosis was 38% (52/137), which agrees well with most of the frequency figures previously reported [2–5]. A 69% incidence of BM involvement has been reported by Barthl et al. [10] in a large series including CLL and hairy cell leukemias. In our study, the frequencies of BM disease in the three major prognostic groups of the NWF were the following: 51% (28/55) for LGML, 32% (18/56) for IGML and 23% (6/26) for HGML. As regards the prognostic value of BM involvement, the survival curves obtained grouping patients into LGML, IGML and HGML were not significantly affected by the presence or absence of marrow disease at presentation (Fig. 2). This finding is in agreement with previous reports using the Rappaport [22] or the Kiel classification [10] but differs from the Stanford experience [23]. Our results confirm the lymph node histology as the major determinant of prognosis independently of the bone marrow status. Nevertheless, among patients with BM infiltration at diagnosis, a focal pattern of proliferation and a low extent of marrow disease (< 30% replacement) discriminated groups with better prognosis (Fig. 3).

Peripheral blood involvement by lymphoma was found at diagnosis in 16% (22/137) of all cases and in 42% (22/52) of patients presenting with marrow disease (Table II). This frequency of blood involvement is consistent with the 14% incidence figure found using similar diagnostic criteria [13]. Additional 23 cases showed leukemic spread during clinical course, after a median time of 10 months from diagnosis. Regarding the clinical significance of the leukemic spread in LGML, our analysis does demonstrate that the prognostic importance of blood involvement is different according to the time of its occurrence. In fact, peripheral blood involvement at diagnosis did not affect survival of patients with LGML. This seems to be related to the 'physiological' mechanism of spread of these mature lymphoma cells, the dissemination pattern of which is not invasive and closely resembles the recirculation process typical of their normal counterparts [24]. In contrast, subsequent leukemic conversion heralded a rapid change to a more aggressive disease (Fig. 5). Indeed, a shift to a less differentiated lymph node histology was documented in five patients with late leukemic conversion. In patients with IGML, either initial or subsequent blood involvement was associated significantly with the same poor prognosis. As regards HGML, the median survival of leukemic and non-leukemic cases did not differ statistically.

Two major conclusions can be drawn from this study. First, the presence of BM infiltration *per se* within each of the three major prognostic groups of the NWF seems not to affect survival. Second, whereas leukemic presentation in LGML has no important effect on the outcome of the disease, late leukemic conversion of LGML and leukemic spread of IGML, whenever it occurs, are associated with a worse prognosis.

Acknowledgements

The authors thank miss Giancarla Motta for skillful secretarial help.

References

1. Rappaport H (1966). Tumor of the hematopoietic system. In: Atlas of Tumor Pathology, section 3, fascicle 8. Washington DC: US Armed Forces Institute of Pathology.
2. Dick R, Bloomfield CD and Brunning RD (1974). Incidence, cytology, and hystopathology of non-Hodgkin's lymphomas in the bone marrow. Cancer 33:1382–1398.
3. McKenna RW, Bloomfield CD and Brunning RD (1975). Nodular lymphoma and blood manifestations. Cancer 36:428–440.
4. Stein RS, Ultmann JE, Byrne GE et al. (1976). Bone marrow involvement in the non-Hodgkin's lymphoma. Cancer 37:629–636.
5. Coller BS, Chabner BA and Gralnick HR (1977). Frequencies and patterns of bone marrow involvement in non-Hodgkin lymphomas: Observations on the value of bilateral biopsies. Amer J Hemat 3:105–119.
6. Lukes RJ and Collins RD (1974). Immunological characterization of human malignant lymphomas. Cancer 34:1488–1503.
7. Foucar F, McKenna R, Frizzera G and Brunning RD (1982). Bone marrow and blood involvement by lymphoma in relationship to the Lukes-Collins classification. Cancer 49:888–897.
8. Lennert K, Mohri N, Stein H and Kaiserling E (1975). The histopathology of malignant lymphoma. Br J Haemat (suppl) 31:193–203.
9. Lennert K, Mohri N, Stein H et al. (1978). Malignant lymphomas other than Hodgkin's disease. Histology-Cytology-Ultrastructure. Immunology. Berlin, Heidelberg, New York: Springer Verlag.
10. Bartl R, Frisch B, Burkhardt R et al. (1982). Assessment of bone marrow histology in the malignant lymphomas (non-Hodgkin's). Correlation with clinical factors for diagnosis, prognosis, classification and staging. Br J Haematol 51:511–530.
11. Brusamolino R, Magrini U, Canevari A et al. (1983). Low-grade malignancy non-Hodgkin's lymphomas: Prognostic relevance of their clinicopathologic heterogeneity. Tumori 69:331–338.
12. Schnitzer B, Loesel LS and Reed RE (1970). Lymphosarcoma cell leukemia: A clinicopathologic study. Cancer 26:1082–1096.
13. Come SE, Jaffe ES, Andersen JC et al. (1980). Non-Hodgkin's lymphomas in leukemic phase: Clinicopathologic correlations. Amer J Med 69:667–674.
14. Fram RJ, Skarin AT, Rosenthal DS et al. (1983). Clinical, pathologic and immunologic features of patients with non-Hodgkin's lymphoma in a leukemic phase. A retrospective analysis of 34 patients. Cancer 52:1220–1228.
15. Mathé G, Rappaport H, O'Connor GT and Torlini H (1976). Histological typing of neoplastic diseases of haematopoietic and lymphoid tissues. In: WHO International Histological Classification of Tumors, n. 14 Geneva World Health Organization.
16. Mathé G, Misset JL, Gil-Delgado M and De Vassal F (1978). Leukemic (or stage V) lymphosarcoma. In: Mathé G, Seligmann M and Tubiana M (Eds.). Recent Results in Cancer Research, Lymphoid Neoplasias. II. Clinical and Therapeutic Aspects, pp. 88–107. Berlin, Heidelberg, New York: Springer Verlag.
17. Morra E, Lazzarino M, Orlandi E et al. (1984). Leukemic phase of non-Hodgkin's lymphoma. Hematological features and prognostic significance. Hematologica 69:15–29.
18. The Non-Hodgkin's Lymphoma Pathologic Classification Project. (1982). National Cancer

224

Institute sponsored study of classifications of non-Hodgkin's lymphomas. Cancer 49:2112–2135.

19. Magrini U, Castello A, Bossi A and Ascari E (1978). Allestimento della biopsia osteomidollare. In: Introzzi P. (Ed.). Trattato italiano di medicina interna. III, pp. 2323–2327. USES, Firenze.

20. Berkson J and Gage RP (1950). Calculation of survival rates for cancer. Proc Staff Meet Mayo Clin 25:270–278.

21. Gehan EA (1965). A generalized Wilcoxon test for comparing singly censored samples. Biometrika 52:203–223.

22. Straus DJ, Filippa DA, Liebermann PH et al. (1983). The non-Hodgkin's lymphomas. A retrospective clinical and pathologic analysis of 499 cases diagnosed between 1958 and 1969. Cancer 51:101–109.

23. Jones SE, Rosenberg SA and Kaplan HS (1972). Non-Hodgkin's lymphomas. I: Bone marrow involvement. Cancer 29:954–960.

24. Galton DAG, Catowsky D and Wiltshaw E (1978). Clinical spectrum of lympho-proliferative diseases. Cancer 42:901–910.

4. Clonal blood B-cell excess in relation to prognosis in untreated non-leukemic patients with non-Hodgkin's lymphoma (NHL)

C. LINDEMALM, H. MELLSTEDT, P. BIBERFELD,
M. BJÖRKHOLM, B. CHRISTENSSON, G. HOLM
and B. JOHANSSON
Radiumhemmet, Department of Radiobiology and Department of Pathology, Karolinska Hospital, Department of Medicine, Danderyd Hospital and Department of Clinical Immunology, Huddinge Hospital, Stockholm, Sweden

Non-Hodgkin's lymphoma (NHL) is a heterogeneous group of diseases which in the majority of cases are of B-cell origin [1]. An excess of B-cells carrying the same light chain isotype as the lymph node tumor cells (monoclonal B-lymphocytes) is often present in the blood of patients with normal lymphocyte counts indicating leukemic spread. This is not only seen in patients with advanced clinical stage, but sometimes also in patients with Stages I and II diseases [2–4]. Similar findings have been reported in other B lymphoproliferative disorders, such as multiple myeloma, Waldenström's macroglobulinemia and monoclonal gammopathy of undetermined significance [5, 6]. If the monoclonal B-lymphocytes belong to the tumor cell clone, the disease is apparently more disseminated than indicated by the clinical stage as determined by usual staging procedures. Such a dissemination may have prognostic implications. In this report, we describe the relation between circulating monoclonal B-lymphocytes and prognosis in non-leukemic NHL patients.

Materials and methods

Patients

The study enrolled 128 newly diagnosed and previously untreated, non-leukemic ($< 4.0 \times 10^9$ lymphocytes/l) NHL patients. The male/female ratio was 66/62 and the median age was 60 years (range 20–87 years). No patient had a concurrent non-lymphoid malignancy. The median observation time at follow-up was 37 months (range 8–84 months). The Kiel nomenclature [1] was used for histologic classification (Table I). Lymphomas referred to the group of low-grade malignancies were: lymphocytic lymphomas (LL);

immunocytomas (IC), centroblastic/centrocytic (CB/CC) and centrocytic (CC). High grade malignancies included centroblastic (CB), lymphoblastic (LB, immunoblastic (IB), and undifferentiated (NOS) lymphomas. Staging was accomplished by clinical evaluation, routine blood laboratory tests, computed tomography of the abdomen and spleen, X-rays of the chest, and bone marrow biopsies. Staging laparotomy was not performed routinely. The Ann Arbor staging classification was used [7].

Patients in Clinical Stages I and II with lymphomas of low grade malignancy, and patients in Clinical Stage I with lymphomas of high grade malignancy were treated by radiotherapy to a target dose of approximately 40 Gy, fractionated over 4 weeks. Patients in advanced stages were given cytostatic drug treatment. Low grade lymphoma patients received COP chemotherapy (cyclophosphamide, vincristine, prednisone) or chlorambucil/prednisone. Patients with high grade malignant lymphomas received either the CHOP combination (cyclophosphamide, doxorubicin, vincristine, prednisone) or CHOP and methotrexate with leucovorin rescue.

Complete remission (CR) was defined as disappearance of all tumor masses and signs of active disease, as ascertained by repeated staging procedures.

Control donors

Blood lymphocytes from 72 healthy persons were used as controls. The male/female ratio was 1:1 and the mean age was 50 years (range 30–75). All controls had normal blood lymphocyte counts. None had signs of infectious or inflammatory disease.

Table I. Clonal B-cell excess in blood of NHL patients in relation to histology and clinical stage

Histology	Clinical Stage				Total	
	I	II	III	IV		
LL	—	—	—	3/3	3/3	(100%)
IC	0/7	0/1	1/3	13/15	14/26	54%
CB/CC	3/11	0/3	3/11	4/11	10/36	28%
CC	1/3	—	1/1	1/2	3/6	(50%)
CB	3/12	1/3	0/3	0/3	4/21	(19%)
LB	1/1	—	1/1	0/1	2/3	(67%)
IB	0/5	—	0/1	1/4	1/10	(10%)
NOS	2/8	0/2	0/1	7/12	9/23	(39%)
Total	10/47 21%	1/9 (11%)	6/21 (29%)	29/51 57%	46/128	36%

Blood lymphocyte preparation

Lymphocytes were purified from heparinized venous blood. The leukocyte-enriched supernatant obtained after sedimentation in gelatin was treated with iron powder. Phagocytic cells were removed by application of a magnetic field. Lymphocytes were further purified by floatation on a Ficoll-Isopaque gradient to remove remaining red blood cells [8]. The lymphocyte suspensions contained > 98 % lymphocytes.

SmIg$^+$ lymphocytes in blood

SmIg$^+$ lymphocytes were identified by direct immunofluorescence (IFL) with F(ab')$_2$ fragment of polyspecific fluorescein conjugated rabbit anti-human Ig serum (Kallestad Lab, Austin, Texas, USA) and rabbit antisera against human κ or λ light chains (Dako, Copenhagen, Denmark).

Before staining, lymphocytes were incubated in serum free medium for 30 min at 37 °C, and washed three times at 37 °C to remove absorbed Ig [9]. Membrane fluorescence was examined in a fluorescence microscope (Zeiss standard fluorescence RA microscope or Leitz Dialux 20 with epi-elumination), and 400 cells were counted.

Preparation of tissue specimens and identification of immunoglobulins on lymph node tissues

Unfixed biopsy material was divided into three parts. One part was fixed in B5 fixative [10] for conventional histologic examination and PAP staining. Another part was frozen in streaming CO_2 and stored at − 70 °C. The frozen biopsies were sectioned at about 5 μm and air dried at room temperature. Unfixed cryosections were used for direct IFL. For indirect IFL dried sections were fixed in cool acetone for one minute. The third part was minced to produce a cell suspension for single cell study by IFL.

SmIg and cytoplasmic Ig were evaluated by direct IFL with F(ab')$_2$ fragments of monospecific anti-human Ig antibodies (Kallestad Lab, Austin, Texas, USA). In addition, immunohistochemical staining by the PAP method was used for detection of immunoglobulins in paraffin-embedded material (antisera and PAP complexes, Dako A/S, Copenhagen, Denmark) [10].

Statistical methods

To test the hypothesis of two means being equal against the two-sided alter-

228

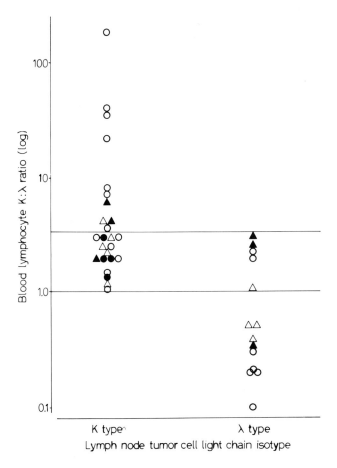

Figure 1. Blood lymphocyte $\kappa:\lambda$ ratio in 39 NHL patients where a simultaneous immune phenotyping of lymph node tissue was performed; ○ indicate low grade malignancy; △ indicate high grade malignancy.
Open symbols Stages I and II and filled symbols Stages III and IV; area within horizontal bars indicate normal range.

native, the Student's t-test was used. Survival curves were constructed according to Peto et al. [11]. Statistical significance of the differences between the curves was assessed using the logrank test [11].

Results

At diagnosis, the ratio between κ-bearing and λ-bearing lymphocytes was outside the normal range (1.0–3.3) [6] in 36% of the patients, suggesting the presence of circulating monoclonal B-lymphocytes (Table I). In all cases

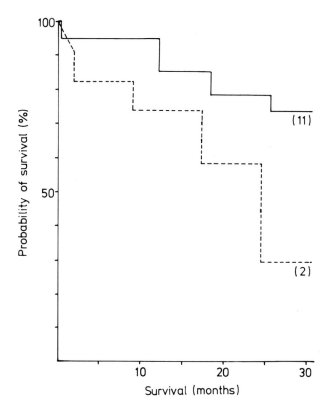

Figure 2. Survival of patients with CB/CC lymphoma in relation to blood lymphocyte $\kappa:\lambda$ ratio. Patients with a normal $\kappa:\lambda$ ratio —— (*n = 26*). Patients with an abnormal $\kappa:\lambda$ ratio (clonal B cell excess) – – – – (*n = 10*). The difference is statistically significant (*p = 0.02*).

where immune phenotyping on lymph node tissue was performed, the clonal blood B-cell excess was of the same light chain isotype as that found on the tumor lymph node cells (Fig. 1). Of the patients with low grade malignant lymphomas, 42% exhibited a monoclonal blood B-cell fraction; the corresponding figure was 28% in patients with high grade malignant lymphomas. A clonal B-cell excess was commonly found in Clinical Stages III and IV (49%), but circulating monoclonal B-cells were also identified in 11 (20%) Stages I and II patients. Median survival for all patients was 24.8 months (range 1–84 months). Patients with Clinical Stages I and II survived significantly longer than patients with Stages III and IV ($p < 0.001$). Patients with low grade malignant lymphoma survived significantly longer than those with high grade malignant lymphoma ($p < 0.01$).

No significant difference in survival could be demonstrated between patients with a clonal B cell excess and patients with a normal $\kappa:\lambda$ ratio.

This was also true when high and low grade diseases were analyzed separately with regard to clonal excess and prognosis. However, in the group of CB/CC patients, those with a normal $\kappa:\lambda$ ratio survived significantly longer than those with an abnormal ratio ($p = 0.02$; Fig. 2), which was true also when CB/CC lymphoma patients in advanced Stages (III-IV) were analysed separately ($p < 0.01$). In the other histopathologic groups no significant correlation between the presence of monoclonal blood B-lymphocytes and survival was observed.

Clonal B-cell excess was also analyzed in 18 patients in first clinical complete remission (CR). Four of these patients had a $\kappa:\lambda$ ratio outside the normal range, but no other signs of active disease. They all relapsed within a median time of 3 months from test (range 2–12 months). Their initial histopathology and stage were CB/CC I A ($n = 2$), CC I A ($n = 1$) and CB III A ($n = 1$). However, only 4 of the remaining 14 patients with a normal $\kappa:\lambda$ ratio have relapsed (median time to relapse 4 months, range 2–12 months). In the latter group, the relapsing patients were CB/CC I A and IV B ($n = 2$), IC I A ($n = 1$) and CC I A ($n = 1$).

Discussion

A clonal excess of B-lymphocytes in blood, i.e. $\kappa:\lambda$ lymphocyte ratio outside the normal range (monoclonal B-lymphocytes), was analyzed in 128 adult, previously untreated, non-leukemic NHL patients. The presence of monoclonal B-lymphocytes in the blood probably indicates a spread of tumor B-cells into the circulation. The assumption that monoclonal blood B-lymphocytes belong to the tumor clone is based on the following findings: i) clonal blood B-cells carry the same light chain isotype as the tumor lymph node cells; and ii) there is a close correlation between a clonal B-cell excess and the presence of idiotypic Ig structures on circulating B-cells in various B-lymphoproliferative disorders including leukemic NHL [6].

A clonal B-cell excess in non-leukemic NHL patients has been reported in 20–60% of the patients [2, 3, 12]. Using the Kiel classification, monoclonal B-lymphocytes were seen more often in low grade (42%) than in high grade (28%) malignant lymphoma, which is in good accordance with the findings of other authors adopting the same classification system [13]. A clonal B-cell excess was also more frequent in Stages III and IV (49%) than in Stages I and II (20%). Thus, a substantial number of patients with limited disease had circulating monoclonal B-cells.

The presence of a clonal B-cell excess was strongly associated with a poor survival in CB/CC lymphomas irrespective of stage. The lack of correlation to survival in the other histopathologic subgroups may have several explanations. The expected survival for patients with lymphocytic lymphomas and immunocytomas is long (median > 5–7 years), and the observation period in this report may thus be too short to identify a difference in survival. In the group of high grade malignancy (as well as in LL and IC), other factors may have greater prognostic effect, hence the presence of monoclonal B-cells might not influence survival. Furthermore, dissemination of tumor cells into the blood stream may not necessarily imply bad prognosis. In studies on solid tumors, the appearance of neoplastic cells in the blood did not always indicate late development of metastatic foci [14].

The fact that the four patients who had clonal B-cell excess while in clinical complete remission did relapse is of great interest. These patients represent different histologies (CB/CC, CC and CB respectively). Although seen in a small number of patients, these preliminary observations suggest that the presence of circulating monoclonal B-cells might be of prognostic importance. Such patients should be followed carefully.

In conclusion, clonal blood B-cell excess in non-leukemic NHL may be a prognostic factor in some histopathologic subgroups. The method may also be a useful diagnostic procedure in establishing complete remission and for monitoring the disease. However, further studies are warranted to fully elucidate the clinical significance of circulating monoclonal B-cells.

Acknowledgements

This study was supported by grants from the Cancer Society in Stockholm, the Swedish Cancer Society, the Karolinska Institute Foundations, the Kaleb Karlström Foundation. We thank Mrs. Margret Wahlström and Miss Eva Gustavsson for technical assistance and Miss Eva-Britt Carlsson for preparing the manuscript.

References

1. Lennert K (1981). Histopatologie der Non-Hodgkin Lymphoma nach der Kiel Klassifikation. Berlin, West-Germany: Springer Verlag.
2. Ault KA (1979). Detection of small numbers of monoclonal B-lymphocytes in blood of patients with lymphomas. N Engl J Med 300:1401–1405.
3. Lindemalm C, Mellstedt H, Biberfeld P et al. (1983). Blood and lymph node T-lymphocyte subsets in non-Hodgkin lymphomas. Scand J Haematol 30:68–78.
4. Gajl-Peczalska KJ, Bloomfield CD, Coccia PF et al. (1975). B- and T-lymphomas. Analysis of blood and lymph node in 87 patients. Amer J Med 59:674–685.
5. Bast EJEG, van Camp B, Reynart R et al. (1982). Idiotype blood lymphocytes in monoclonal gammopathy. Clin Exp Immunol 47:677–682.
6. Mellstedt H, Holm G and Björkholm M (1984). Multiple myeloma, Waldenström's macroglobulinemia and benign monoclonal gammopathy. Characteristics of the B-cell clone,

immunoregulatory cell populations and clinical implications. Adv Cancer Res 41:257–290.

7. Carbone PP, Kaplan HS, Musshoff K et al. (1971). Report of the Committee on Hodgkin's Disease Staging Classification. Cancer Res 31:1860–1861.

8. Holm G, Pettersson D, Mellstedt H et al. (1975). Lymphocyte subpopulations in peripheral blood of healthy persons. Clin Exp Immunol 20:443–447.

9. Pettersson D, Mellstedt H and Holm G (1978). IgG on human blood lymphocytes studied by immunofluorescence. Scand J Immunol 8:535–542.

10. Mason DY and Biberfeld P (1980). Technical aspects of lymphoma immunohistology. J Histochem Cytochem 28:731–741.

11. Peto R, Pike M, Armitage P et al. (1977). Design and analysis of randomized clinical trials requiring prolonged observation of each patient. II. Analysis and examples. Br J Cancer 35:1–39.

12. Ligler FS, Smith RG, Kettman JR et al. (1980). Detection of tumor in the peripheral blood of non-leukemic patients with B cell lymphomas: Analysis of clonal excess. Blood 55:792–801.

13. Lindh J, Lenner P, Roos G (1984). Monoclonal B-cells in peripheral blood of non-Hodgkin's lymphoma. Correlation with clinical features and DNA content. Scand J Haematol 32:5–11.

14. Wood S (1974). Mechanism of establishment of tumour metastatis. In: Joakim HL (Ed.). Pathology Annual. New York: Appleton-Century-Crofts.

5. Patterns of survival
in advanced non-Hodgkin's lymphoma

T. A. REICHERT[1], R. A. CHRISTENSEN[2], A. A. BARTOLUCCI[3]
and C. WALKER[1]
*[1] Division of Hematology/Oncology, Duke University Medical Center,
Durham, North Carolina, [2] Entropy Limited, Lincoln, Massachusetts
and [3] Statistical Center, SECSG, University of Alabama, Birmingham,
Alabama, USA*

In the development of clinical experience, certain factors come to be associated empirically with an extreme prognosis (for example, very long or very short survival). This clinical impression can be quantitated by examining the capacity such factors have to separate the patient population into two or more sub-groups each with a distinct and different survival experience. Those which univariately separate the sample population into statistically significant groupings rightfully assume a greater role in subsequent clinical thinking. Much clinical research has been devoted to comparing the survival experience of patient populations divided into subgroups by combinations of factors which make especially good clinical sense. Unfortunately, even the number of clinically sensible combinations is very large; and the testing of so multiple a hypothesis has its own pitfalls.

Multivariate statistical techniques are often used to sort out those factors which are truly dominant from those which merely correlate with other factors. However, the only multivariate technique in common use in clinical medicine, the Cox proportional hazards model [1], has, as its objective, the description of the survival of all of the patients in the entire sample. Since the factors selected by this procedure are intended to characterize all patients of all prognoses, they may or may not be useful in delineating the extremes of prognosis.

We employ in this study, an information theory guided, computer search and evaluation procedure [2] which discovers the largest sub-groupings for which survival is as extreme as possible. When applied to the data of two sequential clinical trials conducted by the Southeastern Cancer Study Group (SEG) in patients with advanced stage non-Hodgkin's lymphoma (NHL), simple combinations of clinical features were discovered which predict accurately the survival of subgroups of similarly defined and treated patients from independent clinical experience. We call such combinations of features, patterns of prognosis. The patterns which are found to characterize survival in NHL are not only clinically sensible, but seem to offer new insight into long standing points of controversy in these diseases.

Materials and methods

Between January 1973 and February 1977, 404 eligible patients with NHL, nearly all of advanced stage, were entered by the members of the SEG into protocol SEG-NHL-349 which was designed to test the relative efficacies of two multi-agent chemotherapeutic regimens, BCOP (carmustine, cyclophosphamide, Oncovin, and prednisone) and COP. Of the 404 patients entered into the study, 368 were evaluable. Records of 22 clinical and laboratory parameters (missing data < 1%) were obtained on 334 patients (91%) from all 20 institutions participating in the study. The results of this trial were presented in a report [3] which provides details of eligibility, stratification, staging, study design, and definitions of remission status. With the exception of an early survival advantage for BCOP induction in the histologic sub-group of diffuse histocytic lymphoma, not ultimately significant, no survival or response difference was evident between the two therapies in any defined patient cohort. A second clinical trial (SEG-317) comparing BCOP versus CHOP (Hydroxydaunorubicin) in 270 evaluable patients with unfavorable histology, advanced stage NHL, for whom the same data is available has just been reported [4].

In this study, we divided the data from the 334 patients of SEG-349 (BCOP vs. COP) randomly into two groups. The first (224 patients) was used for model development purposes; and the second (110 patients) was reserved for testing the model developed. The division was stratified on the basis of four conditions: sex (M, F), age (< 60 yrs, $\geqslant 60$ yrs), hemoglobin (< 12 g/dl, $\geqslant 12$ g/dl) and histology (favorable, unfavorable).

Initial estimates of survival time were taken as the interval between on-study date and date of death or last report (if alive). Revised estimates for individual times of survival were obtained using a self-consistent decensoring procedure (SCD) [5] on the entire model development subsample. The SCD estimates lead to a survival curve indistinguishable (largest difference < 3%) from that produced by the Kaplan-Meier (K-M) procedure [6].

The entropy minimax technique [2] was used to generate and to evaluate combinations of patient data features in search of a characterization of extremes of survival. A large number of reports of applications has recently been assembled [7].

Results

Fig. 1 shows the survival curve for the 224 patients assigned to the model development group. This group is divided into two sub-groups labeled favorable and unfavorable histology corresponding to low-grade versus intermediate plus high-grade histologies as defined by the Working Formu-

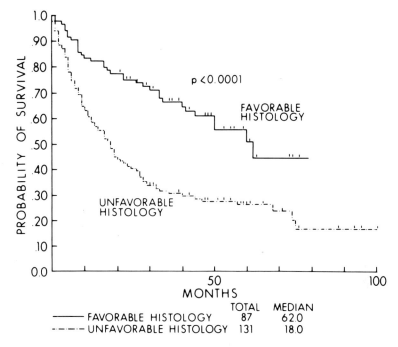

Figure 1. Survival of patients with favorable and unfavorable histology NHL from the model-development group of SEG-349.

lation [8]. The two curves are typical of similar studies, with the favorable histology group showing a continual pattern of relapse, while the unfavorable histologies show a much more marked early decline followed by a shallow, perhaps flat, late portion. The two survival curves come together in this study after about nine years.

Several different overlapping subgroups of patients of clinical significance were analyzed separately. These were: favorable histology; unfavorable histology; complete responders (all histologies); total responders (CR + PR) (all histologies); and all patients (all histologies). In every case, a good prognosis pattern was found combining 'A' symptoms, high Karnofsky status and either a normal serum transaminase (SGOT) level or a normal spleen (by palpation and/or scan).

In all groupings, except for favorable histology disease, a poor prognosis pattern defined by the logical combination of low Karnofsky status ($< 70\%$) or night sweats could be reliably identified.

Summarizing these results, the following patterns may be stated:
#1) Good Prognosis — Karnofsky status $\geqslant 80$ and 'A' Symptoms and SGOT < 36 U/L
#2) Poor Prognosis — Karnofsky status < 70 or Night sweats
#3) Intermediate Prognosis — All remaining.

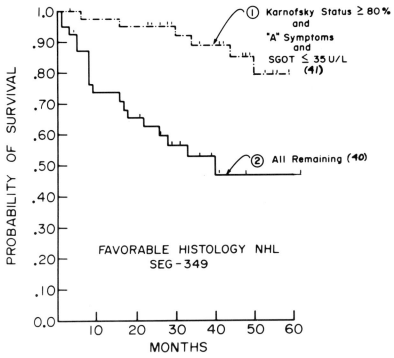

Figure 2. Survival of patients with favorable histology NHL from the model-development group of SEG-349 by pattern of prognosis.

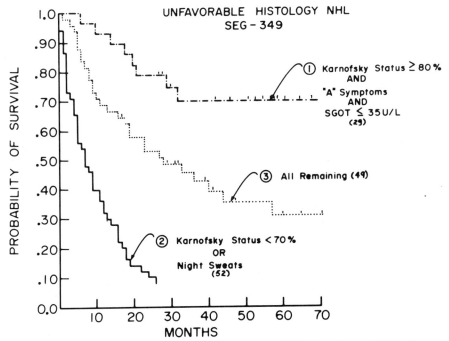

Figure 3. Survival of patients with unfavorable histology NHL from the model-development group of SEG-349 by pattern of prognosis.

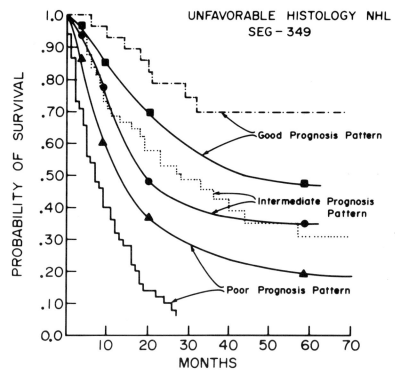

Figure 4. Observed survival of patients (1972-1977) with unfavorable histology NHL treated with BCOP/COP and predicted survival curves for future patients derived from these observations for each prognostic pattern.

In the group limited to favorable histology patients (81 patients in the model-building group), only 15 patients (0.18) match the poor prognosis pattern, #2. The survival curve for these 15 patients could not be separated from that of pattern #3, the remainder group. Thus, we can say that the survival of patients with unfavorable histology NHL appears to be characterized by all three patterns given above, while that of patients with favorable histology disease can be reliably described by the same pattern for good prognosis patients (#1) plus pattern #3 (all other patients).

The survival curves of the subgroups defined by these patterns are presented in Fig. 2 and 3. Patients matching the good prognosis pattern (#1) make up about 50% of patients with favorable histology disease, but only 25–35% of those with unfavorable histology disease. Patients matching the poor prognosis pattern make up 25–45% of those with unfavorable histology disease in SEG experience. No other combination of features provides a separation of these patients into subgroups which are as large and as extreme in survival.

The predicted survival curves for each subgroup of unfavorable histology

238

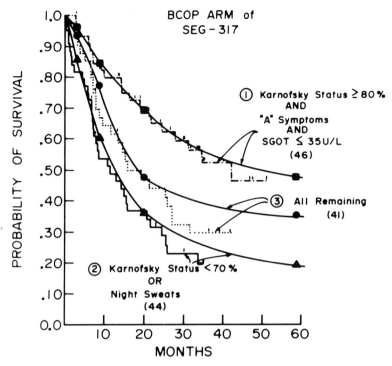

Figure 5. Observed survival of patients (1977-1982) with unfavorable histology NHL treated with BCOP compared with survival predicted by entropy minimax for each pattern of prognosis.

are presented together with the K-M estimates of the observed survival curves from SEG-349 in Fig. 4. Note the especially large deviation of the predicted curve for the poor prognosis subgroup from that observed. These predictions were tested against the survival of similar patients matching these patterns from the subgroup of 110 patients of SEG-349 reserved to the test group. The survival curves for each subgroup in the test group match the predicted curves well, but each such subgroup is quite small. A more definitive test of these predictions is afforded by the recent availability of the data from the clinical trial subsequent to SEG-349, SEG-317 (CHOP vs. BCOP). The K-M estimates of the survival curves for each subgroup of the 131 evaluable patients treated with BCOP are presented in Fig. 5. The agreement with the predicted curves is very good; and is especially gratifying in the poor prognosis subgroup. Thus, these patterns predict future survival for new patients better than actuarial survival curves observed for patients in past experience.

The fact that the good prognosis patterns are the same in both favorable and unfavorable histology disease suggests a homogeneity in a subset of these diseases not previously noted. Returning to the data of the earlier trial,

SEG-349, (Fig. 2 and 3) we note that the survival experience for the good prognosis patients with favorable histology disease appears very similar to that for good prognosis patients with unfavorable histology disease. In fact, these curves are not significantly different ($p = 0.28$). Moreover, the complete response rates are similar (0.70 for unfavorable histology; 0.58 for favorable histology patients). If we examine the survival experience of the good prognosis patients with regard to their complete response to therapy, we find that neither histologic subgroup shows a significant difference ($p = 0.96$, unfavorable histology; $p = 0.22$, favorable histology). Thus, good prognosis patients enjoy the same long survival independent of histology and initial response to therapy.

Discussion

Portlock and Rosenberg [9] hypothesize that patients with favorable histology disease who are 'relatively asymptomatic' need not be treated prior to the onset of symptoms, based on their observation that the survival curve for such patients, who are observed until treatment is required, is no different from that of similarly characterized patients treated with multi-agent chemotherapy in an investigational protocol. They describe a cohort of 44 patients who were followed prospectively without therapy until treatment was required for palliation of symptoms. Seven of the 44 patients had tumors with histology which was diffuse, poorly differentiated lymphocytic lymphoma, a histology not universally designated favorable. All 44 patients were 'relatively' asymptomatic, though specific criteria for inclusion in this category are never rigidly defined. All of the SEG patients in the good prognosis subgroups are asymptomatic in a defined sense. The survival curves presented here completely overlap those of Portlock and Rosenberg. Could it be that reservations with respect to treatment may extend even beyond the group suggested by Portlock and Rosenberg?

More certainly, clinical trials, the populations of which contain a large fraction of good prognosis patients, will enjoy very favorable overall survival experiences, possibly independent of the therapy employed, when compared to trials with a less fortunate mix of patients. In the SEG trial of BCOP vs. CHOP cited above, 1/3 of the patients in the BCOP arm matched each of the three patterns. Despite the randomized, prospective design, 0.43 of the patients in the CHOP arm were members of the poor prognosis subgroup while only 0.27 were members of the good prognosis subgroup. The CHOP arm survival experience was marginally better than that for BCOP ($p = 0.049$) but the true difference between the two regimens is greater than this apparent difference because of the imbalance in prognostic subgroups.

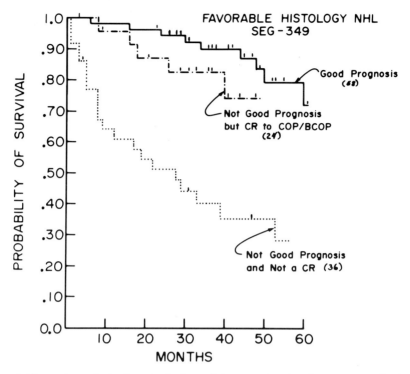

Figure 6. Comparison of actual survival of complete responders to others among patients with favorable histology NHL (SEG-349) who were not of good prognosis; and to the survival of good prognosis patients.

Several authors have suggested that patients with favorable histology disease who obtain a complete response to initial therapy have a significantly longer survival than those who do not so respond [10]. This issue has seen some controversy in the specific instance of nodular mixed histology and the therapy, C-MOPP (cyclophosphamide, Oncovin, procarbazine and prednisone) [11–14]. Those patients, with favorable histology disease but not of good prognosis, do derive significant survival benefit from a complete response to initial therapy (Fig. 6). This benefit is almost completely confined to those patients who do not match the poor prognosis pattern, #2. Patterns which predict response to therapy differ from those prognostic for survival, but the tendency to complete response is strongly correlated with survival. Thus, clinical trials of therapies more or less equivalent to COP/BCOP for which the patient population contains a large fraction of patients not matching the good prognosis pattern for survival will tend to find a significant difference between the survival of patients with and those without a complete response to therapy. Similarly, trials using a patient mix weighted *toward* good prognosis will not find such a difference. This effect will be heightened in small samples. Clinical heterogeneity so dominates histologic diversity that prognostic subgroupings based on features such as those cited here must first be accounted before reliable and consistent results will be obtained from studies subgrouping patients on the basis of histology.

References

1. Cox DR (1972). Regression models and life-tables. J Roy Stat Soc B 34:187–202.
2. Christensen R (1984). Entropy minimax. In: Singh M (Ed.). Encyclopedia of Systems and Control. Oxford: Pergamon Press (in press).
3. Durant JR, Gams RA, Bartolucci AA and Dorfman RF (1977). BCNU with and without cyclophosphamide, vincristine and prednisone (COP) and cycle-active therapy in non-hodgkin's lymphoma. Cancer Treat Rep 61:1085–1096.
4. Gams RA, Rainey M, Bartolucci AA and Dandy M. Phase III study of BCOP vs. CHOP in unfavorable categories of malignant lymphoma. J Clin Oncol (in press).
5. Christensen RA, Eilbert R, Reichert TA (1984). Self-consistent estimates of individual survival expectancy from censored data. (Submitted for publication June, 1984).
6. Kaplan EL and Meier P (1958). Nonparametric estimation from incomplete observations. Amer Stat Assoc J 53:457–481.
7. Christensen RA (1981). Entropy Minimax Sourcebook, Vol. IV, Chap. 14, p. 355: Applications. Lincoln, MA.: Entropy Limited.
8. The Non-Hodgkin's Lymphoma Pathologic Classification Project (1982). National Cancer Institute sponsored study of classifications of non-Hodgkin's lymphomas. Cancer 49:2112–2135.
9. Portlock CS and Rosenberg SA (1979). No initial therapy for Stage III and IV non-Hodgkin's lymphomas of favorable histologic types. Ann Intern Med 90:10–13.
10. Diggs CH, Wiernik PH and Ostrow SS (1981). Nodular Lymphoma: Prolongation of survival by complete remission. Cancer Clin Trials 4:107–114.
11. Anderson T, Bener RA, Fisher RI et al. (1977). Combination chemotherapy in non-Hodgkin's lymphomas: Results of long-term follow-up. Cancer Treat Rep 61:1057–1066.
12. Longo D, Hubbard Wesley M, Jaffe E et al. 1981). Prolonged initial remission in patients with nodular mixed lympoma (NML). Proc Amer Soc Clin Oncol 22:521.
13. Bitran JC, Golomb HM, Ultmann JE et al. (1978). Non-Hodgkin's lymphoma, poorly differentiated lymphocytic and mixed cell types: Results of sequential staging procedures, response to therapy and survival of 100 patients. Cancer 42:88–95.
14. Glick JH, Barnes JM, Ezdinli EZ et al. (1981). Nodular mixed lymphoma: Results of a randomized trial failing to confirm prolonged disease-free survival with chemotherapy. Blood 58:920–925.

V. Special clinical entities

1. Acquired Immune Deficiency Syndrome (AIDS): Basic findings

D. L. LONGO[1], R. G. STEIS[1], H. MASUR[2], H. C. LANE[3],
O. PREBLE[4], A. S. FAUCI[3], and E. P. GELMANN[1]
*Medicine Branch, National Cancer Institute, [1] Critical Care Medicine
Department, Clinical Center, [2] Laboratory of Immunoregulation,
National Institute of Allergy and Infectious Diseases, and
[3] Department of Pathology, The Uniformed Services University of
the Health Sciences, Bethesda, Maryland, USA*

The AIDS syndrome, an almost uniformly fatal, transmissable new disease characterized by profoundly depressed cellular immunity, is manifest clinically by serious, life-threatening opportunistic infections and neoplasms [1]. Over 3000 cases have been reported in the United States and more than 20 countries have identified individuals who have this syndrom, as defined by the Center for Disease Control. There are four major risk groups: male homosexuals and bisexuals (71%), heterosexual drug abusers (17%), Haitians (5%), and hemophiliacs (1%). It appears that the disease is spread through sexual activity or intravenous administration of contaminated material. A large number of opportunistic pathogens which are rare in other populations cause significant morbidity and mortality in this group of patients. Such pathogens include cytomegalovirus, *Candida albicans, Pneumocystic carinii, Mycobacterium avium-intracellulare, Cryptococcus neoformans, Crytosporidium, Toxoplasma gondii,* and Epstein-Barr virus. The immune system is profoundly affected in this disease with an absolute decrease in T-lymphocytes, particularly the subset that subserves the helper/inducer function and is distinguished by its reactivity with the monoclonal antibody OKT4. Recent isolation of HTLV-III from AIDS patients [2], has raised expectations that strategies to boost natural immunity to the virus through a vaccine, or to block retroviral replication with rifampicin or a congener, may prevent the disease.

Two types of malignancy occur with increased frequency in victims of AIDS: Kaposi's sarcoma [3], and malignant lymphomas of several histologic types (Burkitt's lymphoma [4], immunoblastic lymphoma [5], lymphoblastic lymphoma [6], and Hodgkin's disease [7]). The lymphoma subtypes have diverse cells of origin including B-cells, T-cells, and dendritic cells. Patients have rarely both Kaposi's sarcoma and lymphoma.

The male homosexual risk group also suffers an increased incidence of squamous cell carcinoma of the tongue and cloacagenic carcinoma of the rectum. Recognition of the increased incidence of these tumors in male homosexuals, however, predated the appearance of the AIDS syndrome [1] and, therefore, these tumors are probably not AIDS-related, but occur in a common risk group.

Nearly 35% of AIDS patients have developed Kaposi's sarcoma and 30% of those patients have died. The incidence of Kaposi's sarcoma varies among the risk groups, reaching about 50% in male homosexual AIDS victims, but less than 10% in the other risk groups. Nearly 40% of AIDS victims have developed a malignancy including lymphoma and Kaposi's sarcoma. This is more than twice the incidence of malignancy in patients with other primary and secondary immunodeficiency states [8]. The incidence of malignancy is 15.4% in the Wiskott-Aldrich syndrome, 11.7% in ataxia-telangiectasia and only 2.4% in selective IgA deficiency, the most common human immune deficiency. Malignancy occurs in 6% of kidney transplant patients and 8% of heart transplant patients as a result of the iatrogenic immunosuppression. The types of tumors occurring in immunodeficient patients vary with the cause of the immunodeficiency. In primary immunodeficiency states, lymphoma accounts for 68% of neoplasms, leukemia 17%, and all forms of carcinoma only 19% [9]. Kaposi's sarcoma is rare in primary immunodeficiency patients. On the other hand, lymphoma accounts for 26% of the tumors in iatrogenically immunosuppressed patients. Kaposi's sarcoma (5.5% of all tumors) is the fifth leading malignancy in these patients, occurring more commonly than a number of more prevalent tumors.

The histopathology of Kaposi's sarcoma is the same in both the non-epidemic and epidemic (or AIDS-associated) forms. There is vascular proliferation (vascular spaces are often not endothelial lined) and the spindle-shaped neoplastic cells, imbedded in reticulin fibers, are identified as being of endothelial origin by virtue of cytoplasmic binding of antibody to factor VIII and in vitro proliferation in response to endothelial growth factor. Skin lesions are blue to brown nodules or plaques, often with scaling when present on the lower extremities. Although 90% of victims of non-epidemic Kaposi's sarcoma have lesions confined to skin, almost 75% of AIDS patients have disease disseminated to visceral organs [1]. About 5% of AIDS patients with Kaposi's sarcoma will have only organ disease and no skin lesions. Lymph nodes and the gastrointestinal tract are most commonly involved, but unusual sites of disease such as urethra, conjunctivae, and auditory canal are also seen. Lung involvement occurs in only about 15% of patients but can result in serious physiologic compromise. The diagnosis of organ involvement in epidemic Kaposi's sarcoma is exceedingly difficult on clinical examination since lymphadenopathy in these patients need not be due to Kaposi's sarcoma, gastrointestinal involvement may be inconspicuous, and the differential diagnosis of pulmonary nodules and infiltrates is a lengthy procedure in these patients. Biopsies must be performed when Kaposi's sarcoma involvement is suspected in nodes or lung, and upper and lower gastrointestinal endoscopy is the only reliable diagnostic procedure to evaluate the gastrointestinal tract. Because tumor involvement of most organs is submucosal, biopsies of abnormalities seen at endoscopy are often negative on histologic examination. Therefore, visual inspection is the benchmark of gastrointestinal disease. No segment of the gastrointestinal tract is spared from involvement by Kaposi's sarcoma.

Since the vast majority of patients with the nonepidemic form of Kaposi's sarcoma have localized disease, localized therapy with x-rays or electron beam radiation is effective. Those patients with more advanced disease have shown high response rates to a variety of single agents and combination chemotherapy programs [1]. However, the rarity of the tumor has meant that most treatment reports involve small numbers of patients. Among transplant recipients developing Kaposi's sarcoma, complete responses have been seen in 63% (5/8) of patients whose only treatment was the cessation of immunosuppressive drugs. This implies that reversal of underlying immune suppression might also be efficacious in AIDS patients with Kaposi's sarcoma. The median survival of patients with nonepidemic Kaposi's sarcoma is about 13 years and the common causes of death are heart failure, second malignancy, sepsis from infected skin lesions, and hemorrhage. Up to 37% of patients develop a second tumor; 7–17% develop lymphomas (Burkitt's, Hodgkin's, Sezary's) and nearly 10% developed leukemias (acute and chronic lymphocytic, acute myeloblastic) [10].

Treatment of the epidemic form of Kaposi's sarcoma has not been very successful. Nearly 100 patients in three different studies have received alpha interferon. Krown et al. initially reported results of recombinant leukocyte A interferon (Hoffman-LaRoche) in 13 patients with AIDS-associated Kaposi's sarcoma [11], and have subsequently entered a total of 32 patients on study. Groopman et al. reported results in 20 patients of recombinant alpha-2 interferon (Schering) [12], which differs in a single amino acid from leukocyte A interferon. The response rate to interferon in these two reports is 30–40%, with rare complete responses. Responses are short-lived if therapy is stopped, and can be maintained only a few months if therapy is continued. There is no evidence that interferon therapy in these patients reversed any immune dysfunction and no antiviral effects were noted. In general, higher doses seemed somewhat more effective than lower doses. The median time to response was about 10 weeks. It is very important to note that most patients in both studies had T4/T8 ratios > 0.4, few had opportunistic infections, and nearly all were recently diagnosed and had small volumes of disease.

We have used lymphoblastoid interferon, a mixture of several molecules with alpha interferon properties purified from the Namalva cell line (Wellferon, Burroughs-Wellcome), to treat 30 patients with AIDS-associated Kaposi's sarcoma. We treated 10 patients for 28 days at each of the following dose levels: 7.5 MU/m^2/day, 15 MU/m^2/day, and 25 MU/m^2/day. The highest dose level was toxic (intolerable fatigue, weakness, depression) and dose reduction was required in 75% of the patients. There were 3 partial and 4 minor responses (response rate 11–24%). Dose level did not appear to affect response rate. During therapy most patients had a 30–50% fall in absolute lymphocyte count that returned to pre-therapy levels after stopping therapy. We measured circulating interferon levels and examined the *in vivo* and *in vitro* response of the interferon-inducible enzyme 2'-5' oligioadenylate (2–5 A) synthetase before, during, and after interferon therapy. We found that: 1) many patients had significantly elevated baseline levels of 2–5 A synthetase independent of their baseline level of serum interferon; 2) 2–5 A synthetase levels in most patients failed to increase after *in vitro* exposure to interferon, or after *in vivo* interferon administration; and 3) it was not possible to predict antitumor response on the basis of either *in vitro* or *in vivo* rises in 2–5 A synthetase. This indicates that interferon's antiproliferative effect in responding patients results from a different mechanism. In our study, response correlated with higher numbers of OKT4+ lymphocytes and the absence of prior opportunistic infection. Patients with elevated levels of acid-labile alpha interferon before therapy were more likely to have progressive disease on therapy. Thus, it appears that interferon therapy works best in patients who need treatment the least.

Two small non-randomized chemotherapy series have been reported using single agents (vinblastine or etoposide) and combinations (doxorubicin, bleomycin, and vinblastine) [13, 14]. In general, patients with more aggressive disease were given the combinations. Apparently higher incidence of treatment-related morbidity and mortality has been noted in these patients. However, there have been no studies in which patients comparable to those who were treated on the interferon trials have received chemotherapy. Although responses to chemotherapy are common, 30% of all reported cases have died and the projected 2-year survival of AIDS patients with Kaposi's sarcoma is 30%. There have been no long-term disease-free survivors. The causes of death in the majority of epidemic Kaposi's sarcoma patients are opportunistic infections, and irreversible cachexia and wasting. Tumor-related deaths are only about 25% of the total.

Because only a minority of epidemic Kaposi's sarcoma patients appeared to die from progressive malignancy, we decided to try aggressive 6-drug combination chemotherapy in patients whose tumor appeared to be a major threat to their life. We put together two 3-drug regimens with reported high response rates in non-epidemic Kaposi's sarcoma in the hope that the drugs, which act in diverse ways, would be noncrossresistant. We gave doxorubicin, bleomycin and vinblastine on day 1, actinomycin D, vincristine, and dacarbazine on day 8, and bleomycin on day 15 of a 28-day cycle. The median Karnofsky score of the 14 patients entered on study was 50. The median total T4-cells was 182. In our experience, once the number of T4-cells drops to 200, the majority of patients die within 6 months. Thus, the patients in this study had an extremely poor prognosis, from both an immunologic and an oncologic point of view. Nevertheless, there were 3 complete, 9 partial, and 1 minor response in 14 patients (overall CR + PR = 86%). Nine patients have died, but only 2 died from their tumor, and none of the deaths were treatment-related.

Thus, Kaposi's sarcoma in AIDS patients demonstrates a wide spectrum of disease but it appears that opportunistic infection is a greater threat to life than the tumor. If the tumor produces localized symptoms, radiation therapy can be palliative. However, if the tumor appears to represent a threat to life in its pace of progression or its sites of involvement, systemic chemotherapy can be effective at controlling the Kaposi's sarcoma.

Several other approaches to the treatment of epidemic Kaposi's sarcoma are under evaluation such as gamma interferon, interleukin-2, and plasmapheresis. Preliminary data on small numbers of patients are not encouraging that any of these approaches will be beneficial to a significant fraction of patients.

In contrast to AIDS patients with Kaposi's sarcoma, those who develop malignant lymphoma require aggressive management. Such lymphomas are usually rapidly progressive unfavorable histologic subtypes that represent a major threat to life. Central nervous system (CNS) involvement is common; distinguishing this involvement from toxoplasmosis or multifocal leukoencephalopathy may be difficult without brain biopsy. CNS involvement requires radiation and systemic combination chemotherapy. Physicians managing patients who develop malignant lymphoma should make a vigorous attempt to induce complete remission with combination chemotherapy regimens successful in the particular histologic subtypes (CHOMP for Burkitt's lymphomas [15], APO for lymphoblastic [16], ProMACE-MOPP for immunoblastic lymphoma [17], and MOPP for Hodgkin's disease [18]). Ultimate success in controlling malignancies associated with AIDS probably depends on reversing the underlying immune dysfunction.

References

1. Fauci AS, Macher AM, Longo DL et al. (1984). Acquired immune deficiency syndrome: Epidemiologic, clinical, immunologic and therapeutic considerations. Ann Intern Med 100:92–106.
2. Gallo RC, Salahuddin SZ, Popovic M et al. (1984). Frequent detection and isolation of cytopathic retroviruses (HTLV-III) from patients with AIDS and at risk for AIDS. Science 224:500–503.

3. Friedman-Kien AE, Laubenstein LJ, Rubinstein P et al. (1982). Disseminated Kaposi's sarcoma in homosexual men. Ann Intern Med 96:693–700.

4. Ziegler JL, Miner RC, Rosenbaum E et al. (1982). Outbreak of Burkitt's-like lymphoma in homosexual men. Lancet 2:631–633.

5. Snider WD, Simpson DM, Aronoyk KE et al. (1983). Primary lymphoma of the nervous system associated with acquired immune deficiency syndrome. N Engl J Med 308:45.

6. Ciobanu N, Andreeff M, Safai B et al. (1983). Lymphoblastic neoplasia in a homosexual patient with Kaposi's sarcoma. Ann Intern Med 98:151–155.

7. Longo DL, Steis RG and Gelmann EP. Hodgkin's disease in Aids. (In Preparation).

8. Penn I. (1982). The occurrence of cancer in immune deficiencies. Curr Prob Cancer 6:#10, 1–64.

9. Filipovich AH, Spector BD and Kersey J (1980). Immunodeficiency in humans as a risk factor in the development of malignancy. Prev Med 9:252–259.

10. Safai B, Mike V, Giraldo G et al. (1980). Association of Kaposi's sarcoma with second primary malignancies: Possible etiopathogenic implications. Cancer 45:1472–1479.

11. Krown SE, Real FX, Cunningham-Rundles S et al. (1983). Preliminary observations on the effect of recombinant leukocyte A interferon in homosexual men with Kaposi's sarcoma. N Engl J Med 308:1071–1076.

12. Groopman JE, Gottlieb MS, Goodman J et al. (1984). Recombinant alpha-2 interferon therapy for Kaposi's sarcoma associated with the acquired immunodeficiency syndrome. Ann Intern Med 100:671–676.

13. Lewis B, Abrams D, Ziegler JL et al. (1983). Single agent or combination chemotherapy of Kaposi's sarcoma in acquired immune deficiency syndrome. Proc Amer Soc Clin Oncol 2:59.

14. Laubenstein LJ, Krigel RL, Hymes KB et al. (1983). Treatment of epidemic Kaposi's sarcoma with VP-16-213 (etoposide) and a combination of doxorubicin, bleomycin, and vinblastine (ABV). Proc Amer Soc Clin Oncol 2:228.

15. Magrath IT, Spiegel RJ, Edwards BK et al. (1981). Improved results of chemotherapy in young patients with Burkitt's, undifferentiated, and lymphoblastic lymphoma. Proc Amer Soc Clin Oncol 22:520.

16. Weinstein HJ, Cassady JR and Levey R (1983). Long-term results of the APO protocol (vincristine, doxorubicin [adriamycin] and prednisone) for treatment of mediastinal lymphoblastic lymphoma. J Clin Oncol 1:537–541.

17. Fisher RI, DeVita Jr VT, Hubbard SM et al. (1983). Diffuse aggressive lymphomas: Increased survival after alternating flexible sequences of ProMACE and MOPP chemotherapy. Ann Intern Med 98:304–309.

18. DeVita Jr VT, Simon RM, Hubbard SM et al. (1980). Curability of advanced Hodgkin's disease with chemotherapy. Ann Intern Med 92:587–595.

2. Malignant lymphoma in homosexual men: Relationship to Acquired Immune Deficiency Syndrome (AIDS)

F. M. MUGGIA, A. DANCIS, C. ODAJNYK, B. RAPHAEL,
J. C. WERNZ, R. L. KRIGEL, L. J. LAUBENSTEIN, and
D. M. KNOWLES
*Rita and Stanley H. Kaplan Cancer Center, New York University,
New York, New York, USA*

The definition of AIDS has encompassed the diagnosis of opportunistic infection (OI) or Kaposi's sarcoma (KS) arising in certain populations without any previously known immunologic defects [1]. As of April 2, 1984, 3954 patients fulfilling the criteria for AIDS had been reported to the Centers for Disease Control in Atlanta, Georgia. The largest single risk group identified consists of males with homosexual or bisexual practices constituting 71.3% of the total cases, followed by intravenous (iv) drug users, Haitians, and hemophiliacs. Malignancies other than KS, particularly lymphomas have been well known to complicate a variety of genetically determined or induced immunodeficiency states [2–4]. B-cell proliferations including primary central nervous system (CNS) high grade lymphomas are represented with greater than expected frequency; however, Hodgkin's disease and the whole spectrum of acute leukemias, also have been linked to immunodeficiencies.

Because of this probable relationship between immunodeficiency and lymphomas we have become interested in studying the occurrence of malignant lymphoma among homosexual men. We report here on the changing incidence of lymphomas during the current AIDS epidemic, and on the various pathologic and clinical features that are emerging. A preliminary description of the patients has appeared in abstract form [5], with a full report to follow [6]. The discussion will focus on the specific features which characterize the emergence of lymphomas in relation to immunodeficiency and viral oncogenesis.

Materials and methods

Between March 1982 and December 1983 all patients with malignant lymphoma diagnosed at New York University (NYU)—Bellevue Hospital Medical Center among men acknowledging to engage in homosexual practices were registered with the Hematology and Oncology services, and subjected to further study. This included pretreatment evaluation employing the usual lymphoma staging procedures plus a search for clinical or laboratory features of AIDS [7]. We have also applied the definition of pre-AIDS (Table I) to the retrospective characterization of these patients. Patients with other risk factors leading to neoplasia such as renal transplantation were excluded. Pathologic diagnoses were classified in accordance to the non-Hodgkin's Lymphoma Classification Project [8] and staging in accordance to the Ann Arbor definitions [9].

A therapeutic protocol for high grade lymphomas and special studies to be performed on all patients has been recently instituted (Table II).

In an effort to assess whether the occurrence of these lymphomas repre-

Table I. Findings and conditions suspected to precede AIDS (Pre-AIDS)*

Clinical:	Extrainguinal lymphadenopathy ($> 1 \, cm^2$ in chains in two sites or $> 3 \, cm^2$ in one) Oral thrush in the absence of antibiotics Fever > 1 week, unexplained Weight loss $> 10\%$, unexplained Diarrhea, fatigue, night sweats > 1 week, unexplained
Laboratory:	Absolute lymphocytopenia and decrease T helper cells T helper/T suppressor $= 1$ Absent delayed hypersensitivity Unexplained leukopenia and/or thrombocytopenia Elevation of at least one immunoglobulin isotype Reactive hyperplasia on lymph node biopsy Elevated beta-2-microglobulin Elevated acid labile interferon

[a] The National Institutes of Health Task Force on AIDS defines 'lesser AIDS' as subjects manifesting any one clinical feature and any 2 laboratory findings. Other terms: AIDS related complex (ARC), AIDS prodrome, lymphadenopathy syndrome, prison acquired lymphadenopathy syndrome (PALS)

Table II. Special studies and therapeutic protocol

1. Staging: cerebrospinal fluid cytology, abdominal computerized tomography, bone marrow aspiration and biopsy
2. AIDS Evaluation: Includes viral serologies, beta-2 microglobulin, quantitative immunoelectrophoresis, functional T-cell studies
3. Tumor marker studies (T- and B-cell monoclonal antibody panel)
4. Tumor cytogenetics
5. Tumor DNA for immunoglobulin gene rearrangement
6. Therapy (high grade lymphomas): cyclophosphamide/vincristine, alternating with methotrexate/cytosine arabinoside infusions, and intrathecal prophylaxis with the last two drugs

sented an unusual clustering phenomenon or bore some relationship to the AIDS epidemic we reviewed the incidence of high or intermediate grade lymphomas among single men diagnosed since 1976 and appearing in our combined tumor registry of New York University Hospital and the adjoining Bellevue Hospital. The latter services the indigent population of New York City as well as individuals who become ill while detained in city prisons. We also assessed the incidence of KS among both hospitals.

Results

Demographic characteristics (Table III)

Eighteen homosexual men with lymphoma were encountered from March 1982 to December 1983: four had Hodgkin's disease and fourteen had non-Hodgkin's lymphoma (NHL). The patients with NHL fell within three groups: immunoblastic (4 patients), Burkitt's (4 patients) and miscellaneous types (6 patients) including one unclassified primary brain lymphoma. Further demographic features will be described in relation to AIDS. The

Table III. Hodgkin's and Non-Hodgkin's lymphoma in homosexual men (NYU)

Case Number	Pathology	Initial site of involvement (Stage)
I.	Hodgkin's disease	
1	Nodular sclerosis	Cervical nodes (IIA)
2	Nodular sclerosis	Neck, Abdomen (IIIB)
3	Mixed cellularity	Tonsil (IA)
4	Mixed cellularity	Axillary nodes (IIA)
II.	Non-Hodgkin's lymphoma	
1	Immunoblastic	Thigh (IE)
2	Immunoblastic	Small Bowel (IE)
3	Immunoblastic	Small Bowel (IV)
4	Immunoblastic	Small Bowel (IV)
5	Burkitt's	Paraspinal, bone marrow, CNS (IV)
6	Burkitt's	Axillary node, bone marrow, CNS (IV)
7	Burkitt's	Cervical node, bone marrow, CNS (IV)
8	Burkitt's	Mandible (IE)
9	Lymphoma (? type)	Primary CNS
10	Small cleaved	Bone marrow (IV)
11	Lymphoplasmacytoid	Bone marrow, large bowel (IV)
12	Small cleaved	Cervical node, lung (IV)
13	Large uncleaved	Ascites (IV)
14	Large cleaved	Lung (IV)

high frequency of extranodal presentations, particularly in the immunoblastic category is noteworthy. The median age of these patients was 39 (range 20 to 74 years).

Comparative Incidence (Table IV)

Over the initial 4 year period beginning 1976, only 10 single men with the diagnosis of high or intermediate grade lymphomas were identified and no patients with KS, CNS lymphomas or Burkitt's lymphomas within our demographic group were noted. Moreover, the median age of these patients was substantially older than the study population and subsequent cohorts. During the 2 year period preceding the current study population our registry discloses 15 patients with lymphoma fulfilling our demographic constraints which represents a threefold annual increase. A lower median age, extranodal disease and Burkitt's lymphoma also become apparent. The first cases of KS in this subset were also identified. During the 2 years in which we identified and studied the current group of homosexual men, 23 other male patients were diagnosed to have high or intermediate grade lymphoma. A striking number of these had extranodal presentations or the Burkitt's histology; one patient had a primary CNS lymphoma. The staggering number of KS patients is also documented. These changes are further illustrated in Fig. 1. Unfortunately, demographic data is incomplete to delineate further the relationship of these incidence changes to sexual practices, iv drug use, or other considerations.

Relationship to AIDS

Within each histologic subtype we have analyzed the relationship of the occurrence of lymphoma to findings of AIDS or pre-AIDS.

Table IV. High or intermediate grade lymphoma in single men (comparison with KS)

Time period	1976–1979	1980–1981	1982–1983
Number patients	10	15	23
Number extranodal	3	7	20
Median age	55	33	37
Burkitt's lymphoma	0	2	5
Primary CNS lymphoma	0	0	1
Kaposi's sarcoma	0	19	145 *

[a] Data to June 1983.

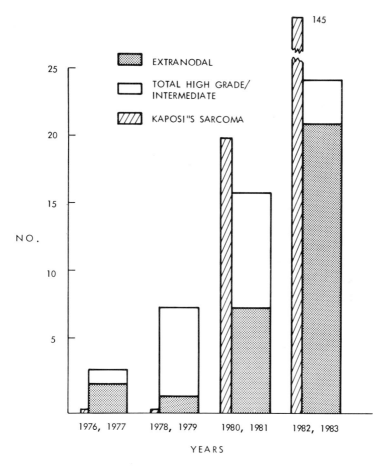

Figure 1. Lymphomas in single men (NYU/Bellevue hospitals).

Two homosexual men with the diagnosis of Hodgkin's disease, nodular sclerosis type manifested signs indicative of AIDS concomitantly or within the first chemotherapy treatment cycle. One patient had simultaneous KS, while the other two developed *Pneumocystis carinii* pneumonia (PCP). The other two patients with mixed cellularity Hodgkin's had unusual features fulfilling pre-AIDS criteria in spite of their stages IA and IIA of disease. Both have experienced intermittent fevers, weight loss and diarrhea while their lymphoma has come under complete control with radiation. One of these patients, moreover, has had persistent neutropenia since presentation, and the other had generalized adenopathy which receded and was followed by the development of axillary lymph node enlargement as part of Hodgkin's disease.

One of the four patients with immunoblastic lymphomas presented initially with OI thus fulfilling the AIDS criteria. The remaining three had pre-AIDS manifestations and one also had a subsequent OI. Two had long standing lymphadenopathy and in one patient this was also accompanied by fever and diarrhea and subsequently by development of a small bowel lymphoma; the other patient had hyperplastic lymph node biopsies and subsequently also an immunoblastic lesion in his thigh. The fourth patient had unexplained neutropenia and thrush several months prior to an acute abdominal event leading to the discovery of a localized lymphoma of the small bowel.

Of the Burkitt's patients two presented de novo with no AIDS or pre-AIDS symptoms; one of these patients presented with a Stage I jaw tumor while the other had disseminated disease involving cervical lymph nodes, bone marrow and CNS. The other two patients did have the pre-AIDS hallmark of lymphadenopathy which included also neutropenia in one.

The six other patients with a variety of NHL diagnoses include four patients with KS and lymphadenopathy who subsequently were documented to have a lymphoplasmacytoid lymphoma of bone marrow and large bowel, a small cleaved lymphoma of the bone marrow, a large uncleaved lymphoma in ascitic fluid and a large cleaved lymphoma of the lung, respectively. This last patient also had PCP prior to manifesting the lymphoma. The fifth patient had an unclassified lymphoma of the frontal lobe diagnosed in the course of treatment of PCP; he died two months later of cryptoccocal pneumonia shortly after completing a course of whole brain irradiation and steroids. The last patient, age 74, with a small cleaved lymphoma in the marrow, lung and lymph nodes may represent a coincidental occurrence.

Discussion

The occurrence of malignant lymphomas during the AIDS epidemic has been recently recognized [10–16]. In homosexual men, moreover, a syndrome of generalized lymphadenopathy which subsequently may culminante in the development of a malignant lymphoma has been described [17–19]. Other abnormalities have also aroused interest because of possible early identification of pathogenetic mechanisms leading to AIDS (Table I). Among these are clinical signs and symptoms and laboratory features which have been sporadically identified in association with malignant lymphoma; for example, lymph node hyperplasia, autoimmune thrombocytopenia and leukopenia, and elevated beta-2-microglobulin levels. Among the current report, we note the concomitant occurrence of KS with NHL in four instances; and with Hodgkin's disease in 1 instance, an association noted in the classic descriptions of KS [20] and in KS complicating renal transplantation [21].

In addition to the clinical and laboratory manifestations of AIDS and pre-AIDS certain patterns characterize these seemingly epidemic lymphomas of homosexual men. In our experience Burkitt's lymphomas and extranodal presentations of immunoblastic lymphoma predominate. However, Hodgkin's disease and other forms of NHL also occur. An association that is not merely coincidental is suggested by the concomitant diagnosis of KS, other manifestations of AIDS, and a background of lymphadenopathy. A compilation of data from six institutions including ours extends these observations [22]. In this larger experience of 90 homosexual men ages 20 to 61 (median 37) 62% were high grade, 29% intermediate grade and 7% low grade lymphomas. All except two had extranodal lymphoma most commonly involving bone marrow, CNS, bowel and mucocutaneous sites. All but fifteen of the patients had some features of pre-AIDS or AIDS. Generalized lymphadenopathy was present in 33 (37%), whereas concomitant opportunistic infections, KS, or both together occurred in 23, 10 and 9 patients respectively. As might be expected, patients with these AIDS manifestations had a particularly short course, and the diagnosis of lymphoma not infrequently (in thirteen instances) took place at autopsy. The actuarial survival of patients otherwise diagnosed is also considerably shorter than composite survival curves from 1175 patients of comparable histologic grade reported by the non-Hodgkin's Lymphoma Pathologic Classification Project [8, 22].

One must strongly suspect a relationship between these malignancies, immune deficiencies, and viral oncogenes. In genetically determined immune deficiencies, the propensity to develop lymphoid and malignancies of various types has not been thoroughly characterized by current histologic and staging criteria [2–4]; however, all histologies are represented including Hodgkin's disease [23]. Certain chronic disorders of the immune system such as Sjogren's syndrome and celiac disease have also been associated with malignant lymphomas, mimicking some animal models. Of additional interest are the iatrogenic lymphomas which have been associated with renal [24] or cardiac transplantation [25, 26]. Because of carefully controlled circumstances, these last conditions have been the subject of increasing scrutiny by modern techniques to delineate their pathogenesis, beyond the obvious immunologic factors, and use of immunosuppressive drugs. Specifically, oncogenetic mechanisms and associated viruses are being studied.

Most helpful in identifying clonal lymphoid proliferations have been the detection of immunoglobulin gene rearrangements in biopsy tissues by the Southern Blot hybridization technique. In cardiac transplant recipients such technique has revealed that hyperplastic specimens in fact contain monoclonal cell populations typical of B-cell lymphomas even when surface markers are not expressed [27–29].

These techniques as well as more extensive monoclonal antibody subtyping of lymphomas will hopefully shed some light on the presumed viral etiology of these tumors. The human T-cell leukemia/lymphoma virus (HTLV-1) was the first human retroviral isolate linked to a clinical disease manifested by cutaneous T-cell neoplasias, hypercalcemia, osteolytic lesions and a defined geographic distribution [30]. Such a discovery stimulated much interest because of the parallel to naturally occurring leukemias or lymphomas in numerous animal species caused by retroviruses (also known as type C or RNA tumor viruses). Of special interest is the feline leukemia virus which in addition to leukemia can produce an aplastic picture reminiscent of AIDS [31]. Recent discovery of HTLV-3 or a lymphadenopathy associated retrovirus (LAV) in the majority of patients with AIDS and pre-AIDS have propelled these viruses as the etiologic vectors responsible for the AIDS epidemic, and must be studied for their possible role in neoplasia.

Finally, the role of Epstein-Barr virus (EBV) in specifically bringing about lymphoid malignancies under various clinical circumstances is being intensively studied. This virus was initially implicated in the African Burkitt's lymphoma by serologic techniques (elevated titres of antibodies to Epstein-Barr viral capsid antigen), by study of Epstein-Barr nuclear antigen in tumor cells, and by DNA-hybridization probes. It has been less frequently implicated in American Burkitt's lymphomas, but has attracted renewed attention by studies linking EBV to lymphoid proliferation in transplant recipients, following infectious mononucleosis and in CNS lymphomas [32–38]. We propose to study the role of EBV in lymphomas occurring in patients with AIDS and pre-AIDS since serologic evidence for EBV's presence (as well as other viruses such as CMV) is extensive [7]. Moreover karyotypic studies should further elucidate whether and how the immunoglobulin gene rearrangements involving translocation of the c-myc oncogene previously described in Burkitt's lymphoma [39] occur in these patients. These new concepts coupled with the increasing recognition of the factors contributing to Epstein-Barr virus immortalization and replication [40, 41] promise to delineate further the findings of this recent epidemic of lymphoid neoplasia, Kaposi's sarcoma and other AIDS-related manifestations occurring in homosexual men.

Acknowledgements

Supported by Cancer Center Core Support Grant No. P30CA-16087.

References

1. Muggia FM (1983). Description of an emerging epidemic: The Acquired Immune Deficiency Syndrome (AIDS). Jpn J Cancer Chemother 10:2429–2441.
2. Gatti RA and Good RA (1971). Occurrence of malignancy in immunodeficiency disease. Cancer 28:89–98.
3. Spector BD, Perry AS and Kersey JH (1979). Genetically determined immunodeficiency diseases and malignancy: Report from the Immunodeficiency Cancer Registry. Clin Immunol Immunopath 11:12–29.
4. Levine AS (1984). Viruses, immune dysregulation and oncogenesis: Inferences regarding the cause and evolution of AIDS. In: Friedman-Kien AE and Laubenstein LJ (Eds.). AIDS, The Epidemic of Kaposi's Sarcoma and Opportunistic Infections. New York: Masson Publishing Co.
5. Dancis A, Odajnyk C, Krigel RL et al. (1984). Association of Hodgkin's and non-Hodgkin's lymphomas with the Acquired Immunodeficiency Syndrome (AIDS). Proc Amer Soc Clin Oncol 3:61.
6. Odajnuk C, unpublished.
7. Friedman-Kien AE, Laubenstein LJ, Rubinstein P et al. (1982). Disseminated Kaposi's sarcoma in homosexual men. Ann Intern Med 96:693–700.
8. The Non-Hodgkin's Lymphoma Pathologic Classification Project (1982). National Cancer Institute Sponsored Study of Classification of Non-Hodgkin's Lymphomas. Cancer 49:2212–2235.
9. Carbone PP, Kaplan HS, Musshoff K et al. (1971). Report of the Committee of Hodgkin's Disease Staging Classification. Cancer Res 31:1860–1861.
10. Ziegler JL, Miner RC, Rosenbaum E et al. (1982). Outbreak of Burkitt's-like lymphoma in homosexual men. Lancet 2:631–633.
11. Doll DC and List AF (1982). Burkitt's lymphoma in a homosexual (letter). Lancet 1:1026–1027.
12. Chaganti RSK, Thanwor SC, Koziner B et al. (1983). Specific translocation characterize Burkitt's-like lymphoma of homosexual men with Acquired Immunodeficiency Syndrome. Blood 61:1265–1268.
13. Levine AM, Meyer PR, Beganany MR et al. (1984). Development of B-cell lymphoma in homosexual men. Ann Intern Med 100:7–13.
14. Ciobanu N, Andreeff M, Safai B et al. (1983). Lymphoblastic neoplasia in a homosexual patient with Kaposi's sarcoma. Ann Intern Med 8:151–155.
15. Snider WD, Simpson DM, Aranoyk KE et al. (1983). Primary lymphoma of the nervous system associated with Acquired Immunodeficiency Syndrome. N Engl J Med 308:45.
16. Case records of the Massachusetts General Hospital (Case 32 – 1983). N Engl J Med 309:359–369.
17. Ioachim HL, Lerner CW and Tapper ML (1983). Lymphadenopathies in homosexual men. JAMA 250:1306–1309.
18. Brynes RK, Chan WC, Spira TJ et al. (1983). Value of lymph node biopsy in unexplained lymphadenopathy in homosexual men. JAMA 250:1313–1317.
19. Metroka C, Cunningham-Rundles S, Pollack et al. (1983). Generalized lymphadenopathy in homosexual men. Ann Intern Med 99:585–591.
20. Reynolds WA, Winkelman RK and Soule EH (1965). Kaposi's sarcoma: A clinicopathologic study with particular reference to its relationship to the reticuloendothelial system. Medicine 44:419–438.
21. Harwood AR, Osoba D, Hofstader SL et al. (1979). Kaposi's sarcoma in recipients of renal transplants. Amer J Med 67:759–765.
22. Ziegler JL, Beckstead JA, Volberding PA et al. (1984). Non-Hodgkin's lymphoma in 90 homosexual men: Relationship to generalized lymphadenopathy and Acquired Immunode-

ficiency Syndrome (AIDS). N Engl J Med. (In Press).

23. Buchler SK, Firme F, Fodor G et al. (1975). Common variable immunodeficiency, Hodgkin's disease, and other malignancies in a Newfoundland family. Lancet 1:195–197.

24. Hoover R and Fraumeni JF Jr (1973). Risk of cancer in renal transplant recipients. Lancet 2:55–57.

25. Krikorian JG, Anderson GL, Beber CP et al. (1978). Malignant neoplasms following cardiac transplantation. JAMA 240:639–643.

26. Lanza RP, Cooper DKC, Cassidy MJD and Bernard CN (1983). Malignant neoplasms occurring after cardiac transplantation. JAMA 249:1746–1748.

27. Arnold A, Cassman J, Bakhshi A et al. (1983). Immunoglobulin gene rearrangements as unique clonal markers in human lymphoid neoplasias. N Engl J Med 309:1593–1599.

28. Cleary ML, Wainke R and Sklar J (1984). Monoclonality of lymphoproliferative lesions in cardiac transplant recipients. N Engl J Med 310:477–482.

29. Cleary ML, Chao J, Warnke R and Sklar J (1984). Immunoglobulin gene rearrangement as a diagnostic criterion of B-cell lymphoma. Proc Nat Acad Sci USA 81:593–597.

30. Blattner WA ,Takatsuki K and Gallo RC (1983). Human T-cell leukemia lymphoma virus and adult T-cell leukemia. JAMA 250:1074–1080.

31. HTLV and AIDS (1983). Editorial. Lancet 1:1200.

32. Evans AS, Carvuelho RPS, Frost R et al. (1978). Epstein-Barr virus infections in Brazil. II. Hodgkin's disease. J Nat Cancer Inst 61:19–26.

33. Hesse J, Levine PH, Ebbesen P et al. (1977). A case control study on immunity to two Epstein-Barr virus-associated antigens and to herpes simplex virus and adenovirus in a population-based group of patients with Hodgkin's disease in Denmark. Int J Cancer 19:49–58.

34. Fanto DW, Frizzera G, Gajl-Peczalaska KJ et al. (1982). Epstein-Barr virus induced B-cell lymphoma after renal transplantation: Acyclovir therapy and transition from polyclonal to monoclonal B-cell proliferation. N Engl J Med 306:913–918.

35. Saemundsen AK, Berkel AI, Henle W et al. (1981). Epstein Barr virus carrying lymphoma in a patient with ataxia telangiectasia. Br Med J 282:425–427.

36. Marker SL, Ascher NL, Kalis JM et al. (1979). Epstein Barr virus antibody responses and clinical illness in renal transplant recipients. Surgery 85:433–440.

37. Saemundsen AK, Purtilo DT, Sakamot K et al. (1981). Documentation of Epstein-Barr virus infection in immunodeficient patient with life-threatening lymphoproliferative disease by Epstein-Barr virus complementary RNA/DNA and viral DNA/DNA hybridization. Cancer Res 41:4237–4242.

38. Hochberg FH, Miller G, Schooley RT et al. (1983). Central nervous system lymphoma related to Epstein-Barr virus. N Engl J Med 309:745–748.

39. Dalla Favera R (1982). The human c-myc onc-gene is located on the region of chromosome 8 which is translocated in Burkitt's lymphoma cells. Proc Nat Acad Sci USA 79:7824–7827.

40. Miller G (1984). Epstein-Barr virus immortalization and replication. N Engl J Med 310:1255–1256.

41. Sixby JW, Nedrud JG, Raab-Traub N et al. (1984). Epstein-Barr virus replication in oropharyngeal epithelial cells. N Engl J Med 310:1225–1230.

3. Unusual presentations
of non-Hodgkin's lymphomas in homosexual males

S. A. RIGGS[1], S. KALTER[1], F. CABANILLAS[1],
F. B. HAGEMEISTER[1], W. S. VELASQUEZ[1], B. BARLOGIE[1],
P. SALVADOR[1], P. MANSELL[2], E. HERSH[3] and J. BUTLER[4]
*Departments of [1] Hematology, [2] Cancer Prevention, [3] Clinical
Immunology and [4] Pathology, University of Texas M.D. Anderson
Hospital and Tumor Institute Houston, Texas, USA*

The acquired immune deficiency syndrome (AIDS), defined by the Center for Disease Control as the presence of either Kaposi's sarcoma or opportunistic infection in a high-risk individual such as a homosexual male, Haitian, drug abuser, or hemophiliac [1], reached epidemic levels in certain areas of the United States in 1981. Doll and List [2] and Ziegler [3] described the first cases of lymphomas occurring in immunosuppressed homosexual males. By 1983, it became apparent that this population had a greater than expected incidence of central nervous system (NCS) lymphoma and, consequently, the presence of primary CNS lymphoma was incorporated into the definition of AIDS [1]. Since 1980, we have seen 15 homosexual males with non-Hodgkin's lymphoma, six of whom had CNS involvement.

Materials and methods

The patient population consisted of 15 male lymphoma patients expressing homosexual preferences who were seen in the U.T. M.D. Anderson Hospital clinics since 1980. The pathology was reviewed by one of us (JJB), using both a modified Rappaport classification and the Working Formulation for Clinical Usage [4], as shown in Table I. Routine clinical staging procedures were used. Special studies, including measurement of peripheral blood T-lymphocyte helper – suppressor ratios, delayed skin test hypersensitivity, and immunoperoxidase staining of frozen tissue sections for B- and T-cell markers were performed as described previously [5]. Additional studies, performed when possible, included flow cytometric analyses for cell proliferative activity and aneuploidy, and chromosomal banding techniques. Human T-cell leukemia-lymphoma (HTVL) viral antibody titers [6] were done through the courtesy of Dr. Robert Gallo's laboratory. Therapy varied

Table I. Presenting data of homosexual male lymphoma patients

Pt	Histology	Age	Stage	Extranodal Sites	KS	Preceding Adenopathy	T$_4$/cu mm	T$_4$/T$_8$	Skin Tests
1	DLC	40	IVB	Brain, Lung, Liver	Yes	No	17	.02	Anergic
2	DLC	38	IVB	Brain, Lung	Yes	No	110	.49	Anergic
3	DLC	36	IVB	Brain	Yes	No	8	.03	Anergic
4	DLC	45	IVA	Brain	No	No	69	.16	Hypoergic
5	DLC	33	IVA	Brain	No	No	66	.15	Anergic
6	DUL (SNCC)	28	IVA	Small bowel	Yes	Yes	75	.33	Hypoergic
7	DUL (SNCC)	20	IIIA	—	No	Yes	397	.50	Hypoergic
8	DUL (SNCC)	30	IVB	Marrow, Tonsil	No	Yes	21	.30	Anergic
9	DUL (SNCC)	34	IVB	Small bowel	Yes	Yes	607	.47	Hypoergic
10	DUL (SNCC)	35	IVA	Marrow. Liver, CNS	No	No	341	.38	Hypoergic
11	DUL (SNCC)	44	IIIA	—	No	No	677	.33	Hypoergic
12	UNCL	37	IVA	Marrow, Lung	No	No	333	.80	Anergic
13	WDLL(SL	45	IVA	Marrow, Ear lobes	No	No	—	—	—
14	NPDL(FSCC)	44	IIEA	Kidney	No	No	—	.	—
15	NPDL(FSCC)	42	IVA	Marrow, Liver	No	No	—	—	—

DLC = Diffuse large cell lymphoma
DUL(SNCC) = Diffuse undifferentiated lymphoma (small non-cleaved cell)
UNCL = Unclassified lymphoma
WDLL(SL) = Well differentiated lymphocytic lymphoma (small lymphocytic)
NPDL(FSCC) = Nodular poorly differentiated lymphocytic lymphoma (follicular small cleaved cell)
KS = Kaposi's sarcoma
T$_4$ = T helper lymphocyte (normal >500/cu mm)
T$_4$/T$_8$ = T helper: suppressor ratio (normal >1.0)
Anergic = Reacting to 0/6 antigens
Hypoergic = Reacting to 1/6 antigens

according to clinical status, histologic subtype and extent of disease. Combination chemotherapy and regional radiotherapy were used as shown in Table II.

Results

Of the 15 patients, five had DLC, six had DUL of either the Burkitt's or non-Burkitt's type, one had unclassifiable lymphoma, one had WDLL, and two had NPDL (Table I). Fourteen patients had advanced disease. Unusual sites of extranodal involvement were seen in all groups of patients, including primary brain DLC, tonsillar DUL, and WDLL of the ear lobes.

The median age of the 15 patients was 36 years. Twelve were from Houston or other cities in Texas, although several had recently traveled to San

Table II. Response of lymphoma to treatment

Pt	Histology	Treatment	Response	Survival
1	DLC	MBV	No	Died 1 month
2	DLC	Cranial XRT, VP-16	No	Died 1 month
3	DLC	Cranial XRT, AM	PR	Died 5 months
4	DLC	Cranial XRT	No	Died 3 months
5	DLC	Cranial XRT, CHOP-B	PR	Died 3 months
6	DUL	CHOP-M	CR	30+ months
7	DUL	MCOAP	CR	14+ months
8	DUL	XRT, IMVP-16	CR	Died 12 months
9	DUL	MCOAP	CR	14+ months
10	DUL	Cranial XRT, VAD	PR	Died 3 months
11	DUL	MCOAP	CR	2+ months
12	UNCL	XRT, CHOP-B	CR	8+ months
13	WDLL	CHOP-B	PR	27+ months
14	NPDL	CHOP-B	PR	52+ months
15	NPDL	CHOP-B	PR	30+ months

MBV   = Methotrexate, bleomycin, Velban
VP-16   = Etoposide
AM   = Cytosine arabinoside, methotrexate
CHOP-B   = Cytoxan, doxorubicin, vincristine, prednisone, bleomycin
CHOP-M   = Cytoxan, doxorubicin, vincristine, prednisone, methotrexate
MCOAP   = Methotrexate, cytoxan, vincristine, cytosine, arabinoside, prednisone
IMVP-16 = Ifosfamide, methotrexate, etoposide
VAD   = Vincristine, doxorubicin, decadron
XRT   = Radiotherapy
PR   = Partial remission
CR   = Complete remission

Francisco or New York. Two patients were intravenous drug abusers and most of the remainder used other types of recreational drugs including amylnitrites.

Four of the DLC patients (No. 1, 2, 3, 5) had AIDS, based on a history of opportunistic infections, including *Candida* and *Toxoplasma* brain abscess, *Cryptosporidium* intestinal infection, *Candida* esophagitis, and *Pneumocystis* pneumonia. The diagnosis of AIDS in one DLC patient (No. 4) was based on primary CNS lymphoma alone, and two DUL patients (No. 6, 9) were later classified as having AIDS when they developed KS. The remainder of the DUL patients and the one with unclassified lymphoma (No. 7, 8, 10, 11, 12) had the AIDS-related complex (ARC), defined as the presence of certain clinical and laboratory parameters indicative of an immunocompromised state, occurring in any individual at high risk for development of AIDS. The three remaining patients (No. 13–15) had neither AIDS nor the ARC.

Immunologic testing (Table I) revealed decreased numbers of helper T-lymphocytes, inverted helper – suppressor T-cell ratios, and decreased delayed hypersensitivity in all patients tested. The most profound deficiencies occurred in the LCL patients. All 12 patients tested had elevated IgG viral capsid antigen antibody titers to the Epstein-Barr virus (EBV), 11 of 12 tested had elevated IgG antibody titers to cytomegalovirus (CMV), and several had positive serologic tests for the hepatitis B surface antigen and antibodies to *Toxoplasma gondii*. Three of six patients tested had positive serum antibody titers to HTLV. No Coomb's positive hemolytic anemias, immune thrombocytopenias, or monoclonal gammopathies were seen.

The lymphoma tissue of all 15 patients had the appearance of B-cell neoplasms. Immunoperoxidase studies in all six DUL patients revealed IgG kappa in four, IgG lambda in one, and IgM kappa in one. Chromosome studies performed on lymphoma tissue in four DUL patients revealed t(8; 14) with loss of the Y chromosome in two, t(8; 14) in one, and t(8; 22), +12 in one. Flow cytometry on the tumor tissue of four DUL patients disclosed high proliferative activity, and the patient with the extra No. 12 chromosome had aneuploidy confirmed by DNA index. Four DUL patients had preceding reactive lymphadenopathy, which was consistent in three with the follicular and sinusoidal hyperplasia described in homosexual males [8]. However, severe lymphoid depletion was found terminally in the lymphoid tissue of all patients autopsied, including three with DLC and two with DUL.

Patients' response to treatment is shown in Table II. All DLC patients had poor tolerance to treatment, with no complete remissions documented, and all died within five months of diagnosis. In contrast, five of the six patients with DUL achieved complete remissions and three remain free of active lymphoma at 14, 14, and 30 months. All showed excellent tolerance to intensive combination chemotherapy. One of the latter (No. 6) has been successfully treated with lymphoblastoid interferon for localized KS of the palate and currently has no evidence of active DUL or KS. The four patients with unclassifiable lymphoma, WDLL, and NPDL are all alive with remissions lasting 8, 27, 30, and 52 months; they are also tolerating combination chemotherapy well.

Discussion

The non-Hodgkin's lymphomas, recently noted to be increased in the male homosexual population, strongly resemble those occurring in other severely immunocompromised individuals, including transplant recipients and children with congenital immunodeficiencies. A close analogy can be drawn between renal and cardiac transplant patients, who have up to a 350 times increased incidence of lymphomas of the brain [9], and our group of diffuse large cell lymphoma patients, who had a 100% prevalence of parenchymal brain lesions. In our experience, only five patients with initial brain involvement alone had been seen since 1952, in a clinic where approximately 60 newly diagnosed, previously untreated DLC patients are evaluated each year. Profound T-cell deficiencies, coexisting opportunistic infections, high prevalence of Kaposi's sarcoma, and multifocal lymphoma at diagnosis were probably all contributing factors to the poor tolerance and response to treatment in our homosexual patients with DLC. Appropriate diagnostic radiologic procedures and brain biopsies in homosexual patients with even minor neurologic symptoms are essential because early diagnosis of brain lymphoma, and especially differentiation from infections such as toxoplasmosis, may lead to improved responses of these malignancies to treatment.

In contrast, only one patient with diffuse undifferentiated lymphoma had CNS involvement and this consisted of a peripheral cranial nerve lesion. Extranodal presentation sites (Table I), except the tonsillar lesion, were those generally expected for American DUL [10]. The tonsillar lesion eventually progressed to massive jaw and cervical soft tissue involvement, similar to that seen in children with Burkitt's lymphoma in endemic areas of Africa. Despite serologic evidence of exposure to numerous infectious agents in these DUL patients, tolerance to intensive chemotherapy was better than that of the DLC patients. Absence of serious active infections and lesser degrees of T-cell abnormalities probably accounted for this improved tolerance. Preceding and coexisting reactive lymphadenopathy in the DUL patients suggested good immunologic reserve. High proliferative activity of their lymphoma tissue may have resulted in diagnosis at earlier stages of disease, thus allowing for more effective therapy.

None of the four patients with unclassifiable or indolent (NPDL and WDLL) lymphomas had clinical evidence of severe immunodeficiency. None have developed either opportunistic infections or Kaposi's sarcoma, but we feel that careful monitoring for either of these complications is indicated in this group.

Most of our patients have evidence of exposure to numerous antigenic stimuli, including cytomegalovirus and the Epstein-Barr virus. The role that these and other factors, such as chronic sperm antigenic stimulation, recreational drugs, and exposure to other infectious agents (e.g. hepatitis viruses and the newly described HTLV-3 organism [11]), play in the development of extranodal B-cell malignancies in the homosexual population deserves extensive further investigation. The polyclonal B-cell proliferation which occurs in AIDS patients [12], in the presence of altered T-cell regulatory systems, may occasionally progress to neoplastic transformation if the appropriate stimuli are present. The study of all of these factors, along with continued investigation of the chromosomal defects seen in the lymphoma tissue of some of these patients, could improve understanding of oncogenesis in lymphoproliferative disorders in general.

The unusual presentations of lymphomas in immunosuppressed homosexual males, including the high incidence of large cell lymphoma of the brain, require appropriate diagnostic workups, including brain and lung biopsies. Lymphomas must be distinguished from the lesions of opportunistic infections, which frequently occur in these patients. Earlier diagnosis may lead to improved response to treatment and survival in these patients. We also stress that aggressive combination chemotherapy can be well tolerated and may lead to an improved survival in the patients without severe concomitant opportunistic infections, including those with undifferentiated and indolent lymphomas.

References

1. Selik RM, Haverkos HW and Curran JW (1984). Acquired immunodeficiency syndrome (AIDS) trends in the United States, 1978–1982. Amer J Med 76:493–500.
2. Doll DC and List AF (1982). Burkitt's lymphoma in a homosexual. Lancet 1:1026–1027.
3. Ziegler JL, Miner RC, Rosenbaum E et al. (1982). Outbreak of Burkitt's-like lymphoma among homosexual men. Lancet 2:631–633.
4. Non-Hodgkin's Lymphoma Pathologic Classification Project (1982). National Cancer Institute sponsored study of classifications of non-Hodgkin's lymphomas. Cancer 49:2112–2135.
5. Reuben JM, Hersh EM, Mansell PW et al. (1983). Immunological characterization of homosexual males. Cancer Res 897–904.
6. Gallo RC and Wong-Staal F (1982). Retroviruses as etiologic agents of some animal and human leukemias and lymphomas and as tools for elucidating the molecular mechanism of leukemogenesis. Blood 60:545–557.

7. Curran JW (1983). AIDS — Two years later (editorial). N Engl J Med 309:609–611.

8. Guarda LA, Butler JJ, Mansell P et al. (1983). Lymphadenopathy in homosexual men. Morbid anatomy with clinical and immunologic correlations. Amer J Clin Pathol 79:559–568.

9. Penn I (1977). Development of cancer as a complication of clinical transplantation. Transplant Proc 9:1121–1128.

10. Arseneau JC, Canellos GP, Banks PM et al. (1975). American Burkitt's lymphoma: A clinicopathologic study of 30 cases. Amer J Med 58:314–329.

11. Gallo RC, Salahuddin SZ, Popovic M et al. (1984). Frequent detection and isolation of cytopathic retroviruses (HTLV-III) from patients with AIDS and at risk for AIDS. Science 224:500–503.

12. Lane HC, Masur H, Edgar LC et al. (1983). Abnormalities of B-cell activation and immunoregulation in patients with the acquired immunodeficiency syndrome. N Engl J Med 309:453–458.

4. Immunoproliferative small intestinal disease

P. SALEM, L. EL-HASHIMI, E. ANAISSI, M. KHALIL
and C. ALLAM
Medical Center, American University of Beirut, Beirut, Lebanon

Primary intestinal lymphoma is the most common form of extra-nodal lymphomas in the Middle East, accounting for 50% of all extra-nodal and 75% of gastro-intestinal lymphomas in adults [1]. In the West, this disease is less frequent, accounting for 20% of all extra-nodal, and 30% of gastro-intestinal lymphomas [2]. A new form of this lymphoma, immunoproliferative small intestinal disease (IPSID), has been shown to be geographically confined primarily to Mediterranean and Middle Eastern countries [3, 4]. In most reports, IPSID was studied and compared to primary intestinal lymphomas as encountered in the West. This study is an attempt to further delineate the distinctive features of IPSID and to compare it to other forms of intestinal lymphomas in the Middle East.

Materials and methods

We have reviewed the hospital records and pathology materials of all patients older than 14 years of age who had suspected primary lymphoma of the intestine and/or the mesentery, and who were diagnosed at the American University of Beirut Medical Center between 1961 and 1980. Pathology materials were classified by one of us (C.A.) according to the Kiel classification and the International Working Formulation [5]. Three types of primary intestinal lymphomas were recognized: IPSID, non-IPSID, and lymphoma of undetermined nature (LUN). IPSID was diagnosed when at least one of the following criteria was documented: 1) Presence of alpha heavy chain protein (ACHP) [6], concomitantly with the presence of diffuse cellular infiltrate in the intestinal mucosa, irrespective of its benign or malignant nature; 2) Malignant lymphoma in intestinal or mesenteric nodes in association with a continuous, diffuse, and dense mucosal infiltrate involving long segments of the small intestine. Primary intestinal lymphoma was considered of undetermined nature (LUN) when adequate studies for distinguishing IPSID from non-IPSID were lacking.

Criteria of inclusion

1) All cases of IPSID irrespective of stage, and including the pre-lymphomatous phase (Stage 0); 2) All cases of non-IPSID and LUN with lymphoma confined to the intestine and/or mesenteric nodes (Stages I-II). Patients with Stages III and IV non-IPSID or LUN were excluded from this study because it was difficult to determine the precise site of the primary in these patients. Some of the patients described in this study have been reported [3].

Laboratory studies

Beginning in 1971, all patients with suspected primary intestinal lymphoma underwent immunoglobulin studies and staging laparotomy. Immunoelectrophoresis was performed on agarose (0.75%) in barbiturate buffer using the LKB system. Goat anti-human polyvalent sera, specific anti-IgG, anti-IgA, anti-IgD, anti-Kappa and anti-Lambda were obtained from Meloy Laboratories. Immunoglobulin levels were determined by the single radial immuno-diffusion test using antibody-containing plates purchased from Meloy Laboratories. Studies of urine were performed on a sample of 24-hour collections concentrated 50–100 times through cellophane bags under vacuum. Immunofluorescence and immunoperoxidase studies on involved intestinal tissues were not performed.

Staging laparotomy

This was performed according to a protocol which was previously described [3]. Patients diagnosed prior to 1971 underwent exploratory laparotomy for diagnostic purposes, and staging in these patients was considered inadequate.

Results

Of a total of 77 patients, 32 had IPSID, 27 had non-IPSID and 18 had LUN. Primary intestinal lymphoma was documented in all patients except in two who were considered in Stage 0 IPSID.

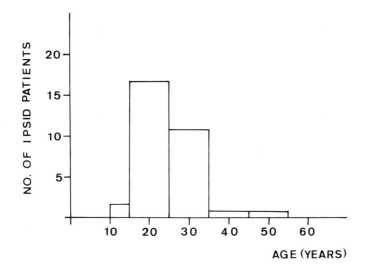

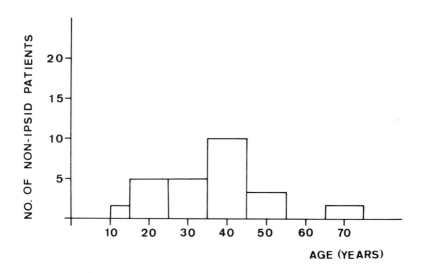

Figure 1. Distribution of patients by age.

Age and sex

There was gradual decrease in incidence with increasing age. IPSID occurred in patients somewhat younger than those with non-IPSID (Fig. 1), with median ages of 25 years (14–46) and 37 years (14–75), respectively. Male to female ratio was 1.7/1 in the entire series, 1.2/1 in IPSID, and 2.1/1 in non-IPSID.

Clinical presentation

Abdominal pain was the most common complaint, occurring in approximately two-thirds of the patients, with no conspicuous difference in incidence or severity between IPSID and non-IPSID (Table I). At presentation, IPSID patients generally had chronic diarrhea, weight loss, emaciation, and clubbing of fingers and toes. Diarrhea was usually associated with malabsorption and its duration, prior to diagnosis, ranged between 3 and 120 months with a median of 18. Non-IPSID patients commonly presented with a palpable abdominal mass and complications such as intestinal obstruction, perforation or bleeding.

Gross pathologic findings

IPSID
Thirty IPSID patients underwent laparotomy; diagnosis was made by peroral multiple intestinal biopsies in the remaining two patients. At laparotomy, gross tumor was lacking in 18, with normal intestinal appearance in 7, and segmental thickening and/or dilation of the intestine in 11 (entire length of the small intestine in four, upper small intestine in six, and ileum in one). Twelve patients had gross tumors in the small intestine (nine), both the small and large intestines (two), or both the stomach and small intestine (one). The proximal one-third of the small intestine was the most common site of involvement. Gross disease was confined to the duodenum and/or proximal jejunum in 77% of the patients who had either gross tumors or intestinal abnormalities. Multiple tumors were found in seven patients.

Non-IPSID
All patients with non-IPSID underwent exploratory laparotomy and all

Table I. Presenting features

	IPSID %	NON-IPSID %	LUN %	Total %
Clinical Features				
Abdominal pain	68	69	63	67
Weight loss	81	30	38	53
Chronic diarrhea	84	7	38	47
Abdominal mass	20	66	50	42
Intestinal obstruction, bleeding or perforation	10	46	25	26
Clubbing of fingers	39	0	6	18

except two were found to have gross tumors. In the two patients who had no tumors, the primary lesion was described by the surgeon as a localized area of intestinal thickening in the jejunum. In the 25 patients who had tumors, the disease was confined to the small intestine in 20 and to the large intestine in one; it involved both small and large intestines in three, and the entire gastro-intestinal tract, from the stomach to the colon, in one. The ileo-coecal region was the most common site of involvement, and was involved in 60% of the patients who had gross tumors. Of note, lymphoma confined to the proximal small intestine was found in 40% of the non-IPSID patients.

Microscopic findings

IPSID

Cellular infiltrates in the mucosa (MCI) were described in all patients, and involved the entire length of the small intestine in the 18 patients who had adequate sampling at laparotomy. There were 4 types of MCI. Diffuse lymphoplasmacytic or plasmacytic (DLP) MCI occurred in 16 patients and was apparently benign in eight. Follicular lymphoid (FL) MCI was described in 10 patients, of whom six had follicular lymphoid hyperplasia, and four had follicular lymphoma. Mixed MCI (DLP in the most superficial layers of the mucosa, and FL in the deeper layers) was found in three patients who had follicular lymphoma in the mucosa. Non-specific MCI (increased cellularity with predominantly normal-looking lymphocytes, plasma cells, and eosinophils) was noted in three patients.

Table II. Pathologic subtypes of lymphoma (Working Formulation)

Lymphoma	IPSID	NON–IPSID	LUN	Total
Low Grade				
Small lymphocytic plasmacytoid	12	—	—	12
Others	5	—	2	7
Intermediate Grade				
Diffuse large cell	2	5	4	11
Diffuse small cleaved cell	2	3	2	7
Diffuse small + large cell	3	3	2	8
High Grade				
Large cell immunoblastic	6	12	7	25
Small non-cleaved cell	—	4	1	5
	30	27	18	75

Of the 30 patients with IPSID who had lymphoma, the lymphoma was mostly of low grade malignancy (Table II). The intestinal lymphomatous infiltrate was confined to the mucosa and submucosa except in patients with gross tumors where the lymphoma penetrated all layers of intestine at the site of tumor. When the mucosal infiltrate was DLP, the lymphoma was usually small lymphocytic plasmacytoid; when it was FL, the lymphoma was of intermediate or of high grade malignancy.

Non-IPSID

In contrast to IPSID, lymphoma in non-IPSID was confined to the site of tumor or gross abnormalities. The type of lymphoma was either of intermediate or high grade malignancy (Table II). All layers of the intestinal wall were involved except in one patient whose disease was restricted to the mucosa and submucosa.

Stage

Our previous staging classification [3] was modified to emphasize that Stage 0 required adequate staging laparotomy and AHCP documentation (Table III). Stage should be considered unknown without proper staging. Twenty-seven patients with IPSID underwent adequate staging; of these, two were in the prelymphomatous phase (Stage 0) and 20 had a lymphoma limited to the intestine and/or mesenteric nodes. Of nine Stage I patients, four had lymphoma in mesenteric nodes without intestinal involvement (Table IV). Of the five Stage III patients, three had lymphoma in peripheral nodes, and two had lymphoma in retroperitoneal nodes. None of our IPSID patients had documented Stage IV. Stages III and IV were excluded from the study when the lymphoma was non-IPSID or LUN as described in Materials and Methods. The overwhelming majority of non-IPSID patients were in Stage II, and none had lymphoma confined to mesenteric nodes.

Table III. Definition of Stage in IPSID

Stage	
0	Diffuse benign-appearing mucosal cellular infiltrate + aHCP without evidence of lymphoma by staging laparotomy
I	Malignant lymphoma either in intestine (Ii) or in mesenteric nodes (In) but not in both
II	Malignant lymphoma in both intestine and mesenteric nodes
III	Involvement of retroperitoneal or extra-abdominal nodes
IV	Involvement of non-contiguous extranodal tissues

Table IV. Stage distribution

	IPSID	NON-IPSID	LUN	Total
Stage				
0	2	0	0	2
Ii	5	6	3	14
In	4	0	2	6
II	11	20	11	42
III	5	Excl	Excl	5
IV	0	Excl	Excl	0
Inadequate staging	5	1	2	8
	32	27	18	77

Immunoglobulin studies

AHCP was studied in the serum and intestinal fluids of 24 patients. Among the nine patients in whom these studies were positive, MCI was apparently benign in eight (DLP: 7, FL: 1) and malignant in one who had DLP infiltrate and small lymphocytic plasmacytoid lymphoma. Among the patients who had documented AHCP, five had small lymphocytic plasmacytoid lymphoma, two had immunoblastic lymphoma (including the case with FL infiltrate), and two had pre-lymphomatous Stage 0 IPSID.

Discussion

Our study indicates that IPSID is a distinct disease entity associated with characteristic clinical, pathologic, and immunologic features. Clinically, patients with IPSID presented with chronic diarrhea, weight loss, and emaciation. Those with non-IPSID presented with an abdominal mass or complications, such as intestinal obstruction, bleeding, and perforation. IPSID is a generalized mucosal disease which is either benign or malignant, while non-IPSID is a localized transmural disease which is always malignant. At laparotomy, none of the non-IPSID patients were free of macroscopic intestinal abnormalities (92.5 % had gross tumors) vs 23 % of the IPSID patients (40 % had gross tumors). The presence of a tumor in the ileo-cecal region was noted in 60 % of the non-IPSID patients, but in none of the IPSID patients. Histo-pathologically, the features were most distinctive and diagnostic. IPSID was always associated with cellular infiltrates confined to the mucosa and submucosa of the entire length of the small intestine which probably accounts for chronic diarrhea and malabsorption. In non-IPSID, this MCI was lacking. Sites distant from the primary lesion were free of lymphomatous infiltrate and the lymphoma mostly involved all layers of the intestinal wall. This explains why patients with non-IPSID are predisposed to bleeding, perforation, and obstruction. In addition, IPSID was commonly associated with small lymphocytic plasmacytoid lymphoma (12/30). This lymphoma was lacking in non-IPSID.

Probably the best single diagnostic criterion of IPSID is the synthesis and secretion of an abnormal IgA immunoglobulin (AHCP) which is devoid of light chains [6]. This abnormal protein could be detected in the serum, urine, intestinal fluid, or abnormal cells. Patients with suspected IPSID whose serum and intestinal fluid are free of AHCP, should have immunofluorescence and immunoperoxidase studies performed on tissues removed from involved intestinal segments for the detection of intra-cellular AHCP. Since these studies were not done in our patients, the presence of AHCP could not be ruled out in the 15 patients who had negative serum and/or intestinal fluid and its specificity for IPSID could not be ascertained.

It was previously emphasized that the cellular infiltrate which is associated with IPSID is characteristically plasmacytic or lymphoplasmacytic [4, 7]. Ten of our IPSID patients had FL infiltrate; all had continuous and uninterrupted MCI along the entire length of the small intestine with clinical and radiologic features that were identical to those with IPSID and DLP infiltrate; ACHP was positive in one. This pattern of IPSID has been reported without, however, AHCP positivity [8, 9]. Immunofluorescence and immunoperoxidase studies should be conducted in a larger number of patients to determine whether the FL pattern represents the non-secretory form of IPSID.

Acknowledgements

This study was supported by the Lebanese National Council for Scientific Research.

References

1. Anaissie E, Geha S, Allam C et al. Non-Hodgkin's lymphoma. A study of 417 patients from the Middle East. (In preparation).
2. Bradly LW and Osbel SO (1980). Malignant lymphoma of the gastrointestinal tract. Radiology 137:291.
3. Salem PA, Nassar VH, Shahid MJ et al. (1977). Mediterranean abdominal lymphoma, or immunoproliferative small intestinal disease. Cancer 40:2941–2947.
4. Khojasten A, Haghshenass M and Haghighi P (1977). Immunoproliferative small intestinal disease. A third-world lesion. N Engl J Med 308:1401–1405.

5. The Non-Hodgkin's Lymphoma Pathologic Classification Project (1982). National Cancer Institute sponsored study of non-Hodgkin's lymphomas. Summary and description of a working formulation for clinical usage. Cancer 49:2112–2135.
6. Seligmann M, Danon F, Hurez D et al. (1968). Alpha-chain disease: A new immunoglobulin abnormality. Science 162:1396–1400.
7. Rappaport H, Ramot B, Hulu N et al. (1972). The pathology of so-called Mediterranean abdominal lymphoma with malabsorption. Cancer 29:1502–1511.
8. Nassar VH, Salem PA, Shahid MJ et al. (1978). Mediterranean abdominal lymphoma or immunoproliferative small intestinal disease. Part II Pathologic aspects. Cancer 41:1340–1354.
9. Rambaud J-C, DeSaint-Louvent P, Marti R et al. (1982). Diffuse follicular lymphoid hyperplasia of the small intestine without primary immunoglobulin deficiency. Amer J Med 73:125–132.

VI. Treatment of Hodgkin's disease

1. The current status of the Stanford randomized clinical trials of the management of Hodgkin's disease

S. A. ROSENBERG

Stanford University School of Medicine, Stanford, California, USA

Randomized trials designed to improve the management of patients with Hodgkin's disease were initiated at Stanford University in 1962. These studies tested different irradiation programs for patients with Clinical Stages (CS) I, II and III disease. In 1967 the study for patients with Stages IA and IIA was modified utilizing more extensive radiation fields and as of July 1968 routine diagnostic exploratory laparotomy and splenectomy.

In 1968 a new series of studies for Stages IB to IV were initiated. Exploratory laparotomy was used for all patients and combined modality programs employing MOPP as an adjuvant after radiotherapy were studied. In 1970, several modifications of these trials were made so that patients with Pathologic Stage (PS) IA and IIA disease were randomized to treatment with combined modality approaches.

In 1974, the third major revision in the Stanford clinical trials was initiated. These series of randomized trials tested MOPP as an adjuvant after minimal involved field irradiation for PS IA and IIA; a less toxic alternative to MOPP, the PAVe regimen, as an adjuvant or in combined modality programs for intermediate stages of the disease; and the use of combined modality regimens for Stage IV disease. In addition, a major change in scheduling of combined modality therapy was introduced; instead of giving all of the radiotherapy first and the chemotherapy later, or vice versa, the two treatment modalities were alternated. A further improvement in freedom from relapse rates for all patients was documented.

In 1980, the fourth major change in the Hodgkin's disease studies was initiated and are ongoing [1]. These current protocols build on the lessons learned from the earlier trials, particularly with respect to the serious long term morbidities of the combined modality programs. New prognostic factors were appreciated and the morbidity of therapy, both acute toxicity and late treatment complications, became major concerns and targets for improvement.

Statistical methods

All curves are actuarial, utilizing the Kaplan-Meier method [2]. Survival curves include deaths from all causes. Freedom from progression (FFP) events include disease recurrences and or extension following complete remission as well as failure to achieve complete remission, when an alternate or salvage treatment plan was decided upon. The actuarial curves begin with the date the patient was first seen at Stanford. All patients are considered evaluable. If patients died without clinical or autopsy evidence of Hodgkin's disease, they were censored in the FFP data, at the time of their death, but are included as events in the survival curves. The differences between actuarial curves were tested for significance by both the Gehan [3] and Cox [4] methods.

Treatment plans and results

The studies, initiated in 1962, utilized bipedal lymphography, bone marrow biopsy and chest tomography as routine staging procedures. Patients with Stages I and II disease, both A and B (without and with systemic symptoms) were randomized to involved field (IF) or extended field (EF) radiotherapy. For these purposes, the mediastinum was considered 'adjacent' to the neck on either side, and the paraaortic plus spleen field was considered 'adjacent' to the mediastinum. After 20 years the actuarial freedom from progression (FFP) rates favor the EF treatment with borderline significance with no difference in the actuarial survival between the two groups. Though patients were not stratified by systemic symptoms prior to randomization, it was observed that patients with systemic symptoms did poorly following IF therapy [5]. A significant advantage of the EF therapy in FFP could be demonstrated for patients with Stages IB and IIB with a borderline advantage in survival (Fig. 1).

Patients with Stage III disease above and below the diaphragm, were treated for the first time with high dose, total lymphoid irradiation in 1962. Patients were randomized to receive 1650 rad to involved fields or total lymphoid irradiation (TLI), to doses of 4400 rad to involved sites and 3500–4400 rad to uninvolved sites. The TLI fields were the mantle and inverted-Y radiation fields, which were developed in the course of these trials. Patients with A or B disease were combined. After randomizing the first 30 patients on this trial, it was appreciated that the higher dose TLI irradiation was safe and well tolerated, and the lower dose irradiation arm was experiencing a high relapse rate. Thereafter all Stage III patients were treated with TLI until the trial was terminated in 1968.

Fig. 2 shows the results of these studies. Minimal differences in survival

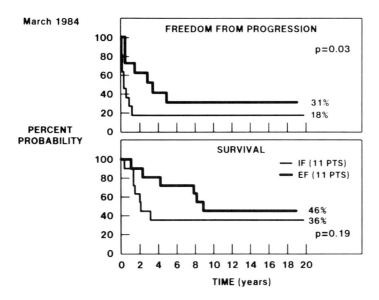

Figure 1. Hodgkin's disease, CS IB and IIB: Actuarial curves of freedom from progression and survival comparing involved field (IF) and extended field (EF) irradiation.

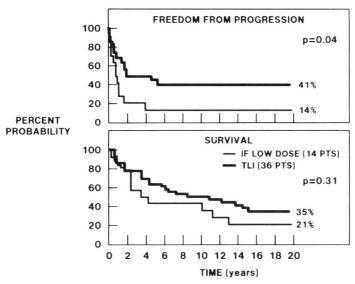

Figure 2. Hodgkin's disease, CS III: Actuarial curves of freedom from progression and survival, comparing involved field (1650 rads) and total lymphoid irradiation (3500–4400 rad).

have been demonstrated. However the FFP advantage was evident for the higher dose treatment, and for the first time long term relapse-free survival, in approximately 40% of patients, was achieved with irradiation alone for patients with Stage III disease.

284

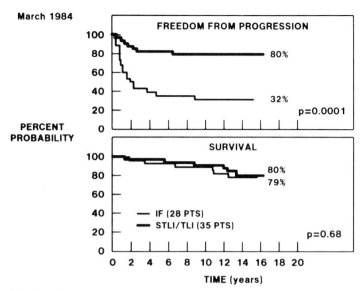

Figure 3. Hodgkin's disease. PS IA and IIA: Actuarial curves of freedom from progression and survival, comparing involved field (IF) and subtotal or total lymphoid irradition (STLI/TLI).

By 1967, the important prognostic difference between asymptomatic and symptomatic patients was evident and different management programs were tested for patients without (A) or with (B) systemic symptoms. Because of the frequent appearance of upper abdominal disease as a site of first extension after involved field mantle irradiation, and the frequent pattern of low neck and abdominal disease, without mediastinal involvement, a new study was devised. Staging laparotomy was utilized routinely after June 1968. The trial compared involved field (IF) radiotherapy to a minimum of subtotal lymphoid radiotherapy (mantle and paraaortic with splenic pedicle fields) in patients with Pathologic Stages IA or IIA disease. Total lymphoid irradiation was used for males and for women who did not wish to preserve fertility. Results of this study are shown in Fig. 3. A significant improvement in FFP resulted from the new definition of extended fields. However, a survival advantage has not been demonstrated, even 17 years after the initiation of the trial. The probable explanation for the lack of a survival advantage is the success of salvage treatment programs with subsequent irradiation and/or MOPP chemotherapy which were employed for patients relapsing after involved field irradiation. Since less than one in three patients enjoyed prolonged FFP following the involved field treatment, it was concluded, that subtotal or total lymphoid irradiation, was the treatment of choice for patients with PS IA and IIA Hodgkin's disease.

In 1968, the value of the MOPP chemotherapy program developed at the National Cancer Institute [6] became evident and trials were developed to

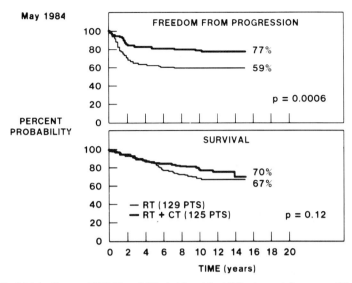

Figure 4. Hodgkin's disease. PS I, II and III: initiated in 1968. Actuarial curves of fredom from progression and survival comparing irradiation alone (XRT) and irradiation followed by adjuvant MOP(P) chemotherapy (CM).

test the value of combined modality therapy in patients with poorer prognoses. Patients staged with routine laparotomy and splenectomy with PS IB through IIIB disease were treated with total lymphoid irradiation either alone or followed by six cycles of MOPP.

In 1970, patients with PS IA and IIA were included in the adjuvant MOPP trial and treated either with a mantle field for favorable patients or subtotal lymphoid irradiation for less favorable patients.

The results of 254 patients in these studies are shown in Fig. 4. The MOP(P) adjuvant program, prednisone withheld in patients who had received mediastinal irradiation, provided an improvement in FFP for the entire group of patients, which was evident by two years following therapy. A survival advantage, for the entire group, was not suggested until six years after therapy, and even at 12 years is only of borderline significance (p(Cox) = 0.09).

However the results were different for the various stages of the disease. Adjuvant MOP(P) improved the FFP, but not the survival for patients with PS IA and IIA; did not improve the FFP or survival for patients with PS IB and IIB; improved the FFP *and* the survival for patients with PS IIIA; improved the FFP and possibly the survival (p(Cox) = 0.18) for patients with PS IIIB disease. Irradiation alone was not satisfactory for patients with PS IIIB disease. The 51% FFP and survival rate for PS IIIB patients treated with combined modality therapy cannot be interpreted as superior to MOPP chemotherapy alone, by comparison to the NCI results [7]. However the results of TLI alone for patients with PS IB-IIB and PS IIIA were quite good with 73% and 70% of these groups enjoying fifteen year FFP after irradiation alone.

In May 1974 the third major revision of the Hodgkin's disease trials was initiated. The new protocols were based upon the six year data of the adjuvant MOP(P) trials. The objectives of these trials were to attempt to reduce treatment morbidity by utilizing involved field radiotherapy followed by adjuvant MOP(P) for all patients with PS IA and IIA; to attempt to reduce the acute toxicity of the adjuvant with a new MOP(P)-like adjuvant regimen, PAVe (procarbazine, Alkeran, and vinblastine) for patients with intermediate prognoses, PS II_E and IIIA. For patients with poorer prognoses, PS IIIB, and IV_L, the chemotherapy regimens (MOP(P) or PAVe) were utilized in split course or alternating combined modality protocols. The alternating treatment plan was devised so that the patient's disease control would have the benefit of good local therapy with irradiation and good systemic therapy with chemotherapy without prolonged time interruptions from either.

For patients with PS I-IIB disease the studies continued to compare TLI to TLI followed by adjuvant MOP(P) because no survival or FFP differences had been demonstrated and it was thought desirable to increase the patient numbers to be more confident of the conclusion.

After enrolling 237 patients in these studies certain conclusions became evident.

1. Adjuvant MOP(P) could replace irradiation of occult disease in patients with PS IA-IIA disease (Fig. 5).
2. PAVe chemotherapy, as an adjuvant or as a component of combined modality programs was as effective as MOP(P).
3. PAVe chemotherapy had significantly less acute toxicity and morbidity than the MOP(P) regimen [8].
4. The split course, or alternating treatment regimen for patients with PS IIIB disease resulted in a significant improvement in FFP and probably survival when compared retrospectively to the experience with TLI alone or TLI followed by adjuvant MOP(P) (Fig. 6) or when compared to the experience with MOPP alone at the NCI [8].
5. The new treatment regimens tested in the 1974–80 studies resulted in improved FFP for *all* patients of all stages, when compared to earlier studies (1968–74) and to the studies in which only patients with CS I-III disease were included (1962–67).

Rationale for current studies

The late serious treatment complications of the combined modality therapy

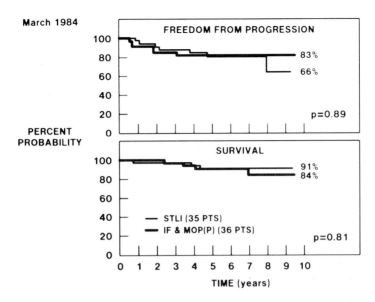

Figure 5. Hodgkin's disease, PS IA and IIA: Actuarial curves of freedom from progression and survival, comparing subtotal lymphoid irradiation (STLI) alone and involved field (IF) irradiation with MOP(P) chemotherapy.

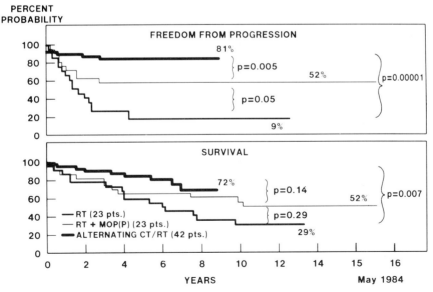

Figure 6. Hodgkin's disease , PS IIIB: Actuarial curves of freedom from progression and survival comparing alternating combined modality regimen to irradiation alone (TLI) and irradiation followed by chemotherapy (TLI & MOP(P).

288

of AML and sterility, make the routine use of MOP(P) or PAVe adjuvant chemotherapy an unacceptable alternative to wide-field irradiation alone. If an equally or relatively effective adjuvant regimen could be developed which is devoid of the serious long term sequelae it would become more acceptable to radically reduce radiation fields and perhaps dose in the treatment of even the most favorable patients. To be acceptable, however, the adjuvant would have to be relatively well tolerated as regards acute toxicity, and have little or no potential of inducing AML or sterility. No such adjuvant regimen has been reported. The Milan ABVD program was considered as an adjuvant regimen because to date no AML and only a low incidence of male sterility has been reported in ABVD-radiotherapy combined modality studies [9]. However, the ABVD program, has serious acute toxicity, including nausea, vomiting, and hair loss, primarily due to doxorubicin and dacarbazine and has the potential of inducing serious long term cardiotoxicity due to doxorubicin.

For these reasons it seems important to develop a relatively mild but effective adjuvant regimen. It was decided to use a combination of at least three agents with demonstrated activity in the disease, each of which has had no record of inducing AML or sterility. The regimen devised, was a combination of vinblastine, bleomycin and methotrexate (VBM). The new adjuvant regimen is being tested only in patients who are pathologically staged, who have the best prognoses, and who have received full dose irradiation to involved fields for known disease. This approach is a logical next step following earlier Stanford studies. Patients with favorable PSIA, IIA, IB, IIB and IIIA are treated with the new management plan, stratifying three groups (Figs. 7, 8).

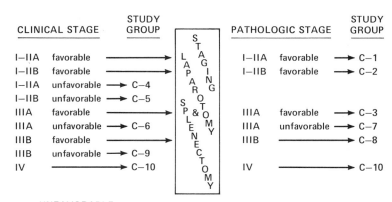

Figure 7. Stanford Hodgkin's disease trials, initiated in 1980, showing stratified groups.

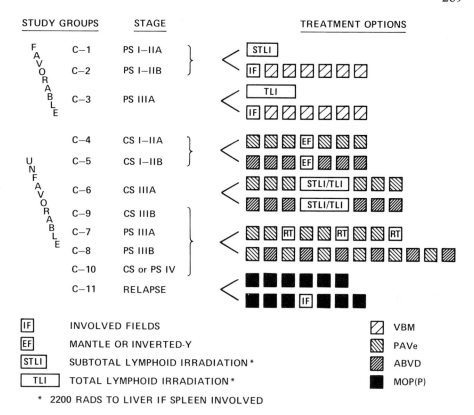

Figure 8. Stanford Hodgkin's disease trials: Schematic representation of randomized treatment options on current trials, initiated in 1980.

For patients with intermediate prognoses, new prognostic factors have emerged which identify patients who require combined modality therapy to achieve high cure and survival rates. Patients with large mediastinal masses, greater than 1/3 the transverse diameter of the thorax, extensive splenic involvement with five or more tumor nodules and multiple extranodal sites (E-lesions) fall within this category. The new trials compare the PAVe regimen to the ABVD regimen, plus radiotherapy of variable extent related to stage, primarily searching for differences in survival and in major long term complications of therapy. Laparotomy is not performed on patients whose relatively unfavorable prognoses already are an indication for chemotherapy in their management. The occurrence of AML, or sterility in men and women, and impairment of cardiac and pulmonary function and bone marrow reserve is being studied prospectively in these patients.

For patients with the poorest prognoses, PS IIIB and IV, the trial compares the Stanford 'best' approach of alternating PAVe and TLI to the Milan 'best' regimen of alternating MOPP/ABVD [10]. However initially

290

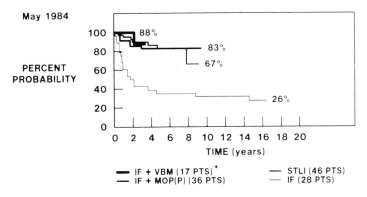

* INCLUDES 3 PATIENTS WITH IIIA

Figure 9. Hodgkin's disease, PS IA and IIA. Actuarial curves of freedom from progression comparing adjuvant VBM (includes three PS IIIA patients), subtotal lymphoid irradiation (STLI), adjuvant MOP(P) and involved field irradiation (IF) groups.

PAVe/ABVD was utilized instead of MOPP/ABVD because of the results of the Stanford studies in which PAVe and MOPP have proved to be equivalent, with PAVe less toxic in combined modality studies.

Preliminary results of the current studies

As of May 1, 1984, 101 patients have been enrolled on the current studies. Because there are 10 stratified groups, it was anticipated that results would have to be analyzed by combining groups with the same, or very similar therapeutic questions.

The C-1, 2 and 3 studies address the same question, whether the new VBM adjuvant can control occult disease as well as irradiation and result in less acute and long term toxicity than MOP(P) chemotherapy. Fig. 9 shows the results of patients enrolled on these studies to date and compares them to the same or similar patients treated on past protocols. There has been one relapse and no deaths in the 16 patients in the VBM adjuvant group. With short term follow-up, the VBM adjuvant appears to be as effective as MOP(P), as used in prior studies. It is too early, however, to be confident of this conclusion. It is already evident that both men and women will maintain fertility after the VBM therapy.

The C-4, 5 and 6 studies compare PAVe and ABVD in combined modality management programs. To date there are no differences between these groups in disease control. The major differences expected will be in treatment complications, acute and long term. It is too early to draw conclusions about the relative toxicities of PAVe and ABVD in combined modality regimens.

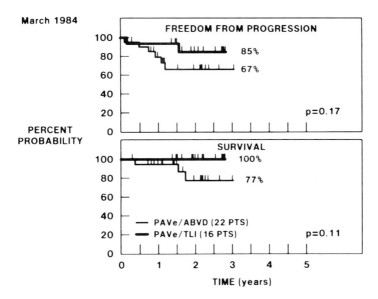

Figure 10. Hodgkin's disease: PS III and IV unfavorable disease settings. Actuarial curves of freedom from progression and survival comparing PAVe/ABVD chemotherapy to PAVe/TLI combined modality treatment groups.

The preliminary results of the C-7, 8, 9 and 10 studies are shown in Fig. 10. There has been a disappointing high failure rate in the PAVe/ABVD treatment group, with 6 of 16 patients failing to achieve a complete remission or recurring after therapy. There have been 3 deaths in this group, 2 of disease and 1 suicide. This is compared to only 2 of 22 patients who have recurred after the PAVe/TLI alternating program with no deaths to date. Though the differences observed are not statistically significant it has been decided to change the PAVe/ABVD regimen to MOPP/ABVD. It is possible that the PAVe program is less effective than MOPP, and the need to confirm the Milan MOPP/ABVD experience argues for the change to that regimen at this time.

Conclusions

The Stanford studies of the treatment of Hodgkin's disease have been significant for many reasons. Both patients and investigators have been willing to test new diagnostic and treatment methods. The careful attention to the details of protocol therapy, randomization between only acceptable treatment options, high quality patient care to provide the best possible salvage therapies and management of complications and patience in interpreting the data have all lead to general advances in the care of patients with Hodgkin's disease at Stanford and elsewhere.

Acknowledgements

These studies were supported, in part, by grants CA-05838, CA-34233, CA-09287 and CA-21555 from the National Cancer Institute, National Institutes of Health. Dr. Rosenberg is an American Cancer Society Professor of Clinical Oncology.

References

1. Rosenberg SA, Kaplan HS, Hoppe RT et al. (1982). The Stanford randomized trials of the treatment of Hodgkin's disease: 1967–1980. In: Rosenberg SA and Kaplan HS (Eds.). Malignant Lymphomas: Etiology, Immunology, Pathology, Treatment, pp. 513–522. New York: Academic Press.
2. Kaplan ES and Meier P (1958). Non-parametric estimation from incomplete observation. Amer Stat Assoc J 53:457–480.
3. Gehan EA (1965). A generalized Wilcoxon test for comparing arbitrarily singly-censored samples. Biometrika 52:203–233.
4. Cox DR (1972). Regression models and life tables. J Roy Stat Soc B 34:187–220.
5. Kaplan HS (1980). Hodgkin's Disease, 2nd ed. Cambridge, London: Harvard University Press.
6. DeVita VT Jr, Serpick AA and Carbone PP (1970). Combination chemotherapy in the treatment of advanced Hodgkin's disease. Ann Intern Med 75:881–895.
7. DeVita VT Jr (1981). The consequences of the chemotherapy of Hodgkin's disease: The 10th David A. Karnofsky Memorial Lecture. Cancer 47:1–13.
8. Wolin EM, Rosenberg SA and Kaplan HS (1979). A randomized comparison of PAVe and MOP(P) as adjuvant chemotherapy for Hodgkin's disease. In: Salmon SE and Jones SE (Eds). Adjuvant Therapy of Cancer. II, pp. 119–127. New York: Grune and Stratton.
9. Santoro A, Bonfante V, Bonadonna G et al. (1981). Therapeutic and toxicologic effects of MOPP vs ABVD combined with radiotherapy in Hodgkin's disease. In: Salmon SE and Jones SE (Eds). Adjuvant Therapy of Cancer. III., pp. 85–91. New York: Grune and Stratton.
10. Santoro A, Bonadonna G, Bonfante V and Valagussa P (1982). Alternating drug combinations in the treatment of advanced Hodgkin's disease. N Engl J Med 306:770–775.

2. The current status of NCI trials in Hodgkin's disease

R. C. YOUNG[1], D. L. LONGO[1], E. GLATSTEIN[1], P. L. DUFFEY[1], C. F. WINKLER[1], P. H. WIERNIK[2], and V. T. DEVITA, Jr.[1]
[1] National Cancer Institute, Bethesda, Maryland and
[2] Montefiore Medical Center, Bronx, New York, USA

The development of effective therapies for all stages of Hodgkin's disease represents one of the most remarkable achievements of modern cancer treatment. What was once considered a uniformly fatal disease has been transformed in the last several decades into one of the most curable malignancies with which we deal. Nevertheless, there are several major areas where improvements in the management of Hodgkin's disease are needed and several of these areas have been the central focus of ongoing clinical trials at the National Cancer Institute (USA).

In no area of Hodgkin's disease treatment have the successes been more apparent than with modern mega-voltage radiation therapy in the management of early stage disease. In the hands of experienced physicians, such therapy has produced cure rates in the range of 75–90% depending upon the particular site, stage and extent of disease [1, 2]. Unfortunately, this means that 10–25% of patients relapse from radiation-induced complete remissions and although chemotherapy can salvage approximately half of such patients, it does so at a cost of some risk of induced second malignancies [3, 4]. Furthermore, successful radio-therapeutic management of early stage disease demands considerable technical expertise and access to sophisticated equipment necessary to achieve results of the type quoted above. Such expertise and equipment is not always easily available to all patients presenting with early stage disease and, as a consequence, compromised therapy design and outdated equipment are used with results nowhere near those quoted for the most successful published radiation therapy series. As an example, a recent patterns of care study in the United States has identified differences in adjusted relative relapse rates of 0% to 11% for infield or marginal recurrences and from 10% to 39% for any relapse among large radiation therapy institutions treating Hodgkin's disease. The vast majority of these differences related to inadequate technology and inaccurate treatment portals [5]. Thus, the search for more easily standardized effective therapy is warranted.

Combination chemotherapy is curative in advanced disease [6] and can salvage many patients who relapse after radiation therapy [7]. Furthermore, the initial experience with MOPP in the treatment of early stage disease in a developing nation where radiation therapy was not available, indicated very high complete remission rates 7/7 (100%) [8]. Follow-up indicated that of the 12 patients who presented with Stage I-IIIA disease and were treated with initial chemotherapy, two were lost to follow-up, in remission, one relapsed and the remaining 9 (75%) were in sustained initial remission for 35-78 months [9]. The investigators concluded that MOPP chemotherapy alone resulted in prolonged, sustained remission in the majority of early stage patients. Furthermore, Pavlovsky et al. have demonstrated equivalent complete remission rates, duration of remissions, and overall survival at 48 months follow-up for 47 patients with Clinical Stage IA-IIA disease treated with combination chemotherapy alone compared to chemotherapy plus radiotherapy [10].

For the above reasons we are comparing MOPP alone to radiation therapy as initial treatment of early stage disease. Those patients who have Pathologic Stage (PS) I (central), II-A, II-B with or without extranodal involvement will be randomized. Early in the trial, those patients who had PS IIIA$_1$ were also randomized, but now such patients are simply treated as advanced stage disease. Peripheral Stage I patients, since their prognosis is so good, are not randomized but receive radiation therapy alone as an integrated part of the trial.

Because the morbidity of the two treatments is significant, important parameters for comparison include not only complete remission frequency, survival, and disease-free survival, and freedom from second relapse but also acute and chronic toxicities and effectiveness of salvage. Toxicity parameters being followed include serious infectious episodes, lung and cardiac toxicity, radiation myelitis, sterility, thyroid dysfunction and subsequent second malignancies.

At present, 88 patients have been treated in this trial, 67 as a part of the randomized portion of the trial and 21 patients with early disease entered directly on the radiation therapy portion of the study. Initial results indicate almost universal complete remissions regardless of the type of initial treatment used. It is too early at this point to make definitive conclusions regarding disease-free survival, survival and relative incidence of early and late toxicities for the two approaches.

Another subset of patients with Hodgkin's disease for whom presently available therapy has been less than optimal are those with massive mediastinal disease at initial presentation. While the involvement of the mediastinum is common, the presence of mediastinal enlargement greater than 1/3 of the total radiographic chest diameter is seen in only about 20% of all cases. Unfortunately, these patients have a significantly worse freedom from relapse than patients of the same stage similarly treated who do not have massive mediastinal disease. For example, among early stage patients treated with radiation therapy at the Joint Center in Boston, 9/18 patients with massive mediastinal disease relapsed compared to 5/93 without massive involvement (50% vs. 5%) [11]. Similar results have been reported from the Royal Marsden Hospital where 53% vs. 14% have relapsed [12]. Likewise, chemotherapy in this group has also been associated with a high relapse rate when used alone. In a preliminary examination of our results with MOPP alone in such patients, approximately 35% remained continuously disease-free after chemotherapy. As a result, we are presently treating such patients with alternating monthly cycles of MOPP-ABVD [13] after radiation ports are designed by simulation to include the entire original extent of disease. After six cycles of chemotherapy, initial trial design called for the administration of 1500 rad to the original tumor volume before reducing the size of the mediastinal field to the size of the residual tumor mass. Because of some combined modality pneumonitis from this approach, we have reduced the initial dose to the original tumor volume to 1050 rad. Following delivery of this dose level, thin lung blocks are inserted and the residual mediastinal volume receives a total of 3500 to 4500 rad. The rationale for such an approach for mantle field irradiation is to minimize the marginal and pulmonary relapses, which are so frequent in this subset of patients [14]. At present 26 patients with massive mediastinal Stages IIA-IV Hodgkin's disease have been entered. Preliminary results indicate a high (85%) complete remission rate in patients treated with this combined modality approach but further follow-up will be required to assess the more important parameters of disease-free survival and overall survival. Toxicity from this aggressive combined modality approach has been significant albeit acceptable and includes combination therapy-related pneumonitis, subclavian venous thrombosis, and granulocytopenia with fever.

Although the treatment of advanced Hodgkin's disease with MOPP has dramatically altered the prognosis in these patients, further progress is still required. Nearly half of the victims of advanced-stage disease die prematurely. The 20% of patients who are induction failures have a median survival of less than one year. Furthermore, those patients who achieve complete remission, but relapse promptly (< 1 yr), have a consistently poor prognosis. Salvage therapy for these two groups of patients has been generally unimpressive [15]. The best results are those reported by Santoro et al. [16] using ABVD. Even in this trial, only a projected 20% of all MOPP resistant patients remain in remission at 5 years. Other studies using the same regimen for salvage have achieved even poorer results. The current NCI trial for advanced disease patients (Stages IIIA, IIIB and IV) is aimed at testing the Goldie-Coldman hypothesis that early exposure of the tumor to two combinations of non-cross resistant drugs is more likely to result in cure than conventional cyclic four-drug treatment. The most impressive data to support clinical relevance of this concept come from the trials of MOPP/ABVD by Santoro and colleagues in advanced Stage IV Hodgkin's disease [13]. Complete remission was documented in 71% of MOPP-treated patients and in 92% of those treated with MOPP-ABVD. Although 5 year survivals were not significantly different, disease-free survival was better (84% vs. 54%) for MOPP-ABVD [13]. Updated results [17] still indicate improved disease-free survival (79% vs. 44%) and a significant difference in overall survival (82% vs. 61%) at 7 years has emerged.

The current NCI study in advanced disease compares MOPP to MOPP alternating with CABS (lomustine, doxorubicin, bleomycin and streptozotocin) chemotherapy. The choice of CABS was based upon early experience with an identical regimen known as SCAB which achieved complete remission in 35% of MOPP-resistant patients [18]. This remission rate was somewhat less than the salvage rate of ABVD reported above but superior to ABVD given by four other groups [15]. Furthermore, in a small number of untreated patients with advanced disease, CABS (SCAB) was as active as MOPP in inducing complete remissions [19].

There is some theoretic basis for using two nitrosoureas in Hodgkin's disease. Both are active and early trials with streptozotocin demonstrated activity in many patients who had failed previous carmustine therapy [20]. This suggests that different nitrosoureas may act at different sites. Furthermore, nitrosoureas with high alkylating and low carbamoylating activity (e.g. chlorozotocin and streptozotocin) are less marrow toxic [21]. Thus, the use of lomustine and streptozotocin together may increase the alkylating activity of the regimen without increasing marrow toxicity substantially. This MOPP versus MOPP/CABS trial is one of the few ongoing studies comparing MOPP to another alternating non-cross resistant chemotherapy regimen in the absence of radiation therapy. Seventy-nine patients have been randomized in the trial, 36 to MOPP alone and 43 to MOPP-CABS. Initial complete response rates are high ($\cong 85\%$) for both regimens and median survivals in both groups exceed 80% at 4 years for either treatment. In light of these extremely good results for both regimens, it is noteworthy that patients with Stage III-IV disease who present with massive mediastinal disease are treated on the previously described study and are not included in this study. Since such patients have historically been included in advanced disease chemotherapy trials and have a somewhat poorer prognosis overall, this may contribute to the improved survival seen in both arms of the present trial. It should not, however, preferentially effect one arm rather than the other.

One of the most encouraging consequences of the widespread use of effective therapy in Hodgkin's disease has been the steady decline in the death rate in the United States despite a slowly rising incidence of the disease. Even with the progress already made, many challenges remain.

The high incidence of second malignancy associated with the use of combined modality therapy suggests that we should restrict its use to subsets of patients with a poor prognosis for initial control, such as the group with massive mediastinal disease. We need improvement, or at the very least, expansion of available options for the treatment of early stage patients. The definition of alternative therapies would at a minimum reduce the risk of second malignancies seen in early-stage patients currently receiving combined modality treatment (e.g., those with Stage IB, IIB or IIIA). Other complications of successful chemotherapy such as sterility continue to deserve study. We have recently initiated a trial of a synthetic analog of luteinizing hormone releasing hormone (LHRH), which is capable of suppressing release of gonadotropin, thereby suppressing gonadal function and hopefully halting spermatogenesis in males and follicle growth in women. Possibly, this might protect against the toxic effects of chemotherapeutic drugs on these proliferating target tissues.

Finally, one of the great problems we all face in the further improvement of the treatment of Hodgkin's disease relates, in part, to the success of present day treatment. As treatment has improved, the next improvements in remission rates from 80% to 95% will require study of many more patients to achieve statistical significance. Second, as treatment has improved and effective therapies are widely available, practicing physicians prefer to retain Hodgkin's disease patients rather than refer them for study. These problems have actually slowed recent progress in clinical trial research in this disease. Nevertheless, important questions remain and require answers before safe, effective and consistently successful therapy will be available for all patients with Hodgkin's disease.

References

1. Kaplan HS (1970). On the natural history, treatment, and prognosis of Hodgkin's disease. Harvey Lectures 1968–1969, New York: Academic Press.
2. Hellman S, Mauch P, Goodman RL et al. (1978). The place of radiation therapy in the treatment of Hodgkin's disease. Cancer 42:971–978.
3. Arseneau JC, Sponzo RW, Schnipper LE et al. (1972). Nonlymphomatous malignancies complicating Hodgkin's disease: Possible association with intensive therapy. N Engl J Med 287:1119–1122.
4. Coleman CN, Williams CJ, Flint A et al. (1977). Hematologic neoplasia in patients treated for Hodgkin's disease. N Engl J Med 297:1249–1252.
5. Kinzie JJ, Hanks GE, MacLean CJ and Kramer S (1983). Patterns of care study: Hodgkin's disease relapse rates and adequacy of portals. Cancer 52:2223–2226.
6. DeVita VT, Simon RM, Hubbard SM et al. (1980). Curability of advanced Hodgkin's disease with chemotherapy. Long-term follow up of MOPP treated patients at the National

Cancer Institute. Ann Intern Med 92:587–595.

7. Canellos GP, Young RC and DeVita VT (1972). Combination chemotherapy for advanced Hodgkin's disease in relapse following extensive radiotherapy. Clin Pharmacol Ther 13:750–754.

8. Ziegler JL, Bluming AZ, Faso L et al. (1972). Chemotherapy of childhood Hodgkin's disease in Uganda. Lancet 2:679–680.

9. Olweny CLM, Katangole Mbidde E, Kiire CL et al. (1978). Childhood Hodgkin's disease in Uganda: A ten year experience. Cancer 42:787–792.

10. Pavlovsky S, Dupont J, Jimenez E et al. (1984). Randomized study of chemotherapy alone vs. chemotherapy plus radiotherapy in Clinical Stage IA-IIA Hodgkin's disease. In: Cavalli F, Bonadonna G, and Rozencweig M (Eds). Malignant Lymphomas and Hodgkin's Disease: Experimental and Therapeutic Advances, pp 337–343. Boston: Martinus Nijhoff.

11. Mauch P, Goodman R and Hellman S (1978). The significance of mediastinal involvement in early stage Hodgkin's disease. Cancer 42:1039–1045.

12. Velentjas E, Barrett A, McElwan TJ and Peckham MJ (1980). Mediastinal involvement in early stage Hodgkin's disease. Eur J Cancer 16:1065–1068.

13. Santoro A, Bonadonna G, Bonfante V and Valagussa P (1982). Alternating drug combinations in the treatment of advanced Hodgkin's disease. N Engl J Med 306:770–775.

14. Kun LE, DeVita VT, Young RC et al. (1976). Treatment of Hodgkin's disease using intensive chemotherapy followed by irradiation. Int J Radiat Oncol Biol Phys 1:619–626.

15. Longo DL, Young RC and DeVita VT (1982). Chemotherapy for Hodgkin's disease: The remaining challenges. Cancer Treat Rep 66:925–936.

16. Santoro A and Bonadonna G (1979). Prolonged disease-free survival in MOPP-resistant Hodgkin's disease after treatment with adriamycin, bleomycin, vincristine and dacarbazine (ABVD). Cancer Chemother Pharmacol 2:101–105.

17. Bonadonna G, Viviani S, Bonfante V et al. (1984). Alternating chemotherapy with MOPP/ABVD in Hodgkin's disease. Updated results. Proc Amer Soc Clin Oncol 3:254.

18. Levi JA, Wiernik PH and Diggs CH (1977). Combination chemotherapy of advanced previously treated Hodgkin's disease with streptozotocin, CCNU, adriamycin and bleomycin. Med Pediatr Oncol 3:33–40.

19. Diggs CH, Wiernik PH, Kaplan RD et al. (1981). Treatment of Hodgkin's disease with SCAB — an alternative to MOPP. Cancer 47:223–248.

20. Schein PS, O'Connell MJ, Blom J et al. (1974). Clinical antitumor activity and toxicity of streptozotocin. Cancer 34:993–1000.

21. Wheeler GP, Schabel FM and Trader MW (1981). Synergistic antileukemic activity of combinations of two nitrosoureas. Cancer Treat Rep 65:591–599.

3. Current status of the Milan trials for Hodgkin's disease in adults

G. BONADONNA, A. SANTORO, P. VALAGUSSA, S. VIVIANI,
R. ZUCALI, V. BONFANTE and A. BANFI
Istituto Nazional, Per lo Studio e la Cura dei Tumori, Milan, Italy

During the past decade, trials for Hodgkin's disease in adult patients carried out at the Milan Cancer Institute mainly focused on the development and evaluation of non-cross-resistant drug regimens [1]. This approach was based on the limitations of MOPP and MOPP-derived regimens in achieving cure in Stage III and IV Hodgkin's disease as well as on the low salvage rate observed with retreatment in complete responders relapsing within 12 months from first complete remission (CR). Both events were attributed to selective resistance to two or more drugs in a single multidrug combination [2, 3]. An additional trial was specifically designed to compare iatrogenic effects resulting from regimens with (MOPP) and without (ABVD) alkylating agents and procarbazine. These drugs are responsible for inducing sterility and cancerogenesis [1, 4].

Previous publications [1, 5–8] provided details on rationale and background studies for designing the ABVD regimen (adriamycin, bleomycin, vinblastine, and dacarbazine). Initial results concerning salvage chemotherapy in MOPP-resistant patients and cyclic delivery of MOPP/ABVD in Stage IV Hodgkin's disease were very promising. Lack of drug-induced leukemia and sterility in ABVD-treated patients was a most encouraging observation [1, 4, 9]. The scope of this paper is to update our findings on salvage chemotherapy, alternating non-cross-resistant regimens and comparative toxicity of MOPP vs ABVD.

Salvage chemotherapy in relapsing patients

As a general policy, relapses following CR lasting for more than 12 months were retreated with the same drug combination. For shorter CR or treatment failure, second-line chemotherapy consisted of non-cross-resistant regimens. Chemotherapy was administered to induction of CR plus two additional cycles for a minimum of 6 cycles. Consolidation with radiotherapy limited to nodal sites of initially bulky disease was given to most patients. CR was not maintained. Patients were pathologically restaged if they presented with extra-nodal invasion, particularly with bone marrow or liver involvement. Patients were considered evaluable if the treatment program was completed or if the disease progressed while on therapy. Our results have been recently updated [10].

Retreatment with the same regimen yielded CR in 78% of 18 patients given different forms of primary chemotherapy (MOPP 7/9, ABVD 4/5, MOPP/ABVD 3/4). The median relapse-free survival (RFS) was longer than 42 months and survival in CR exceeded 51 months. Table I summarizes essential findings observed in 71 consecutive patients given ABVD as soon as they were considered to be MOPP-resistant. Our present results confirm a previous report on a smaller series of patients [7]. At 7 years, about 50% of the patients in CR remain continuously disease-free and no patients relapsed beyond the third year. Total survival analysis further indicates that ABVD can salvage 25% of all MOPP-resistant patients. In 16 ABVD-resistant patients, salvage MOPP induced CR in 25% and PR in 6%. The median RFS was 10 months and the survival in CR less than 3 years.

Since February 1980, patients resistant to both MOPP and ABVD given either in sequence or alternating fashion were treated with CEP chemotherapy. This triple drug regimen consisted of lomustine (80 mg/m^2 p.o. on day 1), etoposide (100 mg/m^2 p.o. from day 1 through 5), and prednimustine (60 mg/m^2 p.o. from day 1 through 5); treatment was recycled on day 29. Our findings in 40 patients (Table II) expand our initial observations with this regimen [1].

We are currently testing the efficacy of two alternating regimens as salvage chemotherapy. Preliminary results reveal that ABVD/CEP induced CR in 61% of 18 MOPP-resistant patients with a median duration in excess of 20 months whereas MOPP/CEP achieved CR in 3 of 5 cases with a median duration of 10 months [10].

Table I. Salvage ABVD in 71 MOPP-resistant patients

	%	*p*-value
Partial remission	14	
Complete remission	55	
Symptoms: A/B	79/36	0.01
Extent: Nodal/Extranodal	69/42	<0.05
Response to MOPP: CR/non CR	77/33	<0.01
At 7 years: RFS	46	
Survival of CRs	51	
Total survival	27	

Table II. Results of salvage therapy with CEP

	Total (40 cases)	M ⇄ A (28 cases)	M/A (12 cases)
Partial remission (%)	25	21	33
Complete remission (%)	35	39	25
RFS, median (mo.)	17	17	6
Survival CRs, median (mo.)	> 30	> 30	> 6
Survival, median (mo.)	30	16	> 8

M: MOPP   A: ABVD

Alternating MOPP/ABVD

The cyclic delivery of two equally effective and non-cross-resistant regimens was carried out on the basis of clinical results with salvage ABVD in MOPP-resistant patients and the following considerations: (a) a major cause of chemotherapy failure is selection and overgrowth of drug-resistant tumor cells, and (b) tumor cell burden and the mix of drug-sensitive and drug-resistant cells represent the crucial prognostic variables. The first prospective randomized trial was restricted to patients with Pathologic Stage IV disease [1, 5, 6, 8], and the 7-year results were recently reported [11]. Table III presents the main patient characteristics and Table IV the 7-year overall results. Comparative RFS and total survival are illustrated in Fig. 1 and 2.

Essentially, present findings further underline the superiority of the alternating regimen, but also a significant improvement in survival over MOPP. An analysis by subgroups fails to demonstrate a difference in RFS or survival between age groups (≤ 40 and > 40 years) among those patients given

Table III. Alternating chemotherapy vs MOPP in Stage IV. Main patient characteristics.

	MOPP (43 cases)	MOPP/ABVD (45 cases)
Male patients	63	49
Age > 40 years	35	36
Nodular sclerosis histology	58	53
Bulky lymphoma	33	40
Systemic symptoms (B)	70	69
> 3 nodal sites	60	73
Multiple extranodal	23	16
Prior radiotherapy	28	29

Data are in percent

302

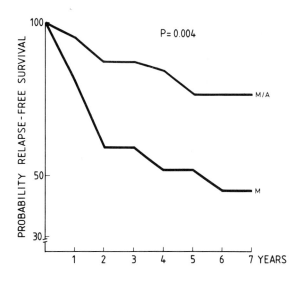

Figure 1. Alternating chemotherapy vs MOPP in Stage IV. Comparative 7-year relapse-free survival.

MOPP/ABVD. The alternating regimen induced CR in all patients older than 40 years whereas, in patients treated with MOPP only, the CR rate was superior in those younger than 40 years. With both treatments, females did better than males in terms of RFS and survival, in spite of similar CR rates, and nodular sclerosis histology showed better RFS compared to other histologic subgroups, which were mainly represented by the mixed cellularity type. MOPP/ABVD yielded superior RFS results in patients with B symptoms than in the others; in contrast, there was no particular RFS difference between these subgroups when treated with MOPP. MOPP/ABVD produced comparable CR rates (88.9%) and RFS in patients with and without bulky disease whereas, in the MOPP treated group, the corresponding CR rates were 57.1% vs 82.8%.

Table IV. Alternating chemotherapy vs MOPP in Stage IV. Comparative 7-year overall results

	MOPP (%)	MOPP/ABVD (%)	*p*-value
Complete remission	74.4	88.9	0.14
Freedom from progression	35.1	68.1	0.001
Relapse-free survival	44.4	76.8	0.004
Survival of CRs	73.2	90.3	0.038
Total survival	61.1	82.3	0.043

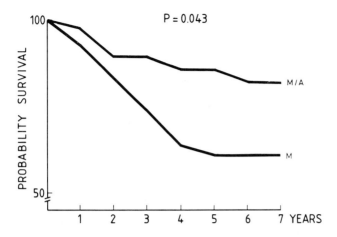

Figure 2. Alternating chemotherapy vs MOPP in Stage IV. Comparative 7-year overall survival.

The efficacy of cyclic MOPP/ABVD through difference sequences is currently tested in a prospective randomized study activated in July 1982. The control arm consists of MOPP/ABVD alternating after each full monthly cycle of either regimen (MM/AA) while, in the experimental arm, half-cycle of MOPP (mechlorethamine and vincristine on day 1, procarbazine and prednisone from day 1 through 7) is alternated within a month period with half-cycle of ABVD given on day 15 (MA/MA). Theoretically, this new alternating-sequence therapy seems more in accordance with the Goldie and Coldman hypothesis [3] and should further improve the RFS achieved in our previous study. This clinical trial is being performed in high-risk groups including Stages IA-IIA bulky disease, Stage IIB, III (A and B), and IV (A and B). Its completion will require a large number of patients. CR is followed by two additional cycles as consolidation chemotherapy. Complete

Table V. Comparative complete remission rate between two sequences of alternating chemotherapy

	MM/AA	MA/MA
Total evaluable [a]	36	40
Complete remission (%)	89	93
'A' symptoms	90	87
'B' symptoms	89	96
Bulky disease	77	88
Non-bulky disease	100	96

[a] As of March 1984

responders receive low dose radiotherapy (2500 rad) to the areas with bulky lymphoma at the start of chemotherapy. The CEP regimen, with or without irradiation, is reserved for patients not achieving CR following 6 cycles of either alternating sequence chemotherapy. Table V summarizes the very preliminary comparative results. Current findings would suggest that MA/MA might be more efficacious than the classical MM/AA sequence, at least in patients with 'B' symptoms and bulky lymphoma.

MOPP vs ABVD within a combined modality therapy

In September 1974, a prospective randomized study with multimodal therapy was started in patients with Pathologic Stages IIB, IIIA, and IIIB disease. The specific intent was to compare the iatrogenic morbidity of MOPP to that of ABVD within a combined modality setting. As detailed in earlier publications [1, 5, 6], all entries were untreated and, after pathologic staging, were randomly allocated to receive three cycles of either MOPP or ABVD, administered according to the classical dose schedules. In the absence of tumor progression, treatment was continued with high-energy irradiation (subtotal nodal irradiation in patients with Stages IIB, III_SA, or III_SB with no para-aortic adenopathy; total nodal irradiation in patients with Stages IIIA or IIIB and retroperitoneal adenopathy). The doses of radiotherapy were 3500 rad to the involved lymphoid areas and 3000 rad to adjacent uninvolved areas. About one month from the end of radiotherapy, treatment was completed with three additional cycles of either chemotherapy program. Although the CR rate was significantly higher in the ABVD group

Table VI. Comparative 5-year results of combined modality therapy

	MOPP group (113 cases)	ABVD group (116 cases)	*p*-value
Complete remission (%)	81.4	92.2	0.03
'A' symptoms	96.6	96.9	
'B' symptoms	76.2	90.5	0.03
Relapse-free survival (%)	80.9	90.7	0.09
'A' symptoms	74.2	100.0	<0.02
'B' symptoms	77.3	88.6	
Total survival (%)	69.9	84.9	0.12
'A' symptoms	74.8	93.4	
'B' symptoms	68.1	81.3	

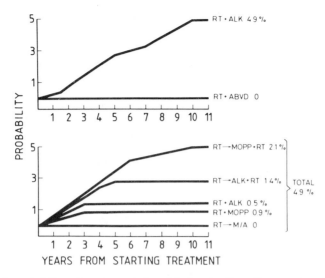

Figure 3. Risk probability of treatment-induced leukemia. Top: Comparative risk in patients receiving radiotherapy (RT) plus alkylating agents (ALK) vs RT plus ABVD.
Bottom: Contribution of different types and sequences of treatment modalities including alkylating agents.

than in the MOPP group, the overall RFS and survival rates were similar between the two combined modality treatments (Table VI).

As far as toxicity is concerned, there is no evidence that ABVD plus radiation induced cardiomyopathy attributable to doxorubicin nor extensive pulmonary fibrosis attributable to bleomycin. However, a detailed comparative analysis on heart and lung toxicity is still ongoing. Table VII reports the comparative incidence of gonadal dysfunction in patients less than 45

Table VII. Comparative gonadal dysfunction: MOPP vs ABVD

	MOPP	ABVD
Males, total evaluable	29	24
azoospermia (%)	97	33
oligospermia (%)	0	21
recovered/reassessed	3/21	13/13
median time to recovery (mo.)	36	10
Females, total evaluable	37	24
amenorrhea > 6 mo. (%)	16	0
<30 years	0/23	
≥30 years	6/14	
recovery	1/6	

years of age who received subtotal nodal irradiation. In both sexes, but particularly in male patients, gonadal dysfunction was definitely less in the ABVD group compared to the MOPP group. More importantly, gonadal damage was fully reversible only in males treated with ABVD [12].

The incidence of chemotherapy-induced second neoplasms in patients treated with regimens containing alkylating agents and/or procarbazine (e.g. MOPP) vs ABVD has been published [9]. Updated findings concerning the incidence of acute leukemia in patients with Hodgkin's disease and given different forms of therapy are displayed in Fig. 3. Results of this analysis confirm the absence of treatment-induced leukemia following ABVD administered either alone or with radiotherapy.

Conclusions

Major progress in advanced Hodgkin's disease was made by combination chemotherapy. Results of MOPP and MOPP-derived regimens revealed a high curative potential and became an essential reference point to design new treatment strategies [1]. Alternating chemotherapy with MOPP/ABVD represents a step further in the control of Hodgkin's disease. The overall superior results achieved with MOPP/ABVD versus MOPP alone substantiate the hypothesis that selection and overgrowth of drug resistant tumor cells is indeed the crucial prognostic factor. MOPP alternated with ABVD was superior to MOPP alone in patients older than 40 years and in the presence of nodular sclerosis histology, bulky disease in the mediastinum and systemic symptoms. Full evaluation of the more recent study testing two different sequences of MOPP/ABVD is premature. However, there is already a trend in favor of half MOPP alternated with half ABVD in bulky disease, which represents a clinical situation probably characterized by a high proportion of tumor cells resistant to one or more compounds included in a single polydrug regimen.

In conclusion, as compared to single drug combination, the alternation of two equally effective and non-cross-resistant regimens, such as MOPP and ABVD, appears to yield superior results in advanced Hodgkin's disease. As far as toxicity is concerned, drug regimens not including alkylating agents and procarbazine, e.g., ABVD, may be devoid of some important side effects notably sterility and secondary leukemia.

References

1. Bonadonna G (1982). Chemotherapy strategies to improve the control of Hodgkin's disease. The Richard and Hinda Rosenthal Foundation Award Lecture. Cancer Res 42:4309–4320.

2. Skipper HE and Schabel FM Jr. (1984). Tumor stem cell heterogeneity: Implications with respect to classification of cancers by chemotherapeutic effect. Cancer Treat Rep 68:43–61.

3. Goldie JH and Coldman AJ (1984). The genetic origin of drug resistance in neoplasms: Implications for systemic therapy. Cancer Res (in press).

4. Bonadonna G, Santoro A (1983). Drug selection in the treatment of Hodgkin's disease. Haematol Oncol 1:3–12.

5. Bonadonna G and Santoro A (1982). ABVD chemotherapy in the treatment of Hodgkin's disease. Cancer Treat Rev 9:21–35.

6. Bonadonna G, Santoro A, Bonfante V and Valagussa P (1982). Cyclic delivery of MOPP and ABVD combinations in Stage IV Hodgkin's disease: Rationale, background studies, and recent results. Cancer Treat Rep 66:881–887.

7. Santoro A, Bonfante V and Bonadonna G (1982). Salvage chemotherapy with ABVD in MOPP-resistant Hodgkin's disease. Ann Intern Med 96:139–143.

8. Santoro A, Bonadonna G, Bonfante V and Valagussa P (1982). Alternating drug combinations in the treatment of advanced Hodgkin's disease. N Engl J Med 306:770–775.

9. Valagussa P, Santoro A, Fossati-Bellani F et al. (1982). Absence of treatment-induced second neoplasms after ABVD in Hodgkin's disease. Blood 3:488–494.

10. Santoro A, Bonfante V, Viviani S et al. (1984). Salvage chemotherapy in relapsing Hodgkin's disease. Proc Amer Soc Clin Oncol 3:254.

11. Bonadonna G, Viviani S, Bonfante V et al. (1984). Alternating chemotherapy with MOPP/ABVD in Hodgkin's disease: Updated results. Proc Amer Soc Clin Oncol 3:254.

12. Viviani S, Santoro A, Ragni G et al. (1984). Gonadal toxicity after combination chemotherapy for Hodgkin's disease. Comparative results of MOPP versus ABVD. (In press).

4. Indications for combined modality therapy in patients with Hodgkin's disease

A. ZABELL and E. GLATSTEIN
Radiation Oncology Branch, Division of Cancer Treatment, National Cancer Institute, Bethesda, Maryland, USA

In the last 4 decades, the study of Hodgkin's disease has gone through a remarkable revolution. It began with an assumption of incurability. Treatment was usually palliative in intent, although the disease was known to be responsive to radiation. The classic studies of Peters, Kaplan, and others elucidated the natural history of the disease, in particular its orderly spread, propensity to remain in nodes and the spleen, and its likelihood for microscopic involvement in clinically and radiographically negative nodal groups. It was, however, the development of megavoltage x-ray equipment that allowed the delivery of wide field high-dose radiation with acceptable toxicity and curative intent. Subsequently, the development of effective combination chemotherapy made cure possible for patients whose advanced disease was not amenable to treatment by radiation. Today, cure rates for 'early stage' disease treated by radiation are over 80% as reported by many groups [1–3], and cure in advanced stage disease with combination chemotherapy is about 50% [4].

The decades of the seventies and eighties have seen a trend towards decreasing therapy for favorable presentations of disease, and more 'aggressive' therapy for those patients with a high likelihood of relapse with standard treatments. Such 'aggressive' therapy has evolved in the general direction of alternating putatively non-cross-resistant drug regimens, or the ultimate in non-cross-resistant regimens, combined modality therapy with combination chemotherapy and radiation therapy. The purpose of this paper is to discuss the current status of this approach.

Efficacy of combined modality therapy

Results of combined modality therapy with low dose (approximately 2000 rad) radiotherapy in pediatric Hodgkin's disease have been most impressive. Long-term relapse free survival of > 90% have been reported, all stages included. Data are so spectacular that little interest has surfaced among investigators to alter this approach in any major way. Yet, one must acknowledge that the superb results achieved with combined modality therapy are not necessarily superior to those obtained with MOPP alone in this age group. Clear data on this issue are lacking.

The Stanford group has generated the largest series of trials testing radiation versus combined modality treatment in adult patients with Hodgkin's disease. In 230 Pathologic Stages I and II patients, no subgroup could be identified in which there was statistically improved 5-year or 10-year actuarial survival with the use of combined modality treatment [5]. Prolonged 5-year disease-free survival was found in patients with mediastinal involvement (86% vs 73% $p = 0.05$), with no overall survival gain. Relapse was especially high in those patients with massive mediastinal involvement, greater than one-third of the thoracic diameter, 7/14 vs 1/49. There was a suggestion of increasing relapse rate with larger mediastinal involvement. Freedom from relapse was 81% with minimal mediastinal involvement and 45% with extensive involvement.

Similar data were reported at the Joint Center for Radiation Therapy where 9/18 patients with massive involvement relapsed versus 5/93 with lesser involvement [6]. The Royal Marsden Hospital found a 53% relapse rate among patients with massive involvement, compared to 14% in patients without such involvement. Similarly, Thar et al., observed more frequent pulmonary and pleural involvement in patients with mediastinal masses greater than 6 cm in diameter (2/43 or 5% versus 10/14 or 71%); local control was worse in patients with this finding [8]. Chemotherapy also fails to control the disease in a majority of these patients. At NCI, using MOPP, the complete remission rate was 33% in patients with massive mediastinal involvement compared to 80% in those with lesser involvement and complete remissions were not always durable [9].

Relapses following radiation treatment tend to follow one of three patterns in patients with massive mediastinal disease: mediastinal recurrence within the treated volume, marginal recurrences at the edge of the treated volume or diffuse pulmonary or pleural recurrences. Relapses following combination chemotherapy tend to occur in previously involved nodes, especially at sites of bulky disease. The use of transmission lung blocks delivering 1500–1600 rad to the lung appears to decrease the frequency of pulmonary recurrences when used prophylactically in patients with hilar disease at presentation [10].

A major problem which develops with radiation in patients with massive mediastinal disease is the need to shield adequate volumes of the heart and lungs. With appropriate shielding, the incidence of pericarditis and pneumonitis is under 3%. Data from Stanford indicate that treatment of the entire pericardium to doses greater than 3000 rad or daily doses in excess of

150 rad to an entire lung result in major risks of pericarditis or pneumonitis (50% and 25% respectively) [10].

A shrinking field technique and appropriately timed treatment breaks allow tumor shrinkage and may permit adequate heart and lung shielding. It has been noted, however, that prolonging treatment times in excess of 34 days for the mantle field may yield an increased relapse rate in patients with bulky mediastinal disease [10].

The rationale for combined modality therapy in patients with massive mediastinal involvement is clear. Neither radiation nor chemotherapy is particularly successful in this group of patients. The use of chemotherapy should produce tumor shrinkage and allow for more adequate shielding of normal tissues. The use of initial radiation eliminates the risks of intubation and general anesthesia noted in these patients [11] and allow for planned staging laparotomy after completion of the mantle field, if deemed necessary. In a practical sense, however, the decision to use combined modality treatment obviates the need for a staging laparotomy.

Given the high salvage rates reported for chemotherapy in patients failing initial radiation therapy, it is not surprising that there are only few data to suggest that the planned use of combined modality treatment significantly increases long-term survival. Levi et al. reported that extralymphatic involvement with Hodgkin's disease (the E lesion of the Ann Arbor staging) conveys a poorer prognosis than disease limited to nodes [12]. The majority of their E patients had pulmonary involvement (12 lung only, 3 with lung plus other, 3 other). Failures were seen in 10/18 (56%) patients with E lesions versus 16/84 (19%) in the others. Following radiation therapy, the corresponding relapse rates were 9/11 (82%) and 14/49 (29%) respectively. Among patients who received limited field irradiation plus MOPP chemotherapy, there were 1/7 (14%) relapses with E lesions and 2/36 (6%) with only nodal disease. Overall and disease-free survival was significantly improved at 3 years in the group undergoing combined modality treatment.

By contrast, the Stanford group reported that 5 of 54 (9%) patients with E lesions relapsed after radiation. This was not significantly different from 37 of 264 (14%) patients with nodal disease. At 10 years, the radiation and combined modality groups did not differ significantly with respect to survival and disease-free survival [13].

The question as to whether E lesions by themselves represent a clear indication for combined modality treatment is still controversial and the answer probably is dependent upon the radiotherapeutic technique that is used. Levi et al., employed a shrinking field technique to shield as much lung as possible, and lacked the benefits of modern simulation techniques. In doing so, peripheral areas of tumor often received no more than 2000 rad, especially in patients with bulky mediastinal disease. This appears to account for the fact that 6 of 7 patients with bulky disease had marginal recurrence. Additionally, thin lung blocks were not used to deliver treatment to areas of possible microscopic disease. The Stanford group routinely used simulation and thin lung blocks which delivered 1500–1600 rad to the uninvolved lung parenchyma, and avoided the use of the shrinking field technique.

Anatomic distribution of disease in Stage III patients might be of prognostic significance. Desser et al., subgrouped 52 patients with Stage III disease into III_1 (involvement of spleen, celiac nodes, splenic nodes, portal nodes) and III_2 (involvement of para-aortic or iliac nodes plus or minus the above nodes) [14]. Survival at 5 years was 93% in Stage III_1 and 57% in Stage III_2 ($p < 0.05$). Relapse-free survival was also significantly higher in Stage III_1. Radiation alone was as effective in Stage III_1 as combined modality treatment (2 relapses, 1 death in 11 patients versus 3 relapses, 0 deaths in 11 patients). In Stage III_2, 14/17 relapsed and 8/17 died after total nodal irradiation versus 1/10 relapse and no deaths after combined modality treatments. Twelve of fourteen relapses after radiation were extra nodal. A major drawback of this study was its inclusion of both Stages IIIA and IIIB patients for whom very different outcomes would be predicted, especially when treated by radiation alone.

A collaborative university report looked at the anatomic substages of Stage IIIA [15]. Again, survival and disease-free survival were higher in Stage $IIIA_1$ than in Stage $IIIA_2$ (respectively 94% versus 65%, and 74% versus 46%). The combined modality group had improved disease-free survival compared to the radiation only group in Stage $IIIA_1$ (96% versus 63%) and in Stage $IIIA_2$ (76% versus 32%). A significant difference in survival was seen only in Stage $IIIA_2$ (84% versus 56%). Survival was excellent in Stage $IIIA_1$ in both arms (100% versus 91%).

A Stanford study on 171 patients with pathologically staged IIIA disease yielded quite different results [16]. Freedom from relapse was statistically improved in the combined modality arm compared to the radiation arm. When analyzed by substage, however, this effect was only seen in Stage $IIIA_1$, not in Stage $IIIA_2$. Radiation treatment yielded equal disease-free survival in Stages $IIIA_1$ and $IIIA_2$. The only factors with prognostic significance for disease-free survival using radiation alone were the presence of extensive splenic involvement (> 4 nodules) or more than 4 sites of disease at presentation. Adjuvant chemotherapy improved disease-free survival significantly only for those patients with Stage $IIIA_1$ and those with extensive splenic involvement. There were no identifiable prognostic factors for survival in this study. Adjuvant chemotherapy had no impact on survival in any subgroup.

Lack of prognostic significance for involvement of para-aortic nodes (Stage $IIIA_2$) was also noted by others. Thus, Krikorian et al., failed to detect any difference in survival or disease-free survival between Stage IIA infra-diaphragmatic and supradiaphragmatic presentations [17].

The disparity among these studies can perhaps be explained by differences in radiation techniques. Stanford has consistently used higher doses, routinely treated the pulmonary hila, and prophylactically treated the lung (with hilar involvement) and the liver (whenever splenic involvement was documented).

Various studies suggest that combined modality therapy may be superior to chemotherapy alone and is clearly superior to radiation alone in Stage IIIB. At the present time, however, there are no data that convincingly demonstrate any major advantage for combined modality treatment over MOPP alone in advanced Stage III and IV Hodgkin's disease.

The Yale University group has treated 123 Stages III, IV A, B patients with six months of combination chemotherapy followed by 1500–2000 rad to sites of initial disease followed by 4 months of chemotherapy [18]. Complete remissions were noted in 84% of the patients. The 5-year disease-free and overall survival rates were 74% and 80% respectively. Sixty-one of these patients were treated after relapse from prior radical irradiation. These impressive results with low doses of irradiation after combination chemotherapy need confirmation.

At the Joint Center for Radiation Therapy, patients with Stages IIB or IIIB disease were treated with either radiation alone or 2 to 3 cycles of MOPP followed by extended field irradiation to a dose of 3500–4000 rad followed by chemotherapy to a total of 6 cycles [19]. In Stage IIB, there were no failures in 12 combined modality patients and 2 failures in 11 patients treated with radiation. These data were not statistically different. In Stage IIIB, there were 2/19 failures in the combined modality group and 4/7 in the radiation group, suggesting that radiation alone may be adequate in Stage IIB, but definitely not in Stage IIIB.

At NCI, 28 patients were treated with 6 cycles of MOPP followed by extended field irradiation to 4000 rad [20]. Tolerance to radiation was poor as evidenced by inability to complete radiation or prolonged delays in treatment secondary to marrow suppression. There was a high frequency of pneumonitis, pericarditis, and soft tissue damage. Four patients died of treatment-induced complications and 2 remained alive with considerable morbidity. The disease-free survival was 61% with a median follow-up of 48 months. This was not statistically different from the results found in patients treated with MOPP alone at the same institution. Also noted was a 14% marginal recurrence rate compared to 4% in patients treated in the same institution with radiation alone. Possibly, this could result from the attempt to spare as much normal lung as possible when administering radiation therapy after chemotherapy.

Stanford conducted a randomized trial in Stage IIIB disease testing total nodal radiotherapy with or without MOPP [21]. Freedom from relapse was improved in the combined modality group, but was not different from that achieved with MOPP alone at NCI. It was clear that radiation therapy alone was not a viable treatment in Stage IIIB.

A more recent Stanford study evaluated alternating chemotherapy and radiation in Stage IIIB [21]. Early results showed improved survival and disease-free survival when compared to the above combined modality group and to radiation only.

Toxicities of combined modality treatment

It is important to appreciate that both radiation therapy and chemotherapy carry the risk of treatment related complications, and that combined modality treatment is likely to carry even greater long-term risks. It is also important to consider these risks when selecting any treatment, but especially so in the case of combined modality treatment. Mauch et al., reviewing data from the Joint Center for Radiation Therapy, have shown that infectious complications of treatment increase with larger volumes of radiation treatment, and increase still further with the use of combined modality therapy [22].

Sterility, as a complication of MOPP chemotherapy, is seen in the vast majority of treated males and in about 50% of treated females. The incidence of sterility in radiation treated patients is lower, but poorly quantified. The incidence of sterility can be decreased by sparing the pelvis with the use of so-called sub-total nodal therapy. In females, the use of oophoropexy at the time of staging laparotomy can remove the ovaries from the treatment volume and the use of double blocking can further reduce the gonadal dose. Fertility can be maintained in about 70% of young women receiving radiation to the pelvis. In males, use of a gonadal shield can accomplish the same goal [23].

Over 300 cases of acute leukemia in treated Hodgkin's disease patients have been reported in the literature. In over 1000 cases treated by radiation, only one has developed this complication. The actuarial incidence of leukemia varies between 12.7% at 10 years [24] and 20.7% at 17 years [25]. These data and data from CALGB indicate that patients over 40 to 50 years of age are at the greatest risk [26].

At present, the data are not adequate to determine the relative risks of chemotherapy alone versus combined modality therapy or to indicate if sequencing is of importance. Risk of leukemogenesis is comparable after combined modality treatment and after salvage chemotherapy following relapse from initial radiation treatment. An increased risk of developing undifferentiated lymphomas after treatment for Hodgkin's disease also exists, but has been less well documented [24].

Conclusions

Improvements in disease-free survival with combined modality therapy have to be tempered by concerns over treatment related leukemia and by acknowledging the considerable success of 'salvage' chemotherapy at the time of relapse after radiotherapy for 'early' stage Hodgkin's disease. No available data convincingly favor combined modality treatment over MOPP alone for advanced stages. Reasonable indications exist for pediatric patients, adults with massive mediastinal disease, probably other instances in which masses larger than 8 cm are present, and perhaps some patients with E lesions. Other poor-risk subpopulations need further identification before such treatment can be recommended in the non-study setting. Delineation of such subgroups has been somewhat hindered by failure in many reports to analyze data by detailed staging features.

References

1. Rosenberg SA, Kaplan HS, Glatstein E and Portlock CS (1978). Combined modality therapy of Hodgkin's disease. Cancer 42:991–1000.
2. Glatstein E (1977). Radiotherapy for Hodgkin's disease. Past achievements and future progress. Cancer 39:837–843.
3. Goodman RL, Piro AJ and Hellman S (1976). Can pelvic irradiation be omitted in patients with pathologic Stage IA and IIA Hodgkin's disease? Cancer 37:2834–2839.
4. DeVita VT, Simon RM, Hubbard SM et al. (1980). Curability of advanced Hodgkin's disease with chemotherapy: Long term follow-up of MOPP treated patients at NCI. Ann Intern Med 92:587–595.
5. Hoppe RT, Coleman CN, Cox RS et al. (1982). The management of Stage I-II Hodgkin's disease with irradiation alone or combined modality therapy: The Stanford experience. Blood 59:455–465.
6. Mauch P, Goodman R and Hellman S (1978). The significance of mediastinal involvement in early stage Hodgkin's disease. Cancer 42:1039–1045.
7. Velentjas E, Barett A, McElwain J et al. (1978). Mediastinal involvement in early stage Hodgkin's disease. Eur J Cancer 42:1039–1045.
8. Thar TL, Million RR, Hausner RT et al. (1979). Hodgkin's disease Stage I and II: Relationship of recurrence to size of disease, radiation dose, and number of sites involved. Cancer 43:1101–1105.
9. DeVita VT, Young RC and Chabner BA. Unpublished data.
10. Carmel RJ, Kaplan HS (1976). Mantle irradiation in Hodgkin's disease. An analysis of technique, tumor irradiation and complications. Cancer 37:2812–2825.
11. Piro AJ, Weiss DR and Hellman S (1976). Mediastinal Hodgkin's disease: A possible danger for intubation anesthesia. Int J Radiat Oncol Biol Phys 1:415–419.
12. Levi JA and Wiernik PH (1977). Limited extra nodal Hodgkin's disease: Unfavorable prognosis and therapeutic implications. Amer J Med 63:365–372.
13. Torti FM, Portlock CS, Rosenberg SA and Kaplan HS (1981). Extra-lymphatic Hodgkin's disease: Prognosis and response to therapy. Amer J Med 70:487–492.
14. Desser RK, Golomb HM, Ultman JE et al. (1977). Prognostic classification of Hodgkin's disease in pathologic Stage III based on anatomic considerations. Blood 49:883–893.

15. Stein RS, Golomb HM, Diggs CH et al. (1980). Anatomic substages of Stage IIIA Hodgkin's disease. Ann Intern Med 92:159–165.
16. Hoppe RT, Rosenberg SA and Kaplan HS (1980). Prognostic factors in pathologic Stage IIIA Hodgkin's disease. Cancer 46:1240–1246.
17. Krikorian JG, Portlock CS, Rosenberg SA and Kaplan HS (1979). Hodgkin's disease occurring below the diaphragm. Cancer 43:1866–1871.
18. Farber LR, Prosnitz LR and Cadman EC (1980). Curative potential of combined modality therapy for advanced Hodgkin's disease. Cancer 46:1509–1517.
19. Goodman R, Mauch P, Piro A et al. (1977). Stage IIB and IIIB Hodgkin's disease: Results of combined modality treatment. Cancer 40:84–89.
20. Kun LE, DeVita VT, Young RC et al. (1976). Treatment of Hodgkin's disease using intensive chemotherapy followed by irradiation. Int J Radiat Oncol Biol Phys 1:619–626.
21. Hoppe RT, Portlock CS, Glatstein E et al. (1979). Alternating chemotherapy and irradiation in the treatment of advanced Hodgkin's disease. Cancer 43:472–481.
22. Mauch P, Rosenthal D, Canellos G et al. Reduction of fatal complications from combined modality therapy in Hodgkin's disease. (Submitted for publication).
23. Fraass BA, Kinsella TJ, Harrington FS and Glatstein E. Peripheral dose to the testes: The design and clinical use of a practical and effective gonadal shield. Int J Radiat Oncol Biol Phys (in press).
24. Coleman CN, Kaplan HS, Cox R et al. Leukemias, non-Hodgkin's lymphomas and solid tumors in patients treated for Hodgkin's disease. Cancer Surveys (in press).
25. Coltman CA, Dixon DO (1982). Second malignancies complicating Hodgkin's disease: A Southwest Oncology Group 10 year follow-up. Cancer Treat Rep 66:1023–1033.
26. Glicksman AS, Pajak TF, Gottlieb A et al. (1982). Second malignant neoplasms in patients successfully treated for Hodgkin's disease: A Cancer and Leukemia Group B study. Cancer Treat Rep 66:1035–1044.

5. Combined modality treatment of Hodgkin's disease confined to lymph nodes. Results 14 years later

J. P. DUTCHER and P. H. WIERNIK
Albert Einstein College of Medicine, Montefiore Medical Center, New York, New York, USA

Although extended field radiotherapy can cure most patients with Hodgkin's disease confined to lymph nodes, a significant number of potentially curable patients given radiotherapy alone relapse and ultimately die of their disease. Combination chemotherapy produces complete remission and prolonged disease-free survival in the majority of patients with advanced disease [1–4]. This study was initially designed following a pilot investigation which demonstrated the feasibility of a combined modality approach to the treatment of early Hodgkin's disease, confined to lymph nodes [5, 6]. We are reporting 14 years of follow-up data from this study [7], begun at the Baltimore Cancer Research Center of the NCI (now the University of Maryland Cancer Center).

Materials and methods

Patients

Eighty-seven previously untreated patients with Hodgkin's disease in Pathologic Stages IA, IIB, and IIIA were assigned at random to receive extended field radiotherapy (RT) alone or followed by six cycles of MOPP [1] combination chemotherapy at standard doses (RT + C). Patients were stratified according to extent of disease prior to randomization and were entered into the study from January 1970 to January 1974. Thirteen patients were excluded from subsequent long-term analysis. The specific reasons for exclusion are detailed in a prior publication [7]. Thus, 74 patients are available for long-term analysis, 41 patients received RT and 33 had RT + C. The RT group consisted of 35 patients with nodular sclerosis histology (85%), five with mixed cellularity (12%) and one with lymphocyte predominant pattern (3%). The RT + C group included 23 patients with nodular sclerosis (70%), seven with mixed cellularity (21%) and three with lymphocyte predominant histology (9%). Of 46 evaluable patients with less than Stage IIIA disease, 29 received RT only, and 17 received RT+C. Of 28 evaluable patients with Stage IIIA disease, 12 received RT only, and 16 received RT+C.

Treatment

Radiotherapy was delivered employing a Theratron 80 cobalt unit. The general radiotherapy treatment plan has been described [8]. A midline dose of approximately 4,000 rad delivered in fractions of 180 to 200 rad/day, five days a week, was achieved. The heart was treated in its entirety if a mediastinal mass was present. Whenever mediastinal disease was present, the whole pericardial silhouette was subjected to at least 2,000 rad before insertion of additional shielding. Hilar and parenchymal lung involvement was identified in the anterior and posterior treatment positions; in the case of hilar disease, a full dose to both hilar areas was given, and in the case of infiltrative E stage disease associated with a large mediastinal mass, at least 1,500 rad were given to the involved lung. If the lung involvement with E stage infiltrative disease was less than 15 percent of the total lung field, 4,000 rad were always given to the involved area. When a large mediastinal mass was present, a 10 to 14 day rest period was allowed after a cumulative dose of 2,000 rad to allow for maximal shrinkage of the mass before new lung blocks were designed and radiotherapy was resumed.

Patients with Stage I or II disease randomized to RT alone were given 4,000 rad to an upper mantle field as described, weighted 2/3 anteriorly. In addition, 4,000 rad to the high periaortic nodes was administered if mediastinal involvement was present. Patients with Stage I or II disease randomized to RT+C were given radiotherapy to the upper mantle only. Stage IIIA patients randomized to RT alone were treated through upper mantle and periaortic ports. The pelvic nodes were irradiated only when the lower abdominal nodes were involved. A wing over the splenic bed was added to the periaortic port only when spleen or splenic nodes were pathologic.

Table 1A. Relapses and deaths — (Study 7107)

Stage	RX	No. treated		No. relapsed (alive)		Died (with HD)	
I-II A-A$_E$	RT	29	$p=0.5$	9	(5)	7 (3)	p=ns
I-II A-A$_E$	RT+C	17		1	(1)	0	
III A-A$_E$	RT	12	$p=.008$	7 [a]	(2)	5 (5)	$p=0.16$
III A-A$_E$	RT+C	16		1	(1)	6 (0)	

[a] 2 late (112, 118 mo.)   6/1/84

Table IB. Causes of death

Cause	RT alone (N = 41)		RT+CT (N = 33)		
Hodgkin's disease	8		0		$(p = 0.013)$
Second neoplasm	3		3		
AMML	1		1		
Sarcoma	2		0		
Lung	0		2		
Cardiac	0		3		$(p = ns)$
Suicide	1		0		

6/1/84

Table II. Second neoplasms – Study 7107

Hodgkin's disease			Second neoplasm	
Stage	Histology	Type	Months after HD treatment	Outcome
Radiotherapy alone				
I A	MC	Fibrosarcoma of chest wall (in RT port)	131	Died of sarcoma
II A	NS	Basal cell cancer	76	NED
II A	NS	AMML	10	Died of AMML
II A_E	NS	Craniopharyngioma	0	Died of HD
II A_E (lung)	NS	Osteosarcoma of lung (in RT field)	131	Dies of sarcoma
Radiotherapy plus chemotherapy				
III A	NS	Adenocarcinoma of lung	53	Died of lung cancer
III A	MC	In situ cervical cancer	50	NED
III A	MC	AMML	45	Died of AMML
III A	MC	Small cell carcinoma of lung	111	Died lung cancer

6/1/84

Patients with Stage IIIA disease randomized to RT+C were given irradiation to the upper mantle and, in addition, to any intra-abdominal site of pathologically documented Hodgkin's disease. Adjuvant chemotherapy consisted of six courses of MOPP as originally described [1], except that prednisone was given in each course.

Table III. Long-term treatment-related morbidity; study 7107 – 74 patients

Gastrointesinal	4 (Stage IIIA; 3RT, 1 RT+C)
Bowel obstruction	2
Small bowel necrosis	1
Chronic diarrhea	1
Endocrine	54 (25 RT+C, 29 RT)
Taking synthroid, hypothyroid, elevated TSH	
Cardiovascular	35
Transient pericarditis after RT	11
Symptomatic constrictive pericarditis	11 [a]
Asymptomatic constriction	8 (4 RT, 4 RT+C)
Myocardial infarction	5 (2 RT, 3 RT+C)
Pulmonary	
Chest X-ray evidence of paramediastinal or other fibrosis	100%
Clinically compromised pulmonary function	0

[a] 8 had pericardectomy

6/1/84

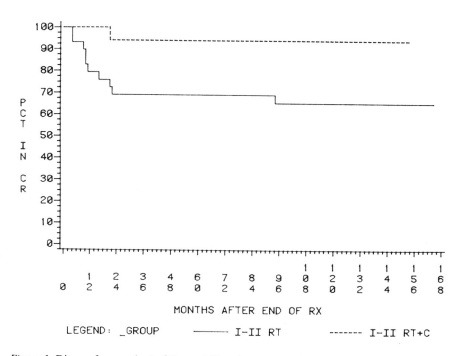

Figure 1. Disease-free survival of Stages I-II patients comparing RT vs. RT+C, ($p<0.04$). BCRC Protocol 7107 for Hodgkin's disease.

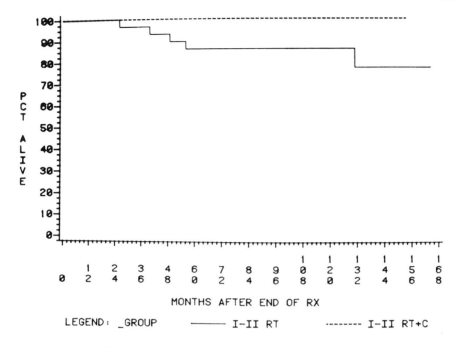

Figure 2. Survival of Stages I-II patients with one suicide in the RT group censored, ($p=0.07$, NS).
BCRC Protocol 7107 for Hodgkin's disease.

Results

Relapse and survival

As of June 1, 1984, follow-up in this study ranges from $8.4+$ to $14+$ years (median $11.4+$ years) from the end of all treatment. Relapse and survival data are presented in Tables I-III and Fig. 1-4. No patient had a relapse with a different histology. Nine of 29 RT alone patients (31 %) with less than Stage IIIA disease have relapsed. None of six Stage IA RT alone patients have relapsed, nor did the one Stage IIB patient. However, five of 18 Stage IIA patients (28 %), both Stage IIA_E (lung) patients and both Stage IIB_E (lung) patients have relapsed from four to 22 months (median 10 months) after completion of treatment. This is in contrast to one relapse (Stage IIA) among 17 patients (6 %) with less than Stage IIIA disease treated with RT+C ($p<0.05$). There were no relapses in Stage IIB patients, one Stage IIA_E (lung) patient, or one Stage IIB_E (lung) patient (RT+C group).

Three RT alone relapsed patients whose disease was less than Stage IIIA

322

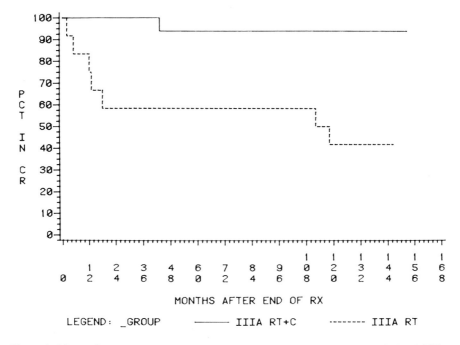

Figure 3. Disease-free survival of Stage IIIA patients comparing RT vs. RT+C, ($p < 0.005$). BCRC Protocol 7107 for Hodgkin's disease.

have died of Hodgkin's disease (2 Stage IIB$_E$ (lung), one Stage IIA). A fourth relapsed patient died of acute leukemia at 50 months from initial treatment. She had evidence of active Hodgkin's disease at death and for most of the 40 months prior to death. A fifth RT alone patient with Stage IIA$_E$ (lung) disease relapsed at 22 months but remained in remission for 109 months following retreatment with chemotherapy. He died at 131 months, of osteo-sarcoma of the lung, still without evidence of Hodgkin's disease. The other five relapsed patients with Stages I-IIA-A$_E$ are alive. Two other RT alone patients in the early stage group who did not have a relapse of Hodgkin's disease have died. One disease-free Stage IIA patient committed suicide at 60 months, and a second Stage IA patient died of a chest wall fibrosarcoma in the radiation port at 131 months after his initial treatment with RT alone.

Among 12 Stage IIIA-A$_E$ patients treated with RT alone, five of nine with Stage IIIA (55%) have relapsed. Two were late relapses, at 112 and 118 months after initial treatment. Two of three RT alone Stage IIIA$_E$ (lung) patients have relapsed (67%). Sixteen Stage IIIA-A$_E$ patients were treated with RT+C and one has relapsed, (Stage IIIA). He remains in remission at

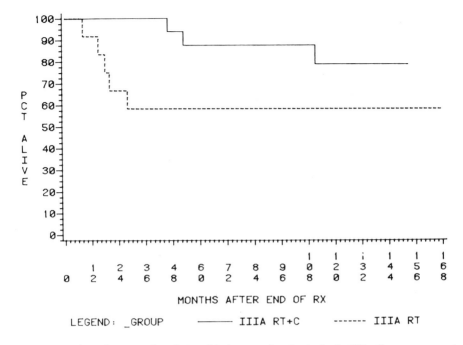

Figure 4. Survival of Stage IIIA patients with three cardiac deaths in the RT + C group censored, (*p* = 0.008, NS).
BCRC Protocol 7107 for Hodgkin's disease.

127 months after treatment. The difference in relapse rate between the two treatment groups is significant ($p < 0.008$). Five Stage IIIA-A_E patients, treated with RT alone have died, all of Hodgkin's disease. The two Stage IIIA patients with late relapses remain alive in subsequent remissions. Six Stage IIIA-A_E patients treated with RT + C have died, three of heart disease at 54, 67 and 84 months following initial treatment (all were older than 45 years). The patient who died at 54 months, a 51 year old woman, had had a pericardiectomy 26 months prior to death for severe radiation-related pericarditis. A fourth patient died of acute leukemia at 46 months following initial treatment. Two other patients died of lung cancer, one of non-small cell lung cancer (at 53 months) and one of small cell lung cancer (at 111 months). None had evidence of Hodgkin's disease.

Thus, there have been no deaths from Hodgkin's disease or any other cause in RT + C patients whose disease was less than Stage IIIA. The death rate in that group is different from that of RT alone patients with the same stages of disease ($p < 0.05$). None of the RT + C Stage IIIA-A_E patients has died of Hodgkin's disease, compared to five of twelve treated with RT alone ($p = 0.016$).

Salvage therapy

Sixteen RT alone and 2 RT+C patients have relapsed. Both RT+C patients responded to salvage chemotherapy and are disease-free at 84+ and 122+ months following relapse. Two RT patients refused treatment for relapse, two received radiotherapy for relapse and achieved complete remission, two received combined modality therapy for relapse and achieved complete remission and 10 patients received chemotherapy for relapse, with 8 achieving complete remission. Thus, 12 of 14 (85%) RT patients were salvaged after relapse. Two of the RT alone relapses were late (112, 118 months), both in patients with Stage IIIA disease. Both patients are currently disease free at 39+ and 49+ months following salvage chemotherapy. Six of the ten patients salvaged after initial relapse have died of Hodgkin's disease (60%). A seventh patient died of osteosarcoma of the previously involved and irradiated lung and of respiratory failure. Only three relapsed RT patients remain alive and disease-free after salvage therapy for a median of 150+ months; two of them have had second relapses.

Second neoplasms

Nine second malignancies were observed in this study, an overall incidence of 12% (Table II). One RT and one RT+C patient died of acute myelomonocytic leukemia, 49 and 45 months after completion of initial therapy, respectively. Two RT+C patients died of carcinoma of the lung, one of adenocarcinoma at 53 months after initial therapy, and one of small cell carcinoma at 111 months. A craniopharyngioma was found at autopsy in one patient who died of Hodgkin's disease. Two other patients have died of sarcomas; one at 131 months of a fibrosarcoma of the chest wall and one of osteosarcoma of the lung at 131 months, both within radiation fields. Two others are currently free of all disease after treatment for in situ cervical carcinoma (RT+C) and another (RT) for a basal cell carcinoma developing within a radiation field.

Long-term treatment-related morbidity

The immediate toxicities of RT and RT+C in this study have been reported [8], as have initial reports of late-appearing complications which may be therapy related [9–15] (Table III).

Radiation-related cardiovascular disease
Some evidence of radiation-related pericardial disease was found in 35 of
the 74 (47%) evaluable patients. This includes 11 patients with transient
pericarditis immediately following radiotherapy [9, 10]. Subsequent follow-
up of the additonal patients has revealed a high incidence of both symptomatic (11 patients) and asymptomatic (8 patients, 4 RT, 4 RT+C) pericardial constriction, 8 of whom required pericardiectomy [11, 12]. Five patients have had myocardial infarctions and three have died (2 RT, 3
RT+C). Four of the five were older than 45 years. One patient who died
was a 51 year old woman who had previously undergone a pericardiectomy
for constriction. One of the two patients remaining alive is a 32-year old
woman. One patient in each treatment group had a subclavian vein thrombosis at 18 and 22 months after radiotherapy. Another RT alone patient had
vascular insufficiency in the upper extremity at 104+ months post radiotherapy and due to subclavian arterial narrowing as a consequence of radiotherapy. Another patient (RT+C) is being evaluated for similar symptoms
at 126+ months following radiotherapy.

Radiation-related hypothyroidism
Hypothyroidism is a well-recognized complication of upper mantle irradiation [13, 14]. Our previous reports have indicated that either chemical
hypothyroidism (significant rise in TSH with or without decreased thyrox-
ine) or clinical hypothyroidism (elevated TSH, significant depression in T4,
and signs or symptoms of hypothyroidism) developed in 54 patients (73%)
treated in this study [14]. Twelve patients developed clinical (8 RT, 4
RT+C), and 42 developed chemical hypothyroidism (18 RT, 24 RT+C).
Interestingly, at least one young female patient who was initially felt to be
infertile following treatment (RT for Stage IIA disease), has had two children on thyroid replacement.

Pulmonary complications
In virtually all patients there is some evidence of paramediastinal or other
fibrosis evident on chest radiographs after radiotherapy. Although no patient in continuous complete remission has clinically compromised pulmonary function, objective evidence of some pulmonary compromise can be
detected with systematic pulmonary function testing [15]. One patient who
relapsed after RT alone, but responded to salvage chemotherapy developed
progressive respiratory deterioration over several years, and died of an
osteosarcoma of the lung. One young male patient (RT alone) underwent
thoracotomy for bleb resection after two spontaneous pneumothoraces. The
lung was found to be fibrotic in the area of the blebs, and this necessitated a
larger resection than originally planned.

Gastrointestinal complications
Four patients (3 RT alone, 1 RT + C) with Stage IIIA disease (all laparotomy staged) have had gastrointestinal complications. Two patients developed a small bowel obstruction at 86 and 130 months after initial treatment. One required surgical lysis of adhesions and has had no further problems and the other required a colostomy for obstruction after a five year history of abdominal pain. A third patient suffers from chronic diarrhea after RT + C. The fourth patient (RT alone) had extensive radiation necrosis of the small bowel requiring resection of more than half of the small bowel. She has suffered from malabsorption and malnutrition and has been maintained on chronic hyperalimentation for ten years.

Infectious complications
There have been no significant infections to date. Specifically, there have been no postsplenectomy pneumococcal or hemophilus infections [16]. In seven patients (all RT + C), localized Herpes zoster developed sometime during follow-up, but none has occurred during the past five years [17].

Discussion

This report confirms and extends our preliminary observations [7, 8] on RT + C for Hodgkin's disease confined to lymph nodes. The subgroups of patients that benefited most from RT + C were patients with large mediastinal masses and E-stage disease of the lung, and those with Stage IIIA disease. Subsequent studies have determined that those Stage IIIA patients who benefit most had Stage $IIIA_2$ [18].

Although most of the acute, short-term toxicities of RT + C are due to chemotherapy, this study with its long follow-up continues to demonstrate significant, long-term chronic complications secondary to RT. These complications could be avoided if radiation exposure could be reduced or eliminated. The results of subsequent investigation by us, updated in this volume, suggest that results comparable to RT + C may be achieved with chemotherapy alone [19].

References

1. DeVita VT Jr, Serpick AA and Carbone PP (1970). Combination chemotherapy in the treatment of advanced Hodgkin's disease. Ann Intern Med 73:881–895.
2. DeVita VT Jr, Simon RM, Hubbard SM et al. (1980). Curability of advanced Hodgkin's disease with chemotherapy. Ann Intern Med 92:587–595.

3. Coltman Ca Jr. (1980). Chemotherapy of advanced Hodgkin's disease. Semin Oncol 7:155–173.
4. Diggs CH, Wiernik PH and Sutherland JC (1981). Treatment of advanced untreated Hodgkin's disease with SCAB — An alternative to MOPP. Cancer 47:224–228.
5. Brace K, Serpick AA, Block JB et al. (1973). Combination radiotherapy and chemotherapy in the treatment of early Hodgkin's disease. Oncology 27:484–489.
6. Wiernik PH and Lichtenfeld JL (1975). Combined modality therapy for localized Hodgkin's disease. A seven year update of an early study. Oncology 32:208–212.
7. Wiernik PH, Gustafson J, Schimpff SC et al. (1979). Combined modality treatment of Hodgkin's disease confined to lymph nodes. Amer J Med 67:183–192.
8. O'Connell MJ, Wiernik PH, Brace KC et al. (1975). A combined modality approach to the treatment of Hodgkin's disease. Cancer 35:1055–1065.
9. Ruckdeschel JC, Chang P, Martin RG et al. (1975). Radiation-related pericardial effusions in patients with Hodgkin's disease. Medicine 54:245–249.
10. Martin RG, Ruckdeschel JC, Chang P et al. (1975). Radiation-related pericarditis. Amer J Cardiol 35:216–220.
11. Applefeld MM, Cole JF and Pollock SH (1981). The late appearance of chronic pericardial disease in patients by radiotherapy for Hodgkin's disease. Ann Intern Med 94:338–341.
12. Applefeld MM, Slawson RG, Spicer KM et al. (1982). Long-term cardiovascular evaluation of patients with Hodgkin's disease treated by mantle radiation therapy. Cancer Treat Rep 66:1003–1013.
13. Fuks Z, Glatstein E, Marsa GW et al. (1976). Long-term effects of external radiation on the pituitary and thyroid glands. Cancer 37:1152–1161.
14. Schimpff SC, Diggs CH, Wiswell JG et al. (1980). Radiation-related thyroid dysfunction: Implications for the treatment of Hodgkin's disease. Ann Intern Med 92:91–98.
15. Schlossberger NM and Wiernik PH (1980). The pulmonary function of post-therapy Hodgkin's disease patients. Proc Amer Assoc Cancer Res and Amer Soc Clin Oncol 21:468.
16. Schimpff SC, O'Connell MJ, Greene WH et al. (1973). Infections in 92 splenectomized patients with Hodgkin's disease. Amer J Med 59:695–701.
17. Ruckdeschel JC, Schimpff SC, Smyth AE et al. (1977). Herpes zoster and impaired cell-associated immunity to the varicella-zoster virus in patients with Hodgkin's disease. Amer J Med 62:77–85.
18. Stein RS, Golomb HM, Wiernik PH et al. (1982). Anatomic substages of Stage IIIA Hodgkin's disease: Follow-up of a collaborative Study. Cancer Treat Rep 66:733–741.
19. O'Dwyer PJ, Wiernik PH, Stewart MB, and Slawson RG (1985). Treatment of early stage Hodgkin's disease: A randomized trial of radiotherapy plus chemotherapy versus chemotherapy alone. In: Cavalli F, Bonadonna G, and Rozencweig M (Eds). Malignant Lymphomas and Hodgkin's Disease: Experimental and Therapeutic Advances, pp 329–336. Boston: Martinus Nijhoff.

6. Treatment of early stage Hodgkin's disease: A randomized trial of radiotherapy plus chemotherapy versus chemotherapy alone

P. J. O'DWYER, P. H. WIERNIK, M. B. STEWART,
and R. G. SLAWSON
University of Maryland Cancer Center (formerly Baltimore Cancer Research Center), Baltimore, Maryland, USA

In 1976, extended field megavoltage radiation had become standard therapy for Hodgkin's disease confined to lymph nodes [1, 2]. While essentially all patients with Stage I disease are cured by this technique, it has become apparent that a significant number of patients with more advanced disease relapse after treatment with radiotherapy alone. This is especially true of Stage IIIA disease [3], and those with large mediastinal masses with or without extranodal extension into lung [4, 5], but among all Stages I and II, relapse rates as high as 27% have been reported [6]. The recognition that combination chemotherapy could prolong both duration of second remission and survival in patients relapsing after radiation therapy [6, 7], prompted the evaluation of several combined modality regimens as initial treatment in patients with Stages I to IIIA disease [8–12]. The apparent benefits of this approach in terms of remission duration [9], and the growing awareness of undesirable long-term toxic effects of combined modality therapy [13], prompted the present study. Interim analyses have been presented previously [14, 15].

Materials and methods

This study was conducted at the Baltimore Cancer Research Center (now the University of Maryland Cancer Center) with patients entered between June 1976 and November 1978. Thirty-six patients with previously untreated Hodgkin's disease, Stages IB to IIIA were randomized to treatment with extended field radiotherapy followed by MOPP (mechlorethamine, vincristine, procarbazine, and prednisone) [16] or MOPP alone. A full staging evaluation was performed on all patients prior to entry. This included complete blood count and differential white cell count, SMA 12 biochemical screen, chest x-ray, lung tomography for patients with mediastinal or lung involvement identified on the chest film, Technetium liver-spleen scan,

[67]Gallium scan, bipedal lymphangiography (LAG), and laparotomy. The following procedures were followed at laparotomy: splenectomy; biopsy of all suspicious nodes on LAG with confirmation by intraoperative abdominal x-ray; biopsy of porta hepatis, splenic pedicle, mesenteric and high periaortic lymph nodes bilaterally; in the absence of suspicious nodes on LAG, random biopsies of bilateral periaortic and iliac nodes; biopsy of suspicious hepatic lesions discovered at operation or by scans, or in the absence of such lesions, random wedge biopsy of both lobes; and iliac crest bone marrow biopsy in patients staged as IIIA on the basis of clinical findings. Staging designations are reported according to the conventions of the Ann Arbor conference [17], and pathologic classification follows that of Lukes and Butler [18].

Radiotherapy was administered according to the following plan. Patients with disease on one side of the diaphragm received radiation to the central lymphatic regions on that side, plus the next adjacent area across the diaphragm. Those with involvement on both sides of the diaphragm were irradiated through both mantle and inverted Y ports, with a four to eight week interval between fields. The mantle field was treated with 4000 rad midplane dose in 20 fractions using a ^{60}Co source or a linear accelerator. X-rays were delivered through parallel opposing ports, weighted two-thirds anteriorly. Where a mediastinal mass greater than one-third the chest diameter was present, approximately 1500 rad were delivered to both entire lung fields. Lead blocks were then applied as radiotherapy continued. Blocks were cut once or twice during treatment as the mass regressed. The inverted

Table I. Patient characteristics

	MOPP+RT		MOPP	
Total number of patients	19		17	
Total evaluable	17		15	
Sex (M/F)	9/8		7/8	
Mean age (range)	26.9 (15-62)		26.8 (14–55)	
Stage	IB	1		
	IIA	8	IIA	8
	IIB	4	IIB	1
	IIIA	4	IIIA	6
Histology	NS	7	NS	11
	MC	7	MC	5
	LD	1	LP	1

NS = Nodular Sclerosing
MC = Mixed Cellularity
LD = Lymphocyte Depleted

Y field was treated similarly with 4000 rad in 20 fractions. Adjuvant chemotherapy consisted of six courses of MOPP – mechlorethamine 6 mg/m^2 i.v. days 1 and 8, vincristine 1.4 mg/m^2 i.v. days 1 and 8, procarbazine 100 mg/m^2 p.o. days 1 to 14, and prednisone 40 mg/m^2 days 1 to 14. Prednisone was omitted on alternate cycles, beginning with the second. Each course was administered on a 28-day cycle, provided that the toxicity of the previous cycle had resolved. Postponement of treatment for a week was allowed when there was a reasonable expectation of the patient tolerating full doses at that time. Dose modifications were based on white blood cell and platelet count nadirs in the previous course.

Four patients, two from each group, were inevaluable. One patient died of unrelated cause before treatment began. One was originally diagnosed as having lymphocytic lymphoma, but was thought to have Hodgkin's disease based on retroperitoneal node histology. While he had a complete response to combined modality treatment, he relapsed in six months with clear-cut nodular poorly-differentiated lymphocytic lymphoma. Two patients, one from each group, refused to continue therapy at an early stage. The characteristics of the evaluable patients are shown in Table I.

Complete remission is defined as complete regression of all measurable lesions, and suppression of all other evidence of active disease. Partial remission is defined as a $\geq 50\%$ reduction of the sum of the products of perpendicular diameters of all areas of measurable disease, without progression of any lesion, or the appearance of new lesions.

The analysis was conducted up to 12/31/1983, and represents a median follow-up of 73.5 months. Remission duration and survival are reported from the date of first treatment.

Results

Response rate and duration

Of the 17 patients in the combined modality (RT+C) treatment group, 16 (94%) entered complete remission, while one had a partial remission. Twelve of the 15 patients in the chemotherapy alone (C) group had a complete remission, one a partial remission, and two patients failed to respond. On subsequent treatment with radiotherapy, the partial responder and one of the two non-responders achieved a complete remission.

The median duration of complete remission in the RT+C group is 72.5+ months, and in the C group (initial complete responders) 69.5+ months. There is no statistically significant difference between the curves (Gehan-Wilcoxon, $p = 0.30$; logrank, $p = 0.53$). A plot of freedom from second relapse which includes the patients in the C group who achieved complete remission following radiotherapy, also demonstrates a lack of difference between the groups (Gehan-Wilcoxon, $p = 0.61$; logrank, $p = 0.59$). Median survival of all patients is 73+ months for the RT+C and 74+ months for the C group. There is no significant difference between the Kaplan-Meier survival curves (Gehan-Wilcoxon, $p = 0.33$; logrank, $p = 0.32$).

Analysis of failures

Radiotherapy and chemotherapy
The patient who failed to achieve complete remission, a 17-year old female with Stage IIA, mixed cellularity Hodgkin's disease, showed progression in four months and died of refractory disease at 21 months. Two patients relapsed: one at 38 months (a 25-year old male with Stage IIIA, nodular sclerosing who died at 48 months), and one at 70 months. Three patients in this group died without known recurrence of Hodgkin's disease, one of unknown causes at 44 months. A 62-year old male (Stage IIA, mixed cellularity) was diagnosed with non-small cell lung cancer 37 months after beginning treatment: he died of that tumor at 57 months. The third patient was a 29 year old female whose chemotherapy was repeatedly interrupted because of hepatitis, later diagnosed as chronic active hepatitis and treated with prednisone and azathioprine. Three months after beginning the latter drug, she developed a urinary tract infection which progressed to Gram-negative septic shock, to which she succumbed at 28 months.

Chemotherapy
One non-responder failed all subsequent therapies and died at 57 months. The other non-responder, and a patient who achieved partial remission, are both disease-free following radiotherapy. The latter, a 21-year old male with Stage IIA nodular sclerosing, developed persistent pancytopenia after abdominal irradiation, followed by the appearance of overt acute non-lymphocytic leukemia 78 months after beginning treatment. Three patients in this group have relapsed at 18, 19 and 24 months. One failed to respond to radiotherapy and died at 25 months. Two were rendered disease-free by radiotherapy, one of whom has relapsed again at 63 months.

Long-term toxicity

Morbidity during the period of follow-up is tabulated (Table II). Viral and fungal infections occurred more frequently in the RT+C group (6 versus 2 episodes); all resolved uneventfully. Toxicity directly attributable to radia-

Table II. Morbidity during years of follow-up, by treatment

	MOPP	MOPP & RT
Infectious		
Aseptic meningitis	0	2
Herpes Zoster		
– local	1	2
– disseminated	0	1
Varicella	1	0
Actinomyces	0	1
Infective endocarditis	1	0
Late gram negative sepsis	0	1
Endocrine		
Hypothyroidism	1	2
Infertility [a]	1	0
Radiation – Related		
Radiation myelitis	0	2
Constrictive pericarditis [b]	0	2
Neoplastic		
Acute myelocytic leukemia [c]	1	0
Squamous cell lung cancer	1	1
Other		
Chronic active hepatitis	0	1
Polyclonal gammopathy	1	0

[a] Few patients had sperm counts performed
[b] Hemodynamically significant
[c] Patient had partial response to MOPP; complete response induced by radiation; after a preleukemic phase, patient developed overt leukemia 6 yrs after presentation

tion was notable, affecting four of 17 patients. Constrictive pericarditis resulted in limited exercise capacity in two patients. Hypothyroidism occurred in two patients treated with radiotherapy. There were three second neoplasms during the years of follow-up: one patient from each group was diagnosed as having squamous cell lung cancer: one has died of that disease, the other remains disease-free 11 months following surgery. One patient from the C group developed acute non-lymphocytic leukemia. As noted above, this patient received both chemotherapy and salvage radiotherapy.

Discussion

After six years of follow-up, this pilot study demonstrates that in the initial treatment of patients with early-stage Hodgkin's disease, MOPP alone is as effective as combined radiotherapy-MOPP in terms of remission duration and survival. The equivalence of the duration of freedom from second relapse is a further indication that patients who relapse from MOPP alone may be successfully salvaged by the use of radiotherapy at that time, perhaps obviating the need for initial radiotherapy.

The survival for all patients is 75 months (78%), which compares favorably with previous studies evaluating combined modality therapy [8–12]. A slight trend in favor of the chemotherapy alone arm may be explained by the occurrence in the RT+C group of two deaths which are probably unrelated to Hodgkin's disease: the first, a patient who died of unknown causes seven months after his last visit (at which time he was clinically free of disease); the second, a patient discussed above, who developed gram-negative sepsis and was treated at a local hospital. Censoring these two patients renders the survival curves for the two study groups virtually identical. As Rosenberg points out [8], freedom from second relapse may be a more meaningful predictor of ultimate survival than duration of initial complete remission. In this study, 80% of the C group and 65% of RT+C group (or 75% if one excludes the two patients discussed above) are alive and free of disease at six years.

In the randomized trials of combined modality versus radiotherapy which have been reported to date, the advantage of the former has been clearly demonstrated in the duration of initial complete remission [8–12]. Overall survival advantage has been observed with combined modality therapy for patients with large mediastinal masses and/or generalized abdominal nodal involvement [19, 20]. Long term toxicity has, however, been a concern in the management of these patients. The risk of second neoplasms, leukemias [21] and lymphomas [22], seems to be increased in patients exposed to combined modality therapy, especially in those patients who receive chemotherapy as salvage therapy [23]. Infectious complications, particularly with the varicella-zoster virus, were a prominent feature of the initial combined modality studies at Stanford [24] and elsewhere [25]. Other investigators have reported hypothyroidism in association with mantle radiation [26]. The cardiotoxicity of mantle radiation has previously been described [27]; its full extent has only recently been appreciated [28]. Future cardiac evaluation of patients treated with currently standard mantle techniques will be important in discerning the relative importance of the newer techniques versus those used in this early study.

All these long-term toxicities were observed in the present study. Infectious episodes were more frequent in the combined modality group, while hypothyroidism was observed in both. Constrictive pericarditis of a degree that was clinically significant occurred in two of the patients treated with mantle irradiation. Finally, the patient who developed secondary ANLL was treated with both modalities. These data suggest strongly that the therapeutic index of chemotherapy alone in the initial treatment of early stage Hodgkin's disease is superior to that of combined modality therapy. Trials are currently in progress at the National Cancer Institute to compare chemotherapy and radiotherapy in early-stage Hodgkin's disease.

References

1. Peters MV (1950). A study of survivals in Hodgkin's disease treated radiologically. Amer J Roentgenol 63:299–311.
2. Kaplan HS (1980). Hodgkin's disease: Unfolding concepts concerning its nature, management and prognosis. Cancer 45:2439–2474.
3. Hoppe RT, Rosenberg SA, Kaplan HS and Cox RS (1980). Prognostic factors in pathological Stage IIIA Hodgkin's disease. Cancer 46:1240–1246.
4. Levi JA and Wiernik PH (1977). Limited extranodal Hodgkin's disease: Unfavorable prognosis and therapeutic implications. Amer J Med 63:365–372.
5. Timothy AR, Sutcliff SBJ, Stansfeld AG et al. (1978). Radiotherapy in the treatment of Hodgkin's disease. Br Med J 1:1246–1249.
6. Weller SA, Glatstein E, Kaplan HS and Rosenberg SA (1976). Initial relapses in previously treated Hodgkin's disease. I. Results of second treatment. Cancer 37:2840–1846.
7. Mintz U, Miller JB, Golomb HM et al. (1979). Pathologic Stage I and II Hodgkin's disease, 1968–1975. Relapses and results of retreatment. Cancer 44:72–79.
8. Rosenberg SA, Kaplan HS, Glatstein EJ and Portlock CS (1978). Combined modality therapy of Hodgkin's disease. Cancer 42:991–1000.
9. Wiernik PH, Gustafson J, Schimpff SC and Diggs C (1979). Combined modality treatment of Hodgkin's disease confined to lymph nodes. Results eight years later. Amer J Med 67:183–193.
10. Andrieu JM, Montagnon B, Asselain B et al. (1980). Chemotherapy-radiotherapy association in Hodgkin's disease, Clinical Stages IA, II$_2$A: Results of a prospective clinical trial with 166 patients. Cancer 46:2126–2130.
11. Hagemeister TB, Fuller LM, Velasquez WS et al. (1982). Stage I and II Hodgkin's disease: Involved-field radiotherapy versus extended field radiotherapy versus involved-field radiotherapy followed by six cycles of MOPP. Cancer Treat Rep 66:789–798.
12. Nissen NI and Nordentoft AW (1982). Radiotherapy versus combined modality treatment of Stage I and II Hodgkin's Disease. Cancer Treat Rep 66:799–803.
13. Arseneau JC, Sponzo RW, Levin DL et al. (1972). Non-lymphomatous malignant tumors complicating Hodgkin's disease. N Engl J Med 287:1119–1122.
14. Wiernik PH, Slawson RG, Burks LC and Diggs CH (1979). A randomized trial of radiotherapy (R) and MOPP (C) versus MOPP alone for Stage IB to IIIA Hodgkin's disease. Proc Amer Soc Clin Oncol 17:314.
15. O'Dwyer PJ, Wiernik PH, Finlay R and Ungerleider RS (1983). A randomized trial of radiotherapy (RT) and MOPP (C) vs MOPP alone for Stages IB-IIIA Hodgkin's disease. Proc Amer Soc Clin Oncol 2:214.
16. DeVita VT, Serpick AA and Carbone PP (1970). Combination chemotherapy in the treatment of advanced Hodgkin's disease. Ann Intern Med 73:881–895.
17. Carbone PP, Kaplan HS, Musshoff K et al. (1971). Report of the Committee on Hodgkin's Disease Staging Classification. Cancer Res 31:1860–1861.
18. Lukes RJ and Butler JJ (1966). The pathology and nomenclature of Hodgkin's disease. Cancer Res 26:1063–1081.

19. Wiernik PH and Slawson RG (1982). Hodgkin's disease with direct extension into pulmonary parenchyma from a mediastinal mass: A presentation requiring special therapeutic considerations. Cancer Treat Rep 66:711–716.
20. Stein RS, Golomb HM, Wiernik PH et al. (1982). Anatomic substages of Stage IIIA Hodgkin's disease: Followup of a collaborative study. Cancer Treat Rep 66:733–741.
21. Coleman CN, Williams CJ, Flint A et al. (1977). Hematologic neoplasia in patients treated for Hodgkin's disease. N Engl J Med 297:1249–1252.
22. Krikorian JG, Burke JS Rosenberg SA and Kaplan HS (1979). The occurrence of non-Hodgkin's lymphoma following therapy for Hodgkin's disease. N Engl J Med 300:452–458.
23. Bonadonna G (1982). Chemotherapy strategies to improve the control of Hodgkin's disease: The Richard and Hinda Rosenthal Foundation Award Lecture. Cancer Res 42:4309–4320.
24. Moore MR, Bull JM, Jones SE et al. (1972). Sequential radiotherapy and chemotherapy in the treatment of Hodgkin's disease: A progress report. Ann Intern Med 77:1–9.
25. Schimpff SC, O'Connell MJ, Greene WH and Wiernik PH (1975). Infections in 92 splenectomized patients with Hodgkin's disease. Ann Intern Med 59:695–701.
26. Glicksman AS and Nickson JJ (1973). Acute and late reactions to irradiation in the treatment of Hodgkin's disease. Arch Int Med 131:369–373.
27. Stewart HR, Cohn KE, Fajardo LF et al. (1967). Radiation-induced heart disease: A study of twenty-five patients. Radiology 89:302–310.
28. Applefeld MM, Slawson RG, Spicer KM et al. (1982). Long-term cardiovascular evaluation of patients with Hodgkin's disease treated by thoracic mantle radiation therapy. Cancer Treat Rep 66:1003–1013.

7. Randomized study of chemotherapy alone vs. chemotherapy plus radiotherapy in Clinical Stages IA-IIA Hodgkin's disease

S. PAVLOVSKY, J. DUPONT, E. JIMÉNEZ,
F. SACKMANN-MURIEL, C. MONTERO and G. GARAY
Grupo Argentino de la Leucemia Aguda (GATLA) and Grupo Latinoamericano de Tratamiento de Hemopatias Malignas (GLATHEM), Buenos Aires, Argentina, and San José, Costa Rica

Major radiotherapy centers or collaborative groups report 5-year survival rates of 80–90% or higher in patients with Stages I-IIA Hodgkin's disease [1–4]. These results have been achieved with megavoltage equipment, variable irradiated fields (involved field to total lymphoid) and doses between 3,500 and 4,400 rad. Adjuvant chemotherapy has significantly increased relapse-free survival compared with irradiation alone (87–92% vs 66–79% at 5 years). However, 5-year survival rates are identical. Comparisons at 10 or more years remain to be determined [1, 2, 4].

In a previous study of GATLA [5], a group of 47 patients with Clinical Stages I-IIA Hodgkin's disease were treated, from 1972 to 1977, with involved field radiotherapy followed by maintenance chemotherapy. Overall and relapse-free survival rates were 73% and 79%, respectively. These percentages were similar (62% and 76%) to those obtained with 6 cycles of the same chemotherapy without radiotherapy in 50 patients with Clinical Stages III-IVA. Subsequently, we initiated a randomized study comparing combination chemotherapy with cyclophosphamide, vinblastine, procarbazine and prednisone (CVPP) vs CVPP plus involved field radiation therapy. The purpose of this report is to present the current results of this trial in Clinical Stages I-IIA disease.

Materials and methods

From April 1979 to December 1983, 103 untreated patients with Clinical Stages I-IIA Hodgkin's disease were randomized to receive either 6 cycles of CVPP or 6 cycles of CVPP plus radiation therapy (CVPP+RT). Results were evaluated in April 1984. Eligibility criteria included histologically confirmed Hodgkin's disease according to Lukes and Butler. Staging was assessed on the basis of clinical history, physical examination, chest roent-

338

genogram, bilateral lymphangiography and/or abdominal CAT scan, and bilateral bone marrow biopsy. Staging laparatomy was not performed, spleen and liver enlargement being considered signs of tumor involvement. A total of 53 patients were treated with CVPP and 50 with CVPP+RT. All entries were evaluable.

The distribution of patients according to age, histology (lymphocyte predominance and nodular sclerosis versus mixed cellularity and lymphocyte depletion), and mediastinal involvement is presented for each group in Table I. There were more children (15 years of age or less) in the CVPP group and more young adults in the CVPP+RT group. However, the number of patients of more than 45 years was similar in both groups.

Chemotherapy consisted of six monthly cycles of CVPP (cyclophosphamide 600 mg/m^2/iv on day 1, vinblastine 6 mg/m^2/iv on day 1, procarbazine 100 mg/m^2 p.o. and prednisone 40 mg/m^2 p.o. both given daily, day 1 through 14). Radiotherapy was administered to the lymph node areas involved at diagnosis. A total of 3,000 rad were given between the third and the fourth cycle of chemotherapy.

Patients were evaluated at the end of 6 cycles of chemotherapy and areas of known involvement before chemotherapy were re-examined. If these areas were tumor-free and if there was no clinical, radiologic or CAT scan evidence of Hodgkin's disease, the patient was considered to be in complete remission (CR). Evaluation included bone marrow and hepatic biopsies, if necessary. Patients were considered in partial remission (PR) when tumor reduction greater than 50% was observed for at least two months.

The statistical analysis of the curves was performed by the life table method and comparisons were done with the logrank test. The Chi-square test was used to analyze response rates and prognostic factors.

Table I. Features at diagnosis in CS I-IIA Hodgkin's disease according to treatment schedule

Feature		CVPP	CVPP+RT
Total		53	50
Age	≤15 yrs	30	15
	16–45 yrs	18	29
	>45 yrs	5	6
Histology	LP-NS	31	22
	MC-LD	22	28
Mediastinal Involvement	+	19	15
	−	34	35

Results

Complete remission was obtained in 46 (86%) of 53 patients treated with CVPP and in 46 (92%) of 50 patients who received CVPP+RT (Table II). Among patients with mediastinal involvement, the complete remission rate was 86% with CVPP compared to 93% with CVPP+RT. In those patients without mediastinal involvement, the corresponding figures were 97% and 91%, respectively (Table III).

In the CVPP group, 40/46 complete responders are still free from relapse vs 41/46 in the combined modality group. The 4-year disease-free survival rate is 85% for the CVPP patients and 84% for the others (Fig. 1). One patient in each group died in complete remission. Four of five patients who relapsed in the CVPP group had lymph node relapse in the site previously involved, compared with 2 of 4 in the CVPP+RT group. The remaining relapses occurred in the liver (one) and the lung (two).

There were 2/53 deaths in the CVPP arm vs 6/50 with CVPP+RT; the corresponding 4-year survival rates are 94% and 85%, respectively (Fig. 2). This difference is not significant. Of the 13 CVPP patients whose disease failed to respond or relapsed, two died (one of disease progression and one in complete remission), seven are being treated for active disease and four are in complete remission. There were nine such patients in the CVPP+RT

Table II. Response in Hodgkin's disease CS I-IIA according to treatment schedule

Treatment	CR No	%	PR	Null	Died (<6 mo)	Total
CVPP	46	86	5	2	—	53
CVPP+RT	46	92	—	3	1 [a]	50

[a] Died of septic shock

Table III. Response in CS I-IIA Hodgkin's disease according to mediastinal involvement and treatment

Mediastinal	CVPP No. Pts	CR No.	%	CVPP+RT No. pts	CR No.	%
Positive	19	13	68	15	14	93
Negative	34	33	97	35	32	91

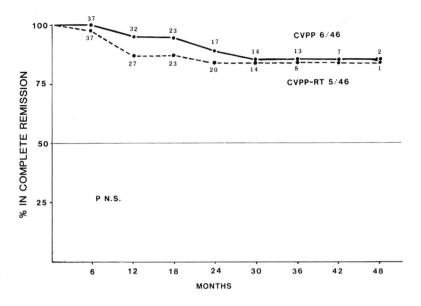

Figure 1. Duration of complete remission in CS I-IIA Hodgkin's disease according to treatment.

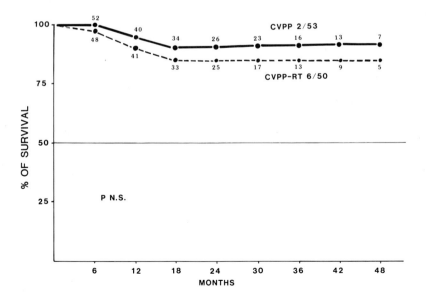

Figure 2. Survival in CS I-IIA Hodgkin's disease according to treatment.

arm: four died of disease progression, one died of sepsis during induction, one died in complete remission, and three are alive, two with active disease and one in complete remission.

No differences were observed in terms of WBC nadirs or episodes of leucopenia during treatment. One patient in the CVPP+RT group died from infection complications during induction. The median treatment duration was 6 months for CVPP and 8 months for CVPP+RT (Table IV).

Discussion

The introduction of combination chemotherapy in the past decade has greatly improved the prognosis of the advanced stages of disease [5–7]. The 5-year survival with Stages III-IV disease is 50% to 70% [6, 7]. The long-term survival with Stage IIIA disease treated with chemotherapy alone has been reported to be 75% to 94% which is not different from results achieved in Stages I-IIA patients with radiotherapy alone [5, 6]. In the original report of De Vita et al. [6], all the 23 asymptomatic patients with Stages III-IV disease achieved complete remission and 94% remained in complete remission at 10 years.

Treatment in the early stages of disease without radiation therapy is still considered unethical by many [1, 7, 8]. However, world-wide, only a small proportion of patients can be treated in well-equipped and well-organized radiation therapy centers with well-trained personnel. In recent years, some studies using chemotherapy alone in early stages of Hodgkin's disease have been performed. Three studies report 10-year survival rates of 80 to 100% with the use of combination therapy (MOPP or equivalent) in children with early stage Hodgkin's disease [9–11].

The present randomized study compared CVPP chemotherapy alone vs the same combination plus radiation therapy, 3,000 rad to areas involved at diagnosis. The percent of complete remission was similar in both treatment

Table IV. Toxicity

	CVPP	CVPP+RT
No. patients		
Nadir WBC	2900	2790
No. episodes <2000WBC	12	14
No. episodes <1000WBC	2	—
Died on treatment		1
Infection		1
Median time on treatment (mo)	6	8

342

groups. Patients with mediastinal involvement had a lower rate of complete remissions with chemotherapy alone (68 vs 93%). Several authors report worse results in Stages I-IIA disease with mediastinal involvement treated with radiation therapy alone [7, 8, 12]. They suggest the use of combination therapy in patients with large mediastinal involvement. In our study, the rate of complete remission in patients without mediastinal involvement is 97% for those treated with CVPP and 91% for those treated with CVPP+RT.

The durations of complete remission and survival are similar, at 48 months, for chemotherapy alone or the combined modality option. We conclude from this preliminary analysis that combination therapy with CVPP is as effective as CVPP+RT in Clinical Stages I-IIA Hodgkin's disease. Longer follow-up is needed to establish the relative merits of these approaches. In a special subgroup of patients with mediastinal involvement, the combined modality therapy is more effective in inducing complete remission.

Acknowledgements

We gratefully acknowledge the statistical assistance of Daniel Goldar and the typographic assistance of Marta O'Brien.

Supported in part by Grant N01-C027391 from the Pan American Health Organization/National Cancer Institute, NIH and FUNDALEU (Argentina Foundation Against Leukemia).

Appendix

The following institutions and investigators participated in the study: Instituto de Investigaciones Hematológicas 'Mariano R. Castex', Academia Nacional de Medicina, Buenos Aires, Argentina (S. Pavlovsky, G. Garay, C. Scaglione, J. Dupont, S. Bruno); Instituto Municipal de Hematología, Hospital Ramos Mejía, Buenos Aires, Argentina (M. Morgenfeld, N. Somoza); Centro de Educación Médica e Investigación Clínica, Buenos Aires, Argentina (A. Suarez, R. Cachione, E. Egozcue); Hospital Escuela 'Gral. San Martín, Buenos Aires, Argentina (C.A. Barros, J. Pileggi, H. de Maria, C. Ruso, M. Curuchet, R.J. Boccaci, R. Kvicala); Policlínica 'Mariano R. Castex', Buenos Aires, Argentina (M. Palau, S.C. de Sica); Instituto 'Gran San Martín', Buenos Aires, Argentina (L. Bergna, R. Tur); Hospital 'Teodoro Alvarez', Buenos Aires, Argentina (F. Cavagnaro, R. Bezares, L. Palmer, E. Morgenfeld, A. Diaz, P. Francica); Hospital 'Clemente Alvarez', Rosario, Argentina (J. Saslavsky, J.M. Lein); Hospital Bancario, Buenos Aires, Argentina (M. Tezanos Pinto, C. Marin, C. Rodríguez Fuchs, L. Carreras); Hospital Ferroviario Central, Buenos Aires, Argentina (E. Quiroga Micheo, S.I. Calabria, S. de Rudoy); Hospital Israelita, Buenos Aires, Argentina (M.O. Dragosky, M.A. Sorrentino, H.H. Murro); Hospital Durand, Buenos Aires, Argentina (A.B.S. Huberman, S. Goldstein, J. Chilelli, F. Helt, N. Shilton, A. Starosta); Hospital Ferroviario, Mendoza, Argentina (J. Sanguedolce, M. Arce-Sosa, R. Bianchi, T.Y. Rodríguez); Hospital Nacional de Niños 'Dr. Carlos Saenz Herrera', San José, Costa Rica (E. Jiménez, F. Lobo, J.M. Carillo); Hospital México, San José, Costa Rica (C. Montero, V. Pérez, R. Cordero); Hospital de Niños, Buenos Aires, Argentina (F. Sackmann-Muriel, J. Braier, B. Diez); Hospital Central, Mendoza, Argentina (L. Pérez Polo, V. Labanca, A. Gray, E. Boris, D. Ramos); Hospital Regional, Neuquén, Argentina (R. Raña, A.S. Palacios, T. Sniechowsky, M. Pasanisi).

References

1. Hoppe RT, Coleman CN, Cox RS et al. (1982). The management of Stage I-II Hodgkin's disease with irradiation alone or combined modality therapy: The Stanford experience. Blood 59:455–465.
2. Nissen NI and Nordentoft AM (1982). Radiotherapy vs combined modality treatment of Stage I and II Hodgkin's disease. Cancer Treat Rep 66:799–803.
3. Bergsagel DE, Alison RE, Bean HA et al. (1982). Results of treating Hodgkin's disease without a policy of laparatomy staging. Cancer Treat Rep 66:717–731.
4. Andrieu JM, Montagnan B, Asselain B et al. (1980). Chemotherapy-radiotherapy association in Hodgkin's disease, clinical Stages IA-III: Results of a prospective clinical trial with 166 patients. Cancer 46:2126–2130.
5. Pavlovsky S, Morguenfeld M, Somoza N et al. (1981). Long term follow-up of two chemotherapy protocols in Hodgkin's disease. Medicina (Buenos Aires) 41(Supl):15–21.
6. DeVita VT, Simon RM, Hubbard SM et al. (1980). Curability of advanced Hodgkin's disease with chemotherapy long term follow-up of MOPP-treated patients at the National Cancer Institute. Ann Intern Med 92:587–595.
7. Kapp DS, Prosnitz LR, Farber LR et al. (1983). Patterns of failure in Hodgkin's disease: The Yale University experience. Cancer Treat Symposia 2:145–156.
8. Fuller LM and Hagemeister FB (1983). Diagnosis and management of Hodgkin's disease in adults. Cancer 51:2469–2476.
9. Olweny CLM, Katongole-Mbidde E, Kiire C et al. (1978). Childhood Hodgkin's disease in Uganda. A ten years experience. Cancer 42:787–792.
10. Ekert H and Waters KD (1983). Results of treatment of 18 children with Hodgkin's disease with MOPP chemotherapy as the only treatment modality. Med Pediat Oncol 11:322–326.
11. Jacobs P, King HS, Karahus C et al. (1984). Hodgkin's disease in children. A ten year experience in South Africa. Cancer 53:210–213.
12. Schomberg PJ, Evans RG, O'Connel MJ et al. (1984). Prognostic significance of mediastinal mass in adult Hodgkin's disease. Cancer 53:324–328.

8. Chemotherapy alone versus combined modality therapy for Stage III Hodgkin's disease: A five-year follow-up of a Southwest Oncology Group study (SWOG-7518) USA

P. N. GROZEA[1], E. J. DEPERSIO[2], C. A. COLTMAN, Jr.[3],
C. J. FABIAN[4], F. S. MORRISON[5], D. O. DIXON[6] and
S. E. JONES[7]

[1] *University of Oklahoma Health Sciences Center, Oklahoma City,
Oklahoma;* [2] *Wenatchee Valley Clinic, Wenatchee, Washington;*
[3] *University of Texas Health Science Center, San Antonio,
Texas;* [4] *University of Kansas Medical Center, Kansas City, Kansas;*
[5] *University of Mississippi Medical Center, Jackson, Mississippi;*
[6] *M.D. Anderson Hospital and Tumor Institute, Houston, Texas;*
and [7] *University of Arizona Health Sciences Center, Tucson, Arizona*

The relapse-free survival (RFS) rate for Stage III Hodgkin's disease treated by conventional total nodal irradiation (TNI) alone (early 1970's) was disappointingly low [1–4]. The development of successful combination chemotherapy by National Cancer Institute workers [5] led SWOG, in 1971, to· devise a single arm study (SWOG-160, CAR-1) consisting of three MOPP cycles followed by TNI in Pathologic Stages IIB, IIIA, and IIIB Hodgkin's disease. This trial, which was completed in 1975, achieved a complete response (CR) rate of 88 % and an actuarial 5-year survival and RFS of 78 % and 68 % respectively [6]. Improvement in survival and promising results obtained on another SWOG study with the addition of low dose bleomycin (LDB 2 mg/m^2) to MOPP [7, 8] prompted SWOG to initiate, in October 1975, a randomized trial of chemotherapy (CT) alone compared to CT plus TNI for Stages IIIA and IIIB Hodgkin's disease with LDB added to the CT regimen (SWOG-7518, CAR-2) [9, 10] (Fig. 1 and Table I).

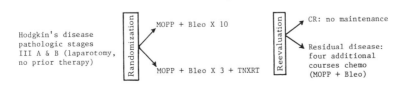

Figure 1. SWOG 7518: Study design.

Table I. MOPP – Bleo schema

Day	1	2 3 4 5 6 7	8	9 10 11 12
Nitrogen mustard (iv)	6 mg/m^2		6 mg/m^2	
Vincristine (iv)	1.4 mg/m^2	(not to exceed 2 mg/injection)	1.4 mg/m^2	
Procarbazine (po)		•— 100 mg/m^2→		•— 100 mg/m^2→
Prednisone (po) [a]		•— 40 mg/m^2→		•— 40 mg/m^2→
Bleomycin (iv) (30 min. after vincristine)	2 mg/m^2		2 mg/m^2	

[a] Cycles 1, 4, 7, 10 (13) of chemotherapy only program
   Cycles 1, (4), (7) of combination chemotherapy + radiation therapy program

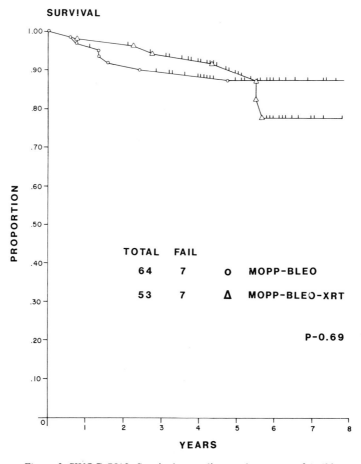

Figure 2. SWOG 7518. Survival according to therapy as of 11/83.

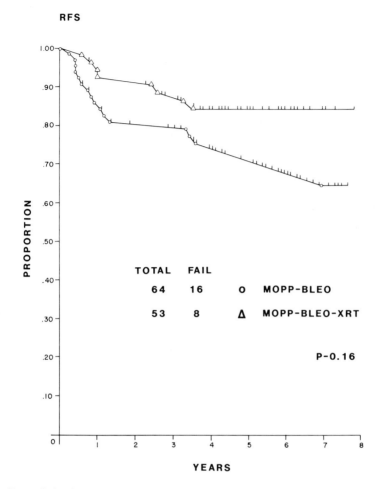

Figure 3. SWOG 7518. Relapse-free survival according to therapy as of 11/83.

Materials and methods

Only patients with exploratory laparotomy established pathologic diagnosis of Stage III Hodgkin's disease with no prior CT or radiotherapy (RT) were eligible. TNI consisted of an upper mantle and inverted Y beginning four weeks after completing chemotherapy, with maximum rest interval to ten weeks. RFS and survival were measured from the time of treatment start. Curves were calculated by the method of Kaplan and Meier [11] and compared by the Gehan modification of the Wilcoxon test [12].

348

Results

By April 1980, at study closing, 137 patients were registered and 117 of these were fully or partially evaluable. Of the 108 evaluable patients, 92% achieved CR, 89% for MOPP-BLEO and 96% for MOPP-Bleo-XRT, $p = 0.27$ (two-sided Chi-square test).

Fig. 2 shows the overall survival for all evaluable patients according to induction treatment, with overall 5-year survival rates estimated at 87% for CT alone and 89% for CT+RT. There have been two late deaths due to marrow failure: one at 4½ years on the CT alone limb and one at 5½ years on the CT+RT limb. Fig. 3 shows the RFS curves by treatment, with a $p = 0.16$ trend in favor of CT+RT. Fig. 4 displays the RFS curves for the pathologic subset nodular sclerosis, by treatment group, with a very strong

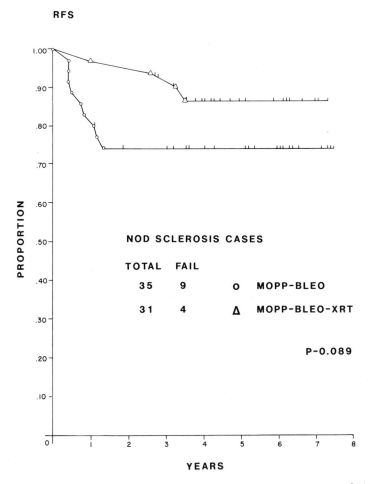

Figure 4. SWOG 7518. Relapse-free survival in nodular sclerosis cases as of 11/83.

statistical trend in favor of the CT+RT group ($p = 0.089$) when considering all fully and partially evaluable patients. When all eligible cases are considered, $p = 0.051$. Nodular sclerosis cases were analyzed for balance in the original pre-treatment characteristics. The CT alone limb was found to have more patients under age 20 (35% vs. 18%), and fewer patients with 'B' symptoms (27% vs. 48%). This imbalance was of approximately the same magnitude as the group as a whole and would not explain the divergence in the pattern of relapses of the nodular sclerosis cases.

The incidence of early and late side effects on the two programs were similar in intensity although they were to some extent qualitatively different. There were comparable degrees of leukopenia and thrombocytopenia considering toxicity grades 3 and 4. There was more neurotoxicity on CT alone and there were two cases of grade 3 pulmonary toxicity on CT+RT. Herpes Zoster infection was detected in 22/60 cases treated with CT+RT, including one fatality and a second case in which Herpes Zoster encephalitis was a contributory cause of death after relapse. This incidence rate (36.7%) compares with the 10/60 (15.6%) rate found on CT alone. On the CT alone limb there was one death due to Pneumococcal sepsis in a patient who was otherwise NED. To date there has been one death due to AML on the combined modality arm. Two new cases have been recently detected, one on each treatment option [13].

Fifty-six percent of patients completed 10 or more cycles of CT alone, 27% had 6-9½ cycles, and 17% received less than 6 cycles. There was less 'percent' drug given to the group of relapsing patients. For the combined modality limb, among patients who completed the mantle, 12/50 (24%) received a dose to the inverted Y that was less than 3000 cGy.

Relapses

On CT+RT, relapses were confined to nodal sites. One patient had a true marginal relapse at the submandibular margin of the field. Two had low doses to the inverted Y (800 and 900 cGy) and another patient represented a protocol violation with blocking abnormalities in the axillae site of relapse. There have been no extra lymphatic relapses. Only 3/7 (43%) of these cases were placed into a durable second CR, two with MOPP alone and one with MOPP and ABVD. On CT alone, 9/12 true relapses were in areas of original disease or a mixture of recurrent and new lymphadenopathy. Four out of twelve of these true relapses included extra lymphatic structures and in one that was the only site of relapse. In 7/9 true relapses the histopathologic cell type was nodular sclerosis. Eight of twelve (75%) were placed into an apparent durable second remission. Six of eight of the second CR's received RT, five alone and one in combination with CT.

Discussion

The most important finding in the study was the pattern of relapses in nodular sclerosis cases. There was a strong statistical trend to better survival on CT+RT in this histological set. A similar effect though has been reported by DeVita et al. [14]. The results of this trial appear to confirm their results and identify the sub-group questioned by Glick [15] for which CT+RT is indicated.

The pattern of relapses on the CT alone limb, occurring mostly in original sites of disease, has obvious implications for treatment of initially involved sites with RT in future studies of combined modality therapy [16, 17].

The toxicities were of predicted levels during the acute MOPP-BLEO phase of therapy, but the finding of two patients having late marrow failure near the 5 year point of the study and three cases to date of AML suggest a late toxicity.

It is generally agreed that the first treatment given to patients with Hodgkin's disease is the most important and that it is necessary to accept some level of risk to cure the disease. With this in mind we recommend: 1) for pathologically staged IIIA and IIIB Hodgkin's disease that the initial therapy be either CT alone, using a combination as effective as MOPP-BLEO, or CT+RT with the exception of nodular sclerosis for which CT+RT is indicated [14] 2) the RT phase of combined modality should be considered to be limited to the original sites of disease or delivered in reduced doses if in TNI form.

Acknowledgements

This investigation was supported in part by the following PHS grant numbers awarded by the National Cancer Institute, DHHS: CA-16957, CA-12644, CA-16385, CA-22411, CA-13612, CA-64919, CA-03096, CA-04920, CA-13238, CA-04915, CA-21116, CA-10379, CA-20319, CA-14028, CA-13392, CA-26766, CA-11233, CA-03389, CA-24433, CA-12014, and CA-16943.

References

1. Johnson RE, Thomas LB, Schneiderman M et al. (1970). Preliminary experience with total nodal irradiation in Hodgkin's disease. Radiology 96:603–608.
2. Goodman R, Rosenthal D, Botnick L et al. (1977). Stage IIIA Hodgkin's disease: Results of treatment with total nodal irradiation. Proc Amer Assoc Cancer Res and Amer Soc Clin Oncol 18:348.

3. Prosnitz LR, Montalvo RL, Fischer DB et al. (1978). Treatment of Stage IIIA Hodgkin's disease: Is radiotherapy alone adequate? Int J Radiat Oncol Biol Phys 4:781–787.

4. Timothy AR, Sutcliffe SB, Stansfeld AG et al. (1978). Radiotherapy in the treatment of Hodgkin's disease. Br Med J 1:1246–1249.

5. DeVita VT Jr, Simon RM, Hubbard SM et al. (1980). Curability of advanced Hodgkin's disease with chemotherapy. Long-term followup of MOPP-treated patients at the National Cancer Institute. Ann Intern Med 92:587–595.

6. Coltman CA Jr., Jones SE, Grozea PN et al. (1978). Bleomycin in combination with MOPP for the management of Hodgkin's disease: Southwest Oncology Group Experience. In: Carter SK, Crooke ST and Umezawa H (Eds.). Bleomycin Current Status and New Developments, pp. 227–242. New York: Academic Press.

7. Jones SE, Coltman CA Jr, Grozea PN et al. (1982). Conclusions from clinical trials of the Southwest Oncology Group. Cancer Treat Rep 66:847–853.

8. Coltman CA Jr, Montague E and Moon TE (1977). Chemotherapy and total nodal radiotherapy in pathological Stage IIB, IIIA and IIIB Hodgkin's disease. In: Salmon SE and Jones SE (Eds.). Adjuvant Therapy of Cancer, pp. 529–536. Amsterdam, Oxford, New York: North-Holland, Publishing Company.

9. Depersio EJ, Grozea PN, Fischer R et al. (1979). Chemotherapy versus chemotherapy plus radiotherapy for Stage IIIA, IIIB Hodgkin's disease. A Southwest Oncology Group study. Int J Radiat Oncol Biol Phys 5:138.

10. Grozea PN, DePersio EJ, Coltman CA Jr et al. (1982). A Southwest Oncology Group Study: Chemotherapy versus chemotherapy plus radiotherapy in the treatment of Stage III Hodgkin's disease. In: Mathe G, Bonadonna G and Salmon S (Eds.). Recent Results in Cancer Research: Adjuvant Therapies of Cancer, pp. 83–91. Berlin, Heidelberg, New York: Springer-Verlag.

11. Kaplan EL, Meier P (1958). Nonparametric estimation from incomplete observations. Amer Stat Assoc J 53:457–481.

12. Gehan EA (1965). A generalized Wilcoxon test for comparing arbitrarily singly-censored samples. Biometrika 52:203–223.

13. Coltman CA Jr and Dixon DO (1982). Second malignancies complicating Hodgkin's Disease: A Southwest Oncology Group 10-year follow-up. Cancer Treat Rep 66:1023–1033.

14. DeVita VT Jr. (1982). Hodgkin's disease: Conference summary and future directions. Cancer Treat Rep 66:1045–1055.

15. Glick JH (1978). The treatment of Stage IIIA Hodgkin's disease: What is the role of combined modality treatment? Int J Radiat Oncol Biol Phys 4:909–911.

16. Coltman CA Jr, Myers JW, Montague E et al. (1982). The role of combined radiotherapy and chemotherapy in the primary management of Hodgkin's disease: Southwest Oncology Group Studies. In: Rosenberg SA and Kaplan HS (Eds.). Malignant Lymphomas, Etiology, Immunology, Pathology, Treatment, pp. 523–536. New York: Academic Press.

17. Cooper D, Prosnitz LR, Kapp DS et al. (1984). Combined modality therapy for treatment of 'poor-risk' Stage IIIA Hodgkin's disease. Proc Amer Soc Clin Oncol 3:251.

9. Chemotherapy plus radiotherapy in Clinical Stage IA to IIIB Hodgkin's disease. Results of the H 77 trial (1977-1980)

J. M. ANDRIEU[1], Y. COSCAS[2], P. CRAMER[3], C. JULIEN[1], M. WEIL[4] and G. TRICOT[5]

[1] Department of Oncology/hematology, Laennec Hospital, Paris,
[2] Department of Radiotherapy, Saint-Louis Hospital, Paris,
[3] Department of Hematology, Saint-Louis Hospital, Paris,
[4] Department of Oncology, Salpetriere Hospital, Paris and
[5] Department of Pathology, Saint-Louis Hospital, Paris, France

Major progress in the treatment of Hodgkin's disease (HD) had been accomplished by the late sixties. Kaplan et al. at Stanford University found that when a very careful staging laparotomy with splenectomy is performed, a majority of patients with Pathologic Stages I and II could be cured by radiotherapy alone [1]. Around the same time, De Vita t al. introduced the MOPP (mechlorethamine, vincristine, procarbazine and prednisone) chemotherapy for the treatment of advanced stages [2]; after 6 cycles of this multiagent chemotherapy, a complete remission was obtained in 60 to 80% of the patients and half of them were probably cured.

In an attempt to improve these results, we decided in 1972 to combine MOPP chemotherapy and irradiation for Clinical Stages (CS) IA to IIIB HD. From 1972 to 1976, 334 patients with CS IA to IIIB were prospectively treated at Saint Louis Hospital. All received 3 or 6 cycles of MOPP plus supra and/or infradiaphragmatic irradiation, according to stage and protocol arm [3, 4].

In 1977, the H 77 trial was activated with the same chemotherapy/radiotherapy sequence, but initial chemotherapy was reduced to a maximum of 3 cycles. Progress reports of these studies were published in 1981 and 1982 [5, 6]. This paper presents updated results as of January 1984.

Materials and methods

From January 1977 to May 1980, 173 patients with CS IA to IIIB were entered. All were clinically staged according to the recommendations of the Ann Arbor Conference. No staging laparotomies were performed.

Treatment programs are described in Fig. 1. The 79 patients with CS IA

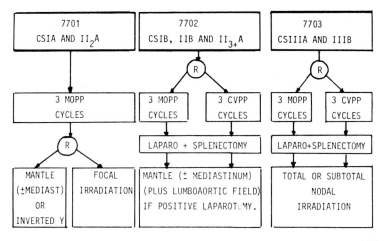

Figure 1. Schematic representation of the H77 treatment programs (1977–1980).

and CS II_2A (i.e. 2 areas involved) followed the randomized trial 7701. Three cycles of MOPP were given first. Patients were then randomized in two groups: the first one received a mantle sparing the mediastinum when it was not involved or an inverted Y in case of initial infradiaphragmatic disease; the other group received only focal field exposure. Forty Gy were delivered to involved areas and 30–35 Gy to contiguous areas.

The 74 patients with CS IB, IIB and CS $II_{3+}A$ (i.e. 3 or more areas involved) followed the randomized program 7702. Three cycles of MOPP or CVPP (lomustine, vinblastine, procarbazine, prednisolone) were given at random. At completion of chemotherapy, patients of both groups with complete or partial remission underwent a control laparotomy with splenectomy. Patients pathologically free of disease received supradiaphragmatic irradiation only; patients who still had splenic or nodal pathologic involvement received an additional lumbo-aortic field.

The 20 patients with CS IIIA and IIIB followed the randomized program 7703. They received 3 cycles of MOPP or CVPP at random. Complete and partial responders then underwent a laparo-splenectomy followed by total or subtotal nodal irradiation (sparing the mediastinum and/or the pelvic areas when not involved). As of April 1979 the post chemotherapy laparo-splenectomy was discontinued and replaced by the irradiation of the spleen.

The remission status of the patients was assessed after completion of chemotherapy and irradiation. Complete remission (CR) and partial remission (PR) were defined as the complete and partial disappearance of initially involved sites. Failure was defined as the persistence, extension or reappearance of the disease at completion of chemotherapy or radiotherapy. The remission status was reassessed every 4 months during the first year, then twice a year until the 5th year and once a year thereafter. Patients with initial failure and those who relapsed were retreated individually by the chemotherapy regimen they had not received (CVPP for MOPP and MOPP for CVPP) preceded or followed by radiotherapy when possible.

Curves for the probability of survival were calculated from the date of diagnosis. Disease-free duration curves were constructed from the date of completion of treatment. All the curves were calculated by the method of Kaplan and Meier; statistical tests for significance between curves were reported using the logrank test.

Results

The initial characteristics of the 173 patients are given in Table I. Seventy-nine patients were allocated to program 7701; all of them entered in CR. Seventy-four patients were randomized into the 7702 program (MOPP 39; CVPP 35). At completion of chemotherapy, the 64 responding patients (CR or PR) underwent a control laparotomy with splenectomy. All of them were found histologically free of occult disease. The 61 patients with supradiaphragmatic disease received therefore supradiaphragmatic irradiation only, and the 3 patients with infradiaphragmatic disease were given an inverted Y. The 64 patients were in CR at the end of irradiation. Nine patients failed at the end of chemotherapy (MOPP 5, CVPP 3); 5 of them were successfully retreated and reached CR; the 4 others died with progressive disease. Another patient who had become icteric and pancytopenic after the second MOPP cycle died shortly thereafter; at autopsy, he had no evidence of HD but an hepatoma was discovered. In summary, 69/74 patients of the 7702

Table I. H 77 Trial. Initial characteristics of the patients

Age (years)			Clinical Stage	
Median	28		IA	42
Min-max	6–65		II_2A	37
			$II_{3+}A$	26
Sex			IB	5
Male	102		IIB	43
Female	71		IIIA	9
			IIIB	11
Histology			Follow-up (mo)	
LP	28			
NS	71		Median	53
MC	55		Min-max	42–84
LD	6			
Uncl	13			

program were in CR at completion of treatment (MOPP 35/39, CVPP 34/35).

Twenty patients were randomized in the 7703 program (MOPP 10, CVPP 10). One patient died after the second course of CVPP because of an accidental overdose of lomustine and the 19 others achieved CR with the scheduled combined-modality therapy; one of them received 3 additional cycles of CVPP after irradiation because of the reappearance of constitutional symptoms after the third MOPP cycle.

A total of 19 patients relapsed after 2 to 60 months of CR (median 12 months). One in situ mediastinal relapse (CS II_2A) was rapidly fatal. Another patient (CS II_2A) with a parasternal infraclavicular relapse at the edge of the irradiation port is still in treatment. Two relapses occurred in a contiguous lymph node area: one patient with bilateral cervical involvement (CS II_2A) who was randomly assigned to focal irradiation relapsed in the left axilla; this would have been irradiated if he had been randomized in the other irradiation arm; another patient (CS IIIB) with disseminated supra and infradiaphragmatic but no mediastinal involvement received an inverted Y plus a mantle sparing the mediastinum. He had a mediastinal relapse after 34 months of CR; both of these patients entered in a second CR with retreatment.

Twelve infradiaphragmatic relapses occurred in the 137 patients with supradiaphragmatic CS I and II. Four were found among the 76 CS IA and II_2A patients and eight others occurred in the 61 CS IB, IIB and $II_{3+}A$ patients who had had, however, a negative post-chemotherapy surgical look and had therefore received no additional infradiaphragmatic irradiation. Four of these relapsing patients died with progressive disease, two are still under treatment and six attained a second still ongoing CR. Three visceral relapses occurred (CS IIB 2, CS III B 1); all 3 were fatal.

Four patients died in first CR: one patient, 32 years old at diagnosis (CS $II_{3+}A$) died of an overwhelming pneumonocal septicemia within 1 month of CR. One patient, 46 years old at diagnosis, (CS IA) died of an oesophagus cancer after 47 months of CR. Two other patients died of an acute non lymphoblastic leukemia. The first (CS IIIB) was 38 years old at diagnosis; she had received 3 MOPP cycles and total nodal irradiation plus 3 CVPP courses (because of the reappearance of constitutional symptoms after MOPP); the leukemia was diagnosed after 29 months of CR; the patient died 14 months later. The second patient (CS IA) was 51 years old at diagnosis; he had received 3 MOPP plus focal irradiation. The diagnosis of leukemia was made after 58 months of CR. The patient expired 1 month later.

The actuarial probabilities of survival (7 years) of the 7701, 7702 and 7703 programs are 93.9%, 83.2% and 80% respectively. The figures for the disease-free duration are 88.6%, 82.5% and 88.8% respectively. No statis-

Table II. H 77 Trial survival and disease-free duration according to clinical stages (CS), sex, age, symptoms

	Survival (%) 'p' at 7 years	Disease-free 'p' duration
CS		
IA	91.8 ⎤ ns	90.3 ⎤ ns
IIA	92.1 ⎤ ns	89 ⎤ ns
IB, IIB	82.6 ⎤ ns	78.7 ⎤ ns
IIIA	88.9 ⎤ ns	88.9 ⎤ ns
IIIB	68.2 ⎦ ns	88.9 ⎦ ns
Sex		
M	87 ⎤ ns	85 ⎤ ns
F	88.7 ⎦	87.5 ⎦
Age (yrs)		
<40	91.1 ⎤ 0.04	87 ⎤ ns
>40	73.3 ⎦	79.8 ⎦
Symptoms		
'A'	91.3 ⎤ 0.04	89.2 ⎤ ns
'B'	80.7 ⎦	79.8 ⎦

tical difference exists between the two arms of each program either for survival or for disease-free duration. The figures are given in Table II for several initial parameters (CS, symptoms, age and sex).

Discussion

Our overall results of 87.8% survival and 85.8% disease-free duration at 7 years support the efficacy of the 3 MOPP (or CVPP) chemotherapy-radiotherapy sequence in the management of HD, CS IA to IIIB.

This policy of treatment has many advantages. With 3 cycles of MOPP or CVPP one can obtain a very high rate of CR (96.5%); all the patients controlled by initial chemotherapy were in CR after radiotherapy. Local eradication rate is very high as well. Only 2 *in situ* or marginal relapses occurred, which is much lower than that expected after irradiation alone where local relapses are particularly frequent in patients with widespread nodal disease [7–10] and/or sizable mediastinal tumors [11–15]. The absence of mediastinal irradiation was advantageous for the 51 patients with supradiaphragmatic CS I and II who had no mediastinal involvement. None of them had a mediastinal relapse thus confirming the results obtained between 1972 and 1976 on a larger group of patients with early HD [3]. Moreover, such patients were not subjected to the iatrogenic consequences of the mediastinal irradiation; this is particularly important for children, the majority of whom have upper cervical presentation with no mediastinal involvement. The 3 MOPP or CVPP cycles are very effective for occult visceral disease. No visceral relapse occurred in patients without constitutional symptoms and only 3 were observed in patients with 'B' symptoms whereas this type of relapse is frequent after irradiation alone, particularly in patients with Stages III and/or 'B' symptoms [16, 17].

However, our policy of treatment has some disadvantages. One fatal overwhelming infection occurred within 2 months following the splenectomy which was carried out after chemotherapy in rearly half of the patients of this trial. It is now well known that the early (operation) and late (infection) mortality of splenectomy is around 2% in adults and probably more in children [18–20]. Approximately 7% of infradiaphragmatic relapses (nodal or splenic) occurred in patients with supradiaphragmatic HD. In CS I and II, occult infradiaphragmatic disease is initially present in around 40%-50% of the cases as proved by systematic staging laparotomies [10, 17, 21]. Out of the 76 CS IA and CS II$_2$A with supradiaphragmatic presentation who achieved a CR after 3 MOPP cycles plus irradiation (trial 7701), 4 infradiaphragmatic relapses occurred (5%), the last after 59 months of CR. We had observed the same infradiaphragmatic relapse rate in 159 patients with supradiaphragmatic CS IA and II$_2$A treated by 3 MOPP plus irradiation between 1972 and 1976 [3]. Out of the 61 patients with supradiaphragmatic CS IB, IIB and II$_{3+}$A, (all with negative post-chemotherapy laparotomy), eight patients relapsed after 2 to 60 months in the lumbo-aortic area which, however, had been explored. We observed the same rate of residual lesions after a 6-MOPP cycle chemotherapy; out of the 63 patients who had a control laparotomy between 1972 and 1976, 4 still had pathologic nodal or splenic disease and 4 others relapsed in the previously explored lumbo-aortic area, the last after 58 months [4]. We can therefore conclude that 6 MOPP cycles are not better at eradicating occult disease than 3 courses of MOPP or CVPP and that the post chemotherapy laparotomy does not identify accurately the small set of patients who still have occult HD either after 6 MOPP or after 3 MOPP or CVPP.

Two acute leukemias occurred in this trial; this corresponds to an actuarial rate of less than 1.5%. It is most likely that this rate will not be higher with a longer follow-up since in our previous trial (1972-1976) [22] after 3 and 6 MOPP cycles performed in 334 patients it did not exceed 1.8% at 10 years. This rate of mortality from leukemia is excessive, particularly in early HD. However, it must be noted that staging laparotomy with splenectomy, which is frequently accepted as the reference staging procedure in early HD, produces a similar percentage of fatal complication [19–21].

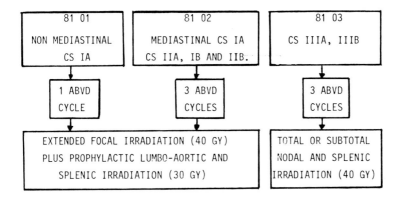

Figure 2. Prospective trial 'P.O.F. 81'.

The last disadvantage of this strategy is male sterility. With 3 MOPP or CVPP cycles azoospermia or severe oligospermia is present in all cases within the first year. However, fertility resumes in around 20% of the cases in the following years. On the other hand, in all women less than 30 at the time of chemotherapy, menses, pregnancy and progeny were normal [23].

In 1981 we designed the POF 81 protocol (Fig. 2). We decided to keep the general philosophy of our previous work, that is, to continue to perform an initial clinical staging only and to associate chemotherapy and irradiation in all stages of the disease. However, we tried to eliminate the disadvantages of the H 77 trial by the following modifications. The initial MOPP or CVPP chemotherapy was replaced by the ABVD combination (3 cycles) which has the same efficacy and gives no secondary leukemia and few gonadal sequellae [24, 25]. Post-chemotherapy laparotomy was discontinued in all stages. In supradiaphragmatic CS IA-IIB disease, it was replaced by a prophylactic short (L3-L4) lumbo-aortic plus splenic irradiation (30 Gy in adults, 20 Gy in children). In the other stages, it was replaced by splenic irradiation included in the infradiaphragmatic port. We abandoned the purely focal fields (with which one relapse occurred) for an extended focal irradiation which encompasses contiguous areas but not the mediastinum when non-involved. In adults the dose is 40 Gy in involved areas and 30 Gy in non-involved ares. In children, when a CR is obtained after ABVD, the irradiation dose is lowered to 25 Gy in involved areas and 20 Gy in non-involved areas.

This POF 81 trial was started in October 1981; as of the first of June 1984, 91 patients with CS IA to IIIB have completed their treatment. All of them are alive in first complete remission.

360

Acknowledgements

This work was supported by 'Ligue de Paris contre le Cancer' and by a grant of A.R.E.M.A.S.

References

1. Kaplan HS and Rosenberg SA (1973). Current status of clinical trials: Stanford Experience 1962-1972. Nat Cancer Inst Monogr 36:363-371.
2. De Vita VT, Serpick AA and Carbone PP (1970). Combination chemotherapy in the treatment of advanced Hodgkin's disease. Ann Intern Med 73:881-895.
3. Andrieu JM, Montagnon B, Asselain B et al. (1980). Chemotherapy-radiotherapy association for Hodgkin's disease Stages IA, IIA. Cancer 46:2126-2130.
4. Andrieu JM, Asselain B, Baule C et al. (1981). La séquence polychimiothérapie MOPP irradiation ganglionnaire sélective dans le traitement de la maladie de Hodgkin, Stade clinique IA-IIIB. Résultats à 8 ans d'un protocole prospectif comportant 334 patients. Bull Cancer (Paris) 68:190-199.
5. Andrieu JM, Casassus P, Coscas Y et al. (1982). Traitement des stades cliniques ganglionnaires intermédiaires et avancés de la maladie de Hodgkin par chimiothérapie courte (3 MOPP ou 3 CVPP) - splénectomie - irradiation limitée. Résultats à 4 ans d'un protocole prospectif (H 7702, 7703) incluant 94 patients. Bull Cancer (Paris) 69:321-329.
6. Andrieu JM, Ozanne F, Dana M et al. (1981). La séquence polychimiothérapie MOPP-radiothérapie sélective ou focale dans la maladie de Hodgkin, Stades Cliniques IA, II2A. Résultats à 4 ans d'un protocole prospectif (H 7701) incluant 79 patients. Bull Cancer (Paris) 68:217-223.
7. British National Lymphoma Investigation (1976). Initial treatment of Stage IIIA Hodgkin's disease. Comparison of radiotherapy with combined chemotherapy. Lancet 2:991-995.
8. Hoppe RT, Rosenberg SA, Kaplan HS and Cox RS (1980). Prognostic factors in Pathological Stage IIIA Hodgkin's disease. Cancer 46:1240-1246.
9. Mauch P, Goodmar RL, Rosenthal DS et al. (1979). An evaluation of total nodal irradiation as treatment for Stage III Hodgkin's disease. Cancer 43:1255-1261.
10. Peckham MJ, Ford HT, McElwain TJ et al. (1975). The results of radiotherapy for Hodgkin's disease. Br J Cancer 32:391-400.
11. Dolginow D and Colby TV (1981). Recurrent Hodgkin's disease in treated sites. Cancer 48:1124-1126.
12. Hellman S, Mauch P, Goodman RL et al. (1978). The place of radiation therapy in the treatment of Hodgkin's disease. Cancer 42:971-978.
13. Lee CK, Bloomfield CD, Godman AI and Levitt SH (1980). Prognostic significance of mediastinal involvement in Hodgkin's disease treated with curative radiotherapy. Cancer 46:2403-2409.
14. Levi JA, Wiernick PH and O'Connell MJ (1977). Patterns of relapse in Stages I, II and IIIA Hodgkin's disease: Influence of initial therapy and implications for the future. Int J Radiat Oncol Phys 2:853-857.
15. Velentjas E, Barrett A, McElwain TJ and Peckham MJ (1980). Mediastinal involvement in early stage Hodgkin's disease. Response to treatment and pattern of relapse. Eur J Cancer 16:1065-1068.
16. Rosenberg SA, Kaplan HS, Glatstein EJ and Portlock CS (1978). Combined modality therapy of Hodgkin's disease. A report on the Stanford trials. Cancer 42:991-1000.
17. Desser RK, Golomb HM, Ultmann JE et al. (1977). Prognostic classification of Hodgkin's disease in pathological Stage III, based on anatomic considerations. Blood 49:883-893.

18. Nordentoft AM, Pedersen-Bjergaard J, Brincker H et al. (1980). Hodgkin's disease in Denmark; A national clinical study by the Danish Hodgkin study group. LYGRA. Scand J Haematol 24:321–334.

19. Aisenberg AC, Linggood RM and Lew RA (1979). The changing face of Hodgkin's disease, Amer J Med 67:921–928.

20. Rutheford CJ, Desforges JF, Davies B et al. (1980). The decision to perform staging laparotomy in symptomatic Hodgkin's disease. Brit J Haematol, 44:347–358.

21. Aisenberg AC and Quazi R (1974). Abdominal involvement at the onset of Hodgkin's disease. Amer J Med 57:850–874.

22. Andrieu JM, Julien C, Casassus P et al. (1983). MOPP plus irradiation for Hodgkin's disease CS IA to IIIB, 10 years later. J Clin Oncol 2:213.

23. Andrieu JM and Ochoa-Molina ME (1983). Menstrual cycle, pregnancies and offspring after MOPP therapy for Hodgkin's disease. Cancer 52:435–438.

24. Bonadonna G, Zucali R, de Lena M and Valagussa P (1977). Combined chemotherapy (MOPP or ABVD) – radiotherapy approach in advanced Hodgkin's disease. Cancer Treat Rep 61:769–777.

25. Santoro A, Bonadonna G, Zucali R et al. (1981). Therapeutic and toxicologic effects of MOPP versus ABVD when combined with RT in Hodgkin's disease. Proc Amer Assoc Cancer Res and Amer Soc Clin Oncol 22:522.

10. Surgical restaging after 3 or 6 courses of MOPP chemotherapy in Hodgkin's disease

C. FERME[1], F. TEILLET[2], M. F. D'AGAY[3] and M. BOIRON[4]

[1] *Département de Médecine Interne et Oncologie. C.M.C. de Bligny, Briis sous Forges;* [2] *Service d'Hématologie-Immunologie, Hôpital Louis Mourier, Colombes;* [3] *Service d'Anatomie Pathologie; and* [4] *Département Hémato-Oncologie, Hôpital Saint-Louis, Paris Cedex 10, France*

A majority of patients with Hodgkin's disease can achieve complete remission and recovery with radiotherapy, combination chemotherapy or both [1–4]. Risks associated with intensive treatments, including the possible occurrence of second malignancies, have led several investigators to evaluate less aggressive therapy. Pretreatment staging laparotomies are used to detect occult disease, especially in the spleen [5–7]. More recently, postchemotherapy surgical restaging has been introduced to identify minimal residual disease and define further therapeutic strategies [8, 9].

Since 1972, chemotherapeutic effectiveness upon occult splenic disease in Clinical Stages IIA, IB, IIB, III has been assessed by surgical restaging following six courses of MOPP and prior to extended field irradiation. However, in 1977, the number of courses of MOPP was reduced to three. Results of surgical restaging after six and after three courses of MOPP as well as the corresponding complete remission rates after extended field irradiation are compared.

Materials and methods

Between 1972 and 1979, 121 patients with Hodgkin's disease, clinically staged IIA, IB, IIB, IIIA-B, previously untreated, received either six or three courses of MOPP before clinical and surgical restaging, followed by irradiation. Luke's criteria were required for patients to be included in this study. The 6 MOPP group was composed of 68 patients treated between 1972 and 1976. The 3 MOPP group was composed of 53 patients treated between 1977 and 1979. Clinical characteristics of both groups are detailed in Table I.

Clinical staging was performed prior to chemotherapy, repeated after radiotherapy and included chest x-rays, tomograms, bipedal lymphangiography, needle bone marrow biopsy, blood tests and liver function. A total of

Table I. Patient characteristics

	Males	Females	Median age	Histologic subtype					Clinical Stage			
				LP	NS	MC	LD	Unclass	IIA	IB-IIB	IIIA	IIIB
6 MOPP No. of pts (%) = 68	43	25	27	2(3)	47(69)	17(25)	2(3)		17(25)	34(50)	5(7)	12(18)
3 MOPP No. of pts (%) = 53	19	34	29	0	33(62)	12(23)	3(6)	5(9)	10(19)	27(51)	8(15)	8(15)

118 patients underwent surgical restaging laparotomy including splenectomy, liver, bone marrow and lymph node biopsies. Three patients with clinically evident disease were not surgically restaged.

Sixty-eight patients were treated with six courses of the MOPP combination (mechlorethamine, vincristine, procarbazine, prednisone), plus a monthly injection of vinblastine for 4 months. Fifty-three received 3 courses of MOPP and within this group, 6 patients with residual disease received, prior to surgical restaging, 3 additional courses of CVPP (CCNU, vincristine, procarbazine, prednisone). One month after surgical restaging, patients underwent extended field irradiation (40 Gray in the involved areas and 30 to 35 Gray in the adjacent regions) according to Clinical Stage (CS) and results of surgical restaging: mantle alone in CS I-II disease with negative surgical restaging (80 patients), mantle plus para-aortic field (18 patients) or inverted Y (20 patients) in CS I-II disease with positive surgical restaging and CS III disease with positive or negative surgical restaging. No maintenance therapy was administered to patients who achieved complete remission.

Complete remission (CR) was defined by the disappearance of all clinical, biological and radiological abnormalities. Partial respone (PR) was defined by a 50% reduction of tumor masses. Failure was defined as the absence of change or an increase of tumor masses. Negative biopsy and absence of splenic involvement defined negative surgical restaging. Histologic involvement of the spleen or biopsy defined positive surgical restaging. Patients were reexamined every six months for the first two years and once a year thereafter. Thirteen patients were lost to follow-up, 4 in group 6 MOPP and 9 in group 3 MOPP.

Results

Results after 6 or 3 courses of MOPP

Overall clinical complete remission rate for the 6 MOPP group was 80%, and 83% for the 3 MOPP group. Partial remission rate was, respectively, 14% and 15% and the failure rate was, respectively, 6% and 2% (Table II).

Upon surgical restaging 83% of 6 MOPP patients were free of residual disease (55 of 66 patients) versus 92% in the 3 MOPP group (52 of 53 patients). Persistent splenic disease was not significantly different between the two groups. Clinical and surgical responses according to histologic subtype, clinical stage and systemic symptoms are detailed in Table III.

A comparison between clinical and surgical restaging confirms the accuracy of the clinical, radiologic and biologic criteria of response to chemo-

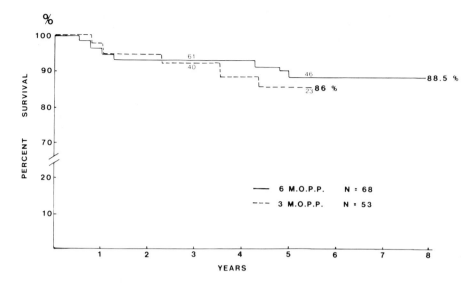

Figure 1. Actuarial survival curves for 121 patients.

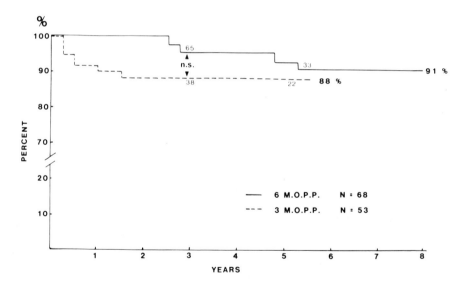

Figure 2. Disease-free survival for 121 patients.

therapy. The incidence of false negative clinical restaging (clinical CR with positive surgical restaging) was 3.5% for the 6 MOPP group, and 2% for the 3 MOPP. Five patients were judged as clinical failures after MOPP, only 2 of these underwent surgical restaging with evidence of persistent disease.

Table II. Therapeutic results

Clinical Stage	MOPP No. courses	Total	Results after MOPP									Results after radiotherapy		
			Clinical status						Anatomic data		False negative (%)	CR	%	Failure
			CR	(%)	PR	%	Failure	%	− LAP	+				
Global	6	68	54	(80)	10	(14)	4	(6)	55	11	(3,5)	64	(94)	4
	3	53	44	(83)	8	(15)	1	(2)	48	4	(2)	51	(96)	2
IIA	6	17	12	(81)	4		1		13	3	(0)	15	(88)	2
	3	10	10						10		(0)	10		
IB-IIB	6	34	29	(85)	4		1		29	4	(7)	33	(97)	1
	3	27	23	(85)	3		1		26	0	(0)	26	(96)	1
III	6	17	13	(76)	2				13	4	(0)	16	(94)	1
	3	16	11	(69)	5		2		12	4	(9)	15	(94)	1

Table III. Clinical and surgical response according to histology, clinical stage and systemic symptoms

	MOPP No. courses	Clinical CR %	Negative surgical restaging %
Nodular	6	77	77
sclerosis	3	88	88
Mixed	6	88	88
cellularity	3	75	83
CS II	6	81	86
	3	91	100
CS III	6	76	76
	3	69	75
A	6	77	86
	3	89	100
B	6	80	82
	3	80	88

Results after MOPP, splenectomy and radiotherapy

Complete remission was obtained in 94% of the patients in the 6 MOPP group and in 96% of those in the 3 MOPP group, following MOPP chemotherapy, laparotomy with splenectomy and extended field irradiation. All patients evaluated as clinical CR after 6 or 3 cycles of MOPP, who underwent surgical restaging, were in CR after irradiation. Fifteen out of eighteen patients clinically evaluated as PR after chemotherapy achieved CR after splenectomy and extended field irradiation. Out of 5 clinically staged failures, 2 patients achieved CR after splenectomy and irradiation (Table II). The overall actuarial survival rate after 66 months is 88.5% for the 6 MOPP group and 86% for the 3 MOPP group (Fig. 1). The relapse free survival period after 66 months for patients who achieved CR is 91% for the 6 MOPP group and 88% for the 3 MOPP group (Fig. 2). Nine patients experienced relapse 6 to 64 months after completion of treatment. Seven of them were clinically staged IB or IIB at initial presentation. Surgical restaging was negative in 6 patients and positive in 3 patients who subsequently relapsed. The sites of relapse were previously irradiated areas in 3 cases and subdiaphragmatic unirradiated areas in 6 cases, with extranodal relapse in 2. There were 11 deaths occurring between 7 and 64 months (one aplasia during initial treatment, 6 failures, 3 relapses, 2 acute non-lymphoblastic leukemia, associated with relapse in one case).

Discussion

To determine the possibility of chemotherapy reduction when combined with irradiation in Hodgkin's disease, we compared clinical and surgical restaging after 3 MOPP versus 6 MOPP courses, prior to extended field irradiation. The complete remission rate was similar after 6 and 3 courses of MOPP and independent of histological subtype, clinical stage and B symptoms. Surgical restaging laparotomy confirmed the accuracy of the clinical response criteria. The false negative rate for clinical restaging after 6 and 3 courses of MOPP was close to 3% and confirmed the concordance between clinical CR and the absence of persistent spleen disease. The actuarial survival and the relapse-free survival at 66 months are similar after 3 or 6 courses of MOPP followed by splenectomy and extended field irradiation. We conclude that 3 courses of MOPP are as efficient as 6 to eradicate occult splenic disease in Clinical Stages IIA, IB, IIB with supradiaphragmatic presentation and to achieve complete remission when combined with irradiation.

References

1. DeVita VT, Simon RM, Hubbard SM et al. (1980). Curability of advanced Hodgkin's disease with chemotherapy: Long-term follow up of MOPP treated patients at NCI. Ann Inter Med 92:587–595.
2. Farber LR, Prosnitz LR, Cadman EC et al. (1980). Curative potential of combined modality therapy for advanced Hodgkin's disease. Cancer 46:1509–1517.
3. Kaplan HS (1980). Hodgkin's Disease, 2nd ed. Cambridge: Harvard University Press.
4. Santoro A, Bonadonna G, Bonfante V and Valagussa P (1982). Alternating drug combinations in the treatment of advanced Hodgkin's disease. N Engl J Med 306:770–775.
5. Glatstein E, True-Blood HW, Enright LP et al. (1970). Surgical staging of abdominal involvement in unselected patients with Hodgkin's disease. Radiology 97:425–432.
6. Kaplan HS, Dorfman RF, Nelson TS et al. (1973). Staging laparotomy and splenectomy in Hodgkin's disease: Analysis of indications and patterns of involvement in 285 consecutive unselected patients. Nat Cancer Inst Monograph 36:291–301.
7. Aisenberg AC and Qasi R (1974). Abdominal involvement at the onset of Hodgkin's disease. Amer J Med 57:870–874.
8. Goodman GE, Jones SE, Villar HV et al. (1982). Surgical restaging of Hodgkin's disease. Cancer Treat Rep 66:751–757.
9. Sutcliffe SB, Wrigley PFM, Timothy AR et al. (1982). Posttreatment laparotomy as a guide to management in patients with Hodgkin's disease. Cancer Treat Rep 66:759–765.

11. Staging laparotomy with splenectomy in Stage I and II Hodgkin's disease. No therapeutic benefit

G. A. GOMEZ[1], L. STUTZMAN[2], P. A. REESE[3], H. NAVA[4],
A. M. PANAHON[5], M. BARCOS[6], T. HAN[1] and
E. S. HENDERSON[1]
*Departments of [1] Medical Oncology, [2] Medicine B, [3] Biomathematics,
[4] Surgical Oncology, [5] Radiation Medicine and [6] Pathology, Roswell
Park Memorial Institute, Buffalo, New York, USA*

During the last two decades, staging laparotomy with splenectomy was adopted by many centers as a routine procedure in the work-up of patients with early stage Hodgkin's disease (HD). This staging procedure determines accurately subdiaphragmatic involvement with HD, thus reduces the extent of radiation therapy (RT). However, despite negative findings at laparotomy, RT continues to be delivered to the upper paraaortic nodes and splenic bed in many centers [1, 2, 3]. Since dissemination of HD in the abdomen appears to begin in the spleen and/or in the lymph nodes of the upper abdomen [4], this routine extention of the RT port to the upper abdomen makes it difficult to assess the role of staging with laparotomy procedure in the prevention of abdominal relapse.

In a prospective randomized study of treatment of patients with Stages I and II HD admitted at this institution, one third of the patients did not have staging laparotomy by study design [5]. The patients in this study received mediastinal or mantle ports (with or without chemotherapy) *minus* the upper paraortic region. Thus, this study offered an opportunity to evaluate if exploratory laparotomy with splenectomy in these patients helped to prevent abdominal relapse, as well as the impact of this surgical procedure in remission duration and survival.

Materials and methods

The present study refers to 104 untreated patients with Stage I and II HD admitted between April 1971 to April 1979 into a prospective randomized study of radiation therapy (RT) or RT followed by chemotherapy (CT). Sections of that study were published elsewhere [6–9]. All of these 104 patients had achieved complete remission (CR) with initial RT and all had presentation above the diaphragm. The follow-up was to July 1983.

The Lukes and Butler criteria were used for histopathologic classification, staging was conducted according to the recommendations of the Ann Arbor Conference. By study design, until 1975, patients were randomly assigned to have staging by laparotomy or by closed techniques [5]. Twenty-eight patients (27%) had closed staging. This included: routine blood and biochemistry profiles, chest x-rays, bipedal lymphangiograms, bilateral bone marrow biopsy, percutaneous liver biopsy, intravenous pyelogram and upper gastrointestinal x-rays. Seventy-six patients (73%) had staging laparotomy. In addition to the above mentioned procedures, these patients had laparotomy with splenectomy and biopsies of iliac, paraaortic, celiac and porta hepatis nodes with placement of metallic clips in biopsy areas, multiple needle and core liver biopsies and core surgical bone marrow biopsy. In females oophoropexy was performed.

Treatment was stratified as follows:

a) *'Good risk' patients* — Patients with nodular sclerosis (NS) or lymphocyte predominant type (LP) HD and without 'B' symptoms were randomly assigned to be treated with RT to the involved field (IF) or IF RT plus CT. When several areas of gross disease were to be treated, a mantle field was used. The lower border of treatment which included mediastinal irradiation was at the line of the insertion of the diaphragm.

b) *'Poor risk' patients* — Patients with mixed cellularity type (MC): or lymphocyte depleted type HD and those with other histologies and with 'B' symptoms were treated with total nodal radiation alone (TNR, mantle, inverted Y plus spleen or spleen pedicle) or TNR followed by CT.

RT was delivered through anterior and posterior fields 5 days per week to a *constant* mid-tumor dose of 3600 rad given in $3\frac{1}{2}$ to 5 weeks. When delivered as part of a large treatment field, the daily dose was 150 rad. When given to smaller fields the daily dose was 200 rad.

The CT program used in this study consisted of 3 courses of vincristine, 1.4 mg/m^2 iv push on days 1, 8, 57, 64, 113 and 120, given simultaneously with oral procarbazine, 100 mg/m^2 for 14 days beginning on days 1, 57 and 113, and 3 courses of vinblastine, 5 mg/m^2 iv push on days 29, 36, 85, 92, 141, and 148, given together with oral prednisone, 40 mg/m^2 and chlorambucil 5 mg/m^2 for 14 days beginning on days 29, 85 and 141. This program was found to produce a CR rate similar to the MOPP regimen in patients with advanced HD [10]. Marginal relapses and localized relapses in non-irradiated lymph node regions were treated with RT. In-field or disseminated relapses were treated with MOPP or analogs, or with RT+CT.

Results are presented for the purpose of this study according to the real staging procedure or treatment received, *not* according to randomization. The duration of remission was calculated from end of RT; survival from onset of treatment. Patients who died in CR were included in the analysis of survival but the duration of remission was censored at that point. Differences between groups of patients were evaluated with the Mantel-Cox test and with the Fisher exact probability test.

Results

As shown in Table I, there were no significant differences in clinical or pathologic features or in treatment distribution between patients staged with or without laparotomy. The number of patients with relapse according to treatment modality and to staging procedure is shown in Table II. With similar follow-up in each group, no significant differences were observed in the proportion of patients relapsing according to whether or not staging laparotomy was done, overall or within each of the treatment modalities.

The number of patients with relapse in the *abdomen,* according to treatment modality and to staging procedure, is shown in Table III. There were no significant differences in the proportion of patients with relapse in the abdomen in the group staged by laparotomy (12%) and in those staged by

Table I. Comparison of clinical features at presentation according to staging procedure

Laparotomy (76 pts)			No laparotomy (28 pts)		*p value*
Males/Females	36/40		15/13		ns
Age range (years)	15–56		15–64		ns
(median)	27		24		ns
Histology: LP	6	(8%)	5	(18%)	ns
NS	56	(75%)	18	(64%)	ns
MC	14	(18%)	5	(18%)	ns
Patients with					
mass >6 cm	32	(42%)	13	(46%)	ns
'E' disease	16	(21%)	5	(18%)	ns
Stage IA	22	(29%)	8	(19%)	ns
IB	1	(1%)	2	(7%)	ns
IIA	40	(53%)	13	(46%)	ns
IIB	13	(17%)	5	(18%)	ns
Treatment: IF RT	34	(45%)	10	(36%)	ns
IFRT+CT	27	(35%)	11	(39%)	ns
TNR	12	(16%)	3	(11%)	ns
TNR+CT	3	(4%)	4	(14%)	ns

LP : Lymphocyte predominant
NS : Nodular sclerosis
MC : Mixed cellularity
ns : Not significant
For other abbreviations – See text

Table II. Number of patients with relapse/total number of patients according to staging procedures and treatment modality

	IF RT	IF RT+CT	TNR	TNR+CT	Total
Laparotomy	19/34 (56%)	4/27 (15%)	8/12 (67%)	1/3 (33%)	32/76 (42%)
No Laparotomy	6/10 (60%)	1/11 (9%)	1/3 (33%)	1/4 (25%)	9/28 (36%)
Total	25/44 (57%)	5/38 (13%)	3/15 (60%)	2/7 (29%)	41/104 (39%)

Table III. Relapse in the abdomen according to staging procedures and treatment modality (number of patients with relapse/total number of patients)

	IF RT	IF RT+CT	TNR	TNR+CT	Total
Laparotomy	6/34 (18%)	3/27 (11%)	0/12	0/3	9/76 (12%)
No Laparotomy	1/10 (10%)	0/11	0/3	0/4	1/28 (3%)
Total	7/44 (16%)	3/38 (8%)	0/15	0/7	10/104 (10%)

closed techniques (3%, $p=0.28$). All ten relapses were observed after treatment with IF RT with or without CT while none of the patients treated with TNR with or without CT had abdominal relapse. Among patients staged by laparotomy, five relapses were both above and below the diaphragm, and four in the abdomen *alone*. The time range to relapse in the abdomen was from 19 to 80 months, the median was 60.5 months. The patient staged by closed techniques relapsed only in the abdomen at 68 months. Three of the ten patients with relapse in the abdomen died, all three had staging by laparotomy and all had had in-field relapse in previously existing large masses.

Fig. 1 shows remission duration and survival in the laparotomy and no laparotomy groups. With similar median follow-up in each group, no significant differences between pairs of curves were detected in remission duration ($p = 0.28$), or in survival ($p = 0.09$). Seven of 13 patients staged by laparotomy died with HD. The other six died of other causes while in CR: three in their first CR (myocardial infarction: one, cerebrovascular accident: one, and non-Hodgkin's lymphoma: one), two with sepsis during salvage or re-salvage chemotherapy, and one died with leukoencephalopathy 30 months after salvage chemotherapy. Three other patients of this group had secondary malignancies successfully controlled (diffuse histiocytic lymphoma, malignant schwannoma and squamous cell carcinoma of the cervix). Death from HD accounted for 2/2 patients staged by closed techniques, no secondary malignancies were observed in this group.

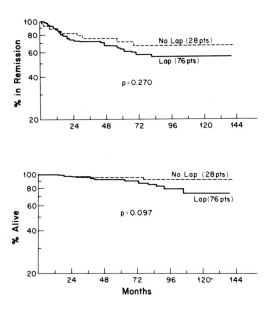

Figure 1. Remission duration and survival in patients with Stages I-II Hodgkin's disease according to staging procedure. Differences in remission and survival were not significantly different. (Reprinted, by permission, from the American Journal of Medicine [9].

Discussion

Our experience [5] and that of others [1–3] showed that unsuspected involvement with HD in the abdomen was found at laparotomy in 1/3 to 1/2 of patients with Clinical Stages I and II. Therefore, relapse in the abdomen would be expected in a substantial proportion of our patients staged by closed techniques. However, only one (3%) such case was observed. This proportion of relapse in the abdomen was not significantly different from that observed in the group staged by laparotomy (12%, see Table III). In addition, staging laparotomy did not improve the duration of remission or survival as compared to closed staging (see Fig. 1). On the other hand relapse in the abdomen, observed as early as 19 months and as late as 80 months, suggests a low probability of success in detecting very early HD by this staging technique, despite serial sections of the spleen and lymph nodes. Strum and collaborators [13] found microscopic foci of HD in long-term survivors apparently 'cured' by treatment that is now considered inferior. That study suggest that at least in some cases, understaging of HD might not prevent long survival and 'cure'.

Similar to other studies [1–3], no relapse in the abdomen was found in the present series after radiation to the paraaortic nodes and the splenic pedicle (or spleen). However, this program of RT was more extensive

(TNR) than what is now considered adequate treatment for these patients. The use of extended mantle has decreased the abdomen relapse virtually to zero [1-3].

Survival did not appear to be affected by relapse in the abdomen. All the patients who died after relapsing in the abdomen also had had in-field relapse in areas of previously existing large tumors, and indeed their abdominal relapses might have been seeded from persistent extra-abdominal sites.

Other studies are now questioning the routine use of staging laparotomy in the planning of treatment of HD [11, 12]. In a large retrospective study, no significant differences in survival were found between patients treated at the Princess Margaret Hospital where staging laparotomy was not used routinely compared to patients treated at the Stanford Medical Center where staging laparotomy was used routinely [12].

Combined modality therapy is recommended by a number of investigators for the treatment of some groups of patients with early stage HD but at high risk of relapse if the treatment offered is RT alone, (i.e., 'B' symptoms, large mediastinal mass, 'E' disease [2, 3, 6]. Obviously, staging laparotomy is not needed in those cases. Staging with lymphangiography, tomodensitometry studies, needle biopsies of bone marrow and scintiscans may suffice for the routine staging in the majority of patients with HD if extended mantle is to be used in their treatment. Patients with equivocal lymphangiograms, or with suspected extranodal involvement in the abdomen might benefit from staging laparotomy since down- or up-staging in those patients might result in a marked difference in the treatment approach.

Acknowledgments

The authors thank the American Journal of Medicine for their permission to reproduce some tables and the figure presented in this study. This research was supported by USPHS Grants CA-16056 and CA5834 from the National Cancer Institute.

References

1. Kaplan HS (1980). Hodgkin's disease, 2nd Ed. Boston: Harvard University Press.
2. Hellman S and Mauch P (1982). Role of radiation therapy in the treatment of Hodgkin's disease. Cancer Treat Rep 66:915-923.
3. Wiernik PH (1982). Combined modality of early stage Hodgkin's disease. In: Wiernik PH (Ed.). Controversies in Oncology, pp. 3-7. John Wiley & Sons.
4. Desser RK, Golomb HM, Ultmann JE et al. (1977). Prognostic classification of Hodgkin's disease in pathologic Stage III, based on anatomic considerations. Blood 49:883-893.

5. Kauffman JH, Mittelman A, Kim U et al. (1979). The place of laparotomy in the staging of patients with Hodgkin's and non-Hodgkin's lymphomas. A randomized study. Abdominal Surg 21:139–147.

6. Gomez GA, Panahon AM, Stutzman L et al. Large mediastinal mass in Hodgkin's disease. Results of two treatment modalities. Amer J Clin Oncol (CCT) (in press).

7. Gomez GA, Friedman M and Reese P (1983). Occurrence of acute non-lymphocytic leukemia in a prospective randomized study of treatment for Hodgkin's disease. Amer J Clin Oncol (CCT) 6:319–324.

8. Gomez GA, Park JJ, Panahon AM et al. (1983). Heart size and function after radiation therapy to the mediastinum in patients with Hodgkin's disease. Cancer Treat Rep 67:1099–1103.

9. Gomez GA, Reese PA, Nava H et al. Staging laparotomy and splenectomy in early Hodgkin's disease. No therapeutic benefit. Amer J Med (in press).

10. Stutzman L and Glidewell O (1973). Multiple chemotherapeutic agents for Hodgkin's disease. JAMA 225:1202–1211.

11. Lacher MJ (1983). Routine staging laporatomy for patients with Hodgkin's disease is no longer necessary. Cancer Invest 1:93–99.

12. Bergsagel DE, Ellison RE, Beau HA et al. (1982). Results of treating Hodgkin's disease without a policy of staging laparotomy. Cancer Treat Rep 66:717–731.

13. Strum SB and Rappaport H (1971). The persistence of Hodgkin's disease in long-term survivors. Amer J Med 51:222–240.

12. Comparison of initial splectomy and spleen irradiation in Clinical Stages I and II Hodgkin's disease

M. HAYAT and P. CARDE

For the EORTC Radiotherapy-Chemotherapy Group, Institut Gustave-Roussy, Villejuif, France

From 1972 to 1976, the EORTC Radiotherapy-Chemotherapy Group carried out its second controlled clinical trial (H2 trial) in Clinical Stages (CS) I and II Hodgkin's disease. Prior to the commencement of this trial, laparotomy with plenectomy had been introduced at Stanford as a new and more appropriate procedure for staging patients with CS I and II [1].

Materials and methods

The H_2 trial design had essentially two aims: first, to compare therapeutic efficacy of spleen irradiation with that of splenectomy, and second to evaluate the prognostic significance in discovering occult disease at the time of laparotomy. In all patients there was the same extended radiotherapy to the mantle field and to para-aortic lymph nodes. For those patients with unfavorable histologic types (mixed cellularity and lymphoid depletion), two adjuvant chemotherapies were randomly compared: vinblastine alone during two years versus vinblastine plus procarbazine during the same period. Details of this protocol have been published [2]. The long follow-up of 300 patients included in this trial is most appropriate for definite results, report of late complications and study of prognostic factors. Nine European centers participated in this trial (see Appendix).

Relapse-free survival (RFS) and survival curves were calculated according to the actuarial method. The logrank test was used to assess the statistical significance of differences in curves. A statistical multivariate analysis of prognostic factors was performed with the Cox model [3].

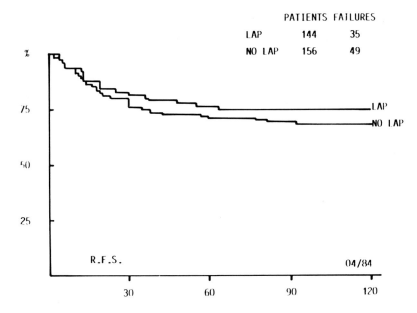

Figure 1. Relapse-free survival of the two randomized groups.

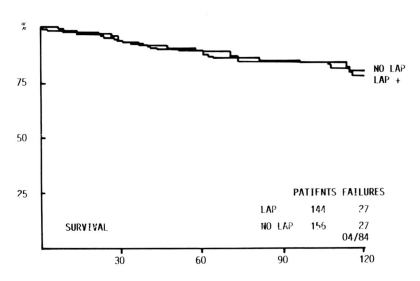

Figure 2. Survival of the two randomized groups.

Results

Overall results

One hundred fifty-six patients were treated by spleen irradiation vs 144 patients treated by splenectomy. The actuarial relapse-free survival and survival at ten years were respectively 73% and 84% in the spleen irradiated group versus 75% and 82% in the group treated by splenectomy. The differences are not statistically significant (Fig. 1 and 2).

Of 52 deaths, only 26 (49%) were due to Hodgkin's disease. Other deaths were due to sequelae of treatments (5 cases), intercurrent diseases (12 cases) and secondary cancer or leukemia (6 cases). Four deaths were due to unknown cause.

Non-lethal complications

It is well known that digestive tract complications may occur many months after abdominal radiotherapy. All the patients of this trial had the same lumbo-aortic radiotherapy; half of them had been randomized to have laparotomy and splenectomy before irradiation. It was interesting to compare the incidence of digestive complications in these two groups. The two main complications registered were small bowel obstruction and gastroduodenal ulcus. Digestive complications were found in 4/152 (2.6%) patients in the group treated by radiotherapy alone versus 25/143 (17.5%) in the other group (Table I). The difference is highly significant ($p < 0.001$). These results indicate that paraaortic radiotherapy following laparotomy is not easily tolerated by the digestive tract. With respect to fertility, 4/148 men over the age of 18 and 12/94 women between the ages of 17 and 45 had children after these treatments.

Table I. H$_2$ Trial: Digestive tract complications

	Radiotherapy alone	Laparotomy followed by radiotherapy	Total
Small bowel obstruction	0/152	8/142	8/294
Gastroduodenal ulcus	4/152	17/142	21/294
Total	4/152 (2.6%)	25/142 (17.5%)	

382

Table II. Prognostic indicators (Cox model)

	Relative Risk	p
Stage II$_2$/Stage I	0.89	ns
Stage II$_3$/Stage I	3.02	<0.001
A + ESR >50 and B + ESR >30/others	2.21	<0.002

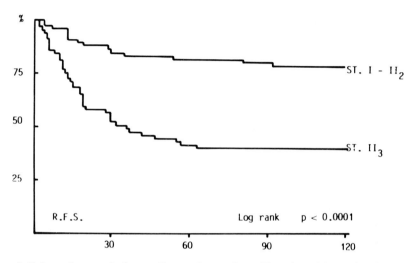

Figure 3. Relapse free survival according to the number of lymph node areas involved.

Prognostic analysis

Numerous prognostic factors were studied: age, sex, mediastinal involvement, stage, number of lymph node areas in Stage II, systemic symptoms, erythrocyte sedimentation rate (ESR). A multivariate analysis with the Cox model was performed only on the group that did not receive any adjuvant chemotherapy. The results of this analysis, summarized in Table II, show the prominent roles of the systemic symptoms and ESR. Although these two parameters are closely related, each of them has an individual prognostic significance. When both are taken into account, their prognostic value is increased. The number of involved lymphatic areas is the third parameter of high prognostic significance. Thus in Stage II cases that had three or more lymphatic areas involved (Stage II$_3$) the risk of relapse is significantly higher than that in stages with two involved areas (II$_2$) (Fig. 3).

Another important prognostic indicator was obtained by laparatomy; 37 patients out 144 (25%) are Pathologic Stage III. Spleen involvement was

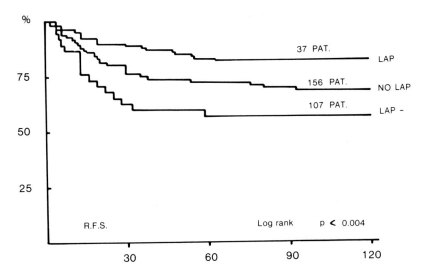

Figure 4. Relapse-free survival according to pathologic stage (Lap+ and Lap−).

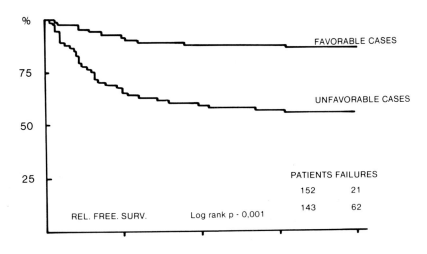

Figure 5. Relapse-free survival according to prognostic subsets of patients.

observed in 33 cases. For this group of Pathologic Stage III patients, RFS at 10 years was 58% versus 85% for the Pathologic Stage II patients. This difference is highly significant ($p < 0.004$) (Fig. 4).

Discussion

When the major prognostic factors are associated, i.e. the number of involved areas and the combination of systemic symptoms and sedimentation rate, it is possible to define two subsets of patients. In the group with favorable prognostic indicators, 10-year RFS was significantly higher than in the group with unfavorable prognosis (Fig. 5).

When these prognostic factors are combined with the information provided by laparotomy it becomes possible to identify a subset of patients for whom the prognosis is excellent and a light treatment is sufficient. For patients with unfavorable prognostic indicators the results are alike whether laparotomy has been positive or negative. For this reason, in the current protocol of the EORTC Radiotherapy-Chemotherapy Group, patients with unfavorable prognostic factors, should not be submitted to laparotomy since whatever the results of laparotomy they would still require a combination of chemotherapy and radiotherapy. Patients with a favorable prognosis are randomly allocated to a group with laparotomy and a group without laparotomy. A light treatment with radiotherapy alone is given to these patients. The para-aortic lymph-nodes and the spleen are irradiated in the group which did not undergo laparotomy.

Appendix

Cooperating centers were Institut Jules Bordet, Brussels, Belgium (J. Henry, J. Lustmann Marechal), Istituto di Radiologia Universita di Firenze, Italy (G. De Giuli, L. Gionini), C.A.C. Reims, France (A. Cattan), St. Radboud Hospital Nijmegen, the Netherlands (Wagener), C.A.C. Caen, France (J.S. Abbatucci), Rotterdams Radio-Therapeutisch Instituut, the Netherlands (B. van der Werf Messing), Antoni van Leeuwenhoek Ziekenhuis, Amsterdam, the Netherlands (K. Breur, M. Burgers), Ziekenhuis Leyenburg, The Hague, the Netherlands (H. Kerkhofs), Institut Gustave-Roussy, Villejuif, France (M. Tubiana, J.L. Amiel).

References

1. Glatstein E, Guernsey JM, Rosenberg SA and Kaplan HS (1969). The value of laparotomy and splenectomy in the staging of Hodgkin's disease. Cancer 24:709–718.
2. Tubiana M, Hayat M, Henry-Amar M et al. (1981). Five-year results of EORTC randomized study of splenectomy and spleen irradiation in Clinical Stages I and II of Hodgkin's disease. Eur J Cancer 17:355–363.
3. Cox DR (1972). Regression model and life tables. J Roy Stat Soc B 34:187–220.

13. Prognostic groups for management of clinically localized Hodgkin's disease

S. B. SUTCLIFFE, M. K. GOSPODAROWICZ, D. E. BERGSAGEL,
R. S. BUSH, R. CHUA, T. C. BROWN and D. F. RIDEOUT
The Princess Margaret Hospital, Toronto, Ontario, Canada

Radiation therapy has conventionally been applied following surgical staging of Hodgkin's disease. However, the risk of occult upper abdominal disease and the need for upper abdominal radiation despite a negative laparotomy are now well recognized. Furthermore, factors other than anatomical stage are increasingly influencing therapeutic choice. The present analysis defines a treatment approach for patients receiving radical irradiation for Clinical Stages (CS) I and II Hodgkin's disease, based upon an analysis of outcome for the period 1968-1977.

Materials and methods

The records of 252 adult patients (≥ 17 years) with biopsy proven CS I and II Hodgkin's disease treated with radical radiation therapy between 1968-1977 at Princess Margaret Hospital (PMH) were reviewed. Pathology was reviewed in all cases and classified by the criteria of Lukes and Butler [1].

Staging investigations included history, physical examination, complete blood count, liver function biochemistry, chest x-ray and bipedal lymphography in all patients. Other investigations were performed as necessary and clinical stage was determined retrospectively according to the Ann Arbor classification [2].

Disease bulk was assessed retrospectively and was classified as 'large' when peripheral nodal masses exceeded 6 cm, or when a mediastinal mass was equal to or exceeded 10 cm on a standard 6 feet P.A. chest x-ray or required a mediastinal port width of ≥ 12 cm in the mid-mediastinum on a simulator film.

Actuarial survival was calculated from the time of first treatment. In the cause-specific survival analysis, patients who died from causes unrelated to Hodgkin's disease were censored. Differences between proportions were determined using Fisher exact test, and multivariate analysis was performed using the logrank method [3].

Patients received involved field radiotherapy, a mantle, or a mantle combined with some upper abdominal irradiation. The majority of the patients received 3500 cGy in 4 weeks, prescribed at mid-plane with compensators to minimize dose variation to $\pm 5\%$ [4]. Treatment was delivered mainly with Co^{60} equipment at extended S.S.D., and port films, shields and compensators were used in all patients received mantle irradiation.

Results

Survival, cause-specific survival and relapse-free rate

The 10-year actuarial and cause-specific survival rates for the 252 CS I-II patients receiving irradiation were 78% and 86%, respectively. The 10 year actuarial relapse-free rate was 61%.

Prognostic factor analysis

The effects of age, stage, histology and disease bulk were studied by multivariate analysis to determine independent prognostic significance in terms of survival and relapse-free rate.

Age, stage and histology each proved to be of independent significance for survival (age, $p < 0.00005$; stage $p = 0.0048$; histology $p = 0.005$) and for relapse-free rate (age, $p = 0.01$; stage, $p = 0.014$; histology, $p = 0.0006$). Disease bulk was not predictive of survival but was predictive of an increased relapse risk ($p = 0.044$); however, this effect was not maintained when patients with large mediastinal masses were excluded from the analysis.

The site of disease relative to the diaphragm (supradiaphragmatic: 228 patients; infradiaphragmatic: 24 patients) predicted neither for survival nor relapse-free advantage.

Twelve of 65 patients with unilateral cervical clinical stage IA disease had nodal involvement above the thyroid cartilage. Relapse occurred in 1 of these 12 patients compared with 19 of 53 with disease in the mid or lower cervical node groups.

In univariate analysis the relapse rates for involved field, mantle and > mantle fields for CS IA disease were 64% ($n = 46$), 81% ($n = 37$) and 33% ($n = 3$); for CS II disease, 40% ($n = 20$), 54% ($n = 84$) and 76% ($n = 38$); and for CS IB and IIB disease, 20% ($n = 5$), 66% ($n = 9$) and 50% ($n = 10$).

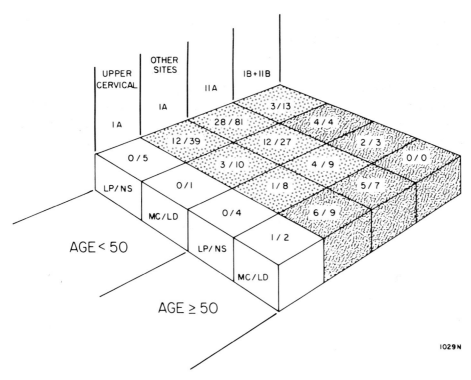

Figure 1. Relapse rates according to age, stage, and histology for patients with supradiaphragmatic Hodgkin's disease, Clinical Stages I and II treated with radical irradiation. LP = lymphocytic predominance; ND = nodular sclerosis; MC = mixed cellularity; LD = lymphocytic depletion.

Prognostic groupings by multifactorial analysis

As age, stage and histology exerted an independent influence upon survival and relapse-free rate, patients with supradiaphragmatic disease undergoing radiation therapy were grouped according to these variables and the combined effect of these factors on relapse-free rate is shown in Fig. 1. Three groups can be defined according to risk of relapse; patients with Stage IA disease and isolated cervical node above the thyroid cartilage notch (Group I; relapse rate 1 of 12), Group II with a relapse rate of approximately 33% (63 of 187 relapsed) and Group III with a relapse rate in excess of 70% (17 of 23 relapsed).

The influence of radiation volume within each prognostic grouping is shown in Table I. Whilst increasing field size had little effect upon relapse rate in Groups I and III, for the Group II which contained the majority of patients, the relapse rates for < mantle, mantle and > mantle fields were 44%, (n = 39) 32% (n = 108) and 27.5% (n = 40), respectively.

Table I. Relapse rates by prognostic grouping according to extent of radiation field

Radiation field	No. Relapses/No. Patients		
	Group I	Group II	Group III
< Mantle	1/10 (10%)	17/39 (44%)	10/14 (71%)
Mantle	0/2 (0%)	35/108 (32%)	5/6 (83%)
> Mantle	0/0 (0%)	11/40 (27.5%)	2/3 (66%)

Group I   : Upper cervical IA
Group II   : Other IA, IIA (<50 yrs or LP/NS if ⩾50 yrs) and IB, IIB (<50 yrs, LP/NS)
Group III : Other IA, IIA (⩾50 yrs, MC/LD) and IB, IIB (⩾50 yrs or MC/LD if <50 yrs)

Prognostic significance of mediastinal and hilar disease

Mediastinal disease was present in 100 of 228 patients with supradiaphragmatic disease; in 14 of 100 the mass was ≥ 10 cm width. Mediastinal involvement did not significantly influence overall survival or relapse rate. By comparison of those with no, small or large mediastinal disease receiving radical irradiation alone, the overall relapse rate was not significantly different; however, those with large mediastinal disease had a significantly higher intrathoracic failure rate ($p = 0.0017$), and 50% of patients failing in the thorax subsequently died of the disease.

Isolated hilar node involvement was uncommon (3 patients), although hilar disease was present in 56 of the 151 patients with mediastinal involvement (37%). The patterns of relapse, intrathoracic relapse and survival were similar for those with and without hilar disease when analyzed according to mediastinal bulk. Thus, no effect of hilar involvement independent of mediastinal disease could be defined.

Infradiaphragmatic disease

No prognostic significance for survival or relapse could be determined according to site of disease relative to the diaphragm. Of the 24 patients with infradiaphragmatic disease, nine had inguinal disease with a normal lymphogram; only one patient relapsed in this group. Four patients had inguino-iliac disease without paraortic involvement by lymphogram criteria; one has relapsed. Ten of the 13 patients with disease confined to the inguino-iliac region remain alive. Eleven patients had abnormal paraaortic nodes; of the 7 who achieved remission, 4 have subsequently relapsed and 5 of the 11 have died of disease.

Discussion

This series of patients treated for CS I and II Hodgkin's disease between 1968-1977 is similar in constitution to that reported from other institutions adopting treatment policies according to pathological stage (PS) of disease [5, 6]. A higher proportion of PMH patients were older (patients ≥ 40 years = 34%). The survival rate for the clinical series is comparable to that achieved following radiation therapy for pathologically staged patients with an actuarial 10-year survival of approximately 80%, and a 14% probability of dying of Hodgkin's disease over the 10-year period. Given that the relapse-free rate of 61% is lower than that of 21–23% reported for surgically staged patients [5, 6], the comparable survival figures reflect the effectiveness of salvage therapy following first relapse.

The relapse rate for this clinically staged series cannot be directly compared with the surgically staged series as the constitution of the two populations by stage is different and in the PMH series the radiation included 'involved fields' and the minority received any upper abdominal irradiation. To address the difference in composition of clinically and pathologically staged series, a theoretical comparison is made in Table II with anticipated cure rates using radiation for Stages I to IIIA, and chemotherapy for Stages IIIB and IV. The overall cure rate of 79.3% for pathologically staged patients presenting with CS I and II disease is almost identical to the 79% survival recorded in our clinical series. Furthermore, the number of patients first cured by irradiation alone in a population of clinically staged patients if treated in the knowledge of pathological stage is 66%; this compares with a figure of 61% for the PMH clinically staged series. Thus the population of

Table II. Actuarial and theoretical predictions for overall and relapse-free survival in Clinical Stage I and II Hodgkin's disease

| | | | Number 'cured' by first treatment | |
	Actuarial survival (96)	Actuarial RFS (%)	xRT	Chemo ±xRT
100 pts with CS I-II				
−70 pts with PS I-II (6)	84	77	54	−
−20 pts with PS IIIA (7)	70	62	12	−
−10 pts with IIIB/IV (8)	65	60	−	6
100 pts with pathologically staged CS I-II	79.3	72	66	6
100 pts with CS I-II at PMH	79	60	60	−

patients who can be cured by irradiation alone is similar irrespective of laparotomy information. The patient population (6%) with occult advanced disease were not correctly identified by our clinical staging techniques and the choice of initial irradiation therapy was inappropriate and a systemic approach would have been preferable.

The use of multiple independent prognostic factors has permitted the identification of patient groups with differing relapse risks with irradiation. Those with isolated high cervical nodal disease have done well even with involved field irradiation. The majority of patients with CS I and IIA disease have a relapse rate which could be reduced by treatment of occult upper abdominal disease, and by so doing relapse rates comparable to those achieved by radiation following surgical staging could be achieved. Those patients of older age ($\geqq 50$ years), with symptomatic disease and unfavorable histologic subtypes (mixed cellularity on lymphocytic depletion), had a high relapse rate with little indication of change by increase in field volume. For this group a policy of combined chemotherapy and irradiation would seem more appropriate.

Patients with bulky mediastinal disease had a high intrathoracic failure rate when treated with conventional upper mantle irradiation. Our subsequent experience has indicated that such patients have a more favorable control rate when treated with initial chemotherapy and subsequent irradiation. Other reports documenting a similar relapse pattern indicate that a combined modality approach or the use of whole thoracic irradiation [9] establish higher control rates for patients with this adverse form of clinical presentation.

References

1. Lukes RJ and Butler JJ (1966). The pathology of nomenclature of Hodgkin's disease. Cancer Res 26:1063–1081.
2. Rosenberg SA (1966). Report of the Committee on the Staging of Hodgkin's Disease. Cancer Res 26:1310.
3. Peto R, Pike MC, Armitage P et al. (1977). Design and analysis of randomized clinical trials requiring prolonged observation of each patient. Brit J Cancer 35:1–35.
4. Leung PMK, Van Dyk J and Robins J (1974). A method of large irregular field compensation. Brit J Radiol 47:805–810.
5. Mauch PM, Lewin A and Hellman S (1982). Role of radiation therapy in the treatment of Stage I-II Hodgkin's disease. In: Rosenberg SA and Kaplan HS (Eds.). Malignant Lymphomas: Etiology, Immunology, Pathology, Treatment, pp. 453–463. Academic Press, New York, N.Y.
6. Hoppe RT, Coleman CN, Cox RS, et al. (1982). The management of Stage I-II Hodgkin's disease with irradiation alone or combined modality therapy: The Stanford Experience. Blood 59:455–465.
7. Hoppe RT, Cox RS, Rosenberg SA and Kaplan HS (1982). Prognostic factors in pathologic

stage III Hodgkin's disease. Cancer Treat Rep 66:743–749.

8. DeVita VT Jr, Simon RM, Hubbard SM et al. (1980). Curability of advanced Hodgkin's disease with chemotherapy. Ann Intern Med 92:587–595.

9. Lee CKK, Bloomfield CD, Goldman AI, et al. (1981). The therapeutic utility of lung irradiation for Hodgkin's disease patients with large mediastinal masses. Int J Radiat Oncol Biol Phys 7:151–154.

14. Management of localized, infradiaphragmatic Hodgkin's disease:
Experience of a rare clinical presentation at St. Bartholomew's Hospital

M. S. DORREEN, P. F. M. WRIGLEY, A. E. JONES,
W. S. SHAND, A. G. STANSFELD and T. A. LISTER
ICRF Department of Medical Oncology, St. Bartholomew's Hospital, London, UK

Hodgkin's disease (HD) confined to infradiaphragmatic sites is uncommon [1-5] and relatively little information regarding the prognosis in this substage is available. An analysis of the outcome of treatment of previously untreated patients with Stages IA-IIB infradiaphragmatic HD referred to St. Bartholomew's hospital, over a 14 year period, is presented.

Materials and methods

Twenty-three consecutive patients referred between January 1969 and the close of 1982, form the basis of this study. Histologic diagnosis was established according to the Rye nomenclature [6]. During the same time period, 165 patients with supradiaphragmatic Stages IA-IIB (Pathologic Stage IA = 51, Pathologic and Clinical Stages IIA-IIB = 114) were also referred for treatment. Selected comparative details are illustrated in Table I.

The criteria of the Ann Arbor conference [7] were used to establish the stage. Bipedal lymphangiography was done in 21/23 patients. Computerized abdominal tomography (CAT scan), alone, was performed in one patient and one patient proceeded directly to laparotomy.

Pathologic staging by laparotomy and splenectomy was formally adopted in 1972 as part of the planned investigation of all patients scheduled to receive radical radiotherapy (RT) [8, 9] and was undertaken in 16 instances. A 17th patient (PS IIA) underwent a diagnostic laparotomy for an 'abdominal malignancy'. Splenectomy was not performed in this case.

Inverted Y Radiotherapy. Treatment from a 4 MeV linear accelerator was delivered through anterior and posterior portals to a target volume which included the splenic pedicle, the paraaortic, iliac, inguinal and femoral lymph nodes. An intravenous pyelogram was performed during initial planning and simulation, to minimize irradiation of renal tissue.

Table I. Patient characteristics compared with supradiaphragmatic Hodgkin's disease

		Infra D	Supra D	
	Stage	I & II	I & II	
Sex	Male	20	83	
	Female	3	82	
	M:F	6.7:1	1:1	
Age (yrs)	Mean	39	32	p<0.05
	Median	37	29	
	Range	20–66	13–72	
Histology	LP	7 (30%)	25 (15%)	
	NS	11 (48%)	110 (67%)[a]	
	MC	4 (18%)	28 (17%)	
	LD	0	2 (1%)	
	U/C	1 (4%)	0	

LP = lymphocyte predominance NS = nodular sclerosis MC = mixed cellularity
LD = lymphocyte depletion U/C = unclassed
Infra D: infradiaphragmatic, Supra D: supradiaphragmatic
[a] In Stage II, the incidence of NS was 75%, a difference significant at p<0.05, in comparison with infradiaphragmatic HD

Shielding blocks were individually moulded from blocks of Cerrobend alloy (Mining and Chemical Products, Ltd., Studley St., Birmingham), with 'beam divergent' edges. In both sexes, the pelvis was shielded in the midline: in women the ovaries were centrally transposed at laparotomy and in men, testicular shielding was provided. Spinal shielding was not used.

A total midplane dose of 3,500 cGy was delivered in 20 fractions over 28 days, with an additional 'boost' of 500 cGy in 3 fractions to peripheral sites of bulk disease. Irradiation of the liver did not form part of the treatment.

Combination chemotherapy. Cyclical combination chemotherapy with mustine, vinblastine, procarbazine and prednisolone (MVPP) was administered, as previously described [10].

Selection of treatment. Between 1969 and 1971, two clinically staged patients received inverted Y RT (Table II). In neither instance was the spleen included within the irradiated field. The broad policy adopted in 1972 prescribed inverted Y for Pathologic Stages (PS) IA and IIA, whereas MVPP was generally reserved for those with extensive disease or with B symptoms. Two patients received both MVPP and inverted Y RT: one was thought to

Table II. Treatment and stage

Treatment	Stage	No. of Patients
Inverted Y	PS IA	4
	PS IIA	6
	CS IIA	1
	CS IIB	1
MVPP	PS IIA	4
	PS IIB	1
	CS IIB	4
MVPP + Inverted Y	PS IIA	1
	PS IA	1

have developed B symptoms after laparotomy; the other had extensive abdominal disease.

Treatment evaluation. Complete remission was defined as the complete resolution of all abnormal signs and symptoms. Actuarial analysis of survival and freedom from relapse was performed, using the life-table method of Kaplan and Meier [11]. Tests of significance were applied using a logrank variance method [12]. Comparisons of patient subpopulations were made using the Student's t-test.

Results

In comparison to the patients with supradiaphragmatic HD, the 23 patients with infradiaphragmatic disease comprised an older population with a striking male predominance (Table I). A distinct subpopulation was formed of patients presenting with 'B' symptoms or with 3 or more sites of disease. This group (Table III) was characterized by an older median age and a lower proportion of lymphocyte predominance histology.

Infiltration of the spleen by HD was found in 9/16 (56%) staging laparotomies (Table IV). Involvement of the spleen correlated both with Stage II disease and number of involved intra-abdominal lymph nodes, being found in all five patients with 2 or more groups of involved abdominal nodes. Although there was considerable overlap in the weights of involved and non-involved spleens, the largest involved spleen weighed 1190 grams.

Complete remission (CR) was achieved in 21/23 (91%) patients: 12/12 following inverted Y RT, 7/9 following MVPP alone and 2/2 patients who received both MVPP and RT.

Details of the three male patients who have relapsed, are given in Table V.

Table III. Prognostic categories

	Group 1 <3 Sites of disease No B symptoms	Group 2 >3 Sites of disease ±B symptoms
Total No.	10	13
Sex	M = 10	M = 10 F = 3
Age (yrs)		
Median	29	41 $p = 0.05$
Range	20–49	22–66
Histology		
LP	5 (50%)	1 (8%) $p = 0.05$
NS	4 (40%)	8 (61%)
MC	1 (10%)	3 (23%)
U/C	0	1 (8%)

Table IV. Pathologic spleen involvement

Incidence:	9/16 (56%)	
CS IA	1/7 (14%)	
CS IIA	8/9 (88%)	
Med weight (range):		
Involved	200 g (100–1190)	
Not involved	155 g (90–200)	

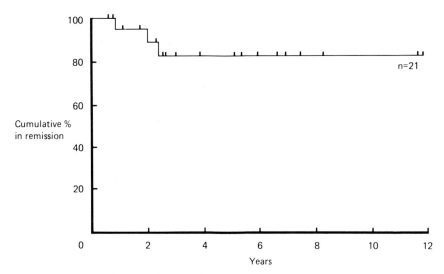

Figure 1. Freedom from relapse (all treatments).

Table V. Details of relapse

Patient	Histology	Stage	Treatment	Site of relapse	Salvage	Outcome	Status
1 Male, 60 years	NS	IIA	Inverted Y	Thoracic + axillary lymph nodes	MVPP	PR	Dead (3 years after relapse)
2 Male, 39 years	NS	IIB	MVPP	Abdominal lymph nodes and spleen	combination CT containing Etoposide	PR	Alive + HD
3 Male, 32 years	MC	IIA	MVPP	Pelvic mass	TNI [a], CT (palliative)	PR	Alive + HD

[a] TNI = total nodal irradiation

Table VI. Complications

Patient	Histology	Stage	Treatment	Complication	Latent interval	Treatment	Status
1 Male, 22 years	LP	IIA	Inverted Y	Pulmonary sarcoidosis	7 years	Prednisolone	NED
2 Male, 30 years	MC	IIB	MVPP	Squamous carcinoma, penis	6 years	Local RT	NED
3 Female, 45 years	U/C	IIB	MVPP	Mycosis fungoides	2 years	PUVA	controlled
4 Male, 33 years	LP	IA	MVPP + RT	Osteonecrosis, femoral head, right hand side	2 years	Total hip replacement	NED

NED = No evidence of disease

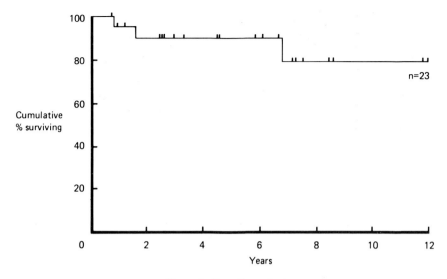

Figure 2. Overall survival.

Two of these had presented originally with bulky HD and the third with B symptoms. Recurrence was confirmed histologically, the histological type being identical, in all cases, to that at presentation. Actuarial freedom from relapse is illustrated in Fig. 1.

Twenty patients remain alive at a minimum follow-up of 1 year. All three deaths occurred from active HD, including the two patients who failed to attain CR and one who relapsed. The predicted 10-year cumulative survival is 79% (Fig. 2).

Four patients developed late complications after treatment (Table VI), although only the occurrence of avascular necrosis was considered to have been directly attributable to the preceding therapy. No patient has developed evidence of renal, bowel or neurological damage resulting from radiotherapy.

Discussion

In keeping with other reports, the occurrence of HD, confined to infradiaphragmatic sites, has been a rare presentation at St. Bartholomew's Hospital where it has accounted for approximately 5% of a total population of around 480 previously untreated patients referred during the period of this study. The results also confirm those of others [3–5] with respect to the older age and higher proportions of lymphocyte predominance and mixed cellularity histology as compared with supradiaphragmatic presentations.

Because of the small numbers, the choice of therapy has been based on

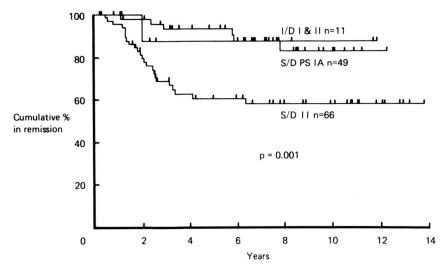

Figure 3. Freedom from relapse after radiotherapy. Infradiaphragmatic (I/D) vs supradiaphragmatic (S/D) disease.

individual considerations. Nevertheless, the broad principles of management appropriate to supradiaphragmatic HD, have held true. At this and at least one other West European center [13], inverted Y RT has been the basis for the management of Stages IA and IIA infradiaphragmatic HD. In contrast, wider field RT has been used at centers in the USA, varying from total nodal irradiation [14, 15] to loco-regional RT for disease confined entirely to peripheral lymph nodes [4, 5, 16]. For more extensive presentations, combined modality treatments with RT and combination chemotherapy have been advocated [4, 5].

In this study, the results of inverted Y RT compare very favorably with those achieved using 'mantle' RT [8, 17] in supradiaphragmatic PS IA (Fig. 3) and in Stage IIA patients with no mediastinal disease [17].

The prognostic importance of splenic involvement with HD remains debatable. By analogy with its reputedly bad outlook in PS IIIA HD [18, 19], the discovery of splenic HD could be considered a feature of adverse prognostic impact. Mauch et al. [4, 5] have managed their infradiaphragmatic presentations with splenic involvement by a combined modality approach. In this study, only 1/4 patients with involvement of the spleen, treated by RT alone, has relapsed. It is not clear how far the effect of splenectomy itself might contribute to the success of RT but the high incidence of splenic HD would indicate a need to pursue the present policy of staging laparotomy with splenectomy in all patients planned for treatment by inverted Y RT.

The selection of MVPP was based on the demonstration of bulky disease,

B symptoms, or both. The CR rate (82%) and the subsequent freedom from relapse (76%) compare favorably with other presentations of localized disease [17, 20]. Nonetheless, the fact that both non-responding and relapsing patients fell within the category of extensive/symptomatic disease must reflect the potentially unfavorable outlook in this group. In contrast to other reports [4, 5, 21], we have not observed the small but striking incidence of HD presenting primarily as bulky, retroperitoneal lymphadenopathy. In these cases, the outlook has been almost invariably fatal, despite intensive therapy.

The incidence of long-term complications has been acceptably small and, in most instances, well controlled. The occurrence of avascular necrosis of the femoral head following therapy, particularly combination chemotherapy and RT, has been well documented [22, 23].

In conclusion, the results of treatment compare favorably with supra-diaphragmatic HD. More specifically, the results suggest that the bulk of disease at presentation is at least as important as its anatomical localization. The use of inverted Y radiotherapy as the initial treatment of pathologically staged patients with 'limited' disease (PS IA or less than 3 sites of disease) seems justified. In all other instances, combination chemotherapy is probably the treatment of first choice.

Acknowledgements

We are indebted to Miss M. Faux for collating and analyzing the data and also to Doreen for typing this manuscript.

References

1. Fuller LM (1966). Results of large volume irradiation in the management of Hodgkin's disease and malignant lymphomas originating in the abdomen. Radiology 87:1058–1064.
2. Fuller LM, Gamble JF, Ibrahim E et al. (1973). Stage II Hodgkin's disease. Significance of mediastinal and nonmediastinal presentations. Radiology 109:429–435.
3. Krikorian JG, Portlock CS, Rosenberg SA and Kaplan HS (1976). Hodgkin's disease, Stages I and II occurring below the diaphragm. Cancer 43:1866–1871.
4. Mauch PM, Lewin A and Hellman S (1982). The role of irradiation in the treatment of Stage I-II Hodgkin's disease. In: Rosenberg SA and Kaplan HS (Eds.). Malignant Lymphomas: Etiology, Immunology, Pathology, Treatment, pp. 453–467. New York: Academic Press.
5. Mauch PM, Greenberg H, Lewin A et al. (1983). Prognostic factors in patients with sub-diaphragmatic Hodgkin's disease. J Haematol Oncol 1:205–214.
6. Lukes RJ, Craver LF, Hall TC et al. (1966). Report of the Nomenclature Committee. Cancer Res 26:1311.
7. Carbone PP, Kaplan HS, Musshoff K et al. (1971). Report of the Committee on Hodgkin's Disease Staging. Cancer Res 31:1860–1861.

8. Sutcliffe SBJ, Wrigler PFM, Smyth JF et al. (1976). Intensive investigation in the management of Hodgkin's disease. Brit Med J 2:1343–1347.

9. Timothy AR, Sutcliffe SBJ, Stansfeld AG et al. (1978). Radiotherapy in the treatment of Hodgkin's disease. Brit Med J 1:1246–1249.

10. Sutcliffe SBJ, Wrigley PFM, Peto J et al. (1978). MVPP chemotherapy regime for advanced Hodgkin's disease. Brit Med J 1:679–683.

11. Kaplan E and Meier P (1958). Nonparametric estimation from incomplete observations. Amer Stat Assoc J 53:457–480.

12. Peto R, Pike MC, Armitage P et al. (1977). Design and analysis of randomised clinical trials requiring prolonged observation of each patient. II. Analysis and examples. Brit J Cancer 35:1–35.

13. Pene F, Henry-Amar M, Le Bourgeois JP et al. (1980). A study of relapse and course of 153 cases of Hodgkin's disease (clinical Stages I and II) treated at the Institute Gustave-Roussy from 1963 to 1970 with radiotherapy alone or with adjuvant monochemotherapy. Cancer 46:2131–2141.

14. Kaplan HS (1980). Hodgkin's disease, 2nd ed. Cambridge: Harvard University Press.

15. Hoppe RT, Coleman CN, Cox RS et al. (1982). The management of Stage I-II Hodgkin's disease with irradiation alone or combined modality therapy: The Stanford experience. Blood 59:455–465.

16. Fuller LM, Madoc-Jones H, Hagemeister FB et al. (1980). Further follow-up of results of treatment in 90 laparotomy-negative Stage I and II Hodgkin's disease patients: Significance of mediastinal and non-mediastinal presentations. Int J Radiat Oncol Biol Phys 6:799–808.

17. Dorreen MS, Plowman PN, Laidlow J et al. (1984). The management of Stage II supradiaphragmatic Hodgkin's disease at St. Bartholomew's Hospital: A retrospective review of 114 previously untreated patients over 14 years. Cancer (in press).

18. Hoppe RT, Rosenberg SA, Kaplan HS and Cox RS (1980). Prognostic factors in pathological Stage IIA Hodgkin's disease. Cancer 46:1240–1246.

19. Hoppe RT, Cox RS, Rosenberg SA and Kaplan HS (1982).Prognostic factors in pathologic Stage III Hodgkin's disease. Cancer Treat Rep 66:743–749.

20. Lister TA, Dorreen MS, Faux M et al. (1983). The treatment of Stage IIIA Hodgkin's disease. J Clin Oncol 1:745–749.

21. Westling P (1965). Studies of the prognosis in Hodgkin's disease. Acta Radiol (Suppl) 245:5–125.

22. Ihde DC, DeVita VT (1975). Osteonecrosis of the femoral heads in patients with lymphoma treated with intermittent combination chemotherapy. Cancer 36:1585–1588.

23. Timothy AR, Tucker AK, Park WM and Cannell LB (1978). Osteonecrosis in Hodgkin's disease. Brit J Radiol 51:328–332.

15. Chemotherapy (MVPP) for Stage IIIB/IV Hodgkin's disease with an assessment of prognostic factors

W. P. STEWARD [1], J. WAGSTAFF [1], I. D. TODD [2]
and D. CROWTHER [1]
Departments of [1] Medical Oncology and [2] Radiotherapy, Christie Hospital and Holt Radium Institute, Manchester, UK

Of all patients presenting with Hodgkin's disease, in excess of 30 % will have Clinical Stage (CS) IIIB or IV disease or will be found to have Pathologic Stage (PS) IIIB/IV disease following staging laparotomy. Prior to the use of combination chemotherapy with mustine, vincristine, procarbazine and prednisolone (MOPP) [1], the prognosis for such patients was bleak. With the advent of the MOPP regimen a high percentage of durable complete remissions could be obtained. The dramatic improvement in survival for these patients has, however, led to a popular misconception that advanced stage Hodgkin's Disease is a readily curable malignancy. Unfortunately, despite drug and dosage alterations, little advance has been made in the 20 years since the introduction of MOPP and 30–40 % of patients will die using currently available therapy [2–4].

In 1968, a new combination of chemotherapy was introduced in which vinblastine was substituted for vincristine in the MOPP regimen and prednisolone was given with every course. These courses (MVPP) were repeated every 6 weeks. This approach has been attended by fewer side effects than MOPP and the complete remission (CR) rate, relapse-free survival (RFS) and overall survival were equally good, if not better [5]. The schedule introduced originally involved 4 years chemotherapy but an approach in Manchester using MVPP to 6 courses beyond CR with a treatment period less than 1 year has been attended by no reduction in efficacy [6]. The aim of achieving minimal exposure to chemotherapy without reducing efficacy was to reduce the potential risk of the development of second malignancies in patients cured of Hodgkins's disease, a risk estimated to be as high as 10 % [7, 8].

Because it has been demonstrated that relapse following CR is attended by poor results using salvage chemotherapy [9, 10], and because relapses following chemotherapy are more frequent in areas where there was previously bulky disease [11], a decision was taken to give radiotherapy to those areas after completion of MVPP.

Materials and methods

One hundred-eighteen patients with histologically confirmed and centrally reviewed diagnosis of Hodgkin's disease were entered between 1975 and 1982. Patient characteristics are shown in Table I. Patients were excluded from entry if their age was outside the range 16–65, they had received previous cytotoxic therapy or they had any pre-existing malignancy. Routine investigations initially included a FBC, ESR, biochemical screen, liver function tests and a chest radiograph. If the results of these investigations and full physical examination resulted in the patients being staged as CS IIIB or IV, CAT scans of the abdomen were performed (if chest x-ray was abnormal, lung CAT scans were usually obtained). Clinical Stages IA-IIIA were referred for staging laparotomy resulting in downstage to PS IIIB or IV in 27 patients.

A clinician's assessment was made as to whether the liver was involved with lymphoma and took into account both physical examination and the results of radiological and biochemical investigations (the elevation of two or more enzymes was taken as being significantly abnormal). It was appreciated that in several cases such an assessment may not have accurately reflected involvement of the liver with lymphoma though confirmation of a clinical impression of involvement was obtained by histologic proof in several instances.

Response was assessed by standard criteria, a complete remission being defined as the disappearance of all known disease and all previously abnormal investigations. Partial remission was a 50% or more decrease in the

Table I. Patient characteristics

	Number	%
Total	118	
Sex: Male	83	70
Female	35	30
Age years (mean)	38	
Stage IIIB	30	25
IVA	21	18
IVB	67	57
Bulk disease	59	50
Pathology LP	12	11
NS	30	25
MC	65	55
LD	11	9
Liver involved	44	37
Bone marrow involved	13	11
Lung parenchyma involved	22	19

sum of the products of perpendicular diameters of measurable lesions, lasting for more than 4 weeks. Progression of disease was defined as the appearance of new lesions or an increase of greater than 25% in the sum of the products of perpendicular diameters of measurable lesions lasting more than 4 weeks. Static disease amounted to neither a 25% increase nor a 50% decrease in the size of measurable lesions.

Several variables were considered in the following analyses, including age, sex, stage, histology, bone marrow and liver involvement, individual liver enzymes, serum albumin and LDH, hemoglobin, lymphocyte count and ESR, bulky disease, B symptoms, performance status and remission achieved. Survival curves were calculated according to the method of Kaplan and Meier [12] and tests for differences in survival distributions were based on the logrank test [13]. Cox's proportional hazards model [14] was used to determine the most significant variables that were related to survival.

Treatment with MVPP was given in cycles every six weeks until CR was achieved, followed by a further 6 cycles to consolidate remission. No more than 10 cycles were given to any one patient. The regimen comprised mustine 6 mg/m^2, vinblastine 6 mg/m^2 both given iv days 1 and 8, with procarbazine 100 mg/m^2 and prednisolone 40 mg both given daily on days 1–14. A FBC was obtained before each course was given. Hematologic toxicity was graded according to the WHO criteria and drug doses were modified if toxicity occurred. Each new cycle was given at full dosage but if the blood count was low, a delay of chemotherapy with subsequent full dosage rather than dose reduction was the preferred option. If, at day 8, Grade 1 toxicity occurred, 50% dose was given. If Grade II toxicity occurred the course was aborted and, when possible, the next cycle was started after a delay of 2–4 weeks. If other evidence of severe toxicity occurred modification of therapy was at the discretion of the physician in charge.

Areas of previous bulky disease (mass $\geqslant 5$ cm) were irradiated at the end of chemotherapy in all patients who achieved CR. Radiotherapy was given with minimal margins around the initial tumor as 8 fractions in 10 days. A dose of 2500 cGy using a 4 MV linear accelerator was prescribed.

Results

A total of 735 courses of MVPP were given to the total patient group with a median of 7 (range 1–10) courses given to each patient. At the time of analysis, the median duration of follow-up was 66 months (range 15–97 months).

The complete response rate was 74% and a further 20 patients (17%) achieved a partial response. The median number of courses of MVPP to the time of CR was 2. The 5-year survival of the total patient group was 73 % and of the 42 patients at risk beyond 5 years, 4 have died (3 of Hodgkin's disease and 1 of acute myelogenous leukemia). The 5-year relapse free survival of the 87 patients achieving a CR was 86 %.

Analysis of 25 variables was performed to identify factors which were of prognostic significance. On logrank analysis, factors found to significantly predict survival were remission achieved ($p < 0.0001$), age ($p = 0.0002$), serum LDH level ($p = 0.004$), stage ($p = 0.008$) and serum AST level ($p = 0.03$). Because the remission status was of paramount importance, factors which could have predicted an increased likelihood of achieving a CR were examined but none were found to be significant. Similarly, when these factors were examined to identify a population which could be predicted to have a prolonged relapse-free survival, none were identified which reached levels of significance.

Because several of the factors may have been inter-related, a Cox's multivariate analysis was done to identify factors of independant significance, and once again achievement of a complete remission was found to be the most important predictor of survival (Table II). Stage III disease became the second most important followed by the serum LDH level and finally the age of the patient (lower values being associated with longer survival). Because, at the time when treatment decisions are made at the patient's first visit, the response status is unknown, and cannot be predicted, a multivariate analysis was repeated without taking remission status into account. Low age, Stage III disease, and female sex became the most accurate predictive model of prolonged survival (Table III).

Table II. Cox multivariate analysis of factors affecting survival

Factor	p-value	Favorable feature
Remission	<0.001	Low value
Stage	<0.001	Stage III
LDH (log)	0.013	Low value
Age (log)	0.036	Low value

Table III. Cox multivariate analysis of factors affecting survival excluding remission status

Factor	p-value	Favorable feature
Age (log)	<0.001	Low value
Stage	0.006	Stage III
Sex	0.036	Female

The toxicity of this regimen was moderate; the majority of the patients experienced nausea and vomiting lasting for 12–24 hours after each injection (worse on day 1). Despite this, in most cases the planned number of courses of MVPP could be given. In only 7 cases was the number of courses reduced and the treatment substituted with alternative regimens, in 4 cases substituting chlorambucil for mustine.

Seven patients died during treatment from causes not directly related to Hodgkin's disease. Of these, three had documented infections, two had cerebrovascular accidents demonstrated at autopsy and two died suddenly at home without undergoing postmortem examination.

Discussion

The results of this study are similar to those from most other institutions treating advanced stage Hodgkin's disease with various combinations of chemotherapy. The complete response rate of 74% is lower than the 80% achieved at the NCI using MOPP [15] but the 5-year survival of 73% compares favorably. In keeping with the experience of others, relapse and death from Hodgkin's disease is uncommon beyond 5 years.

Neurotoxicity is an often distressing side effect associated with the vincristine included in the MOPP regimen and this was not seen in patients on MVPP. In other respects the toxicity was similar.

In common with all other series in which multivariate analysis of prognostic factors has been performed, the most important single factor predictive of prolonged survival in patients with advanced stage Hodgkin's disease is the achievment of CR. We did not, however, confirm the results of some series which have found the presence of B symptoms or different histologic subtypes to be of prognostic significance [15, 16].

In this series radiotherapy was given to sites of previous bulky disease and the possible value of this policy may be borne out by the fact that in no patient was the site of relapse only within areas treated with radiotherapy. For the majority of patients this treatment policy provides prolonged relapse-free survival. Unfortunately, there is still a high proportion of patients who will not be cured and, from a careful analysis of a small group of pretreatment risk factors, those who are unlikely to be treated adequately with this regimen can be identified. Clearly, alternative policies need to be adopted for such patients, possibly with alternating cross-resistant regimens of chemotherapy. Although only one patient has so far developed secondary leukemia, the follow-up of the total patient group is not long enough to allay the fear that the combination of as many as ten courses of MVPP and radiotherapy may result in an unacceptable number of second malignancies. For the group of patients who can be predicted to have a high chance of being cured of Hodgkin's disease, particularly the young patients with Stage IIIB disease, consideration must be made to reducing the amount of treatment.

References

1. DeVita VT and Serpick A (1967). Combination chemotherapy in the treatment of advanced Hodgkin's disease. Proc Amer Assoc Cancer Res 8:13.
2. Frei E III, Luce JK, Gamble JF et al. (1973). Combination chemotherapy in advanced Hodgkin's disease: Induction and maintenance of remission. Ann Intern Med 79:376–382.
3. Moore MR, Jones SE, Bull JM et al. (1973). MOPP chemotherapy for advanced Hodgkin's disease — prognostic factors in 81 patients. Cancer 32:52–60.
4. Bonadonna G, Zucali R, Monfardini S et al. (1975). Combination chemotherapy of Hodgkin's disease with adriamycin, bleomycin, vinblastine and imidazole carboxamide versus MOPP. Cancer 36:252–259.
5. Sutcliffe SB, Wrigley PFM, Peto J et al. (1978). MVPP chemotherapy regimen for advanced Hodgkin's disease. Brit Med J 1:679–683.
6. Crowther D (1981). Hodgkin's disease: A curable malignancy. Clin Radiol 32:241–250.
7. Pederson-Bjergaard J and Larsen SO (1982). Incidence of acute non-lymphocytic leukaemia, pre-leukaemia, and acute myeloproliferative syndrome up to 10 years after treatment of Hodgkin's disease. N Engl J Med 307:965–971.
8. Coltman CA Jr. and Dixon DO (1982). Second malignancies complicating Hodgkin's disease: A Southwest Oncology Group 10-year follow up. Cancer Treat Rep 66:1023–1029.
9. Krikorian J, Portlock GS, Robertson A et al. (1978). Treatment of advanced Hodgkin's disease with adriamycin, bleomycin, vinblastine and imidazole carboxamide (ABVD) after failure of MOPP therapy. Cancer 41:2107–2111.
10. Porzig K, Portlock C, Robertson A et al. (1978). Treatment of advanced Hodgkin's disease with B-CAVe following MOPP failure Cancer 41:1670–1675.
11. Young R, Canellos G, Chabner B et al. (1978). Patterns of relapse in advanced Hodgkin's disease treated with combination chemotherapy. Cancer 42:1001–1007.
12. Kaplan EL and Meier P (1958). Non-parametric estimation from incomplete observations. Amer Stat Assoc J 53:457–481.
13. Peto R and Peto J (1972). Asymptotically efficient rank invariant test procedures. J Royal Statist Soc A. 35:185–207.
14. Cox DR (1972). Regression models and life tables. J Roy Stat Soc B. 34:187–220.
15. DeVita VT, Simon RM, Hubbard SM et al. (1980). Curability of advanced Hodgkin's disease with chemotherapy. Ann Intern Med 92:587–595.
16. Coltman CA (1981). Chemotherapy of advanced Hodgkin's disease. Semin Oncol 7:155–173.

16. Incidence of liver involvement and correlation of biopsy results with Ann Arbor clinical criteria and response to chemotherapy in advanced Hodgkin's disease: A Southwest Oncology Group study

C. J. FABIAN[1], C. M. MANSFIELD[2], D. O. DIXON[3],
S. E. JONES[4], P. M. GROZEA[5], F. S. MORRISON[6], J. K. WEICK[7]
and R. M. O'BRYAN[8]

[1] University of Kansas Medical Center, Kansas City, Kansas;
[2] Jefferson Medical College, Philadelphia, Pennsylvania; [3] Southwest Oncology Group Biostatistical Center, Houston, Texas; [4] University of Arizona Health Science Center, Tucson, Arizona; [5] Oklahoma Medical Research Foundation, Oklahoma City, Oklahoma; [6] University of Mississippi Medical Center, Jackson, Mississippi; [7] Cleveland Clinic Foundation, Cleveland, Ohio; [8] Henry Ford Hospital, Detroit, Michigan, USA

The reported incidence of liver involvement in Hodgkin's disease in laparotomy based series varies from 8–19% [1–6]. The variation is probably related to the proportion of patients in the series with early clinical stage disease. Determination of liver status is critical for patients who are otherwise Stage IIIA or less as it would indicate a definite need for chemotherapy if positive. However, knowledge of liver status, at least at restaging, may be important for later stage patients as well. Assessment of liver involvement by clinical means is fraught with error. Several authors have noted the lack of correlation of liver function tests, liver/spleen scan, and wedge liver biopsy results obtained at laparotomy [1–6]. Correlation of CAT scan of the liver with positive and negative liver biopsies in a sizable cadre of patients has not been done.

Percutaneous liver biopsy series have a lower rate of positivity (5%) than laparotomy series and thus a high false-negative rate has been suggested [7]. Although the incidence of positivity in peritoneoscopy series is higher than percutaneous series, the false-negative rate of peritoneoscopy in Hodgkin's disease is really unclear. The proportion of previously untreated patients in each clinical stage who have biopsy proven liver involvement has not been described. Given this and the difficulty of proper evaluation of the liver, there is a tremendous variation in the vigor with which oncologists pursue initial or restaging evaluation of the liver.

In 1978 the Southwest Oncology Group (SWOG) initiated a large randomized trial in Stage III and IV patients to examine the relative efficacy of low dose involved field radiation as consolidation versus no further treatment after complete remission (CR) had been induced with chemotherapy. Liver biopsies were required for all previously untreated patients entering the study for the first four years.

The following analysis focuses on correlation of several variables regarding liver involvement in Hodgkin's disease most of which have not been adequately studied in a large number of identically treated patients with Stages III and IV Hodgkin's disease:

1) Correlation of percent positive liver biopsies with clinical stage.
2) Correlation of Ann Arbor clinical criteria with liver biopsy results.
3) Correlation of CAT scans with liver biopsy results.
4) Incidence of false-negative percutaneous and laparoscopy obtained biopsies in patients who subsequently have a laparotomy obtained biopsy.
5) Effect of positive Ann Arbor criteria and/or positive liver biopsy on subsequent response to chemotherapy.

Materials and methods

SWOG 7808 was opened in June of 1978 and is currently ongoing. The schema is given in Fig. 1. Doses and scheduling for drug and radiation therapy are given in Tables I and II, respectively. The objective of the study is to evaluate the potential for low dose involved field radiotherapy (LD IF XRT) to prolong duration of CR after this has been induced with six cycles of MOP-BAP chemotherapy (Table I). All patients without prior radiation who attain CR are randomized to receive LD IF XRT (to all initially involved sites except bone marrow) or no further treatment. Patients in partial remission (PR) at the end of six cycles of MOP-BAP, without residual bone marrow involvement, receive LD IF XRT. Patients relapsing after radiation therapy may be entered, but receive only induction chemo-

Table I. MOP-BAP chemotherapy doses

Nitrogen Mustard	6 mg/m^2 iv d 1
Vincristine	1.4 mg/m^2 (maximum 2 mg) iv d 1& 8
Procarbazine	100 mg/m^2 po d 2–7 & 9–12
Prednisone	40 mg/m^2 po d 2–7 & 9–12 cycles 1& 4
Doxorubicin	30 mg/m^2 iv d 8
Bleomycin	2 mg/m^2 iv d 1& 8

Courses are repeated every 28 days for 6 cycles. Patients with impaired marrow reserve defined as age 65, bone marrow involvement plus cytopenia or patients with radiation of 25% bone marrow bearing areas begin treatment at 50% dose reduction of nitrogen mustard, procarbazine and doxorubicin

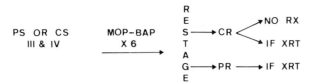

Figure 1. Outline of SWOG 7808. Clinical (CS) or Pathologic (PS) Stage III and IV Hodgkin's patients all receive 6 monthly cycles of MOP-BAP (See Table I for doses) and are restaged. Complete responders (CR) are randomized between no further therapy and low dose involved field radiation (IF XRT) to all previously involved sites. Partial responders all receive radiation therapy to all previously and presently involved sites (See Table II for XRT doses).

Table II. Low dose involved radiation therapy doses

CR	
All previously involved nodes [a]	2000r/150r/fx
Liver	1500r/120r/fx
Lung	1000r/100r/fx
Spleen/pedicle	2000r/125r/fx

PR
As for CR, except for residual, nodal areas receive 2500 rad

[a]   If mesenteric nodes involved, whole abdomen is irradiated to 1500 rad and then identified masses on CAT scan are further boosted to 2000 rad.

Radiation starts 6 weeks after day 1 of the last cycle of chemotherapy if WBC ≥ 3000 and platelets are $\geq 100,000$. Otherwise treatment is delayed until these minimum counts are present. A 3-week rest is advised between irradiation of large volumes or major lymph node areas

therapy and are not part of the randomized consolidation phase of the study.

To be eligible, patients must have Clinical (CS) or Pathological Stage (PS) III or IV Hodgkin's disease, normal renal function tests, no prior history of congestive heart failure, and vital capacity and forced expiratory volume of at least 75% of normal. Patients may not have had prior chemotherapy. Patients not meeting these requirements were considered ineligible. Central lymphoma panel pathology review is required and is complete for approximately 60% of the patients.

Prestudy staging requirements are listed in Table III. Since radiation therapy was to be given to all initially involved sites, including liver, for patients randomized to that treatment, liver biopsy was initially required on all patients without prior radiation therapy. Although liver biopsy via peritoneoscopy or laparotomy was encouraged, the percutaneous method was allowed as well.

Table III. Prestudy staging requirements

CBC, Platelets
BUN, Creatinine, Uric acid
Alk phos, Bilirubin, SGOT, LDH
Pulmonary functions, EKG
Chest x-ray
CAT Scan or Abdomen or Liver Spleen Scan
Staging laparotomy [a] or All of following
Lymphangiogram [b]
Bone Marrow BX
Liver BX (Percutaneous or Peritoneoscopy)

---

[a] Staging laparotomy includes sampling of all lymph node groups, splenectomy, wedge and needle biopsy of the liver, and bone marrow biopsy.
[b] Lymphangiogram is omitted if abdominal and pelvic disease is present on CAT scan, if patient is >65 years of age or has had prior radiation therapy.

In July of 1982 the requirement for liver biopsy was amended so that patients with Clinical Stage IIIA or less, and patients with strong Ann Arbor clinical criteria for a positive liver were no longer required to undergo liver biopsy, although this was encouraged. The rationale for the change in biopsy requirements were: 1) patients with Clinical Stage IIIA or less disease had only a 15% incidence of liver involvement; and 2) patients with overwhelming clinical evidence for liver involvement were often too ill to undergo peritoneoscopy or laparotomy and percutaneous biopsies in these patients were sometimes negative. If these patients were later randomized to radiation therapy, uncertainty arose whether to radiate the liver or not. Pathologic criteria for liver involvement included demonstration of Reed-Sternberg cells or mononuclear varient [2]. Ann Arbor clinical criteria for liver involvement consisted of a) hepatomegaly plus an elevated alkaline phosphatase, b) elevation of two liver function tests (SGOT and alkaline phosphatase) or c) an abnormal liver scan and at least one abnormal liver function test [8]. In most cases the actual radiology reports as well as pathology reports were reviewed in addition to the prestudy forms.

Response status is not determined until six cycles of MOP-BAP and restaging has been completed, unless the patient is removed from study before that time. All initially abnormal tests must be completed at restaging. For the purpose of this analysis complete response rates are those seen after completion of chemotherapy *not* consolidation radiation therapy in patients so treated. Patients with seriously inadequate prestudy or response determination parameters are considered eligible but not evaluable. Patients with designations of early death, lost to follow-up or refused further treatment before a response determination could be made as well as those with an inadequate trial due to toxicity are considered partially evaluable and are included in response determination denominators.

Results

Two hundred fifteen patients underwent a liver biopsy via laparotomy, laparoscopy or percutaneous biopsy (Table IV). Twenty-four percent (52/215) of these biopsies were positive. Incidence of positive liver biopsies in laparotomy staged patients ranged from 15% in Clinical Stage IIIA or less to 48% in patients who were Clinical Stage IVB (Table V). The IIIA or less patients rendered IVB by liver biopsy were not rendered PS IVB by any other means (lung or bone marrow). In fact, overall incidence of liver involvement (24%) in this study was more common than bone marrow involvement (17%).

There was little correlation betwen Ann Arbor clinical criteria and liver biopsy results (Table VI). Fifty-six percent of patients who were liver biopsy positive were clinical criteria negative. Conversely, 21% of patients who were liver biopsy negative were Ann Arbor criteria positive. There was no convenient way of predicting which Ann Arbor criteria positive patients

Table IV. Distribution of type of liver biopsy in 215 patients

LAP	152
LAP alone	114
PC+LAP	29
Laparoscopy+LAP	9
PC+Laparoscopy	63
Percutaneous alone	50
Laparoscopy alone	13

LAP = Laparotomy
PC = Percutaneous

Table V. Incidence of positive liver BX in laparotomy staged patients by clinical stage

% Positive	(No. Patients)	Clinical Stage
15	(9/58)	IIIA
35	(13/37)	IIIB
35	(6/17)	IVA
48	(22/46)	IVB

Table VI. Lack of correlation between liver BX and Ann Arbor clinical criteria

Liver biopsy + AA −	56 % (29/52)
Liver biopsy − AA +	21 % (35/163)

Table VII. Correlation between liver biopsy, CAT and liver scans

	Liver scan neg	CAT scan neg
Pos liver BX	62 % (25/40)	81 % (17/21)
Neg liver BX	69 % (67/97)	87 % (76/97)

would have a positive liver biopsy. Median number of abnormal liver parameters was 3 in the biopsy negative group and 4 in the biopsy positive group. Both liver and CAT scans had a high incidence of false-negative scans. Sixty-two percent of the patients having a positive liver biopsy had a negative liver scan and 81 % having a positive biopsy had a negative CAT scan (Table VII).

Twenty-nine patients had a negative percutaneous biopsy and subsequently had a laparotomy directed biopsy. Twenty-eight percent of the negative percutaneous biopsies (8/29) were found to be positive at laparotomy. Nine patients with a negative peritoneoscopy obtained biopsy underwent subsequent laparotomy. Eleven percent (1/9) of these patients had a positive liver biopsy at laparotomy.

Patients who had either positive Ann Arbor clinical criteria or a positive liver biopsy have complete response rates that are 10–13 % less than patients who are Ann Arbor clinical criteria and liver biopsy negative. However, this difference was not significant. Table VIII gives complete response rates for evaluable patients by Ann Arbor criteria and liver biopsy status. CR rates vary from 61 % for Ann Arbor positive biopsy positive patients to 74 % for Ann Arbor negative biopsy negative patients. Table IX gives complete

Table VIII. Complete response rates by Ann Arbor clinical criteria and liver biopsy status

AA+	Bx+	AA+	Bx− LAP only
61 %	(13/21)	64 %	(14/22)
AA−	Bx+	AA−	Bx− LAP only
62 %	(16/26)	74 %	(58/78)

Table IX. Complete response of all partially and fully evaluable patients by stage to 6 cycles of MOP-BAP

IIIA	77%
IIIB	64%
IVA	62%
IVB	45%

response rates by pathologic stage to six induction cycles of MOP-BAP chemotherapy for all partially and fully evaluable patients in #7808 (whether or not they had an initial liver biopsy). These rates do not include PR converted to CR after radiation consolidation. Complete remission rates range from 77% for Stage IIIA patients to 45% for Stage IVB patients. In this study as well as previous SWOG studies, patients who have their liver biopsied have higher complete response rates than those who do not.

Discussion

Before the Ann Arbor clinical criteria were devised, multiple investigators had noted that neither liver function tests, physical examination or liver scan correlated well with the presence of Hodgkin's disease. Alkaline phosphatase was too sensitive and the liver scan was not sensitive enough [1, 4, 6]. Consequently, in 1971, a combination of parameters was delineated as clinical evidence for Hodgkin's disease in the liver consisting of either: 1) hepatomegaly plus an elevated alkaline phosphatase; 2) elevation of two liver function tests or; 3) an abnormal liver scan and at least one abnormal liver function test. As our results indicate, these criteria are not very sensitive as 56% of patients with negative criteria had positive biopsies. They are also non-specific as 21% of all biopsy negative and 22% of laparotomy biopsy negative were criteria positive.

DeVita et al. found a 5% (4/73) incidence of positive liver biopsies by Menghini needle percutaneous technique [7]. In another group of patients, he found a 16% incidence (6/38) of positive liver biopsies by peritoneoscopy and thus thought there was an unacceptable false-negative rate with the percutaneous technique. We found a 28% false-negative rate (8/29) in patients having a negative percutaneous biopsy who later underwent laparotomy. Eleven percent (1/9) of the patients who had a negative peritoneoscopy followed by laparotomy had a positive biopsy at laparotomy. Although the percent of false-negatives with peritoneoscopy appear smaller than with the percutaneous technique, the number of patients having both peritoneoscopy and laparotomy is too small to draw definite conclusions.

Despite the non-specificity of clinical parameters and high false-negative rate of percutaneous biopsies, large study groups often use clinical as well as a variety of biopsy results to determine liver involvement. Luckily, liver involvement per se does not appear to be an important independent prognostic variable determining response rate as 61% of liver biopsy positive as opposed to 72% of laparotomy biopsy negative patients had a complete response to 6 cycles of MOP-BAP chemotherapy.

This study does point out the frequency of liver involvement in Clinical Stages IIIB (35%), IVA (35%) and IVB (48%) patients. This high incidence underscores the need for aggressive restaging of the liver with laparotomy or possibly laparoscopy when clinical CR has been achieved in IIIB, IVA and IVB patients before discontinuing treatment.

In addition, this study supports the use of staging laparotomy in patients who are Clinical Stage IIIA or less before a patient is treated with non-systemic therapy due to the 15% incidence of a positive liver biopsies in this group of patients.

Acknowledgements

This investigation was supported in part by the following PHS grant numbers awarded by the National Cancer Institute, DHHS: CA-13612, CA-16957, CA-04919, CA-04915, CA-16385, CA-21116, CA-26766, CA-28862, CA-22411, CA-12644, CA-03389, CA-22433, CA-03195, CA-27057, CA-13238, CA-03352, CA-20319, CA-03096, CA-12213, CA-22416, CA-12014, CA-32102.

References

1. Glatstein E, Guernsey JM, Rosenberg SA and Kaplan HS (1969). The value of laporotomy and splenectomy in the staging of Hodgkin's disease. Cancer 24:709–718.
2. Gilver RL, Brunk SF, Hass CA and Gulesserian HP (1971). Problems of interpretation of liver biopsy in Hodgkin's disease. Cancer 28:1335–1342.
3. Bagley CM, Roth JA, Thomas LB and DeVita VT (1972). Liver biopsy in Hodgkin's disease. Ann Intern Med 76:219–225.
4. Lipton MS, DeNardo GL and Silverman S (1972). Evaluation of the liver and spleen in Hodgkin's disease. I. The value of hepatic scintigraphy. Amer J Med 52:356–361.
5. Piro A, Hellman S and Moloney WC (1972). The influence of laporotomy on management decisions in Hodgkin's disease. Arch Intern Med 130:844–848.
6. Kadin ME, Glatstein E and Drofman RF (1971). Clinicopathologic studies of 117 untreated patients subjected to laparotomy for the staging of Hodgkin's disease. Cancer 27:1277–1294.
7. DeVita VT, Bagley CM, Goodell B et al. (1971). Peritoneoscopy in the staging of Hodgkin's disease. Cancer Res 31:1746–1750.
8. Carbone PP, Kaplan HS, Musshoff K et al. (1971). Report of the Committee on Hodgkin's Disease Staging Classification. Cancer Res 31:1860–1861.

17. Second cancers after treatment in two successive cohorts of patients with early stages of Hodgkin's disease

M. HENRY-AMAR

Département de Statistique Médicale, Institut Gustave Roussy, Villejuif, France

In the recent 20 years, the survival of patients with Hodgkin's disease (HD) has increased due to extensive treatment with radiotherapy (RT) and chemotherapy (CT). However, extensive treatment has its price and there is evidence in the literature [1-28] that modern aggressive treatment may induce severe complications such as second cancers (SC). The aim of this study was to compare the risk of SC in two randomized successive cohorts of patients with HD of Clinical Stages I and II that were followed for 7 to 20 years after the end of their initial treatment.

Materials and methods

Patient populations and treatment

From 1964 to 1976, two successive cohorts of patients with HD of Clinical Stages I and II were enrolled in two successive trials (H1 and H2) [29-32] and treated by the members of the Radiotherapy-Chemotherapy Cooperative Group of the European Organization for Research and Treatment of Cancer (EORTC). A histology review committee (R. Gerard-Marchant and J. A. M. Van Unnik) assessed the slides of all the patients. Three hundred and sixty-nine patients were treated according to the H1 protocol (1964-1971) and 300 according to the H2 protocol (1972-1976). In the first trial H1 [29-31], the initial treatment was regional radiation by telecobalt or megavoltage therapy with the use of the mantle field or the inverted Y technique. A total dose of 40 Gy was delivered over 4-week period. No radiation was given on the other side of the diaphragm. Four weeks after the end of irradiation, patients who obtained complete remission were randomly assigned to 2 groups: a) those with no further treatment, or b) those given a weekly injection vinblastine (VLB) for 2 years. In the second trial H2 [32], only patients with supra-diaphragmatic presentations were included. They were treated using the same mantle field technique followed by either paraaortic and spleen irradiation (40 Gy over a 4-week period) or paraaortic irradiation and splenectomy at random. Moreover, patients with mixed cellularity or lymphocytic depleted histologic types were given CT comparing VLB alone to VLB + procarbazine (PCZ) for two years after randomization.

In the event of relapse, the physicians were free to chose the mode of therapy. Localized RT alone was usually given for the first recurrence (H1 and H2 cohorts) or extension of the disease (H1 cohort), and very often followed by VLB. When a second relapse or an extranodal relapse occurred, more extensive CT was administered. Of the 122 patients (H1: 68 patients; H2: 54 patients) with relapse(s) who were treated by extensive CT, 52 (25 + 27) received MOPP alone, 29 (21 + 8) received MOPP plus another drug combination, 17 (11 + 6) received PCZ in combination, and 24 (11 + 13) patients received other alkylating agents in combination. The administered doses were not registered.

Treatment categories

The following 3 categories of treatment intensities were defined, which took into account the total treatment administered: 1) No relapse: initial treatment only; 2) No polychemotherapy for relapse: patients who had relapse(s) and whose relapse(s) were not treated with polychemotherapy; 3) Polychemotherapy for relapse: initial treatment followed by extensive CT for relapse. Extensive CT is defined as a combination of 3 or more drugs used cyclically in a coordinate regimen (no number of cycles specified).

Analysis of the data

The computation of the time at risk for SC was as follows: Patients were classified according to the total treatment received. The time at risk for SC began 4 weeks after the end of RT and ended at the date of death, date of SC occurrence, date of last known status, or May 1, 1984, whichever came first. The analyses of the data described above were considered as time-dependent covariate analyses where the time-dependent covariate is the status of the patients changing at the time of new therapy for relapse. Three approaches were used to estimate the association between treatment and risk: 1) Comparison of cancer incidence between the population of patients with HD and the general population based on the accumulation of person-years of observation. Patients with multiple secondary neoplasms (two in our series) were considered to have had only one SC. The ratio of the number of SC observed among the patients with HD (O) to the expected number

(E) was computed from general population cancer incidence data with the use of age-, sex-, and calendar year-specific cancer incidence rates published in France [33] and Holland [34]. The confidence limits of O/E were obtained with the use of the Poisson distribution of O [35]. The test statistic (O-E)$**$2/E was compared to a Chi-square distribution with one degree of freedom; 2) Comparison of occurrence of SC in the two cohorts based on the Mantel-Haenszel procedure [36]. Cumulative proportions of SC were estimated as a function of time since initial treatment and then compared using the logrank test. The Cox model [37, 38] was used to assess the risk induced by the therapy after adjustment on nuisance variables such as age, sex or clinical stage; 3) Comparison of occurrence of SC in the 3 treatment categories by cohort based on the Mantel-Byar approach [39]. A quantification of the relationship between the time of occurrence of SC and concomitant variables such as age, sex and clinical stage was done by the Cox model. In this model, relative risk (RR) of SC can be estimated when adjusted for variable follow-up periods.

Data were collected, verified and analysed in the Département de Statistiques Médicales, Institut Gustave Roussy, Villejuif, using an interactive database management system (PIGAS) [40].

Results

Type of SC observed

Table I lists the SC observed after the diagnosis of HD. Among the H1 cohort, we observed 21 SC: 14 solid tumors (ST), 3 non-Hodgkin's lymphomas (NHL), and 4 acute leukemias (AL). Among the H2 cohort, we observed 15 SC: 11 ST, 2 NHL and 2 AL. The median time to SC were 10 years (range: 2–16 yr) in the H1 cohort and 6 years (range: 3–10 yr) in the H2 cohort. None of the SC observed in the no polychemotherapy and polychemotherapy groups occurred before the appearance of the relapse. Time lapse to SC ranged from 0 to 12 years (H1) and from 2 to 6 years (H2) after retreatment for relapse. In the H1 cohort, ST include 3 basal cell carcinomas, 1 melanoma, 2 breast cancers, 1 parotid gland cancer, 2 bronchial cancer, 2 esophageal cancers, 1 testicular cancer, 1 bladder cancer and 1 anal cancer; they include 2 basal cell carcinomas, 1 breast cancer, 1 pharyngeal cancer, 2 bronchial cancers, 2 kidney cancers, 2 bowel cancers and 1 anal cancer in the H2 cohort. Of the 6 AL observed, 5 occurred after MOPP therapy and 1 after regional RT alone (H1 cohort). Times to AL were 5, 5, 6, 6 and 10 years after MOPP therapy and 7 years after diagnosis of HD respectively. The AL were classified as M2, M4 (2 patients) and M6 (FAB classification); the other two were initiated with a dysmyelopoietic syndrome. No karyotype analysis was done.

Table 1. SC observed by cohort, treatment categories and localization

	H1 COHORT	H2 COHORT
		Relapse-free patients
SC in a non-irradiated area	Testicular cancer, Basal cell carcinoma Non-Hodgkin's lymphoma Acute leukemia	Basal cell carcinoma (2 patients) Kidney cancer, Anal cancer Non-Hodgkin lymphoma
SC in an irradiated area	Esophageal cancer Breast cancer (2 patients)	Bronchial cancer, Pharyngeal cancer, Breast cancer, Kidney cancer, Bowel cancer (2 patients)
		No-polychemotherapy for relapse
SC in an irradiated area	Basal cell carcinoma Esophageal cancer, Bronchial cancer Parotid gland cancer	Bronchial cancer
		Polychemotherapy for relapse
SC in a non-irradiated area	Melanoma, Anal cancer Non-Hodgkin's lymphoma (2 patients)	Non-Hodgkin's lymphoma
SC in an irradiated area	Basal cell carcinoma, Bronchial cancer	
Possible CT-induced SC	Bladder cancer Acute leukemia (3 patients)	Acute leukemia (2 patients)

Table II. General population comparisons: Risks of SC

Treatment category	No. of patients	Median follow-up time, yr (range)	Type of SC (No.)		RR = O/E	95% confidence limits for RR	p-value
H1 cohort							
No relapse	188	11 (2–20)	Solid T.	(6)	1.66	0.61–3.61	ns
			Leukemia	(1)	12	0.30–67	ns
No polychemotherapy for relapse	113	7 (0–18)	Solid T.	(4)	3.72	1.01–9.54	=0.0192
			Leukemia	(0)			
Polychemotherapy for relapse	68	9 (1–19)	Solid T.	(7)	14	5.70–29	<0.0001
			Leukemia	(3)	250	52–731	<0.0001
All patients	369	10 (0–20)	Solid T.	(17)	3.28	1.91–5.25	<0.0001
			Leukemia	(4)	34	9.24–87	<0.0001
H2 cohort							
No relapse	217	8 (0–12)	Solid T.	(11)	3.30	1.65–5.90	<0.0001
			Leukemia	(0)			
No polychemotherapy for relapse	29	8 (0–11)	Solid T.	(1)	3.35	0.08–19	ns
			Leukemia	(0)			
Polychemotherapy for relapse	54	6 (0–11)	Solid T.	(1)	4.18	0.11–23	ns
			Leukemia	(2)	286	35–1032	<0.0001
All patients	300	8 (0–12)	Solid T.	(13)	3.36	1.79–5.74	<0.0001
			Leukemia	(2)	25	3.03–90	<0.0001

RR = relative risk
NS = not statistically significant at 5% level

422

General population comparisons

The risks of SC relative to the general population (O/E) were calculated among the two cohorts for the overall population and by treatment categories (Table II). In the two cohorts, we observed an excess of SC in the overall population, for both ST and AL. Although this excess is primarily due to the polychemotherapy group in the H1 cohort, this is not true in the H2 cohort where 11 of the 15 SC observed are included in the relapse-free patients group. Moreover, one can note that the O/E ratios for AL are similar in the two cohorts. The results observed were not modified when the 6 skin cancers were omitted from the analysis. Considering the 5 NHL observed, the same conclusions could be drawn from the data as for AL.

Comparison between the two cohorts

The cumulative proportions of SC by cohort are plotted on Fig. 1. In these series the probability of occurrence of SC are 1.8% and 3.5% seven years after the diagnosis of HD in the H1 and H2 cohorts, respectively. Probabilities of occurrence of SC are continuously greater in the H2 cohort than in the H1 cohort but the difference is not statistically significant ($p = 0.11$). As the majority of the SC are included in the relapse-free patients group in the H2 cohort, it is of interest to compare the two groups including relapse-free patients which only represent 61% of the entire group. Using the Cox model to eliminate the influence of age, which had a great influence on occurrence of SC (RR = 6.22, $p < 0.0001$), we found a risk for H2 cohort relative to H1 equal to 3.68 ($p = 0.0416$).

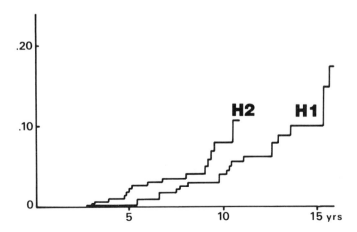

Figure 1. Cumulative proportion of SC by cohort for all types of SC (logrank test: $p = 0.11$).

Comparisons among the 3 treatment categories by cohort

The cumulative proportions of SC by treatment categories are plotted on Fig. 2 and 3 for the H1 and the H2 cohort separately. The risk of SC was significantly higher in the polychemotherapy group than in the other groups ($p = 0.0004$) in the H1 cohort (Fig. 2), whereas the difference observed

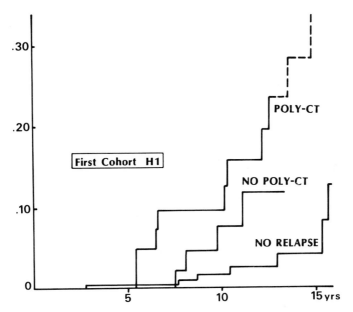

Figure 2. Cohort H1: Cumulative proportion of SC by treatment categories for all types of SC (logrank test: $p = 0.0004$).

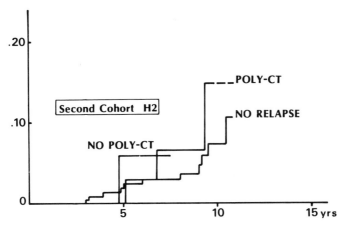

Figure 3. Cohort H2: Cumulative proportion of SC by treatment categories for all types of SC (logrank test: $p = 0.62$).

between the other two groups was not statistically significant. Conversely, we did not observe any significant difference between the 3 treatment categories among the H2 cohort (Fig. 3) but the numbers of SC observed are very small in the no polychemotherapy and the polychemotherapy groups, 1 and 3 respectively. Using the Cox model, the RR of SC was estimated both for polychemotherapy and no polychemotherapy relative to no relapse in the two cohorts separately. All RR estimates were adjusted for the potential confounding effects of sex, clinical stage and age at diagnosis. Table III gives the various RR for a model allowing for all the variables simultaneously. In both cohorts, age had a large influence whereas polychemotherapy had a significant influence on occurrence of SC in the H1 cohort only. The same conclusions were made when all ST or all possible radiation-induced cancers were considered separately.

Table III. Cox model: Relative risk by cohort for a model allowing for all the variables simultaneously

Variables	H1 cohort		H2 cohort	
	RR	p-value	RR	p-value
Sex (F/M)	0.72	ns	1.09	ns
Clinical Stage (II/I)	1.17	ns	0.90	ns
Age (40–70/0–39)	3.80	< 0.001	7.45	< 0.0001
Treatment category:				
No poly-CT/no relapse	1.52	ns	0.96	ns
Poly-CT/no relapse	5.24	< 0.0001	2.64	ns
Global Chi-square	$p < 0.0001$		$p = 0.0023$	

ns = not statistically significant

Discussion

Part of the data reported above have been published [41] but with fewer patients and less follow-up time. The present observations from H1 cohort are very likely nearer to reality than those published in 1983, especially when considering the cumulative proportions of SC. All the conclusions are still in accordance to those previously presented.

Of major interest is the homogeneity of the two cohorts for recruitment, stage, age, sex, and treatment management. Moreover, the patients included were all prospectively followed. The differences between the two cohorts are: 1) the initial paraaortic +/− spleen irradiation which was not performed in the H1 trial; and 2) the relapse treatment which was more often polychemotherapy in the second cohort H2.

Despite the fact that some patients were treated with complementary CT after initial RT, i.e. VLB or VLB + PCZ, there was no statistical difference in observed occurrence of SC among the different sub-groups of patients, especially among the relapse-free patients caregory.

Several conclusions can be drawn from the data. First, in the general population comparisons, the estimated risks of SC are similar in the two cohorts, when considering the overall population. Risks of AL are significantly increased to 200 after polychemotherapy which is consistent with the data of the literature [13, 22]. For the ST results, there are some discrepancies in the results. Risk of ST is significantly increased in the no relapse category in the H2 cohort while it is not different from 1 in the H1 cohort. This may be due to the higher proportion of relapses and the longer delay between initial treatment and SC in the first cohort compared to the second cohort. This is obvious when comparing the cumulative proportions of SC (Fig. 1). Moreover, 3 ST localized in an infra-diaphragmatic irradiated area were observed in the H2 relapse-free patients group, i.e. a left kidney cancer (Grawitz tumor) 10 years after spleen RT, and 2 bowel cancers (sigmoid) 4 and 6 years after RT. No similar localization for ST was observed in the H1 cohort. Secondly, comparison of the three treatment categories pointed out that polychemotherapy for relapse appeared to be the major prognostic factor for SC occurrence in the H1 cohort whereas the increase of the RR is not statistically significant in the H2 cohort (Fig. 2-3, Table III). Anyway, median follow-up time from relapse treatment to date of last known status is rather short in the second cohort and one may object that SC will be observed later. Fig. 3 seems to be in accord with this assertion.

Many papers have emphasized the role of extensive CT used alone or in combination in the development of SC [4-6, 8-25, 27, 28]. RT has also been accused of inducing malignancies [42-44]. Our data are consistent with those of the literature; they demonstrate the existence of a balanced risk between survival probability and therapy-related cancer probability. Although the risk of SC exists, it is always much lower than the risk of relapse, and death, from inadequate treatment. In that perspective, physicians should clearly look at long-term side-effects and avoid aggressive therapy when possible in early stages of HD.

Appendix

Cooperating centres in the Netherlands were Antoni van Leeuwenhoek Ziekenhuis, Amsterdam (M. Burgers, R. Somers); University Hospital, Leiden (P. Thomas); St. Radboud Academic Hospital, Nijmegen (D. Wagener); Rotterdamsch-Radiotherapeutisch Instituut, Rotterdam, (M. Qasim, W. Sizoo); Ziekenhuis Leyenburg, The Hague (H. Kerkhofs); and University

Hospital, Utrecht (H. van Peperzeel). Cooperating centres in Belgium were Institut Jules Bordet, Brussels (J. Henry, J. Lustmann Marechal); Centre René Goffin, La Louvière (J. C. Goffin); Hopital de Bavière, Liège (R. Lemaire); and Academisch Ziekenhuis St. Rafael, Leuven (E. van der Schueren, J. Thomas). The cooperating centre in Italy was Istituto di Radiologia, Universita di Firenze (L. Cionini, G. de Giuli). Cooperating centres in France were Fondation Bergonié, Bordeaux (C. Lagarde); Centre François Baclesse, Caen (J. Abbatucci); Centre Léon Bérard, Lyon (J. Papillon, L. Revol); Centre Antoine Lacassagne, Nice (C. Lalanne, M. Schneider); Hotel-Dieu, Paris (R. Zittoun); Institut Jean Godinet, Reims (A. Cattan); Centre Henri Becquerel, Rouen (H. Piquet); Institut Gustave Roussy, Villejuif (J.L. Amiel, M. Hayat, M. Tubiana); and Institut de Cancérologie et d'Immunogénétique, Hôpital Paul Brousse, Villejuif (G. Mathé).

Acknowledgements

We are grateful to all the physicians who participated in the collection of data. We are also grateful to Mrs. N. Dupouy, Data Manager, Institut Gustave Roussy, for her active collaboration and to A. Kramer, Ph.D., Institut Gustave Roussy, for his assistance in the analysis.

References

1. Berg JW (1967). The incidence of multiple primary cancers. I. Development of further cancers in patients with lymphomas, leukemias, and myeloma. J Nat Cancer Inst 38:741–752.
2. Canellos GP, DeVita VT, Arseneau JC et al. (1975). Second malignancies complicating Hodgkin's disease in remission. Lancet 1:947–949.
3. Rosner F and Grunwald H (1974). Hodgkin's disease and acute leukemia. Report of eight cases and review of the literature. Amer J Med 58:339–353.
4. Arseneau JC, Canellos GP, Johnson R and DeVita VT (1977). Risk of new cancers in patients with Hodgkin's disease. Cancer 40:1912–1916.
5. Brody RS, Schottenfield D and Reid A (1977). Multiple primary cancer risk after therapy for Hodgkin's disease. Cancer 40:1917–1926.
6. Coleman CN, Williams CJ, Flint A et al. (1977). Hematologic neoplasia in patients treated for Hodgkin's disease. N Engl J Med 297:1249–1252.
7. Neufeld H, Weinerman BH and Kemel S (1978). Secondary malignant neoplasms in patients with Hodgkin's disease. JAMA 239:2470–2471.
8. Krikorian JG, Burke JS, Rosenberg SA and Kaplan HS (1979). Occurrence of non-Hodgkin's lymphoma after therapy for Hodgkin's disease. N Engl J Med 300:452–458.
9. Baccarani M, Bosi A and Papa G (1980). Second malignancy in patients treated for Hodgkin's disease. Cancer 46:1735–1740.
10. Borum K (1980). Increasing frequency of acute myeloid leukemia complicating Hodgkin's disease: A review. Cancer 46:1247–1252.

11. Brody RS and Schottenfeld D (1980). Multiple primary cancers in Hodgkin's disease. Semin Oncol 7:187–201.
12. Valagussa P, Santoro A, Kenda R et al. (1980). Second malignancies in Hodgkin's disease: A complication of certain forms of treatment. Br Med J 280:216–219.
13. Boivin JF and Hutchison GB (1981). Leukemia and other cancers after radiotherapy and chemotherapy for Hodgkin's disease. J Nat Cancer Inst. 67:751–760.
14. Nelson DF, Cooper S, Weston MG and Rubin P (1981). Second malignant neoplasms in patients treated for Hodgkin's disease with radiotherapy and chemotherapy. Cancer 48:2386–2393.
15. DeVita VT (1981). The consequences of the chemotherapy of Hodgkin's disease: The 10th David A. Karnofky memorial lecture. Cancer 47:1–13.
16. Brusamolino E, Lazzarino M, Salvaneschi L et al. (1982). Risk of leukemia in patients treated for Hodgkin's disease. Eur J Cancer Clin Oncol 18:237–242.
17. Coleman CN (1982). Secondary neoplasms in patients treated for cancer: Etiology and perspective. Radiat Res 92:188–200.
18. Coltman CA, Dixon DO (1982). Second malignancies complicating Hodgkin's disease: A Southwest Oncology Group 10-year follow-up. Cancer Treat Rep 66:1023–1033.
19. Glicksman A, Pajak TF, Gottlieb A et al. (1982). Second malignant neoplasms in patients successfully treated for Hodgkin's disease: A Cancer and Leukemia Group B study. Cancer Treat Rep 66:1035–1044.
20. Grunwald HW and Rosner F (1982). Acute myeloid leukemia following treatment of Hodgkin's disease. A review. Cancer 50:676–683.
21. Kyle RA (1982). Second malignancies associated with chemotherapeutic agents. Semin Oncol 9:131–142.
22. Pedersen-Bjegaard J and Larsen SO (1982). Incidence of acute non lymphocytic leukemia, preleukemia, and acute myeloproliferative syndrome up to 10 years after treatment of Hodgkin's disease. N Engl J Med 307:965–971.
23. Penn I (1982). Second neoplasms following radiotherapy or chemotherapy for cancer. Amer J Clin Oncol 5:83–96.
24. Valagussa P, Santoro A, Fossati Bellani F et al. (1982). Absence of treatment-induced second neoplasms after ABVD in Hodgkin's disease. Blood 59:488–494.
25. Jacquillat C, Auclerc G, Weil M et al. (1983). Leucémies aigues et tumeurs solides dans l'évolution de la maladie de Hodgkin. Bull Cancer (Paris) 70:61–66.
26. Rosner F (1983). Cancer and secondary leukemia. Bull Cancer (Paris) 70:55–60.
27. Tester W, Kinsella T, Waller B et al. (1983). Second malignant neoplasms (SMN) complicating Hodgkin's disease (HD). Amer Soc Clin Oncol 2:222.
28. Tucker MA, Meadows AT, Boice JD et al. (1984). Secondary leukemia (SL) after alkylating agents (AA) for childhood cancer. Amer Soc Clin Oncol 3:85.
29. Hayat M (1972). EORTC Radiotherapy-Chemotherapy Group: A randomized study of irradiation and vinblastine in clinical Stages I and II of Hodgkin's disease. Preliminary results. Eur J Cancer 8:353–362.
30. van der Werf-Messing B (1973). Morbus Hodgkin's disease, Stages I and II: Trial of the European Organization for Research on Treatment of Cancer. Nat Cancer Inst Monogr 36:381–386.
31. Tubiana M, Henry-Amar M, Hayat M et al. (1979). Long-term results of the EORTC randomized study of irradiation and vinblastine in clinical Stages I and II of Hodgkin's disease. Eur J Cancer 15:645–657.
32. Tubiana M, Hayat M, Henry-Amar M et al. (1981). Five-year results of the EORTC randomized study of splenectomy and spleen irradiation in Clinical Stages I and II of Hodgkin's disease. Eur J Cancer 17:355–363.
33. Schaffer P, Lavillaureix J (Eds.) (1981). Le Cancer dans le Bas-Rhin: Incidence des Nouveaux Cas de 1975 a 1977. Paris: Economica.

428

34. Netherlands Central Bureau of Statistics (Ed.) (1979). Cancer morbidity and mortality 1975–1976. The Hague: Staatsuitgeverij.
35. Schoenberg BS and Myers MH (1977). Statistical methods for studying multiple primary neoplasms. Cancer 40:1892–1898.
36. Mantel N (1966). Evaluation of survival data and two new rank order statistics arising in its consideration. Cancer Chemother Rep 50:163–170.
37. Cox DR (1972). Regression model and life-tables. J Roy Stat Soc 34:187–220.
38. Breslow N (1979). Statistical methods for censored survival data. Environ Health Perspect 32:181–192.
39. Mantel N and Byar DP (1974). Evaluation of response-time data involving transient states: An illustration using heart-transplant data. JASA 69:81–86.
40. Wartelle M, Kramar A, Jan P and Kruger D (1983). 'PIGAS': An interactive statistical database management system. In: Proceedings of the Second International Workshop on Statistical Database Management, pp. 124–132. Los Altos, California, USA.
41. Henry-Amar M (1983). Second cancers after radiotherapy and chemotherapy for early stages of Hodgkin's disease. J Nat Cancer Inst 71:911–916.
42. Hutchison GB (1976). Late neoplastic changes following medical irradiation. Cancer 37:1102–1107.
43. Kohn HI and Fry RJM (1984). Radiation carcinogenesis. N Engl J Med 310:504–511.
44. Rubin P (1984). The Franz Buschke lecture: Late effects of chemotherapy and radiation therapy: A new hypothesis. Int J Radiat Oncol Biol Phys 10:5–34.

18. Late complications of cytotoxic chemotherapy given for advanced Hodgkin's disease

J. H. WAXMAN[1], M. S. DORREEN[2], P. F. M. WRIGLEY[1] and
T. A. LISTER[1]
[1] *ICRF Department of Medical Oncology, St. Bartholomew's Hospital London and*
[2] *Royal Hallamshire Hospital, Sheffield, UK*

The long-term morbidity and mortality of patients with Hodgkin's disease treated with radical radiotherapy, combination chemotherapy or both, have become increasingly apparent with prolonged follow-up of large numbers of patients. The experience at St. Bartholomew's Hospital with the two major long-term problems, second malignancy and infertility, is presented below and compared with that from other centers.

Second malignancy

Materials and methods

Patients
Five hundred and twenty-eight patients were assessed, and constituted all patients alive and not lost to follow-up, 1 to 16 years from their first treatment. The clinical details of the patients who developed second tumors are described in Table I.

Table I. Characteristics of patients developing second malignancies

Sex ratio	Male (15): Female (11)			
Age	At diagnosis		Mean 38 (range 9–60) years	
	At second malignancy		Mean 46 (range 13–65) years	
Original histology	Lymphocyte predominant (6)		Mixed cellularity (7)	
	Nodular sclerosing (11)		Lymphocyte depleted (2)	
Disease stage	IA (3)	IIA (4)	IIIA (2)	IVA (3)
	IIB (4)	IIIB (5)	IVB (5)	

( ) = patient numbers

Treatment

Radiation. Megavoltage therapy to the mantle, inverted Y fields, or both (TNI) was prescribed as previously described for patients for whom radiotherapy was expected to be curative [1].

Chemotherapy. Cyclical combination chemotherapy comprising between six and twelve cycles of mustine, vinblastine, prednisolone and procarbazine [2] every six weeks was prescribed for patients with advanced disease receiving chemotherapy either as primary treatment, or following relapse after irradiation. Details of their treatment is described in Table II.

Combined modality. Treatment with both radiotherapy and chemotherapy as given above within 3 months of each other.

Statistical Methods
Life table analysis was used to calculate the risks of developing a second

Table II. Treatment of patients developing second tumors

Treatment		No. of patients	No. with 2nd tumors
I	RT only	146	6
II	Single course of MVPP	121	6
III	Multiple courses of MVPP	45	1
IV	MVPP+adjuvant RT	49	0
V	MVPP+RT for relapse	167	13
		528	26

Table III. Time interval from diagnosis of Hodgkin's disease to second malignancy

	Years					
	1–2	2–5	5–10	10–15	15+	Total
Leukemia	0	3	1	0	1	5
Non-Hodgkin's lymphoma	1	1	0	1	1	4
Adenocarcinoma	0	0	2	1	1	4
Squamous cell carcinoma	1	0	2	0	1	4
Carcinoma (other)	0	0	2	2	1	5
Glioma	1	0	0	0	0	1
Sarcoma	0	0	2	1	0	3
						26

malignancy [3]. The Chi-square test was applied to compare patient populations.

Results

Twenty-six out of five hundred and twenty-eight (4.9%) patients have developed a second malignancy (4 leukemia) at a minimum of 1 year and maximum of 16 years follow-up (Table III). The frequency of developing second malignancy was 4.1% in patients treated with radiotherapy alone (no leukemias), 5% in those receiving chemotherapy alone (no leukemias) and

Table IV. Second tumors related to the treatment of Hodgkin's disease

Sex	Age	Histo-logy	Stage	Treat-ment	Diagnosis of 2nd tumor	Latent period from treatment	Status
M	35	LP	IIA	I	squamous carcinoma, skin	12 months	alive
M	52	LP	IIA	I	cerebral glioma	17 months	dead
M	65	NS	IA	I	bladder carcinoma, transitional	7 years	dead
F	64	MC	IIA	I	rectal adenocarcinoma	10 years	dead
M	34	LP	IA	I	testicular teratoma	14 years	alive
M	50	NS	IIA	I	lymphoplasmacytoid lymphoma	15 years	alive
F	46	MC	IIB	II	mycosis fungoides	2 years	alive
M	62	LP	IVA	II	immunoblastic lymphoma	$2\frac{1}{2}$ years	dead
M	53	LP	IIIB	II	oat cell carcinoma, bronchus	$6\frac{1}{4}$ years	dead
M	36	MC	IIB	II	squamous carcinoma, penis	$6\frac{1}{2}$ years	alive
M	64	LD	IVB	II	basal cell carcinoma, skin	$9\frac{1}{2}$ years	alive
M	48	NS	IIIB	II	immunoblastic lymphoma	10 years	alive
M	32	NS	IVB	III	myeloproliferative syndrome	9 years	dead
M	57	MC	IIB	V	subacute myeloid leukemia	17 months	dead
M	63	NS	IIA	V	acute myeloid leukemia	2 years	dead
M	43	LD	IIA	V	acute myeloid leukemia	$2\frac{1}{2}$ years	dead
M	64	NS	IVA	V	acute myeloid leukemia	5 years	dead
M	13	LP	IIIB	V	osteogenic sarcoma	4 years	dead
F	31	NS	IVB	V	Kaposi's sarcoma	4 years	dead
F	32	NS	IVA	V	adenocarcinoma, uterus	5 years	alive
F	33	MC	IIIB	V	follicular carcinoma, thyroid	5 years	
					squamous carcinoma, vulva	10 years	alive
F	45	NS	IVB	V	bladder carcinoma, transitional	6 years	alive
F	57	NS	IIB	V	adenocarcinoma, lung: resected	9 years	
					metastatic carcinoma, lung	13 years	dead
M	63	MC	IVB	V	adenocarcinoma, pancreas	11 years	dead
F	33	NS	IIIB	V	in situ carcinoma, vulva	$13\frac{1}{4}$ years	alive
F	26	MC	IIIA	V	fibrosarcoma, uterus	8 years	dead

* See Table II

7.8% in those receiving radiotherapy and chemotherapy for relapse (Table IV). There have been no second malignancies in the group that received combined modality treatment electively, though this is the group with the least patient years at risk.

Those tumors with a high proliferative index tended to present early. Four patients developed leukemia within five years of treatment, whilst the sarcomas and carcinomas tended to present late. The incidence of second tumors was much higher than would be expected in age matched populations. The incidence of acute myeloid luekemia in an age matched population is 0.004%, whereas in the studied group of patients it was 0.9% ($p < 0.0001$). The prospect of survival subsequent to the development of a second tumor was poor; 65% of patients died as its consequence.

The results of 3 major studies are compared to those from St. Bartholomew's Hospital in Table V. All centers show an increased incidence of second malignances, particularly leukemias, and this is most significant in patients treated with both radiotherapy and chemotherapy.

Gonadal function

Materials and methods

Forty six men and 28 women in complete remission of advanced Hodgkin's disease were available for assessment. All were in remission of their disease which had been treated between 1968 and 1978. The patient characteristics are described in Table VI.

Table V. Comparative risk of second malignancy in patients treated for Hodgkin's disease

Authors	Treatment	Patient years	Cancer incidence rates
Arsenau et al. [5]	RT	562	7.1
	CT	371	8.1
	CT + RT	108	28
Canellos et al. [6]	CT	371	11
	CT + RT	265	23
Toland et al. [8]	RT	526	11
	CT	450	20
	CT + RT	81	25
St. Bartholomew's Hospital	RT	915	7.7
	CT	1012	4.9
	CT + RT	1230	9.8

Table VI. Details of patients assessed for gonadal function

	Age (mean) at treatment (years)	Age (mean) at follow-up (years)	Years (mean) after chemotherapy
Men	12–55 (27)	16–61 (34)	2–12.5 (6.5)
Women	17–48 (30)	25–60 (39)	2–12.5 (7.2)

Treatment

Patients whose gonadal function was assessed were treated with 6 to 16 courses of cyclic combination chemotherapy [2] alone, or with chemotherapy and supradiaphragmatic radiotherapy.

Assessment of gonadal function

Semen was collected for analysis after a minimum of three days abstinence. Menstruating women were studied on days 3–5 of their cycle. After basal blood specimens had been obtained for estimation of concentrations of prolactin (mean of three measurements), sex-hormone-binding globulin, testosterone, and 17-B-oestradiol a standard test was performed in which luteinising-hormone-releasing hormone (100 μg) was given. Concentrations of progesterone, were measured on days 20–22 of a cycle if present. Follicle stimulating hormone, luteinising hormone, and prolactin concentrations were measured by specific double antibody radio-immunoassay using MRC standards 69/104, 68/40 and 71/222 respectively. After ether extraction testosterone and oestradiol concentrations were measured by tritiated radio-immunoassay. Progesterone concentration was measured by tritiated radio-immunoassay after hexane extraction. Concentrations of sex-hormone-binding globulin were measured by saturation radio-immunoassay [4].

Results

Men

Serial samples of semen were obtained from 41 men, two to 12.5 years after chemotherapy. Thirty-six men were profoundly oligospermic with total sperm counts of less than 0.6 million. Five men had had counts of between 20 and 88.4 million. Three of this group were initially azoospermic, showing recovery of spermatogenesis two to 10 years after the end of chemotherapy. One patient fathered two normal children. All patients with recovery of spermatogenesis were 20 to 30 years of age at the time that treatment was initiated.

Concentrations of testosterone and sex hormone binding globulin were normal in all patients (Table VII). Three patients had marginally elevated

Table VII. Hormone concentrations in 46 men and 28 women treated for Hodgkin's disease

	Men			Women		
	Range	Mean	Normal Range	Range	Mean	Normal Range
Prolactin (mU/l)	98–1114	273	<360	163–562	289	<360
Sex hormone binding globulin (nmol/l)	16–42	27	17–50	20–>120	56	38–102
Testosterone (nmol/l)	13–33	21	10–38	1–3.2	1.85	0.5–3.0
17 B oestradiol (pmol/l)	<30–205	101	<30–128	<30–525	172	110–1290 premenopausal 37–129 postmenopausal
Progesterone (nmol/l)				<1–42.4	7.33	>33
Luteinizing hormone (U/l) baseline	2.9–28	12	1.4–9.7	2.9–>50	29	2.5–14.1
Minutes after 100 g luteinising hormone releasing hormone:						
20	34–>50	48	13.1–57.6	33–>50	48	15–42
60	29.8–>50	37	11–47.6	46–>50	49	12–35
Follicle stimulating hormone (U/l) baseline	3.7–>25	15	1–7	1.5–>25	18	1–10
Minutes after 100 g luteinising hormone releasing hormone:						
20	6.6–>25	23	1–7	10.7–>25	23	1.2–11.1
60	7.6–>25	24	0.8–5.2	11.7–>25	23	1.2–24.5

Conversion SI to traditional units – Sex-hormone-binding globulin: 1 nmol/l = 5.2 µg/100 ml. Testosterone: 1 nmol/l = 28.8 ng/100 ml. 17 B ostradiol: 1 pmol/l = 26.5 pg/100 ml. Progesterone: 1 nmol/l = 31.4 ng/100 ml concentrations of 17-B-oestradiol, eight patients had elevated prolactin concentrations. Thirty-four men had elevated basal concentrations of both luteinizing hormone and follicle stimulating hormone, two of luteinizing hormone and six of follicle stimulating hormone alone, whilst four had normal gonadotrophin concentrations despite azoospermia in three. All 37 men tested had excessive responses of follicle stimulating hormone and 34 of luteinizing hormone to luteinizing-hormone-releasing hormone. Four of five patients with active spermatogenesis had elevated basal gonadotrophins.

Women

Twenty-two women became amenorrhoeic, and there was no late return of menses if periods had failed to return within 3 months from the completion of treatment. Six patients retained normal menstruation, and five of these women were under 30 at the time of treatment. Two subsequently delivered normal children.

In women with amenorrhoea, both high basal and dynamic gonadotrophins were noted, together with low concentrations of 17 B oestradiol and progesterone (Table VII). Seven women had elevated concentrations of prolactin, two of sex hormone binding globulin whilst testosterone was normal in all of the women studied.

Discussion

The overall incidence of second malignancy following treatment for Hodgkin's disease was 26 of 528 (4.9%) patients. This result compares with those from other major centers.

The development of second primary tumors after treatment for Hodgkin's disease was documented by Arsenau et al. in 1972, in 12 of 425 patients treated at the National Institutes of Health [5]. Canellos et al., updating this report in 1975 described second tumors in 16 of 455 patients, 2 of which were leukemias. In those patients receiving both chemotherapy and radiotherapy the incidence of second tumors was highest, and was 15-fold greater than age matched controls [6]. Brody et al. reported 23 second malignancies in 1028 patients treated at the Memorial Sloan Kettering Cancer Center. In contrast to the previous reports, no second tumors occurred in the group of patients treated with both chemotherapy and radiotherapy [7]. Data from the Southwest Oncology Group were presented in 1978 by Toland et al. [8]. Eighteen second malignancies, 11 of which were leukemias developed in 643 patients and combined modality treatment produced the greatest increase in the incidence of second tumors. In 1981, Boivin and Hutchinson reported 27 second malignancies in 1553 patients of which 6 were leukemias [9]. All leukemias developed in patients treated with both radiation and chemotherapy.

In the patients studied at St. Bartholomew's Hospital, gonadal failure occurred in 88% of the men and 78% of the women. The likelihood of return of spermatogenesis or retention of menses was highest in those patients aged under 30 years at the time of treatment for Hodgkin's disease. There was no late return of menses but occasional recovery of spermatogenesis was noted.

Gonadal failure results in sterility and in women loss of libido and premature osteoporosis. Spitz, in 1943, first described the toxic effects upon the gonad of single agent therapy given for Hodgkin's disease, reporting absent spermatogenesis in 27 of 30 men treated with nitrogen mustard [10]. Twenty-five years later, Sherrins and DeVita described the sterilizing potential of combination chemotherapy given to 10 men treated up to 7 years previously [11]. At review, eight were profoundly oligospermic. Since then, a number of studies have assessed various aspects of the gonadal consequence of chemotherapy given for Hodgkin's disease. Amongst the contentious issues have been the influence of sex, age and remission duration upon the recovery of germ cell function. Chapman et al. prospectively studied 47 men who were treated with MVPP chemotherapy [12]. At presentation 12 of 37 (32%) were oligospermic, and this was unrelated to age, disease stage or the presence of B symptoms. All of these patients were rendered profoundly oligospermic by two courses of chemotherapy [11]. Sanger et al. noted more subtle qualitative abnormalities in men with normal sperm counts, who presented prior to treatment for cryopreservation of semen [13]. In eight of nine patients, post-thawing sperm motility was so low as for those men to be considered sterile.

The ovarian effects of chemotherapy are more difficult to assess than the testicular toxicity. Post-treatment laparotomy has shown a characteristic ovarian appearance with a reduction in follicle numbers and stromal fibrosis. Because some follicles persist the effects of chemotherapy may not be immediately apparent. Horning et al. assessed 34 women with a median age of 23 years treated with either MOPP or MVPP chemotherapy [14]. The median interval from completion of treatment to assessment was 45 months. Menses were retained in 29 women, and in this group their retention was related to age with an increased probability of regular menstruation with age less than 30 years at treatment.

Our study reports a similar incidence of oligospermia and relationship of recovery of spermatogenesis to age, as have other workers. Follow-up is over a greater time interval and demonstrates little long-term recovery. A higher incidence of ovarian failure occurred in the patients treated at St. Bartholomew's Hospital and this may relate to the more prolonged interval between treatment and assessment.

Second malignancy and gonadal failure are the major late complications of the treatment of Hodgkin's disease. Although their consideration is a luxury that relates to a revolution in the management of this condition, both features are of importance. Their avoidance dictates an alteration of current treatment programmes. This may be provided by alternative chemotherapy regimens [15] or by gonadal down regulation during treatment with conventional chemotherapy [16].

References

1. Timothy AR, Sutcliffe SB, Stansfeld AG et al. (1978). Radiotherapy in the treatment of Hodgkin's disease. Br Med J 1:1246-1249.
2. Sutcliffe SB, Wrigley PFM, Peto J et al. (1978). MVPP chemotherapy for advanced Hodgkin's disease. Br Med J 1:679-683.
3. Kaplan EI and Meier P (1958). Non parametric estimation from incomplete observation. Amer Stat Assoc J 57:457-480.
4. Fattah DI and Chard T (1981). Method for measuring sex hormone binding globulin. Clin Chem 27:1277-1279.
5. Arsenau JC, Spouzo RW and Levin DL (1972). Non lymphomatous malignant tumours complicating Hodgkin's disease. N Engl J Med 287:1119-1122.
6. Canellos GP, DeVita VT, Arsenau JC et al. (1975). Second malignancies complicating Hodgkin's disease in remission. Lancet 1:947-949.
7. Brody RS, Schottenfeld D and Reid A (1977). Multiple primary cancer after treatment for Hodgkin's disease. Cancer 40:1917-1926.
8. Toland DM, Coltman CA and Moon TE (1978). Second malignancies complicating Hodgkin's disease: The Southwest Oncology Group experience. Cancer Clin Trials 1:21-33.
9. Boivin JF and Hutchison GB (1981). Leukaemia and other cancers after radiotherapy and chemotherapy for Hodgkin's disease. J Nat Cancer Inst 67:751-760.
10. Spitz S (1948). The histological effects of nitrogen mustard on human tumours and tissues. Cancer 1:383-398.
11. Sherins RJ and DeVita VT (1973). Effect of drug treatment for lymphoma on male reproductive capacity. Ann Intern Med 79:216-220.
12. Chapman R, Sutcliff S, Rees LH et al. (1979). Cyclical combination chemotherapy and gonadal function. Lancet 1:285-290.
13. Sanger WG, Armitage JO and Schmidt MA (1980). Feasibility of semen cryopreservation in patients with malignant disease. JAMA 244:789-790.
14. Horning SJ, Hoppe RT, Kaplan HS et al. (1981). Female reproductive potential after treatment for Hodgkin's disease. N Engl J Med 304:1377-1382.
15. Santoro A, Viviani S, Zucali R et al. (1983). Comparative results and toxicity of MOPP vs ABVD combined with radiotherapy (RT) in PS IIB, III (A, B) Hodgkin's disease (HD). Proc Amer Soc Clin Oncol 2:223.
16. Waxman JH, Lister TA, Ahmed R et al. Effects of gonadal down-regulation with a long acting analogue of gonadotrophin releasing hormone during the treatment of Hodgkin's disease. (In preparation).

VII. Treatment of non-Hodgkin's lymphomas

1. Overview on current strategy of the treatment of non-Hodgkin's lymphomas

E. R. GAYNOR and J. E. ULTMANN
Section of Hematology/Oncology, Department of Medicine, University of Chicago and The University of Chicago Cancer Research Center, Chicago, Illinois, USA

We are currently in the midst of an exciting information explosion regarding the pathophysiology of the malignant lymphomas. Although tremendous advances in our understanding of these diseases have been made in the past ten to fifteen years, our therapeutic approaches to some of these diseases have remained relatively stagnant. This overview will briefly summarize advances in the fields of immunology, cytogenetics, molecular biology, and virology, examine the current status of therapy for the malignant lymphomas, and speculate regarding future trends in therapeutics.

Immunology

Over the past 30 years various histopathologic classification systems have been proposed to group the diverse entities called lymphomas in an orderly manner that would have prognostic and therapeutic significance. The classification system proposed by Rappaport, which categorized the lymphomas according to the presence or absence of a nodular architecture, was one of the most widely used [1]. Though a useful and still widely used classification system, the Rappaport model has not stood the test of time. In the 1960s, it became apparent that there were two major subpopulations of lymphocytes, T-cells and B-cells, and that each of these populations occupies a characteristic area within lymph nodes and spleen. Furthermore, it became evident that the mature lymphocyte was not an end stage cell but rather was a cell that could be 'transformed' by appropriate stimuli to become an effector cell. Lymphomas, the malignant counterparts to the normal cells of the immune system, could be of either T- or B-cell origin; the observed histologic diversity resulted because the lymphomas are clonal expansions occurring at various points in the normal maturation sequence.

Many histopathologic classification schemes for the malignant lymphomas have attempted to integrate the knowledge gained from basic immunology during the 1970s. The Kiel [2] and Lukes-Collins [3] systems are among the most widely used. The recently proposed Working Formulation for Clinical Usage is a very useful system, but is suffers, as do all histopathologic systems, from a lack of reproducibility among various centers [4]. This common problem of reproducibility has been and will continue to be overcome by the use of precise immunologic probes that are able to characterize phenotypically the malignant lymphomas.

Monoclonal antibodies have been used extensively to characterize the morphologically diverse malignant lymphomas at various stages of differentiation. Phenotypic analysis has shown that most lymphomas, both of B- and T-cell origin, are in fact clonal expansions of lymphocytes at a specific stage of differentiation. Characterization of the malignant lymphomas has not only precisely defined the nature of the malignant cells but has allowed refinement of our concept of neoplasia. Formerly, we had regarded lymphomas as abnormal proliferations of malignant cells, with emphasis both prognostically and therapeutically focusing on this abnormal proliferation. With the recognition of the immune system as a network of cells originating from a primitive stem cell, the neoplastic process might be more appropriately viewed from the perspective of differentiation.

As proposed by Magrath, the neoplastic process may be conceptualized in terms of stem cell proliferation and differentiation [5]. Stem cells possess many attributes which include the capacity for self renewal, the ability to respond to a demand for more progeny cells, and the ability to differentiate. Arising ultimately from one stem cell are various subpopulations of cells at varying stages of maturation and differentiation; each subpopulation comprises a compartment. Cell loss from any compartment can result either from maturation (with cells entering the successive compartment) or from cell death. Accumulation of cells at any stage will occur if there is a block in the differentiation process or if the fraction of stem cells that are proliferating is increased. In the latter situation, one would expect that all compartments would increase in size but that the relationship among compartments would not change. Because there is amplification of each successive compartment in the differentiation pathway, the absolute size increase would be much greater in the larger compartments, and the clinical manifestation of a disorder in stem cell proliferation would be mainly or entirely perceived in the largest compartment. The clinically apparent neoplastic process may then be only the tip of the iceberg; therapy directed only at what is clinically apparent may fall far short of cure.

The phenotypic description of both the normal cellular elements and the malignant neoplasms of the immune system have made possible a clearer definition of clinical syndromes. Through the study of surface antigens, we now know that the diffuse histiocytic lymphomas in the Rappaport classification are in fact a group of diseases encompassing at least five subsets. Discovering these subsets has allowed us to recognize that the aggressive tumors of one subset, immunoblastic lymphoma, require more intensive therapy than tumors in other subsets of large cell lymphoma. Further characterization of the various cell populations of the immune system will hopefully enable us to classify patient populations into more precise subsets which will have both therapeutic and prognostic impact.

Cytogenetics

With the introduction of chromosomal banding techniques in the early 1970s and the identification by Rowley of a non-random chromosome translocation t(9; 22) in chronic myelogenous leukemia, the field of cancer cytogenetics took on new impetus [6]. Characteristic chromosomal abnormalities, such as t(15; 17) in acute promyelocytic leukemia, are now frequently observed in certain subclasses of acute nonlymphocytic leukemia. With improved methods of metaphase cell preparations from tumor tissue, scientists have recently discovered that the majority of malignant lymphomas also show clonal chromosomal abnormalities.

Manolov and Manolova first described the 14q$^+$ chromosome in Burkitt's lymphoma in cells obtained from five different biopsy specimens [7]. It was subsequently shown that in most cases the donor chromosome was 8 (8 q−) and that the specific bands involved in the reciprocal translocation wee 8 q 24 and 14 q 32 [8].

Variant translocations in both endemic and nonendemic Burkitt's lymphoma have recently been described [9, 10]. In each of these cases chromosome 8 was involved in a reciprocal translocation; either chromosome 2 or chromosome 22 donated chromosomal material to chromosome 8. These observations suggest that a translocation involving chromosome 8 is the critical chromosomal change in Burkitt's; such a translocation may be important to the development of this malignancy.

Reports from two large series have recently expanded our knowledge of cytogenetic abnormalities in the non-Hodgkin's lymphomas (NHL). Yunis et al. examined biopsy material from 44 patients with NHL [11]. Twenty-seven of these patients had no previous therapy. Of 42 successfully analyzed biopsy specimens, all were found to have clonal chromosome abnormalities. In this study, 16 of 19 patients with follicular lymphoma were found to have t(14; 18). Three of three patients with small non-cleaved non-Burkitt's lymphoma and two of three patients with large cell immunoblastic lymphoma were found to have t(8; 14) as previously described in Burkitt's lymphoma. Results of this study indicate that the extra chromosomal material on chromosome 14 may be derived from different chromosomes; the donor chromosome seems to be chromosome 8 in aggressive histology lymphomas and chromosome 18 in the less aggressive follicular lymphomas. The breakpoint on chromosome 14 appears, however, to be fairly consistently located at band q32. Bloomfield et al. performed chromosome analysis on lymph node biopsy specimens from 94 patients with NHL [12]. Chromosomal abnormalities were noted in 91 of these patients, including all 81 patients with B-cell lymphoma and six of nine patients with T-cell lymphoma. The authors observed seven recurring translocations; all except one of these involved chromosome 14 at band q32. The t(14; 18) as observed by Yunis was seen in 22 patients in Bloomfield's series; all were lymphomas of follicular center origin. Overall the 14q$^+$ anomaly was found in 66% of 90 cases of non-Burkitt's lymphoma including three of nine cases of T-cell lymphoma. No abnormality was restricted invariably to a given histology or immunologic phenotype.

These and other studies prompt many questions: Are karyotypic abnormalities related to the pathogenesis of the lymphomas? Does a consistent breakpoint on chromosome 14 at band 32 confer a proliferative advantage on the cell? Can consistent chromosomal changes predict therapeutic response with our current treatment programs?

Molecular biology — the oncogene

The answers to some of the questions raised by cytogenetic research are beginning to unfold as it becomes possible to probe the DNA sequences which make up the cellular genome. Because consistent breakpoints on chromosomes have been observed and because all of the cells in a tumor have the same chromosomal rearrangement, it is assumed that these chromosomal rearrangements confer a selective advantage on the neoplastic cells. These translocations probably occur at sites in the genome where genes important to neoplastic development are located.

Recent work regarding the consistent chromosome 8 abnormality in Burkitt's lymphoma supports these assumptions. As previously noted, in the majority of cases of Burkitt's lymphoma there is a characteristic reciprocal translocation involving chromosomes 8 and 14. Other less common, or variant, translocations in Burkitt cells involve reciprocal translocations between chromosomes 8q and 22q or between 8q and 2p. Genes coding for immunoglobulin heavy chains have recently been found in band 32 on chromosome 14; in Burkitt cells the 14q+ retains the gene coding for the constant region of the heavy chains, whereas genes coding for all or a portion of the variable region translocate to the 8q− chromosome [13]. In the rare variants, the portion of the short arm of chromosome 2 that contains the gene coding for the kappa light chains translocates in a reciprocal fashion to chromosome 8 [14]. Likewise, the portion of the long arm of chromosome 22 that contains the gene coding for the lambda light chains is involved in a reciprocal translocation with the long arm of chromosome 8 [15].

It now appears that there are DNA sequences in the human genome that are analogous to known retrovirus oncogenes. One such human oncogene is c-myc, which is strongly homologous with v-myc, the transforming sequence of the avian retrovirus, MC-29. There is substantial evidence that chromosomal translocations involving the c-myc oncogene and one of the immunoglobulin loci are very common in human lymphoid malignancies. The insertion of certain retroviral sequences in the vicinity of c-myc can greatly enhance its expression and result in oncogenic transformation. The chromosomal translocations observed in malignant lymphomas may be similarly effective in the activation of the myc oncogene [16].

The c-myc oncogene has been localized to chromosome 8 band 24 in the human genome [17]. In both the common translocation (8; 14) and the variant translocations (8; 22) and (2; 8), this band is involved in the breakpoint in the reciprocal translocation. In the common translocation the myc locus translocates to chromosome 14, while in the variant translocations the myc locus remains on chromosome 8 [18, 19]. In all cases, however, the myc locus is juxtaposed with one of the immunoglobulin gene loci in an immunoglobulin producing cell. This juxtaposition presumably results in c-myc activation.

Cellular oncogenes have been mapped to human chromosomes 1, 2, 3, 5, 6, 7, 8, 9, 11, 12, 15, 17, 20, and 22, and in many instances have been shown to be involved in specific chromosomal translocations within the malignant clone. Although different transforming onc genes may be activated in different types of tumors, the same gene appears to be activated in tumors of the same type whether they are induced by viruses, radiation, or chemicals. Activation of an oncogene is, however, probably only one essential step in a sequence which must be followed to produce the clonal disease. The subsequent progression of the tumor may be further promoted by additional genetic and cytogenetic changes within the malignant clone, some of which may affect other oncogenes.

Virology

Retroviruses are enveloped RNA viruses best known for their ability to cause malignant tumors in various vertebrates. Until very recently there has been no consistent association of a retrovirus with human malignancy. Blaney et al. have now clearly shown that the human T-cell leukemia retrovirus (HTLV) is associated with a subset of adult T-cell malignancies as evidenced by viral specific natural antibodies [20]. The virus has been shown to be an exogenous virus acquired by infection and not transmitted in the germ line. Although T-cell lymphomas encompass a wide variety of diseases, HTLV is most commonly associated with lymphosarcoma cell leukemia, peripheral T-cell lymphoma, and Japanese adult T-cell leukemia/lymphoma. The virus is capable of transforming human cord blood mature T-cells when they are cultivated *in vitro* with malignant cells. Epidemiologic studies indicate clustering of human T-cell lymphoma/leukemia in areas where the HTL virus is endemic.

Japanese researchers have described a very similar, if not identical, adult T-cell leukemia retrovirus (ATLV) in association with a T-cell leukemia/lymphoma endemic in certain areas of Japan [21]. Sera from almost all patients with the disease react specifically with an ATLV associated antigen (ATLA). Furthermore, current evidence suggests that healthy subjects with anti-ATLA sera harbor T-lymphocytes carrying ATLA, which has been shown to be specific for ATLV.

Fukahara et al. recently reported chromosome studies on ATLA (+) cells obtained from healthy donors [22]. Chromosome aberrations were found in three of five anti-ATLA sero-positive healthy subjects. These results suggest that some anti-ATLA sera (+) healthy people have clones of T-lymphocytes with chromosomal abnormalities in their peripheral blood that may be associated with ATLV.

Since 1981, when the acquired immunodeficiency syndrome (AIDS) was initially described, there has been speculation regarding the role of a retrovirus as the causative agent of this disease. The human T-cell leukemia viruses are T-cell tropic agents that are associated in certain instances with proliferation of cells with the T4 antigen. The underlying abnormality in AIDS appears to be a depletion of T4 cells. This predilection of human T-cell leukemia virus for T4 cells supports the idea that the virus may be associated with AIDS. Recently, French and American investigators described a new retrovirus, named HTLV III by Gallo et al., which is strongly associated with AIDS and may in fact be the causative agent of this syndrome [23, 24].

Research efforts in the past several years have confirmed the long-suspected viral etiology of some human malignancies. What remains to be elucidated are the mechanisms by which viruses can initiate the neoplastic process.

Current approaches to therapy

As mentioned earlier, the Working Formulation for Clinical Usage separates the non-Hodgkin's lymphomas into three basic categories: favorable histology, intermediate histology, and aggressive histology. A brief summary of current treatment strategies for each of these subgroups follows.

Favorable histology lymphomas usually occur in middle-aged patients and, in the majority of cases, the disease is advanced (Stage III or IV) at presentation. Approximately 10% of these patients will have local disease which is in true Pathologic Stage (PS) I or II. This small group of patients may be cured with radiotherapy alone and hence many authors recommend involved field radiotherapy (IFRT) for Clinical Stage (CS) I and II disease.

Considerable controversy exists regarding the optimum therapy for advanced disease. Although both total nodal irradiation and intensive combination chemotherapy have yielded excellent response rates, relapses are frequent; the risk of relapse remains high for as long as ten years. Portlock et al. have reported the results of a randomized trial comparing combination chemotherapy, combination chemotherapy plus irradiation, and single alkylating agent therapy [25]. There was no statistical difference in either response rate or survival among the three groups. Furthermore, in a retrospective analysis the same authors reported on a group of patients with lymphoma who for various reasons had received no initial therapy for their disease [26]. When compared with patients randomized to one of the three treatment arms noted above, the authors found no difference in actuarial survival. Thus it may be beneficial to give no initial therapy to some patients with favorable histology lymphomas. However, these patients should be followed closely for progression or complications of their disease.

Some researchers have reported very favorable results for some patients who received combination chemotherapy, particularly those patients with nodular mixed cell histology, although there are conflicting results regarding therapy in this subset of patients [27, 28]. No consistent survival benefit appears to result from intensive therapy in most of these favorable histology lymphomas. While complete remission can be achieved in some instances, late relapses make cure very unlikely in this group of diseases.

Intermediate histology lymphomas include the histologies of diffuse poorly differentiated (DPDL), diffuse mixed (DM), diffuse histiocytic (DHL), and nodular histiocytic (NH) lymphomas. Much progress has been made in improving both the complete remission rate and survival time in patients with diffuse histiocytic lymphoma in the past 15 years. Because NH and DPDL are clearly more aggressive than the favorable histologic subgroups and require intensive therapy, most current clinical trials include DPDL, DM, NH, and DHL.

Current approaches to the intermediate grade lymphomas include both aggressive single combination chemotherapy programs and also alternating or sequential non-cross resistant combination therapy programs. Impressive results, such as a 74% complete response rate with a median survival of 36+ months, have been reported with the ProMACE/MOPP regimen [29].

This approach is unique because the number of cycles of each of the two regimens given depends on the individual patient's tempo of response. Such flexible therapy, tailored to each individual's response, is an attractive option which deserves further exploration.

Unfavorable histology lymphomas comprise a heterogeneous group of rapidly progressive lymphomas which are uniformly fatal in weeks to months if untreated. This category includes some cases of DHL (immunoblastic sarcoma), lymphoblastic lymphoma, and undifferentiated (small cell) lymphomas, both Burkitt's and non-Burkitt's types. Various successful chemotherapeutic approaches have been developed for each of these subtypes.

With newer combination programs such as ProMACE/MOPP [29] and COP · BLAM [30], the response rates and survival statistics are improving for patients with immunoblastic sarcoma. Similar improvements have been noted in the treatment of lymphoblastic lymphoma. Coleman et al. treated 13 patients with an induction program including Cytoxan, Oncovin, doxorubicin, and prednisone, and a consolidation program including L-asparaginase and high dose methotrexate with leucovorin rescue, as well as intrathecal methotrexate [31]. All patients achieved complete response and 61% of the patients are alive at three years. Burkitt's lymphoma is known to be exquisitely sensitive to chemotherapy, with complete response rates of 95% to 100% with high dose Cytoxan alone or in combination with vincristine, methotrexate, adriamycin, and corticosteroids [32]. However, relapse is a significant problem because only 50% to 60% of patients achieve long-term remissions. In non-Burkitt's lymphoma, a rare tumor which in the past had a dismal prognosis, recent results have been encouraging. Newer combination therapy programs like M-BACOD have yielded a 77% CR rate in patients with this histologic subtype [33].

Future trends

Monoclonal antibody therapy

In 1975 Kohler and Milstein described a technique for fusing murine B-lymphocytes with murine myeloma cells that resulted in the production of hybridoma cell lines secreting antibodies of predefined specificity [34]. In 1980 Nadler developed a monoclonal antibody, Ab89, which reacted with the malignant cells of approximately 10% of patients with DPDL and B-cell chronic lymphocytic leukemia (CLL); the antibody did not react with normal hemopoietic tissue [35]. The authors made the important observation that the patient's plasma contained large amounts of circulating antigen that blocked the binding of Ab89 to tumor cells *in vivo*. The following year,

Miller and Levy used a monoclonal antibody to treat a patient who had T-cell lymphoma [36]. The patient initially showed a good response; the circulating Sezary cells cleared and tumor infiltrates in the skin and lymph nodes regressed. However, the patient did not achieve a CR and after seven weeks the tumor began to proliferate despite continued antibody infusion. In 1982, Miller et al. successfully treated a patient who had B-cell PDL that had become resistant to cytotoxic drugs and interferon [37]. An anti-idiotype monoclonal antibody was developed which was specific for the idiotype on the surface membrane of the patient's malignant cells. Circulating IgM idiotype was detected prior to therapy, but after continued monoclonal antibody therapy the idiotype level fell and then disappeared. A complete clinical response was eventually achieved.

Although the previous three studies illustrate that monoclonal antibodies can be therapeutically useful, several problems currently limit the efficacy of monoclonal antibody therapy [38]. First, in several studies, circulating antigen that effectively blocks antibody binding *in vivo* or *in vitro* has been demonstrated. A second problem is antigenic modulation. Apparently the binding of the monoclonal antibody to the cell surface alters the cell membrane so that the antigen forms microaggregates which are not susceptible to antibody attack. An alternate theory is that the binding of antibody to the cell surface antigen causes the antigen-antibody complex to be internalized within the cell. The third, and perhaps most difficult problem, is that these antibodies are not inherently toxic and the mere binding of antibody to the cell surface does not usually affect cell growth. Possibly ways to overcome this problem are: 1) to develop new monoclonal antibodies (such as IgM antibodies) which are more efficient in the activation of complement; 2) to use monoclonal antibody when the body burden of tumor is small (e.g., as an adjunct to cytotoxic therapy); and 3) to develop Ab-drug or Ab-toxin conjugates that are able to specifically kill the tumor cells to which they are directed. Monoclonal technology is less than ten years old; the marked advances that have been made already suggest that monoclonal antibody therapy will be a key factor in future treatment of the malignant lymphomas.

Interferons

The interferons are small, biologically active proteins that appear to have some growth regulating capacity because their anti-proliferative effects are measurable both *in vitro* and in animal model systems. These proteins are known to have profound effects on the immune system, depending on the dose range. Although it is unclear whether interferons work primarily through an antiproliferative effect or through alterations of the immune response, the anti-tumor activity of interferons has been most reproducibly seen in the lymphomas.

In a multi-institutional trial of recombinant leukocyte A interferon (Hoffman La Roche), Sherwin et al. noted significant antitumor activity in favorable histology NHL and mycosis fungoides; the median duration of response was 5+ months in the former and 3+ months in the latter [39]. A similar study by Ozer et al. employing recombinant DNA alpha$_2$ interferon (Schering) noted a partial response in 4 of 10 patients with NPDL and 2 of 10 patients with DHL [40]. As with monoclonal antibodies, current trials with interferon have been restricted mainly to patients with disease which has become refractory to conventional therapy. In the future we may be able to identify subgroups of patients who will benefit from interferon therapy early in the course of their disease, possibly as an adjunct to cytotoxic therapy.

Active specific immunotherapy

The recognition that a specific retrovirus, HTL, is associated with a specific class of leukemia/lymphoma and that this virus and its associated disease are endemic in certain areas of the world suggests that it might be possible to develop a vaccine to the virus that could be administered to the population at risk. Although a clear cut relationship between a given virus and a specific type of lymphoma exists only for the HTL virus, further research in tumor virology may identify further virus/tumor relationships, offering the potential for control of these diseases in much the same way that the viral illnesses of the 1950s and 1960s are now controlled by large-scale immunization programs.

The demonstration of a living etiologic agent is not essential for the successful use of active immunization, for the lymphoma cell itself may provide the antigen against which to immunize. As Oldham points out, research into mechanisms by which tumors evade the immune system has focused primarily on the poor immunogenicity of spontaneous tumors or on the immune competence of the host [41]. Less attention has been given to the possibility that the anatomic characteristics, such as vascular barriers of the tumor, protect tumors from immunotherapy. A major limitation of active specific immunotherapy has been the source and availability of a suitable tumor antigen.

Adoptive immunotherapy

Interleukin 2 (IL-2), a T-cell derived cytokine, was originally identified as a result of its nonspecific enhancing effect on murine thymocyte production.

IL-2 can mediate the growth of T-cells *in vitro*, and therefore it is possible to expand T-lymphocytes from tumor bearing hosts *in vitro*. If we could identify cells with antitumor reactivity or if such cells could be generated from the immune system of the tumor bearing host, these cells could theoretically be cloned *in vitro* and large populations could be generated from single starting cells. With this technique, a hyperimmune lymphoid population with the desired antitumor reactivity could be generated. Rosenberg, who successfully used this approach in an animal system, has demonstrated that the adoptive transfer of sensitive syngeneic lymphocytes can mediate the regression of established transplantable tumors [42].

There are three major challenges to the use of adoptive immunotherapy in humans. It is first necessary to identify the appropriate cell type for use in adoptive transfer. Second, suitable human tumor cell preparations are currently unavailable and such preparations need to be developed. Finally, effective means of blocking suppressor systems which would inhibit the transfused activated cells need to be explored.

Differentiation agents

Various chemicals including cis retinoic acid, dimethylsulfoxide (DMSO) and vitamin D analogues are capable of inducing leukemic cells *in vitro* to differentiate along either granulocytic or monocytic pathways [43, 44]. Recently, a patient with acute promyelocytic leukemia who was treated *in vivo* with cis retinoic acid had a transient increase in mature granulocyte cells both in the bone marrow and peripheral blood [45].

The preceding discussion on the target cell in malignant transformation and the dichotomy in response to chemotherapy seen in lymphomas of favorable and aggressive histologies suggest that differentiating agents may have a role in therapy for certain non-Hodgkin's lymphomas. Might it be possible to induce the malignant cell of an NDPL tumor to differentiate to a transformed cell characteristic of a diffuse large cell lymphoma and then intervene with cytotoxic therapy which is known to be effective in treating large cell lymphomas? If malignant lymphomas are neoplasms which in many instances represent a block in a normal differentiation sequence, the use of differentiating agents in therapy is certainly an area for further research.

Genetic engineering

We now know that most non-Hodgkin's lymphomas have clonal chromosomal abnormalities and that in some cases of Burkitt's lymphoma the chromosomal abnormality involves a part of the genome which contains the myc oncogene. The assumption is that combining the DNA sequences of the oncogene with the DNA sequence of an immunoglobulin may in some way 'turn on' the affected cell, provide a proliferative advantage, and ultimately give rise to the neoplastic clone of cells. If the cell is 'turned on', 'immortalized' or 'deregulated', is there any way to reverse these processes? Might a protein be synthesized which would attach to the involved 'turn on' site and render it inactive? The therapeutic implications of genetic engineering are now speculative; however, once we understand the intricate coding system within the cell, it seems that the next step will be to manipulate that system to our therapeutic advantage.

Conclusion

We have made tremendous therapeutic advances in the past ten years in our management of certain groups of the non-Hodgkin's lymphomas. Paradoxically, the lymphomas which previously were considered 'bad prognosis' are now curable in the majority of cases, while those previously considered 'good prognosis' remain incurable. The challenge before us now is to integrate our newly gained pathophysiologic insights into more effective treatment approaches. Hopefully the next decade will be the era during which the entire spectrum of non-Hodgkin lymphomas will be regarded as highly curable malignancies.

Acknowledgements

Supported in part by The University of Chicago Cancer Research Center; Public Health Service Grants 2P30 Ca-14599-11 (National Cancer Institute) and 5-T-32-AM 07134-09 (National Institute of Arthritis, Diabetes, and Digestive and Kidney Diseases), National Institutes of Health, Department of Health and Human Services; and the Beverly Duchossois, Jean Heiman, and Joanne Heppes Funds.

References

1. Rappaport H (1966). Tumors of the hemopoietic system. Atlas of Tumor Pathology. Section 3, Fasc. 8, pp. 1–442. Washington, DC: Armed Forces Institute of Pathology.
2. Gerard-Marchant R, Hamlin I, Lennert K et al. (1974). Classification of non-Hodgkin's lymphomas. Lancet 2:406–408.
3. Lukes RJ and Collins RD (1975). New approaches to the classification of the lymphomata. Br J Cancer 31 (Suppl. 2):1–28.

4. Non-Hodgkin's Lymphoma Pathologic Classification Project (1982). National Cancer Institute sponsored study of classification of non-Hodgkin's lymphomas. Cancer 49:2112–2136.

5. Magrath IT (1981). Lymphocyte differentiation: An essential basis for the comprehension of lymphoid neoplasia. J Nat Cancer Inst 67:501–514.

6. Rowley JD (1973). A new consistent chromosomal abnormality in chronic myelogenous leukemia identified by quinacrine fluorescence and Giemsa staining. Nature 243:290–293.

7. Manolov G and Manolova Y (1972). Marker band in one chromosome 14 from Burkitt lymphoma. Nature 237:33–34.

8. Manolova Y, Manolov G, Kieler J et al. (1979). Genesis of the 14q+ marker in Burkitt's lymphoma. Hereditas 90:5–10.

9. Van Den Berghe H, Parloir C, Gosseye S et al. (1979). Variant translocation in Burkitt lymphoma. Cancer Genet Cytogenet 1:9–14.

10. Berger R, Bernheim A, Weh HJ et al. (1979). A new translocation in Burkitt's tumor cells. Hum Genet 53:111–112.

11. Yunis JJ, Oken MM, Kaplan ME et al. (1982). Distinctive chromosomal abnormalities in histologic subtypes of non-Hodgkin's lymphomas. N Engl J Med 307:1231–1236.

12. Bloomfield CD, Arthur DC, Frizzera EG et al. (1983). Nonrandom chromosome abnormalities in lymphoma. Cancer Res 43:2975–2984.

13. Kirsch IR, Morton CC, Nakahara K and Leder P (1982). Human immunoglobulin heavy chain genes map to a region of translocations in malignant B-lymphocytes. Science 216:301–303.

14. Malcolm S, Barton P, Murphy C et al. (1982). Localization of human immunoglobulin kappa light chain variable region genes to the short arm of chromosome 2 by *in situ* hybridization. Proc Nat Acad Sci USA 79:4957–4961.

15. Erikson J, Martinus J and Croce CM (1981). Assignment of the genes for human lambda immunoglobulin chains to chromosome 22. Nature 294:173–175.

16. Klein G (1983). Specific chromosomal translocations and the genesis of B-cell derived tumors in mice and men. Cell 32:311–315.

17. Dalla-Favera R, Bregni M, Erikson J et al. (1982). Human c-myc onc gene is located on the region of chromosome 8 that is translocated in Burkitt lymphoma cells. Proc Nat Acad Sci USA 79:7824–7827.

18. Erikson J, Finan J, Nowell PC and Croce CM (1982). Translocation of immunoglobulin-V_H genes in Burkitt lymphoma. Proc Nat Acad Sci USA 79:5611–5615.

19. Lenoir GM, Preudhomme JL, Berheim A and Berger R (1982). Correlation between immunoglobulin light chain expression and variant translocation in Burkitt's lymphoma. Nature 298:474–476.

20. Blaney DW, Jaffe ES, Fisher RI et al. (1983). The human T-cell leukemia/lymphoma virus, lymphoma, lytic bone lesions and hypercalcemia. Ann Intern Med 98:144–151.

21. Yoshida M, Miyoshi I and Hinuma Y (1982). Isolation and characterization of retrovirus from cell lines of human adult T-cell leukemia and its implication in the disease. Proc Nat Acad Sci USA 79:2031–2035.

22. Fukuhara S, Hinuma Y, Gotuh Y and Uchino H (1983). Chromosome aberrations in T-lymphocytes carrying adult T-cell leukemia associated antigens from healthy adults. Blood 61:205–207.

23. Vilmer E, Barre-Sinoussi F, Rouzioux C et al. (1984). Isolation of new lymphotropic retrovirus from two siblings with hemophilia B, one with AIDS. Lancet 1:753–757.

24. Popovic M, Sarngadharan MG, Read E and Gallo RC (1984). Detection, isolation and continuous production of cytopathic retroviruses (HTLV III) from patients with AIDS and pre-AIDS. Science 224:497–500.

25. Portlock CS, Rosenberg SA, Glatstein E and Kaplan HS (1976). Treatment of advanced

non-Hodgkin's lymphoma with favorable histologies: Preliminary results of a prospective trial. Blood 47:747–756.

26. Portlock CS and Rosenberg SA (1979). No initial therapy for Stage III and IV non-Hodgkin's lymphomas of favorable histologic types. Ann Intern Med 90:10–13.

27. Anderson T, Bender RA, Fisher RI et al. (1977). Combination chemotherapy in non-Hodgkin's lymphoma: Results of long term follow-up. Cancer Treat Rep 61:1057–1066.

28. Glick JH, Barnes JM, Ezdinli EZ et al. (1981). Nodular mixed lymphoma: Results of a randomized trial failing to confirm prolonged disease free survival with COPP chemotherapy. Blood 58:920–925.

29. Fisher RI, DeVita VT, Hubbard SM et al. (1983). Diffuse aggressive lymphomas: Increased survival after alternating flexible sequences of ProMACE and MOPP chemotherapy. Ann Intern Med 98:304–309.

30. Laurence J, Coleman M, Allen SL et al. (1982). Combination chemotherapy of advanced diffuse histiocytic lymphoma with the six drug COP-BLAM regimen. Ann Intern Med 97:190–195.

31. Coleman CN, Cohen JE, Burke JS and Rosenberg SA (1981). Lymphoblastic lymphoma in adults: Results of a pilot protocol. Blood 57:679–684.

32. Ziegler JL (1981). Burkitt's lymphoma. N Engl J Med 305:735–745.

33. Skarin AT, Canellos GP, Rosenthal DS et al. (1983). Improved prognosis of diffuse histiocytic and undifferentiated lymphoma by use of high dose methotrexate alternating with standard agents (M-BACOD). J Clin Oncol 1:91–97.

34. Kohler G and Milstein C (1975). Continuous cultures of fused cells secreting antibody of predefined specificity. Nature 256:495–497.

35. Nadler LM, Stashenko P, Hardy R et al. (1980). Serotherapy of a patient with a monoclonal antibody directed against a human lymphoma associated antigen. Cancer Res 40:3147–3154.

36. Miller RA and Levy R (1981). Response of cutaneous T-cell lymphoma to therapy with hybridoma monoclonal antibody. Lancet 2:226–230.

37. Miller RA, Maloney DG, Warnke R and Levy R (1982). Treatment of B-cell lymphoma with monoclonal anti-idiotype antibody. N Engl J Med 306:517–522.

38. Ritz J and Schlossman SF (1982). Utilization of monoclonal antibodies in the treatment of leukemia and lymphoma. Blood 59:1–11.

39. Sherwin S, Foon K, Bunn P et al. (1983). Recombinant leukocyte A interferon in the treatment of non-Hodgkin's lymphoma, chronic lymphocytic leukemia, and mycosis fungoides. Proc Amer Soc Hematol 62:765.

40. Ozer H, Leavett R, Ratanatharathorn V et al. (1983). Experience in the use of DNA Alpha$_2$ interferon in the treatment of malignant lymphomas. Proc Amer Soc Hematol 62:761.

41. Oldham RK (1984). Biologicals and biological response modifiers: Fourth modality of cancer treatment. Cancer Treat Rep 68:221–232.

42. Rosenberg SA (1984). Adoptive immunotherapy of cancer: Accomplishments and prospects. Cancer Treat Rep 68:233–255.

43. Collins SJ, Ruscetti FW, Gallagher RE and Gallo RC (1978). Terminal differentiation of human promyelocytic leukemia cells induced by dimethyl sulfoxide and other polar compounds. Proc Nat Acad Sci USA 75:2458–2462.

44. Breitman TR, Selonick SE and Collins SJ (1980). Induction of differentiation of the human promyelocytic cell line (HL-60) by retinoic acid. Proc Nat Acad Sci USA 77:2936–2940.

45. Flynn PJ, Miller WJ, Weisdorf DJ et al. (1983). Retinoic acid treatment of acute promyelocytic leukemia: *In vitro* and *in vivo* observations. Blood 62:1211–1217.

2. The low grade non-Hodgkin's lymphomas: Current approaches to therapy

S. A. ROSENBERG

Stanford University School of Medicine, Stanford, California, USA

The non-Hodgkin's lymphomas are a diverse group of human neoplasms. Among the ten major histologic subtypes recognized by the current histopathologic classifications are several of the most rapidly progressive and fatal human neoplasms, and also some of the most slowly growing, relatively indolent ones [1]. It is paradoxical that those non-Hodgkin's lymphomas which are the most rapidly progressive are also the types which are increasingly curable by currently available therapies. The slowest growing tumors, which also are highly responsive to therapy, have been the most difficult to eradicate. Because of this difference in curability at the extremes of the histologic subtypes, the term 'low-grade' has been recommended for these relatively indolent lymphomas, rather than the previously used term 'favorable'. In fact, patients with low grade lymphomas have a poorer survival rate beyond ten years than do patients with the remaining non-Hodgkin's

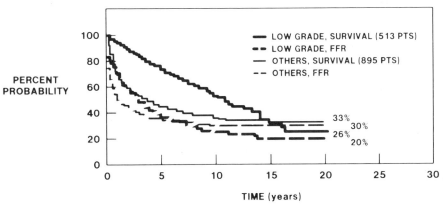

SURVIVAL (-INTERCURRENT DEATHS)   March 1984

Figure 1. Actuarial survival and probability of freedom from relapse (FFR) in non-Hodgkin's lymphomas seen at Stanford University between 1962–1982. Deaths without clinical or autopsy evidence of disease have been excluded (censored at the time of the intercurrent death).

456

lymphomas, all of which have a more aggressive and serious natural history, when untreated (Fig. 1).

The low grade non-Hodgkin's lymphomas are composed of three histologic subtypes, which using the terminology of the working formulation are: follicular, small cleaved cell (FSC), follicular mixed, small and large cell (FM) and small lymphocytic (SL) [1]. The FSC is by far the most common, and corresponds to the nodular, lymphocytic poorly differentiated subtype in the Rappaport classification. The follicular lymphomas are the most common types of non-Hodgkin's lymphomas seen at some United States medical centers, comprising 45% of all primary untreated patients with non-Hodgkin's lymphomas seen at Stanford during a recent international study. During this same period, the follicular subtypes comprised 30% of the non-Hodgkin's lymphomas at two other major United States centers, and only 14% of those seen in Milan, Italy. In Japan, two recent studies found 7% and 18% of non-Hodgkin's lymphomas to be of the follicular subtypes.

Various areas of research, relating to the low grade lymphomas, will be reviewed. The data and observations of Stanford University investigators will be emphasized, though in some areas they are representative of work in the field.

Results of therapeutic trials

The Stanford randomized trials, comparing four different treatment approaches are outlined in Table I [2]. These studies, initiated in 1971, modified in 1974 and closed in 1978 have demonstrated no survival advantage of different therapeutic approaches, with follow-up of six to thirteen years (Fig. 2). All treatment programs, including combination chemotherapy, combined modality treatment, whole body irradiation and single alkylating

Table I. Low grade non-Hodgkin's lymphoma. Stanford randomized trials

1971–1974	Stage IV, 63 pts
	CVP alone CVP/TLI split course Single agent (chlorambucil or Cytoxan)
1974–1978	Stages III, 17 pts and IV, 34 pts
	CVP alone WBI and boost Single agent (chlorambucil or Cytoxan)

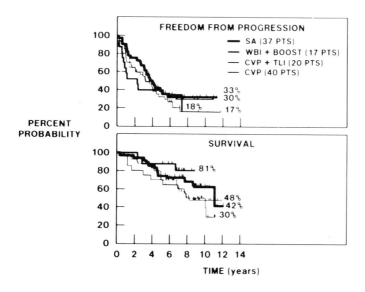

Figure 2. The results of two series of randomized trials of the treatment of advanced low grade non-Hodgkin's lymphomas, initiated in 1971 and modified in 1974. The curves are actuarial and compare single alkylating agent chemotherapy (SA), cyclophosphamide-vincristine-prednisone combination chemotherapy (CVP), whole body irradiation with boost to major involved sites (WBI + BOOST), and combined combination chemotherapy with total lymphoid irradiation (CVP + TLI).

agent therapy have yielded high complete response rates of approximately 80%. Despite these responses, a continuous slow relapse rate has been observed with no evidence for a cured population. The actual survival of these patients has been excellent, however, 76% surviving five years and 55% (actuarially) surviving ten years after treatment initiation (Fig. 3). At about 10 years, 25% of all patients are actuarially free of relapse. It is unlikely that these patients are 'cured' of their disease. Other studies reporting five-year results are comparable (Table II). No curative or superior treatment results have been described [3–10].

Because of the responsiveness of these patients to most forms of therapy, and their excellent survival despite relapse of the disease, randomized controlled clinical trials are essential in comparing different proposed treatment programs.

No initial therapy

The results of therapeutic trials which demonstrate excellent survival despite high relapse rates have made it acceptable to observe selected patients without therapy, until required [11]. A series of 83 such patients has now

Table II. Low grade non-Hodgkin's lymphoma, Stage III & IV, 5-year results

Group	No. Pts	Histologic Subtypes		Stage		Therapy	% Survival	(10 year)	% FFR	(10 year)	Reference
Medical College of Wisconsin	29	SL FSC FM FLC	(1) (20) (4) (4)	III only		TLI	78		61		Cox et al., 1981 [3]
Stanford	66	FSC FM	(42) (24)	III only		TLI (48) TLI+CVP (13) WBI (5)	75	(50)	58	(40)	Paryani et al.,1984 [4]
Hôpital St. Antoine	31	FSC		III & IV		CVP	69		45 (est)		Parlier et al., 1982 [5]
ECOG	97	SL FSC FM FLC	(8) (60) (22) (7)	III & IV		BCVP	62		NA		Oken et al., 1983 [6]
U Washington	16	SL FSC FM	(7) (7) (2)	II III IV	(1) (3) (12)	CHOP×4+TBI or IF	33 (6 yr)		NA		Sullivan et al., 1983 [7]
U Iowa	27	FSC FM	(23) (4)	II III IV	(2) (7) (18)	TBI+CVP	60		27		Corder et al., 1983 [8]
Stanford	114	SL FSC FM	(13) (80) (21)	III IV	(17) (97)	CVP (40) CVP+TLI (20) TBI+Boost (17) Single Agent (37)	76	(55)	35	(25)	Rosenberg et al., 1984 [9]
Stanford	83	SL FSC FM	(21) (44) (18)	III IV	(17) (66)	No initial therapy	75	(65)	40 [a]	(20) [a]	Horning et al., 1984 [10]

[a] Actuarial % not yet requiring therapy

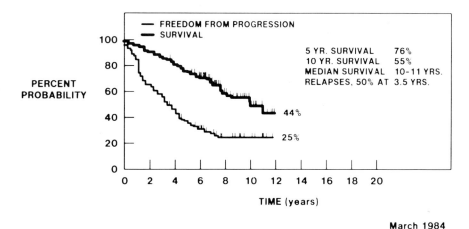

Figure 3. The combined results of 114 patients with advanced low grade non-Hodgkin's lymphomas, receiving the four treatment programs shown in Fig. 2.

been collected at Stanford [10]. These older patients (median age of 57 years), with advanced disease (80% Stage IV), who are asymptomatic and without major threats from the site or bulk of their lymphadenopathy have enjoyed excellent survival (median of 11 years after diagnosis). On the average, these patients who must be observed closely, require some form of therapy, with 50% being treated by three years. In patients with the most common subtype, FSC, the disease progresses somewhat more slowly, with half requiring therapeutic intervention by 50 months. After 10 years, there remain a group of 20% (actuarially) who have yet to require therapy. The FM subgroup differs from the others in this regard, in that all 18 patients of this type have required therapy, with a median time of 11 months.

Those patients approached conservatively with observation initially, have enjoyed as good survival as all patients of these subtypes enrolled on Stanford clinical trials during this period, even correcting for their asymptomatic and non-threatening disease presentations (Fig. 4).

Spontaneous regressions and histologic transformation

Two important clinical and biologic observations have been made in patients with low grade non-Hodgkin's lymphomas. The observation of patients without therapy have facilitated their recognition and interpretation.

Spontaneous regression of the low grade lymphomas is a relatively common event. In patients observed without initial therapy over 20% have experienced a significant spontaneous regression. In the most common FSC

460

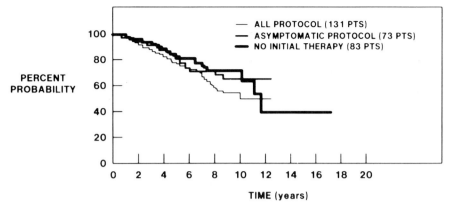

Figure 4. The actuarial survival of 83 patients with advanced low grade non-Hodgkin's lymphomas managed with no initial therapy, compared to 131 patients enrolled on randomized treatment protocols during the same period, including 73 patients of the protocol patients judged to be eligible for the no initial treatment approach.

subtype over 30% will experience such a regression. Spontaneous regressions are not limited to patients who have had no initial therapy. Others who are observed after relapse from chemotherapy or radiotherapy may also spontaneously regress. Of 19 patients reported by Horning to regress without initial therapy, only six have subsequently progressed, and only three of these 19 patients have required treatment of any kind [10]. The mechanism of spontaneous regression is unknown, though it occasionally has been observed after a viral illness (i.e. varicella-zoster infection). It may be that the mechanism of spontaneous regression and of the response to interferon are similar or related.

Another important observation in patients with low grade non-Hodgkin's lymphoma, whether treated or not, is their clinical and histologic transformation to more aggressive non-Hodgkin's lymphomas of intermediate or high grade [12, 13]. With time this transformation occurs, actuarially, in approximately half of all patients with a second biopsy, by 8–10 years. A similar observation has been that follicular lymphomas are rarely found at autopsy, when patients with these lymphomas die as a result of their neoplasm. It remains to be established, with certainty, that the cellular transformation observed morphologically, occurs from the precise clone of neoplastic B-cells found in the original low grade lymphoma. This seems likely from limited immunophenotyping studies available, but more sensitive methods are required.

From a clinical and practical point of view, these transformations present a therapeutic challenge, since they are difficult to treat and to prevent.

Table III. Nodular lymphomas

| IFN | Inst | Dose/schedule | Length | Pt no. | (PrevTx) | Responses | | Duration |
						CR	PR	
rIFNα	Multi	3–50 × 10⁶ u/d	8 w	17	(93)	2	4	2–12 m
rIFNα	BRMP	50 × 10⁶ u/m tiw	12 w	25	(100)	2	13	
rIFNα	Multi	10–25 × 10⁶/m tiw	12 w	11			5	
		Response rate 49%		53		4	22	

Interferon studies

It is of considerable interest that the low grade follicular non-Hodgkin's lymphomas were among the first to be shown to be responsive to the administration of leukocyte interferon. The first three patients of these sub-types treated at Stanford with Cantell interferon all had significant regression of their disease [14]. The responsiveness of these patients to various forms of interferon has been confirmed. Table III summarizes the results of three major trials that used recombinant alpha interferon in patients with low grade lymphomas. Overall the response rates have been approximately 50 percent, usually partial responses, lasting a matter of months, usually less than one year. The mechanism of responses of these neoplasms to interferon has not yet been explained, nor is it known how to incorporate interferon into a treatment program which will have an important impact on these diseases.

Idiotypic monoclonal antibody studies

R. Levy and his colleagues at Stanford have utilized the hybridoma technique towards a better understanding, and perhaps improved management of the low grade B-cell non-Hodgkin's lymphomas [15]. The production of significant quantities of idiotypic specific monoclonal antibodies directed against B-cell neoplasms has been achieved. The initial patient treated with such an antibody has enjoyed a continuous complete remission of his disease for approximately three years. The treatment of additional patients has not been so successful. Of eight patients treated to date, one has had a complete remission, four have had partial remissions and three have had no significant response.

Circulating idiotypic antibody is more common than had been appreciated. This protein if present in sufficient amounts can serve as an effective blocking antibody preventing the therapeutic benefit of the monoclonal antiidiotype. Patients may develop an anti-mouse antibody which limits the anti-tumor effect of the human-mouse hybridoma. Of great interest has been the demonstration of more than one idiotype in immunophenotyping of tumor sections, confirmed as biclonal in immunoglobulin gene rearrangement studies.

Immunoglobulin gene rearrangement studies

The new technique of identifying immunoglobulin gene rearrangements as sensitive specific markers for B-cell neoplasms is providing important new information about the non-Hodgkin's lymphomas, especially the low grade type [16]. The studies by Cleary and Sklar at Stanford are especially relevant [17]. This technique, based on the concepts of Leder, provides a much more sensitive method of identifying small clonal populations of B-cells. It recognizes cells as being of the B-cell lineage even without the expression of surface or secretory immunoglobulins. The technique can recognize as few as one percent clonal cells among a cell population. It is already apparent that low grade B-cell lymphomas are not always monoclonal. Bi-clonal cell populations are being found with surprising frequency in preliminary studies. It is also evident that some low grade to higher grade transformations involve different B-cell clones, or perhaps subclones from a common precursor cell.

This technique promises more than a better understanding of the origin and biology of these neoplasms. It will soon be possible to identify minimal or residual tumor cell populations from tissue, bone marrow and peripheral blood with more sensitivity. The implications for clinical staging and monitoring of clinical trials are obvious and exciting.

Conclusions

The low grade non-Hodgkin's lymphomas present a clinical and biologic challenge to physicians and investigators. These tumors, as suggested by E. Jaffe, have many characteristics, often associated with benign tumors, perhaps peculiar because of the wide distribution of normal B-lymphocytes [18]. The tumors must retain some degree of normal regulation, to be stable for such prolonged periods and to undergo spontaneous regression so often. Their relentless recurrence, despite sensitivity to therapy, their usual normal chromosome number (though abnormal karyotype with 14–18 translocation) [19], their frequent multiclonality and transformation imply fundamental biologic differences of these neoplasms from most others. It may be that responses to human interferon, to anti-idiotype monoclonal antibody, and spontaneous regression are all related to perturbations of the slightly altered lymphoid immunoregulation that characterizes these fascinating human tumors.

Acknowledgements

These studies were supported, in part, by grants CA-05838, CA-34233, CA-09287 and CA-21555 from the National Cancer Institute, National Institutes of Health. Dr. Rosenberg is an American Cancer Society Professor of Clinical Oncology.

References

1. The Non-Hodgkin's Lymphoma Pathologic Classification Project. (1982). National Cancer Institute sponsored study of classifications of non-Hodgkin's lymphomas: Summary and description of a working formulation for clinical usage. Cancer 49:2112–2135.
2. Hoppe RT, Kushlan P, Kaplan HS et al. (1981). The treatment of advanced stage favorable histology non-Hodgkin's lymphoma: A preliminary report of a randomized trial comparing single agent chemotherapy, combination chemotherapy, and whole body irradiation. Blood 58:592–598.
3. Cox JD, Komaki R, Kun LE et al. (1981). Stage III nodular lymphoreticular tumors (non-Hodgkin's lymphoma): Results of central lymphatic irradiation. Cancer 47:2247–2252.
4. Paryani SB, Hoppe RT, Cox RS et al. Role of RT in the management of Stage III follicular lymphomas. J Clin Oncol (in press).
5. Parlier Y, Gorin NC, Najman A et al. (1982). Combination chemotherapy with cyclophosphamide, vincristine, prednisone, and the contribution of adriamycin in the treatment of adult non-Hodgkin's lymphomas: A report of 131 cases. Cancer 50:401–409.
6. Oken MM, Costello WG, Johnson GJ et al. (1983). The influence of histologic subtype on toxicity and response to chemotherapy in non-Hodgkin's lymphoma: An Eastern Cooperative-Oncology Group study utilizing the BCVP regimen. Cancer 51:1581–1586.
7. Sullivan KM, Neiman PE, Kadin ME et al. (1983). Combined modality therapy of advanced non-Hodgkin's lymphomas: An analysis of remission duration and survival in 95 patients. Blood 62:51–61.
8. Corder MP, Leimert JT, Tewfik HH and Lovett JM (1983). Multimodality therapy of favorable prognosis non-Hodgkin's lymphoma. Int J Radiat Oncol Biol Phys 9:1009–1012.
9. Rosenberg SA. Low Grade Non-Hodgkin's Lymphomas: Challenges and opportunities. J Clin Oncol (in Press).
10. Horning SJ and Rosenberg SA (1984). Survival, spontaneous regression and histologic transformation in initially untreated non-Hodgkin's lymphomas of low grade. Proc Amer Soc Clin Oncol 3:253.
11. Portlock CS and Rosenberg SA (1979). No initial therapy for Stage III and IV non-Hodgkin's lymphomas of favorable histiocytic types. Ann Intern Med 80:10–13.
12. Hubbard SM, Chabner BA, DeVita VT Jr et al. (1982). Histologic progression in non-Hodgkin's lymphoma. Blood 59:258–264.
13. Acker B, Hoppe RT, Colby TV et al. (1983). Histologic conversion in the non-Hodgkin's lymphomas. J Clin Oncol 1:11–16.

14. Merigan TC, Sikora K, Breeden JH et al. (1978). Preliminary observations on the effect of human leukocyte interferon in non-Hodgkin's lymphoma. N Engl J Med 299:1449–1453.

15. Miller RA, Maloney DG, Warnke R and Levy R (1982). Treatment of B-cell lymphoma with monoclonal anti-idiotype antibody. N Engl J Med 306:517–522.

16. Korsmeyer SJ, Arnold A, Bakshi A et al. (1983). Immunoglobulin gene rearrangement and cell surface antigen expression in acute lymphocytic leukemias of T-cell and B-cell precursor origins. J Clin Invest 71:301–313.

17. Cleary ML, Chao J, Warnke R and Sklar J (1984). Immunoglobulin gene rearrangement as a diagnostic criterion of B-cell lymphomas. Proc Nat Acad Sci 81:593–597.

18. Jaffe ES (1983). Follicular lymphomas: Possibility that they are benign tumors of the lymphoid system. J Nat Cancer Inst 70:401–403.

19. Yunis JJ, Oken MM, Kaplan ME et al. (1982). Distinctive chromosomal abnormalities in histologic subtypes of non-Hodgkin's lymphomas. N Engl J Med 307:1231–1236.

3. Treatment of diffuse large cell non-Hodgkin's lymphomas

R. I. FISHER, V. T. DEVITA, Jr., D. L. LONGO, D. C. IHDE and
R. C. YOUNG
*Medicine Branch and Naval Medical Oncology Branch, National
Cancer Institute, Bethesda, Maryland, USA*

Advanced stages of diffuse mixed lymphoma, diffuse histiocytic or large cell lymphoma, and diffuse undifferentiated non-Burkitt's lymphoma have traditionally been considered rapidly progressive, fatal diseases. During the 1960s, few of these patients survived for five years [1]. In 1975, it became apparent that combination chemotherapy could achieve long-term disease-free survival in advanced diffuse histiocytic lymphoma [2]. This observation was confirmed soon thereafter [3-6] and, by 1977, it was established that complete remissions, documented by re-evaluation of all initially involved sites, could be obtained in approximately 40-50% of these patients, and that 75-80% of the complete responders would have long-term disease-free survival. In 1983, results of the ProMACE-MOPP treatment program suggested further improvement in these therapeutic results [7]. Several other studies also indicated significantly prolonged survival [8-10]. At present, long-term disease-free survival may be achieved in approximately 60% of all patients with advanced stages of diffuse aggressive lymphomas.

Initial chemotherapy studies

The first generation of NCI studies involved 27 Stage II-IV patients treated with either the C-MOPP regimen or the classical MOPP chemotherapy program [2]. Monthly cycles were repeated for a minimum of 6 cycles or at least 2 cycles after complete clinical remission had been achieved. One month after chemotherapy had been stopped, patients were re-evaluated to determine the status of all previously involved sites. Only patients having no evidence of disease at that point were considered complete responders. Eleven of the 27 patients (41%) achieved complete remission and, with no maintenance chemotherapy, 37% of the patients were alive and disease-free at 5 years. Follow-up now exceeds 10 years and the disease-free survival curve remains essentially flat. There was no significant difference in therapeutic results between C-MOPP (17 patients) or MOPP (10 patients), but the number of patients receiving each regimen was relatively small.

The second generation of NCI studies with combination chemotherapy for the treatment of advanced diffuse histiocytic lymphoma utilized the BACOP chemotherapy regimen [11]. Twelve of 25 patients (48%) with Stage II-IV diffuse histiocytic lymphoma achieved pathologically documented complete remission. These complete remissions also proved durable with few relapses.

Prognostic factors in diffuse aggressive lymphomas

In 1981, we analyzed the prognostic factors associated with long-term survival in all 151 patients with diffuse mixed, histiocytic, or undifferentiated non-Burkitt's lymphoma treated at the National Cancer Institute between 1964 and 1977 [12]. This study indicated that poor prognosis could be expected with a number of characteristics including male sex, constitutional or B symptoms, advanced stage, bone marrow invasion, huge abdominal mass (> 10 cm) with gastrointestinal involvement, hepatic involvement, hemoglobin < 12 g/dl and serum LDH > 250 U. In contrast, classification into diffuse mixed, diffuse histiocytic, or diffuse undifferentiated lymphoma did not provide significant prognostic information. In addition, expert hematopathologists, even at the same institution, had difficulty in consistently separating these histologic subtypes. Therefore, this pathologic subdivision was removed as a critical stratification criterion for clinical trials and the term 'diffuse aggressive lymphomas' was introduced.

The C-MOPP and BACOP studies demonstrated several important conclusions [13]. Essentially all relapses occurred within the first twenty-four months after therapy. Disease-free survival beyond two years was tantamount to cure. In subsequent follow-up, although there has been an occasional late relapse, disease-free survival curves remain flat with 37% long-term disease-free survival. Only patients who achieved pathologically documented clinical remission had long-term disease-free survival. Partial responders included patients in complete clinical remission, but with microscopic residual disease at re-staging evaluation; their survival did not significantly differ from that of the non-responders.

It is important to note that patients in these studies were previously untreated, except for local radiation therapy. The probability of achieving complete remission falls dramatically when relapse occurs after chemotherapy. In fact, there is no evidence at this time that long-term disease-free survival can be obtained in that circumstance.

ProMACE-MOPP clinical trial

Patients received induction therapy with the ProMACE regimen [7] followed by MOPP chemotherapy and late intensification with the ProMACE program. The number of cycles of therapy during each phase of this sequence was determined by the rate of tumor response; the alternate chemotherapy regimen was administered whenever clinically available tumor measurements revealed reduced tumor response. This approach was based on the rationale that a decrease in the rate of tumor response indicated either a reduced rate of cell kill or regrowth of cells that were resistant to the chemotherapy being used in that phase. Details of the carefully structured 'flexi-therapy' induction schedule are presented elsewhere [7].

From September 1977 to August 1981, 79 consecutive patients were entered. The complete remission rate for the entire group of patients was 74%. Median follow-up for this study now exceeds 2½ years. Actuarial analysis predicts that 76% of the complete responders will remain disease-free for more than 3 years and the 4-year survival rate, including all entries, will be 65%. Myelosuppression was dose-limiting and there was a 10% septic death rate. Of note, three of these cases were septic prior to initiation of therapy.

Comparison of chemotherapeutic regimens for diffuse aggressive lymphomas

Comparisons of therapeutic results achieved with the C-MOPP or BACOP regimens versus those obtained with the ProMACE-MOPP program clearly demonstrate a significant improvement with the 'flexi-therapy' sequence. Regardless of the category of patients analyzed, complete remission rates with the ProMACE-MOPP regimen are always higher than those yielded in the previous studies [6]. Survival analyses significantly favor ProMACE-MOPP chemotherapy over the C-MOPP or BACOP programs (Fig. 1).

Table I depicts the pathologic complete remission rate and long-term survival figures for chemotherapeutic regimens commonly used in the treatment of diffuse aggressive lymphomas. In the United States, probably the most commonly utilized chemotherapy for the treatment of diffuse lymphomas is the CHOP regimen (cyclophosphamide, doxorubicin, vincristine and prednisone) [4]. Complete remission rates in CHOP studies have varied depending on whether re-staging of all initially involved sites was performed. None of these studies yielded greater than 60% complete remission rates. Even with pathologic re-staging, more than 50% of the complete responders relapse by two years [4]. This high rate of relapse is in contrast to that seen with any of the other known regimens used for the treatment of this disease. Furthermore, there is no evidence of a significant plateau on the disease-free survival curve following CHOP chemotherapy. As a result fewer than 30% of all patients would be expected to have long-term disease-free survival when treated with CHOP.

SURVIVAL IN DIFFUSE AGGRESSIVE LYMPHOMA

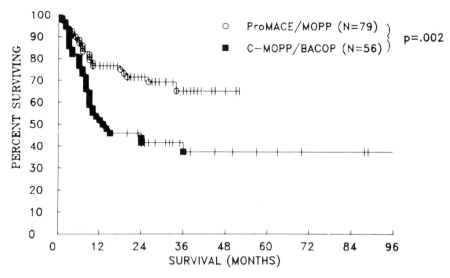

Figure 1. Overall survival of all patients with diffuse aggressive lymphomas treated with either the ProMACE/MOPP or C–MOPP/BACOP regimens.

Table I. Comparison of chemotherapy regimens for aggressive diffuse lymphomas

Regimen (Institution)	No. of patients	Pathologic CR	Long-term survivors
MOPP/C-MOPP (NCI)	24	45%	37%
BACOP (NCI)	32	46%	37%
CHOP (SWOG)	112	58%	< 30%
COMLA (Chicago)	42	55%	48%
COP-BLAM (NYU)	33	73%	TE
M-BACOD (Boston)	101	72%	59%
ProMACE-MOPP (NCI)	79	74%	65%

The highest complete remission rates have recently been reported with ProMACE-MOPP, M-BACOD and the COP-BLAM program [9, 10]. The study of the COP-BLAM program involves a relatively small number of patients and follow-up is too short for long-term predictions. The M-BACOD regimen appears comparable in many regards to the ProMACE-MOPP regimen. Toxicity was also significant with 4–6% of the patients experiencing toxic death. Of note, in the M-BACOD study, patients with diffuse mixed lymphoma were reported separately and, for unclear reasons, experienced a much higher relapse rate [14].

Current NCI trial

Long-term survival rates for patients with diffuse aggressive lymphomas may vary from less than 30% to approximately 60%, depending on the chemotherapeutic regimen utilized. The newer regimens, however, are more complicated and not easily applied to non-research hospitals or to office practice settings. As a result of these limitations, the current NCI study is a prospective randomized trial comparing ProMACE-MOPP with a regimen termed ProMACE-CytaBOM [15]. The ProMACE-MOPP regimen has been changed to give the ProMACE drugs on day 1, MOPP drugs on day 8 and then methotrexate at a dose of 500 mg/m^2 rather than the original 1.5 g/m^2 on day 15. The ProMACE-CytaBOM regimen includes the ProMACE drugs on day 1 and then cytarabine, bleomycin, vincristine and methotrexate on day 8. Both these regimens were designed to allow outpatient administration and to eliminate the need for hospitalization related to methotrexate therapy. At present, 89 patients have been entered. Preliminary analysis indicates a complete remission rate of 70% for ProMACE-MOPP and 80% for Pro-MACE-CytaBOM. There are no statistically significant differences in the complete remission rate or survival between the two regimens at this time. Although it is much too early for definitive conclusions, both regimens appear to be very effective. The septic death rate and the number of hospitalizations for fever or granulocytopenia appear to be significantly reduced. However, the ProMACE-CytaBOM regimen has been associated with approximately a 30% incidence of diffuse interstitial pneumonitis and 7 cases of *Pneumocystis carinii* pneumonia. We have therefore instituted prophylaxis with trimethoprim-sulfamethoxazole for all patients receiving ProMACE-CytaBOM. If longer follow-up proves that the newer treatment programs are as effective as the original regimen, and if we can eliminate *Pneumocystis* infections occurring with ProMACE-CytaBOM, extremely useful treatments would become available for patients with diffuse aggressive lymphomas.

References

1. Jones SE, Rosenberg SA, Kaplan HS et al. (1972). Non-Hodgkin's lymphomas. II. Single agent chemotherapy. Cancer 30:31–38.
2. DeVita VT, Canellos GP, Chabner BA et al. (1975). Advanced diffuse histiocytic lymphoma, a potentially curable disease. Lancet 1:248–250.
3. Berd D, Cornog J, DeConti R et al. (1975). Long term remission in diffuse histiocytic lymphoma treated with combination sequential chemotherapy. Cancer 35:1050–1054.
4. Jones SE, Grozea PN, Metz EN et al. (1979). Superiority of adriamycin containing combination chemotherapy in the treatment of diffuse lymphoma. Cancer 43:417–425.

5. Skarin AT, Rosenthal DS, Maloney WC and Frei E (1977). Combination chemotherapy of advanced non-Hodgkin's lymphoma with bleomycin, adriamycin, cyclophosphamide, vincristine, and prednisone (BACOP). Blood 49:759–770.

6. Sweet DL, Golomb HM, Ultmann JE et al. (1980). Cyclophosphamide, vincristine, methotrexate with leucovorin rescue, and cytarabine (COMLA) combination sequential chemotherapy for advanced diffuse histiocytic lymphoma. Ann Intern Med 92:785–790.

7. Fisher RI, DeVita VT, Hubbard SM et al. (1983). Diffuse aggressive lymphomas: Increased survival after alternating flexible sequences of ProMACE and MOPP chemotherapy. Ann Intern Med 98:304–309.

8. Cabanillas F, Burgess MA, Bodey GP and Freireich EJ (1983). Sequential chemotherapy and late intensification for malignant lymphomas of aggressive histologic type. Amer J Med 74:382–388.

9. Laurence J, Coleman M, Allen SL et al. (1982). Combination chemotherapy of advanced diffuse histiocytic lymphoma with the six drug COP-BLAM regimen. Ann Intern Med 97:190–195.

10. Skarin AT, Canellos GP, Rosenthal DS et al. (1983). Improved prognosis of diffuse histiocytic and undifferentiated lymphoma by use of high dose methotrexate alternating with standard agents (M-BACOD). J Clin Oncol 1:91–97.

11. Schein PS, DeVita VT Jr, Hubbard SP et al. (1976). Bleomycin, adriamycin, cyclophosphamide, vincristine and prednisone (BACOP) combination chemotherapy in the treatment of advanced diffuse histiocytic lymphomas. Ann Intern Med 85:417–422.

12. Fisher RI, Hubbard SM, DeVita VT et al. (1981). Factors predicting long-term survival in diffuse mixed, histiocytic, or undifferentiated lymphoma. Blood 58:45–51.

13. Fisher RI, DeVita VT, Johnson BL et al. (1977). Prognostic factors for advanced diffuse histiocytic lymphoma following treatment with combination chemotherapy. Amer J Med 63:177–182.

14. Canellos G, Skarin A, Rosenthal D et al. (1982). High dose methotrexate combination chemotherapy (M-BACOD) of advanced favorable and intermediate prognosis histology non-Hodgkin's lymphoma. Proc Amer Soc Clin Oncol 1:159.

15. Fisher RI, DeVita VT, Hubbard SM et al. (1984). Randomized treatment of ProMACE-MOPP vs ProMACE-CytaBOM in previously untreated, advanced stage, diffuse aggressive lymphomas. Proc Amer Soc Clin Oncol 3:242.

4. The use of chemotherapy for localized large cell lymphoma. Results from the University of Arizona

S. E. JONES and T. P. MILLER
Section of Hematology and Medical Oncology, Department of Medicine and Cancer Center, University of Arizona Health Sciences Center, Tucson, Arizona, USA

Historically radiotherapy (XRT) alone has been used to treat non-Hodgkin's lymphoma (NHL) of limited extent [1]. The rationale for this approach has included the ability to eradicate tumor in a treatment field and the apparent success of this approach in limited stage Hodgkin's disease (HD). However, it has become clear that the NHL are a diverse group of lymphoid neoplasms clearly distinguishable from HD. The prototype curable NHL is the large cell or 'histiocytic' lymphoma. This differs from HD in that it occurs in older patients, has a high growth fraction with a propensity for rapid hematogenous dissemination, and fails to exhibit the classic radiation dose-response curve [2]. Thus, it is not surprising that many, if not the majority of patients with large cell lymphoma, fail to be cured with radiotherapy alone [1].

During the time that we were learning of the inability of radiotherapy alone to cure large cell lymphoma, effective combination chemotherapy that produced cures in 30–40% of patients with advanced stages of large cell lymphoma became available [3–5]. In 1979, we reported our initial experience with a doxorubicin-based regimen (CHOP = cyclophosphamide, doxorubicin, vincristine, and prednisone) for patients with Stages I or II large cell lymphoma [6]. Our early results suggested that chemotherapy was more effective than radiotherapy alone. Other groups have now confirmed our initial experience [7]. Recently we reported our results with more patients and longer follow-up [8]. In this paper we have further updated our experience utilizing initial chemotherapy (with or without involved field adjuvant radiotherapy) for localized large cell lymphoma.

Materials and methods

Between 1971 and 1983, 49 patients with localized large cell lymphoma received initial chemotherapy. Follow-up extends into 1984 and the median period of follow-up is 41 months. Of the 49 patients, 47 had diffuse large cell and 2 had follicular (nodular) large cell lymphoma.

All patients received chemotherapy with CHOP, except one with pre-existing heart disease who received cyclophosphamide, vincristine, procarbazine, and prednisone (C-MOPP). Patients who received full or nearly full dose chemotherapy were treated with 6–11 courses of CHOP. Elderly patients who received reduced doses of chemotherapy due to bone marrow reserve or those who failed to achieve complete remission (CR) with 3 courses of CHOP received involved field XRT (3600–6000 rad) after chemotherapy. Patients were restaged for residual disease following completion of therapy. Regular examinations were part of the follow-up routine. Relapse was confirmed by biopsy. Retreatment was individualized, but consisted, in general, of reinduction with CHOP, local XRT, and 1 year of further chemotherapy with cyclophosphamide, vincristine, and prednisone (COP). More details on this trial can be found elsewhere [8].

Results

The clinical features, including prognostic factors that are associated with decreased survival, are shown in Table I. Of 49 patients, 30 (61%) received chemotherapy alone and 19 (39%) received adjuvant XRT after chemotherapy. The median time of follow-up is now 41 months.

Forty-eight of 49 patients (98%) have achieved a CR. Seven patients have relapsed (Table II) and 41 patients remain continuously free of disease. Of the 7 patients who relapsed, 6 achieved a second CR and 4 remain alive for 6+ to 36+ months. Although the results of treatment with CHOP plus XRT are somewhat better than CHOP alone (2 relapses in 19 patients compared to 6 relapses in 30 patients), this difference is not significant (Table

Table I. Clinical and treatment features of 49 patients with localized large cell lymphoma

Chemotherapy alone	61%
Chemotherapy + XRT	39%
Stage I (I_E)	37%
Stage II (II_E)	63%
Potentially adverse factors	
Age >65	33%
GI tract involvement	14%
Bulky disease	35%
Extranodal disease	55%
Median age (range)	60 (24–86)

Table II. Treatment outcome in 49 patients with localized large cell lymphoma

	Chemotherapy alone	Chemotherapy plus radiotherapy
No. treated	30	19
% CR	100%	95%
No. relapses	6	2
% Relapse-free survival at 2 years	76%	92%
% Survival at 2 years	96%	95%

II). None of the potentially adverse prognostic factors shown in Table I affected treatment outcome.

Discussion

In the last 10 years we have evaluated the strategy of initial doxorubicin-based combination chemotherapy as primary therapy for patients with Clinical Stages I or II large cell lymphoma. This approach alleviates the need for surgical staging and permits immediate systemic treatment which avoids the 10–20% probability of systemic relapse during local radiotherapy. A 98% CR rate was achieved in 49 consecutive patients. Based on our and other studies [7, 9], the strategy of initial chemotherapy has proven to be an effective means of increasing the cure rate in patients with localized large cell lymphoma.

Two major questions remain. The first is whether adjuvant involved field radiotherapy should be given after initial chemotherapy. In our series the best results were obtained with adjuvant radiotherapy (Table II). However, additional data would be required for firm conclusions.

The second question is what constitutes the best chemotherapy for these patients. In a recent report by the Milan group, chemotherapy with a doxorubicin regimen (BACOP) administered before XRT proved to be superior to COP [9]. Thus, a program like CHOP or BACOP utilizing doxorubicin appears to be the standard for future comparisons. Recently, several groups

Table III. Comparison of 3 treatment regimens for Stage II lymphoma

Regimen (Reference)	No.	% CR	% RFS
CHOP ($\pm$XRT) (current series)	31	97%	84%
M-BACOD [10]	15	87%	80%
ProMACE-MOPP [12]	17	82%	—

have reported apparently even better results employing regimens with other drugs, e.g., M-BACOD or ProMACE-MOPP [10–12]. Although these regimens appear to produce better results than CHOP or BACOP in advanced stage disease, their relative value is less clear in early stage disease. In Table III, we have compared our results for patients with Stage II disease treated with CHOP to those published with M-BACOD or ProMACE-MOPP [10, 12]. There does not appear to be much difference. However this issue, too, could only be resolved by a comparative clinical trial.

References

1. Miller TP and Jones SE (1980). Is there a role for radiotherapy in localized diffuse lymphomas? Cancer Chemother Pharmacol 4:67–70.
2. Fuks Z and Kaplan HS (1973). Recurrence rates following therapy of nodular and diffuse malignant lymphomas. Radiology 108:675–684.
3. DeVita VT, Canellos GP, Chabner BA et al. (1975). Advanced diffuse histiocytic lymphoma, a potentially curable disease: Results with combination chemotherapy. Lancet 1:248–250.
4. McKelvey EM, Gottlieb JA, Wilson HE et al. (1976). Hydroxyldaunomycin (adriamycin) combination chemotherapy in malignant lymphoma. Cancer 38:1484–1493.
5. Jones SE, Grozea PN, Metz EN et al. (1979). Superiority of adriamycin containing combination chemotherapy in the treatment of diffuse lymphoma: A Southwest Oncology Group study. Cancer 43:417–425.
6. Miller TP and Jones SE (1979). Chemotherapy of localized histiocytic lymphoma. Lancet 1:358–360.
7. Cabanillas F, Bodey GP and Freireich EJ (1980). Management with chemotherapy only of Stage I and II malignant lymphoma of aggressive histologic types. Cancer 46:2356–2359.
8. Miller TP and Jones SE (1983). Initial chemotherapy for clinically localized lymphomas of unfavorable histology. Blood 62:413–418.
9. Bonadonna G, Bajetta E, Lattuada A et al. (1984). CVP vs BACOP chemotherapy sequentially combined with irradiation in Stage I-II diffuse non-Hodgkin's lymphomas. In: Jones SE and Salmon SE (Eds.). Adjuvant Therapy of Cancer. IV. New York: Grune and Stratton. In press.
10. Skarin AT, Canellos GP, Rosenthal DS et al. (1983). Improved prognosis of diffuse histiocytic and undifferentiated lymphoma by use of high dose methotrexate alternating with standard agents (M-BACOD). J Clin Oncol 1:91–98.
11. Skarin A, Cannellos G, Rosenthal D et al. (1983). Moderate dose methotrexate (m) combined with bleomycin (B), adriamycin (A), cyclophosphamide (C), oncovin (o) and dexamethasone (D), (m-BACOD), in advanced diffuse histiocytic lymphoma (DHL). Proc Amer Soc Clin Oncol 2:220.
12. Fisher RI, DeVita VT, Hubbard SM et al. (1983). Diffuse aggressive lymphomas: Increased survival after alternating flexible sequences of ProMACE and MOPP chemotherapy. Ann Intern Med 98:304–309.

5. A randomized comparison of two chemotherapy regimes: BACOP vs COPP in the treatment of diffuse histiocytic and mixed lymphoma

J. DUPONT [1], G. CARAY [1], C. SCAGLIONE [1], S. BESUSCHIO [1],
S. BRUNO [1], P. WOOLLEY [2], M. TEZANOS PINTO [1],
P. SCHEIN [2] and S. PAVLOVSKY [1]
[1] Grupo Argentino de la Leucemia Aguda (GATLA), Buenos Aires, Argentina, and [2] T.V. Lombardi Cancer Research Center, Georgetown University, Washington, D.C., USA

Diffuse histiocytic lymphoma (DHL), the paradigm of the aggressive lymphomas, is the most common subtype among the non-Hodgkin's lymphomas. Current therapeutic strategies are based on a long history of clinical trials. Radiation therapy has repeatedly proved insufficient to control high grade lymphomas [1, 2]. DHL is very sensitive to chemotherapy as even single agent treatment may produce complete remission (CR) [3]. Early drug combinations yielded CR rates as high as 44%, but median relapse-free survival was approximately 14 months [4]. Others reported CR rates of 15 to 20% and also found short relapse-free survival [5].

Initial reports from the US National Cancer Institute (NCI) described the potential of the C-MOPP regimen for diffuse histiocytic lymphoma [6]. At the same time, the aggressive nature of the disease and its ability to progress during rest intervals following myelosuppressive chemotherapy was being recognized. The subsequent NCI regimen (BACOP) included bleomycin and prednisone given between cyclic administrations of cyclophosphamide, doxorubicin and vincristine [7]. Clinical results obtained with BACOP were superior to those of C-MOPP, with long-term complete remission rates of 45% vs 40% [8].

Our study was undertaken to randomly compare these regimens. The BACOP vs C-MOPP trial was started in October 1977 and closed in December 1983.

Materials and methods

The study conducted in the framework of a collaborative PAHO-NCI project, was open to patients under 70 years of age with no prior treatment, except for palliative localized radiation therapy, and the diagnosis of diffuse histiocytic lymphoma, diffuse mixed lymphoma or undifferentiated lymphomas at any clinical stage. Ineligibility criteria included severe pulmonary

Table I. Drugs, dose and schedule of BACOP and C-MOPP

BACOP		C-MOPP	
Cyclophosphamide	650 mg/m^2 IV d 1 & 8	Cyclophosphamide	650 mg/m^2 IV d 1 & 8
Doxorubicin	25 mg/m^2 IV d 1 & 8	Vincristine	1.4 mg/m^2 IV d 1 & 8
Vincristine	1.4 mg/m^2 IV d 1 & 8	Procarbazine	100 mg/m^2 PO d 1 to 8
Prednisone	60 mg/m^2 PO d 14 to 28	Prednisone	40 mg/m^2 PO d 1 to 14
Bleomycin	5 mg/m^2 IV d 14 & 20		

disease unrelated to lymphoma, chronic renal impairment, uncontrolled infection or diabetes mellitus.

Routine staging methods consisted of physical examination, blood cell counts, bipedal lymphangiogram, bilateral biopsy of the bone marrow utilizing a Jamshidi needle, and percutaneous liver biopsy. Computed tomography was used when available. Laparotomy was not routinely performed, but nine patients underwent laparotomy due to initial abdominal tumor or gastrointestinal tract involvement. Tissue sections were reviewed in our institution (B.S.) as well as at Georgetown University.

Following stratification by institution (Georgetown vs GATLA) and Clinical Stages II-II vs III-IV), patients were randomly allocated to receive either the BACOP or the C-MOPP induction regimen (Table I). Cycles were repeated at 28-day intervals. Patients who had clinical complete response after 6 cycles were restaged with liver and bone marrow biopsies as well as repeat lymphangiograms and CT scans, even when baseline studies were normal. Patients who were in partial remission after 6 cycles received 2 additional cycles. Treatment was withdrawn after 2 cycles of treatment in non-responders. After completion of treatment, responders were observed monthly for signs of relapse; all patients were to be followed up until death.

Response rates were analyzed with the Chi square test. Life tables were compared with the logrank test.

Results

Of 106 patients entered, 92 were considered evaluable (Table II). Fourteen patients were not evaluable because of follow-up shorter than 8 months (ten), prior malignancy, relapsed lymphoma, drug dosage violation or loss to follow-up during induction therapy (one each).

Fifty-one percent of the patients (25/49) on BACOP and 49% (21/43) on C-MOPP achieved CR. Patients with mixed lymphoma had a lower CR rate (38%) than patients with DHL (54%). A trend to lower CR rate was

Table II. Clinical features of 92 evaluable patients

	BACOP	COPP
Median age	50 Y	54 Y
Range	(20–70 Y)	(19–73 Y)
Male	38	19
Female	11	24
DHL	41	32
DML	8	11
Stage I	—	1
Stage I$_E$	3	1
Stage II	2	4
Stage II$_E$	7	3
Stage III	14	12
Stage IV	23	22
Mediastinum	10	3

Extranodal sites-number of patients (localized and advanced)

	BACOP	COPP
Marrow	3	4
Liver	4	5
Lung	1	1
Bone	5	1
Soft-Tissue	1	—
GI	6	5
Effussion	3	4
Skin	4	2
Breast	1	3
Other	14	8

More than one site is considered separately

observed in the elderly and in patients with multiple extranodal sites or bulky abdominal disease. Among those with Stage I-II disease, the CR rate was 58% with BACOP vs 67% with C-MOPP (Table III). None of these differences were statistically significant. The three patients (2 BACOP; 1 C-MOPP) who presented with initial CNS involvement responded briefly.

Eight of the 25 CR with BACOP and 11 of the 21 with C-MOPP have relapsed. Eleven patients had CNS relapses that were either isolated (2 BACOP; 2 C-MOPP) or that occurred with relapses in other sites (3 BACOP; 4 C-MOPP). Eight initially had cranial palsies, two had lymphomatous meningitis and one had spinal cord compression. All had bulky abdominal disease or extranodal disease at presentation.

At 48 months, 63% of the BACOP patients are projected to remain in first CR vs 40% for the C-MOPP patients (Fig. 1). This difference is not statistically significant. The median CR duration with C-MOPP is 10

478

Table III. Response to induction treatment according to induction scheme and stages

	Stage	CR		PR	Null (> 6 cyc)	Died	Total
		No.	%				
BACOP	I-II	7	58	2	2	1	12
	III	9	64	1	2	2	14
	IV	9	39	4	5	5	23
COPP	I-II	6	67	1	–	2	9
	III	5	42	5	1	1	12
	IV	10	45	6	3	3	22

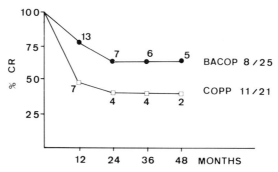

Figure 1. Duration of complete remission from diffuse histiocytic and mixed non-Hodgkin's lymphoma according to treatment.

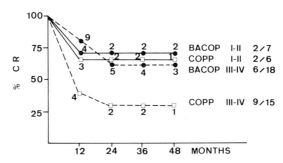

Figure 2. Duration of complete remission from diffuse histiocytic and mixed non-Hodgkin's lymphoma according to stage and treatment.

months. Disease-free survival curves in both treatment groups have plateaued after 24 months. Only one relapse has been observed after 18 months in the BACOP group.

CR duration was affected by Clinical Stage, but not by histology. The probability to remain in CR at 48 months was 67% for Stages I-II, 53% for

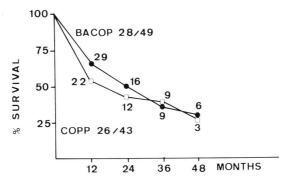

Figure 3. Survival in patients with diffuse histiocytic and mixed non-Hodgkin's lymphoma according to treatment.

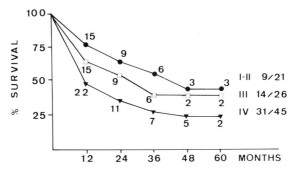

Figure 4. Survival in patients with diffuse histiocytic and mixed non-Hodgkin's lymphoma according to stage. Stage I-II vs Stage IV = $p < 0.05$.

Stage III and 39% for Stage IV patients. Among those with Stages III-IV disease, this probability was 61% with BACOP vs 30% with C-MOPP (Fig. 2). This important and persistent trend did not reach statistical significance.

Expected survival at 48 months was 29% and 28% for the BACOP and C-MOPP arms, respectively (Fig. 3). Median survival was 24 months for BACOP and 14 months for C-MOPP patients. None of these differences are significant.

Clinical Stages I-II patients had longer survival than Stages III-IV patients ($p < 0.05$) (Fig. 4). The median survival times in Clinical Stages I-II, III and IV were 40, 27, and 12 months, respectively. The three patients who had initial CNS involvement lived for 2, 11, and 20 months, respectively. Overall, 51% of the CR patients were alive on the projected curve at 60 months. Fourteen of 46 CR patients died, mostly after remissions of less than 18 months. Median survival of partial responders was 14 months, with only 3 of 19 patients still alive. Response to therapy results in a marked difference in survival ($p < 0.0005$) (Fig. 5).

480

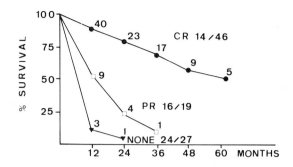

Figure 5. Survival in patients with diffuse histiocytic and mixed non-Hodgkin's lymphoma according to response.
CR vs PR = $p<0.0005$; CR vs No response = $p<0.0005$; PR vs No response = $p<0.005$.

Toxicity

Myelosuppression was most common and predictable. Median WBC nadir was $1600/mm^3$ with BACOP and $2600/mm^3$ with C-MOPP. Hospitalization for suspected or documented infections was required in five patients (4 BACOP; 1 C-MOPP).

One patient in the BACOP arm had documented septal fibrosis complicated with pulmonary candidiasis and subsequently died without evidence of disease. Another patient in the same treatment arm died from liver failure shortly after induction therapy. Repeated liver biopsies showed fatty replacement and incipient fibrosis. She had no clinical or radiologic evidence of active disease. None of the patients developed clinical heart failure during the induction phase and there were no reports of cardiac failure in patients followed up while in CR.

Discussion

Results initially reported with chemotherapy combinations such as BA-COP [7] and CHOP-Bleo [9] were most promising and doxorubicin-containing regimens have even been advocated for standard treatment in the community for patients with aggressive lymphoma [10]. However, there are a number of disappointing reports with CHOP-like regimens. Parlier et al. [11] treated advanced diffuse lymphomas with CVP vs CVP plus doxorubicin. The latter induced significantly more CR (67 vs 25%), but median survival was similar in both groups (26 months for CVP plus doxorubicin vs 24 months for CVP alone). Armitage et al. [12] reviewed their CHOP experience and found a 30% actuarial relapse rate. Relapses were evenly distributed throughout the first 2 years of remission and whether patients will stop relapsing after longer follow-up remains unclear. In addition, the British group reported 39% of CR with CHOP as compared to 23% with total body irradiation [13]. CHOP did significantly better in Stage III patients. There was a leveling off in relapse-free survival, but the median survival in both treatment groups was less than 2 years.

The BACOP regimen developed at NCI appeared to achieve higher CR rate as compared to historical controls treated with C-MOPP [8]. At Sidney Farber, a non-randomized trial also suggested increased response rate and response duration with a BACOP program [14]. In our study, about 50% of the patients achieved complete remission with either BACOP or C-MOPP. Partial responders tended to relapse rapidly, with progression in the original sites of disease and generally short-lasting or no response to secondary therapy.

There was a remarkable trend favoring BACOP over C-MOPP in terms of CR duration, especially in Stages III and IV. This trend was not translated into differences in overall survival; five patients in C-MOPP relapsed and remain alive with disease, while only one relapsed patient in BACOP remains alive. Disease-free survival curves are plateauing with only one late relapse. Overall, CNS relapses occurred in 12% of the patients, but only one-third of these relapses were initially isolated.

Toxicities of the regimens were comparable and generally acceptable, considering the advanced stage of disease in most patients. Only one patient developed pathologically documented bleomycin-related pulmonary fibrosis. Myelosuppression was not a limiting factor. None of the patients experienced doxorubicin-induced congestive heart failure.

Our results are consistent with those of the few trials that also randomly evaluated the role of doxorubicin regimens. BACOP increased response duration but failed to prolong survival. As suggested by other studies, diffuse histiocytic lymphoma might still require a more aggressive therapeutic approach. Most favorable results were recently reported. The ProMACE-MOPP regimen achieved 74% CR in 74 evaluable patients [15]. Only 18% of the CR patients had relapsed at the time of report; median survival was expected to exceed 4 years. Skarin et al. [16], using the M-BACOD regimen that incorporates high-dose methotrexate (HDMTX), obtained 72% CR in 101 patients; the projected 5-year survival rate was 80%. CNS relapses occurred in 5.4% of the patients compared to 18% in their previous report on BACOP. This improved figure was ascribed to HDMTX and better disease control.

Appendix

The following institutions and investigators participated in the study: Insti-

482

tuto de Investigaciones Hematológicas 'Mariano R. Castex', Academia Nacional de Medicina, Buenos Aires, Argentina (S. Pavlovsky, G. Garay, C. Scaglione, J. Dupont, S. Bruno); Centro de Educación Médica e Investigación Clínica, Buenos Aires, Argentina (A. Suarez, R. Cachione, E. Egozcue); Hospital Escuela 'Gral. San Martín, Buenos Aires, Argentina (C.A. Barros, J. Pileggi, H. de Maria, C. Ruso, M. Curuchet, R.J. Boccaci, R. Kvicala); Policlínica 'Mariano R. Castex', Buenos Aires, Argentina (M. Palau, S.C. de Sica); Instituto 'Gral San Martín', Buenos Aires, Argentina (L. Bergna, R. Tur); Hospital 'Teodoro Alvarez', Buenos Aires, Argentina (F. Cavagnaro, R. Bezares, L. Palmer, E. Morgenfeld, A. Diaz, P. Francica); Hospital 'Clemente Alvarez', Roario, Argentina (J. Saslavsky, J.M. Lein); Hospital Bancario, Buenos Aires, Argentina (M. Tezanos Pinto, C. Marin, C. Rodríguez Fuchs, L. Carreras); Hospital Ferroviario Central, Buenos Aires, Argentina (E. Quiroga Micheo, S.I. Calabria, S. de Rudoy); Hospital Israelita, Buenos Aires, Argentina (M.O. Dragosky, M.A. Sorrentino, H.H. Murro); Hospital Durand, Buenos Aires, Argentina (A.B.S. Huberman, S. Goldztein, J. Chilelli, F. Helft, N. Shilton, A. Starosta); Hospital Ferroviario, Mendoza, Argentina (J. Sanguedolce, M. Arce-Sosa, R. Bianchi, T.Y. Rodríguez); Hospital Central, Mendoza, Argentina (L. Pérez Polo, V. Labanca, A. Gray, E. Boris, D. Ramos); Hospital Regional, Neuquén, Argentina (R. Raña, A.S. Palacios, T. Sniechowsky, M. Pasanisi); V.T. Lombardi Cancer Research Center, Georgetown University, Washington, D.C. (P. Woolley, P. Schein).

Acknowledgements

Supported in part by Grant N01-C027391 from the Pan American Health Organization/National Cancer Institute, NIH and FUNDALEU (Argentina Foundation Against Leukemia).

We gratefully acknowledge the statistical assistance of Daniel Goldar and the typographical assistance of Marta O'Brien.

References

1. Glatstein E, Fucks Z, Goffinet DR et al. (1976). Non-Hodgkin's lymphoma of Stage III: Is total lymphoid irradiation appropriate treatment? Cancer 37:2806–2812.
2. Johnson RE, Canellos GP, Young RC et al. (1978). Chemotherapy (Cyclophosphamide, Vincristine, and Prednisone) versus radiotherapy (total body irradiation) for Stage II-IV poorly differentiated lymphocytic lymphoma. Cancer Treat Rep 62:321–325.
3. Jones SE, Rosenberg SA, Kaplan HS et al. (1972). Non-Hodgkin's lymphoma II: Single agent chemotherapy. Cancer 30:31–38.
4. Coltman CA, Luce JK, McKelvey EM et al. (1977). Chemotherapy of non-Hodgkin's lymphoma: Ten years experience in the Southwest Oncology Group. Cancer Treat Rep

61:1067–1078.

5. Portlock C and Rosenberg SA (1976). Combination chemotherapy with cyclophosphamide, Vincristine and Prednisone in advanced non-Hodgkin's lymphomas. Cancer 37:1275–1282.

6. DeVita VT, Canellos CP, Chabner BA et al. (1975). Advanced diffuse histiocytic lymphoma, a potentially curable disease Lancet 1:248–250.

7. Schein PS, DeVita VT, Hubbard S et al. (1978). Bleomycin, adriamycin, cyclophosphamide, vincristine and prednisone (BACOP) combination chemotherapy in the treatment of advanced diffuse histiocytic lymphoma. Ann Intern Med 85:417–422.

8. Fisher RI, DeVita VT, Johnson BL et al. (1977). Prognostic factors for advanced diffuse histiocytic lymphoma following treatment combination chemotherapy. Amer J Med 63:177–182.

9. Rodriguez V, Cabanillas F, Burgess EM et al. (1971). Combination chemotherapy (CHOP-Bleo) in advanced (non-Hodgkin) malignant lymphoma. Blood 49:325–333.

10. Jones SE, Grozea PN, Metz EN et al. (1979). Superiority of adriamycin containing combination chemotherapy in the treatment of diffuse lymphoma. Cancer 43:417–425.

11. Parlier Y, Gorin NC, Stachoeiak J et al. (1981). Adriamycin for the treatment of non-Hodgkin's lymphoma. Sem Hop Paris 57:1685–1690.

12. Armitage JO, Corder MP, Leimert JT et al. (1980). Advanced diffuse histiocytic lymphoma treated with cyclophosphamide, doxorubicin, vincristine and prednisone (CHOP) without maintenance therapy. Cancer Treat Rep 64:649–654.

13. British National Lymphoma Investigation Report (1981). A prospective comparison of combination chemotherapy with total body irradiation in the treatment of advanced non-Hodgkin's lymphoma. Clin Oncol 7:193–200.

14. Skarin AT, Rosenthal DS, Moloney WC and Frei E III (1977). Combination chemotherapy of advanced non-Hodgkin's lymphoma with bleomycin, adriamycin, cyclophosphamide, vincristine and prednisone (BACOP) Blood 49:759–770.

15. Fisher RI, DeVita VT, Hubbard SM et al. (1983). Diffuse aggressive lymphomas: Increased survival after alternating flexible sequences of ProMace and MOPP chemotherapy. Ann Intern Med 98:304–309.

16. Skarin AT, Canellos GP, Rosenthal DS et al. (1983). Improved prognosis of diffuse histiocytic and undifferentiated lymphoma by use of high dose methotrexate alternating with standard agents (M-BACOD) J Clin Oncol 1:91–98.

6. Results of ifosfamide-Etoposide combinations for patients with recurrent or refractory aggressive lymphoma

F. CABANILLAS, F. B. HAGEMEISTER, S. RIGGS,
P. SALVADOR, W. VELASQUEZ, P. MCLAUGHLIN and T. SMITH
*Section of Lymphoma, Department of Hematology, Division of
Medicine and Department of Biomathematics, The University of
Texas System Cancer Center M.D. Anderson Hospital and Tumor
Institute, Houston, Texas, USA*

The prognosis of patients with recurrent or refractory lymphoma is known to be extremely poor. This is particularly true with the aggressive types of lymphoma which correspond to the intermediate and high grade cell types of the International Working Classification [1]. From 1977-1983, we treated 187 patients with recurrent or refractory aggressive lymphoma. The main goal of this study is to assess their response to salvage chemotherapy and their long-term outcome. A secondary goal is to compare the three different treatment programs used during this six-year period, all of which were based on ifosfamide and etoposide (VP-16).

Materials and methods

A total of 187 consecutive patients with the following histologic types were treated: 150 with follicular or diffuse large cell, 16 with diffuse small cleaved, 14 with lymphoblastic, 7 with diffuse small non-cleaved. All but eight of these 187 patients had recurrent or progressive lymphoma after previous chemotherapy regimens that included doxorubicin in all except two. The eight individuals who were treated before progressive or recurrent disease developed were patients who had received first-line doxorubicin combination regimens for a minimum of six courses and had only achieved a partial remission. They were clearly not approaching complete remission and their therapy was changed to the salvage regimen before progressive disease ensued. These eight patients are analyzed separately.

The three salvage regimens as well as the years in which they were utilized and the number of patients in each regimen are shown in Table I. The doses and schedules used in each of these regimens have been published [2-4]. Patients were treated for a minimum of one year or until they developed progressive disease while on therapy. Complete responders received therapy for one year after achievement of complete response (CR), defined as the

Table I. Ifosfamide + VP-16 based salvage combinations at M. D. Anderson Hospital

Year	Acronym	No. Patients	Drugs
1977–80	IMVP-16	33	Ifosfamide, methotrexate, etoposide
1980–81	AIVP-16	24	Amsacrine, ifosfamide, etoposide
1981–83	MIME	122	Mitoguazone, ifosfamide. methotrexate, etoposide

disappearance of all signs and symptoms related to the disease for a minimum of 2 months. Partial remission (PR) was defined as a $\geq 50\%$ reduction in the sum of the product of the diameters of measured lesions lasting for at least one month. Any response less than partial remission including mixed responses, and response $> 50\%$ but lasting less than one month were considered failures. Overall and relapse-free survival were measured from onset of treatment with the salvage regimen until evidence of progressive disease was documented. Survival curves were analyzed by the Gehan modification of the Wilcoxon test [5]. Chi square tests were used to compare response rates.

A stepwise logistic regression procedure had previously been used in patients treated with IMVP-16 and AIVP-16 to determine the combination of patient characteristics important in predicting complete response [6]. This resulted in an equation that related the probability of response to a linear function of regression coefficients times patient characteristics. The form of the equation is as follows:

$$\ln(pi/1 - pi) = a_o + a_l \text{ (characteristic l)} + \ldots + aj \text{ (characteristic j)}$$

where pi is the probability of response for the ith patient, and the a's represent regression coefficients. The stepwise determination of the coefficients allows an ordering of the importance of the factors in the equation. Thus, the first patient characteristic was the most important single characteristic in predicting probability of response, the second characteristic the second most important (assuming the first one was in the equation), and so on. The resulting equation was then used to predict prospectively the response of patients treated with MIME.

Results

Table II depicts the response rate of the 179 patients who were treated with any of our 3 salvage regimens after they had relapsed or progressed on first line therapy. The highest CR rate occurred in the lymphoblastic types and

Table II. Response of aggressive histologic types

Cell type	No.	% CR	% CR + PR	p value
Large cell	142	32	60	
Diffuse small cleaved (DPDL)	16	38	82	
Lymphoblastic	14	50	64	ns
Diffuse small non-cleaved (DUL)	7	43	72	
Total	179	33	63	

the highest overall response rate took place in the diffuse small cleaved (diffuse poorly differentiated lymphocytic in Rappaport's classification). The small number of patients in all but the large cell category makes it difficult to compare adequately response among the different cell types. The CR rate for all cell types was 34% and overall response rate was 63%.

The response rate according to treatment regimen is shown in Table III. The highest CR rate observed was in the amsacrine-containing AIVP-16 regimen. However, the overall response rate for that particular regimen was the lowest. These differences are not statistically significant.

The most frequently observed cell type in this study was the large cell. The response of this particular type according to the treatment regimen used is shown in Table IV. Again, the highest CR rate recorded was in the AIVP-16 regimen but the overall response rate was lowest in that regimen also. A total of 32% CR and 60% overall response rate was seen when all regimens were combined.

In order to detect if there were any differences in response rate related to the number of relapses experienced before treatment with the salvage regimen, Table V was constructed. Here are shown, in addition to the 179 patients previously analyzed, the eight patients who were treated before relapse. These are represented under 0 relapses. The CR rate decreased pro-

Table III. Response according to treatment regimen

Regimen	No.	% CR	% CR + PR	p value
MIME	122	31	64	
IMVP-16	33	33	66	ns
AIVP-16	24	50	54	
Total	179	33	63	

Table IV. Response of large cell lymphomas according to treatment

Regimen	No.	% CR	% CR+PR	p value
MIME	99	31	63	
IMVP-16	28	29	61	
AIVP-16	15	40	40	ns
Total	142	32	60	

Table V. Response according to number of relapses

No. Relapses	No. Patients	% CR	% CR+PR	p value
0	8	88	100	
1	86	44	70	
2	62	27	56	<.05
≥3	31	19	55	

gressively as the number of relapses increased. The overall response rate followed a similar pattern. These differences were highly significant statistically.

A mathematical model was derived from the experience gained with the IMVP-16 and AIVP-16 studies (Fig. 1). This model takes into consideration three prognostic factors determined to be important in predicting response to these salvage regimens. These factors are: quality of response to first line treatment, histologic type (aggressive vs indolent), and presence or absence of central nervous system lymphoma. This regression model was prospectively applied to the patients treated with MIME. In 17 patients treated with MIME, there was not enough information available to calculate the predicted probability of response. This probability was calculated for the remaining 105 patients. These patients were grouped into four prognostic categories for which actual or observed response rate is shown in Table VI. The percent observed response rate increases in proportion to the increase

$$\ln\left(\frac{p}{1-p}\right) = 0.05 - 1.05\,(R-1.78) + 1.38\,(D-1.64) - 2.17\,(C-0.06)$$

Figure 1. Regression equation derived from IMVP-16 and AIVP-16 studies used to predict response to salvage chemotherapy. p = probability of response, R = response to first line treatment (CR = 1, PR = 2, F = 3), D = diagnosis (low grade = 1, high and intermediate grade = 2), C = CNS disease (yes = 1, no = 0).

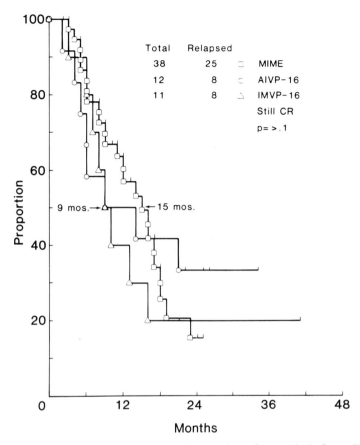

Figure 2. Ifosfamide + VP − 16 based salvage regimens relapse-free survival of complete responders with aggressive histologies according to treatment.

in percent predicted response rate. In the prognostic categories in which < 50 % and 50–74 % response were expected, the observed/expected ratio was > 1.

Table VI. Results of applying regression model to MIME regimen

Ranks of predicted response	No. patients	% Expected response	% Observed response	Observed/ Expected	*p* value
< 50	27	33	39	1.18	
50–74	30	62	70	1.13	.85
75–100	48	82	83	1.01	
Total	105	64	67	1.05	

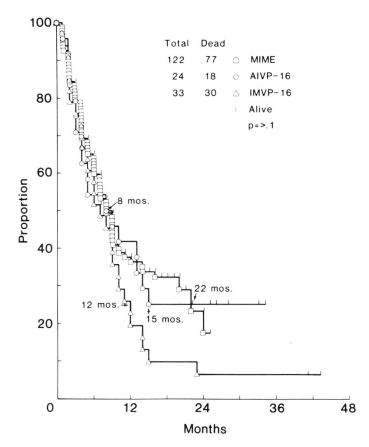

Figure 3. Ifosfamide + VP − 16 based salvage regimens. Survival of aggressive histologies according to treatment.

The relapse-free survival of the 60 patients who achieved CR is depicted in Fig. 2. The median relapse-free survival of the MIME treated patients is 15 months compared to nine months for the other two regimens. This difference, however, was not statistically significant. The survival of the 179 patients treated is shown in Fig. 3. The median survival was 7–8 months for all patients independent of the treatment regimen used.

Discussion

Paradoxically, patients with aggressive types of lymphoma have been found to respond better to salvage combination chemotherapy with ifosfamide-VP-16 regimens than those with the indolent types of lymphoma. We have shown in this study that 33% of all patients with aggressive histologic types can be expected to achieve CR with these combinations. Sixty-three percent can be expected to achieve either CR or PR. AIVP-16 yielded the highest CR rate of the three regimens (Table III) but its overall response was the lowest. In spite of higher CR rate with this regimen, survival did not appear to be prolonged as compared to that seen with MIME (Fig. 3). There is a suggestion that the tail of the AIVP-16 curve is higher than that in the IMVP-16 curve. Similarly, the 25th percentile survival of the MIME treated patients is superior to the IMVP-16 regimen (22 months vs 12 months) but the difference is not statistically significant (Fig. 3). In view of the fact that the CR rate of these three regimens was < 50%, a difference in median survival should not be expected. However, longer follow-up might reveal some important differences in the 25th percentile survival. The median relapse-free survival of the MIME treated patients is 15 months vs 9 months for the other two regimens (Fig. 2). This initial advantage in relapse-free survival is lost later as the slope of the curve so far has not changed significantly, in contrast to the other two treatment groups. The shape of the MIME curve can still change in the future since it contains numerous early censored observations.

The fact that both the overall response and CR rates are higher for patients treated for first relapse should encourage us to use these salvage regimens as early as possible. In fact, the high CR rate seen in the eight patients who were treated when their partial response to first-line treatment had reached a plateau suggests that this might be the best time to utilize these salvage regimens. Another approach might be to utilize these regimens in alternating fashion with other established regimens such as CHOP-Bleo as part of front line therapy.

Finally, we have shown that the regression model derived from the data accumulated in the IMVP-16 and AIVP-16 studies can accurately divide the MIME treated patients into three prognostic categories. The observed response rate for each of these categories is different and changes in proportion to the predicted response rate (Table VI). Applying the model prospectively to MIME, we have found that actual and predicted response rates to MIME are very similar (67% observed vs 64% expected). The accuracy of this model in predicting response to ifosfamide-VP-16 based salvage regimens makes it an important tool in analyzing future clinical trials.

References

1. The Non-Hodgkin's Lymphoma Pathologic Classification Project (1982). National Cancer Institute sponsored study of classifications of non-Hodgkin's lymphomas. Cancer 49:2112–2135.
2. Cabanillas F, Hagemeister FB, Bodey GP and Freireich EJ (1982) IMVP-16: An effective

492

regimen for patients with lymphoma who have relapsed after initial combination chemotherapy. Blood 60:693–697.

3. Cabanillas F, Legha S, Bodey GP and Freireich EJ (1981). Initial experience with AMSA as a single agent treatment against malignant lymphoproliferative disorders. Blood 57:614–616.

4. Cabanillas F, Hagemeister FB, McLaughlin P et al. (1984). MIME combination chemotherapy for refractory or recurrent lymphomas. Proc Amer Soc Clin Oncol 3:250.

5. Gehan EA (1965) A generalized Wilcoxon test for comparing arbitrarily singly censored samples. Biometrika 52:203–224.

6. Cox DR (1970). The Analysis of Binary Data, pp. 87–90. London: Methuen & Co., Ltd.

7. New agents for Hodgkin's and non-Hodgkin's lymphomas

A. C. LOUIE [1], F. CAVALLI [2] and M. ROZENCWEIG [1]

[1] *Bristol-Myers Company, Syracuse, New York, USA and*
[2] *Servizio Oncologico, Ospedale San Giovanni, Bellinzona, Switzerland*

Advances in the treatment of Hodgkin's and non-Hodgkin's lymphomas represent one of the great triumphs of cancer research of the past two decades. A relatively large number of active drugs have been found and their use in a variety of combinations has led to clinically useful responses and cures in substantial numbers of patients with disease too advanced to be considered for radiation therapy. Inspite of these successes, a decreasing but very important fraction of patients fail to respond or progress after successful conventional chemotherapy. Consequently, new therapeutic agents are needed to improve the results of both front-line and salvage regimens.

The very success of conventional chemotherapy and radiation therapy has complicated the search for new agents. New drugs for lymphoma must be active in patients with marked reductions in bone marrow function and other organ system impairments due to extensive prior treatment or lymphomatous involvement. In addition, the new drug must not be cross-resistant with any of the 6 to 10 antineoplastic drugs the patient has generally been already exposed to. Identifying a useful new agent is a challenging task considering these constraints.

Despite these difficulties, new agents continue to be tested for activity in lymphomas. The 1983 edition of the Compilation of Experimental Cancer Therapy Protocol Summaries prepared by the International Cancer Research Data Bank lists 105 lymphoma study protocols. Fifty-three of these trials (50%) utilize one or more new agents for some phase of treatment and 40 trials (48%) are specific for previously treated patients. New cytotoxic agents are tested most frequently. Biologic response modifiers and immunologic manipulations are used in far fewer trials. The surprisingly high percentage of studies utilizing investigational drugs reflects both the level of interest in developing new drugs and the high degree of difficulty in bringing many of these compounds to market.

Two factors which may impact on the probability of response in phase II trials are the likelihood of cross resistance to prior therapy and the probability of suboptimal dosing due to bone marrow impairment. In theory, novel chemotypes should have a lower probability of cross resistance with prior therapy than analogs and the need for dose reductions for real or anticipated myelosuppression should be less for agents with reduced effect on the bone marrow. Consequently, among drugs with equal inherent anti-lymphoma activity, novel chemotypes which are non-myelosuppressive could be expected to have the greatest likelihood of succeeding in early clinical trials. Conversely, myelosuppressive analogs, especially analogs of drugs which are widely used for lymphomas, are likely to have a low probability of success. This article will review a number of new agents which are or might be of interest for the treatment of Hodgkin's and non-Hodking's lymphomas. These agents have been grouped according to whether they are novel chemotypes or analogs and whether they are myelosuppressive or non-myelosuppressive (Table I).

Novel agents with minimal myelosuppression

Gallium nitrate

Gallium nitrate is a novel chemotype with intrinsic activity against non-Hodgkin's lymphomas and modest activity against Hodgkin's disease. It is a group IIIA metal salt with activity against Walker 256 carcinosarcoma [1]. Inflammatory and neoplastic lesions concentrate gallium salts such as iso-

Table I. New agents for Hodgkin's and non-Hodgkin's lymphoma

Novel agents	Analogs
Non-myelosuppressive	
Gallium nitrate	Bleomycin analogs
Mitoguazone	Peplomycin
Spirogerimanium	Tallysomycin S_{10}b
Myelosuppressive	
Amsacrine	Anthracycline analogs
Diaziquone	Aclacinomycin
DFMO	4-demethoxydaunorubicin
Mitoxantrone	4-deoxydoxorubicin
	Platinum analogs
	Carboplatin
	Iproplatin

topic gallium citrate [2]. Clinical studies have been conducted with gallium nitrate since 1978 and phase I studies of gallium nitrate found dose-limiting nephrotoxicity following brief intravenous infusions [3]. Phase II studies have been successful because this drug has minimal myelosuppression and dose-schedule adjustments have reduced the morbidity from nephrotoxicity. Response may be schedule dependent and it will be very important to confirm reports of superior activity for continuous infusions over intermittent schedules.

Warrell et al. [4] performed a phase I-II study in lymphoma patients using a 7-day continuous infusion of gallium nitrate with doses of 200–400 mg/m^2/day. The recommended dose for phase II trials was 300 mg/m^2 × 7 days and nausea was dose-limiting. Other adverse events included reversible non-cumulative nephrotoxicity, hypocalcemia, pulmonary complications (including fever, pleural effusions, and interstitial lung infiltrates), diarrhea, paresthesia, and high frequency hearing loss. Myelosuppression was minimal. Among the 47 patients from both the phase I and phase II groups with bidimensionally measurable lesions, objective responses were found in 5 of 10 DLPD, 6 of 15 DHL, 2 of 5 NLPD, and 3 of 17 Hodgkin's disease patients. A total of 16 patients had objective response for an overall response rate of 34%, and 2 of the 6 responses in DHL were complete responses (CR) lasting 10 and 14+ months. The median duration of response was only 2.5 (1–14+) months. The authors noted that the absence of nausea and myelosuppression made this drug especially useful for patients with extensive prior therapy.

A phase II study using gallium nitrate 700 mg/m^2 every 2 weeks was conducted by the Southwest Oncology Group [5]. Thirty-three of 38 patients were evaluable and responses were seen in 1 of 5 Hodgkin's disease, 6 of 26 (23%) diffuse non-Hodgkin's lymphomas (2 of 10 DHL, 2 of 6 DLPD, 2 of 6 DML, 0 of 2 DLWD, 0 of 2 DUL), and 0 of 5 nodular non-Hodgkin's lymphomas (0 of 3 NLPD, 0 of 1 NML, and 0 of 1 NHL). Every patient had extensive prior therapy and 4 of the 7 responders had never achieved a response with prior combination chemotherapy. Toxic effects included nausea, vomiting and renal toxicity. Myelosuppression was mild with only 5 of 32 (16%) evaluable patients having moderate to life threatening decreases in blood count and 3 of these 5 patients had tumor involvement of the bone marrow with reduced pretreatment blood counts.

The Southeastern Cancer Study Group used the same dose and schedule and reported objective responses in 3 of 15 Hodgkin's disease and 4 of 14 patients with favorable non-Hodgkin's lymphomas [6]. Only 1 of 18 patients with large cell lymphomas, 2 of 16 patients with unfavorable histology lymphomas, and 0 of 10 patients with CLL responded. Decreases in hemoglobin and creatinine clearance were noted and 30% of patients had nausea with or without vomiting. Treatment was generally well tolerated.

Mitoguazone (methylglyoxal-bis[guanylhydrazone])

This drug was first synthesized by Thiele and Dralle [7] in 1898 and was the subject of *in vitro* studies in the late 1950s [8–11]. The mechanism of action has not been established but is believed to be related either to interference with polyamine synthesis or to a direct antimitochondrial effect [12]. By the mid 1960's clinical studies utilizing multiple daily dosing schedules for 5 to 14 days demonstrated activity in lymphomas, acute leukemia, and several solid tumors but at the expense of severe side effects including hypoglycemia which was occasionally fatal, myelosuppression, and ulceration of the skin and gastrointestinal tract. These difficulties led to a general loss of interest for nearly 15 years which ended when studies using weekly schedules were found to be less morbid [12]. More recent studies have confirmed activity for mitoguazone in Hodgkin's and non-Hodgkin's lymphomas inspite of extensive prior therapy. Drug toxicities although troublesome have usually been reversible and are considered acceptable. The absence of major myelosuppression is a useful characteristic and of equal importance is the apparent lack of cross-resistance with other drugs.

The early studies have been well summarized by Warrell and Burchenal [12]. These trials administered mitoguazone at intervals of less than one week, usually on daily schedules of 5, 10, or 14 days duration. Responses were seen in Hodgkin's disease, reticulum cell sarcoma, and mycosis fungoides.

Hart et al. [13] reported one partial response (PR) lasting 5+ months among 2 evaluable Hodgkin's disease patients given mitoguazone by 24 hour infusion. Mucositis was the principal toxicity noted.

Two large phase II trials confirmed activity for mitoguazone in both Hodgkin's and non-Hodgkin's lymphomas. Warrell et al. [14] treated 51 patients with weekly mitoguazone $600 \, mg/m^2$. The treatment schedule was changed to every other week for patients who experienced dose-limiting toxicity. All patients had received extensive prior therapy, with a median of 3 [1–7] prior chemotherapy courses and a median exposure to 8 [4–12] prior chemotherapeutic agents. No complete responses were observed but partial response occurred in 6 of 13 (46%) with Hodgkin's disease, 3 of 13 (23%) with diffuse histiocytic lymphoma, 5 of 10 with DLPD, 2 of 4 with NLPD, and 2 of 6 with mycosis fungoides. The median duration of response was 3 (1–11+) months. Treatment induced myopathy was dose limiting and facial paresthesias could be reduced by prolonged infusion. Other side effects included vomiting, mucositis, myalgia, skin rash, diarrhea, arthralgia, and bronchospasm. The authors concluded that mitoguazone was active against lymphomas, although at the cost of substantial toxicity. They noted that changing from a weekly to an every other week schedule, reduced the treatment morbidity.

The Southwest Oncology Group also used mitoguazone 600 mg/m² weekly to treat extensively pre-treated patients with Hodgkin's and non-Hodgkin's lymphomas [15]. One of 6 (17%) patients with NLPD had a complete response. Partial response occurred in 3 of 10 with Hodgkin's disease, 2 of 13 with DLPD, 2 of 9 with DLWD, 1 of 10 with DHL, 1 of 1 with NML, 1 of 6 with NLPD, 1 of 4 with unclassified lymphoma, and 2 of 2 with mycosis fungoides. No response was seen in a single patient with nodular histocytic lymphoma. Response duration was 26+ weeks for the single patient with CR and 6 (2–36+) weeks for patients with PR. Adverse events were similar to those reported earlier and included nausea, vomiting, anorexia, diarrhea, mucositis, neuralgia, circumoral paresthesia, skin rash and mild hematologic toxicity consisting of anemia in 6, leukopenia in 5 and thrombocytopenia in 1 of the 62 treated patients.

Difluoromethylornithine (DFMO)

DFMO is an irreversible inhibitor of ornithine decarboxylase, the first enzyme of the polyamine synthetic pathway. Inhibition of this enzyme blocks the rate limiting step in the conversion of ornithine to polyamines thought to be important in the control of cell growth and differentiation. Although this drug is myelosuppressive, it is discussed with mitoguazone because it is also a polyamine synthesis inhibitor. DFMO inhibits a number of *in vitro* experimental tumors including L1210 leukemia, rat hepatoma, HeLa cells, and mouse mammary sarcoma. It also inhibits *in vivo* human small cell lung carcinoma grown in nude mice. Phase I studies in which drug was administered every 6 hours for 28 days showed 2.25 gm/m² to be the maximally tolerated dose but produced no responses in Hodgkin's disease (2 patients) or non-Hodgkin's lymphoma (one patient) [16]. The dose limiting toxicity was thrombocytopenia and other side effects included fatigue, anemia, anorexia, diarrhea, and nausea. Although no anti-lymphoma activity has been demonstrated for DFMO, it and other polyamine synthesis inhibitors should be evaluated further because of their unique mechanism of action. Unfortunately, this drug will be difficult to use in patients with impaired bone marrow function because of dose limiting thrombocytopenia.

DFMO has also been combined with mitoguazone. Interest in this drug combination increased after a report of activity in acute lymphocytic leukemia [17]. A phase I trial of DFMO and mitoguazone was conducted by Warrell et al. [18]. No responses were reported for 12 patients with lymphoma treated with this combination and the use of DFMO 4 gm/m² daily and mitoguazone 200–700 mg/m² every 2 weeks produced substantial toxicity. These trials are based upon observations of synergistic cytotoxicity in experimental *in vivo* model systems [19, 20], the possibility that sequential interference of polyamine synthesis could be more effective than use of either drug by itself [18] and evidence of increased mitoguazone uptake following exposure of cells to DFMO [21].

Spirogermanium

Spirogermanium is a novel azaspirane compound in which germanium is substituted for a one carbon moiety in the spirane structure. It is inactive against the usual experimental models used for screening, such as the L-1210 and P-388 leukemias, B-16 melanoma, and Lewis lung carcinoma but is active against Walker 256 carcinosarcoma, 13762 mammary adenocarcinoma, and 11095 prostatic carcinoma [22]. In toxicology studies lethal doses produced generalized seizures in dogs and mice and there was a notable absence of bone marrow toxicity [23]. Phase I studies demonstrated dose-limiting neurologic toxicity which could be diminished by reducing the rate of administration. Although doses and schedules were different among the various phase I studies responses were reported in some [24–26] but not all trials [27, 28] in patients with non-Hodgkin's lymphomas including the diffuse histiocytic and diffuse mixed subtypes. Phase II studies have confirmed activity for this compound against lymphomas. The absence of myelosuppression allows the use of this drug in patients with impaired bone marrow function. The occurrence of central nervous system toxicity, marked by dizziness, paresthesia, and lethargy complicates treatment although these effects can be mitigated somewhat by reducing the rate of administration. It is encouraging that prolonged complete responses were achieved in a few cases in spite of extensive prior therapy.

Evidence of anti-lymphoma activity in phase I trials led to a phase II study conducted at Georgetown University and the Baltimore Cancer Research Center [29]. Spirogermanium $50 \, mg/m^2$ was administered either 3 times per week for one week every three weeks or every other day for 6 doses followed by weekly maintenance doses. Objective responses occurred in 4 of 19 (21%) patients with non-Hodgkin's lymphomas and 1 of 4 (25%) Hodgkin's disease patients. Response durations were 78+ and 61+ weeks for the two complete responders and 13, 10, and 9 weeks for the three partial responders. All but a single patient had received extensive prior treatment and 11 of the 23 patients had received both chemotherapy and radiation therapy prior to entry. There was no evidence of bone marrow toxicity despite the presence of tumor involvement in the bone marrow in 12 of the 23 patients.

Analogs with minimal myelosuppression

Bleomycin analogs: Peplomycin and tallysomycin $s_{10}b$

Peplomycin is an analog of bleomycin which differs only in the terminal amino moiety. It's mechanism of action and activity in experimental tumor systems are similar to bleomycin. Clinical trials performed in Japan and Europe demonstrate objective responses in lymphomas [30].

Mathe et al. [31] reported a broad phase II trial conducted by the E.O.R.T.C. Clinical Screening Group in which peplomycin 5 or 10 mg/m^2/day was given for 5 consecutive days. A total of 21 patients with non-Hodgkin's lymphomas were treated resulting in 2 complete and 5 partial responses. Three partial responses were also seen in 10 patients with Hodgkin's disease. Approximately 30–35% of patients experienced moderate or greater toxicity.

Kimura et al. [32] also reported 7 complete and 5 partial responses among 36 patients with non-Hodgkin's lymphoma and 2 complete and 1 partial response among 7 Hodgkin's disease patients.

Peplomycin, like bleomycin, has intrinsic activity against lymphomas with little impact on the bone marrow. What is unclear from the available data is what effect prior treatment with bleomycin has on the likelihood of response to peplomycin.

Tallysomycin $s_{10}b$ is a bleomycin analog which contains an additional amino sugar (4 amino-4, 6-dideoxy-L-talose), a longer peptide chain and a shorter terminal amino group. Compared with bleomycin this drug has similar activity in experimental tumor systems, mechanism of action, and toxicology. Phase I studies have just been completed and phase II trials are about to begin. It is too early to evaluate the activity of this compound in lymphomas [30].

Novel myelosuppressive chemotypes

Amsacrine

Amsacrine is an amino acridine first described by Cain et al. in 1974 [33, 34]. It entered clinical trials in 1978 and was found in phase I trials to have activity in Hodgkin's disease and CLL [35]. Phase II trials confirmed intrinsic activity for this drug against lymphomas (Table II) but also demonstrated its potential for severe myelosuppression. In every trial myelosuppression was the most prominent toxic event and occasionally persistent leukopenia would lead to major infections. Other common adverse events included nausea, vomiting, and mucositis.

Table II. Activity of amsacrine in lymphoma

	Author (Ref.)	No.	CR	PR	% RR	Remission duration
Hodgkin's Disease	Weick [36]	20	0	4	20	2, 3, 5, 8 mos.
	Bajetta [42]	12	1	6		
	Ahmann [39]	5	0	2		4, 5 mos
	Cabanillas [40)	4	0	0		
	Case [37]	2	0	0		
	Total	43	1	12	30	
Non-Hodgkin's Lymphoma	Weick [36]	51	1	7	16	9 mos. (CR) 1, 1, 3, 4, 4, 12, 33 mos. (PR)
	Bajetta [42]	37	4	6	27	
	Cabanillas [40]	21	3	3	29	8, 14+, 18+ mos. (CR) 1, 3, 5 mos. (PR)
	Case [37]	18	2	8		
	Warrell [38]	15	0	0		
	Ahmann [39]	9	0	3		
	Tan [44]	5	0	1		
	Calabresi [41]	2	0	0		
	DeJager [43]	1	0	1		
	Total	159	10	29	25	

Most of the trials reported for lymphomas have used a single dose of $90-120 \text{ mg/m}^2$ every 3-4 weeks. The largest trial using this dose and schedule was reported by Weick et al. [36] for the Southwest Oncology Group in which 1 CR (9 mos) and 7 PR (4 mos, range 1-33) among 51 (16%) evaluable non-Hodgkin's lymphoma patients and 4 PR (2, 3, 5, 8 mos) among 20 (20%) Hodgkin's disease patients were observed. Case [37] treated patients with a similar dose and schedule and had 2 CR and 8 PR among 18 patients with non-Hodgkin's lymphoma and no response in 2 patients with Hodgkin's disease. Warrell et al. [38] using the same dose and schedule, 120 mg/m^2 every 3 weeks, reported no responses in 15 non-Hodgkin's lymphoma patients. Nine patients were treated by Ahmann et al. [39] and 33% had objective responses.

A smaller number of patients have been treated with amsacrine $30-40 \text{ mg/m}^2 \times 3-4$ days. Using this schedule Cabanillas et al. [40] achieved 3 complete (8, 14+, 18+ mos) and 3 (1, 3, 5 mos) partial responses in 21 (29%) patients with non-Hodgkin's lymphoma and no response among 4 patients with Hodgkin's disease. Calabresi et al. [41] had no response in 2 patients with non-Hodgkin's lymphoma. Bajetta et al. [42] reported that amsacrine doses of 90–120 mg/m^2 given every 3 weeks produced objective responses in 50% of Hodgkin's disease and 23% of non-Hodgkin's lymphoma patients. In a later trial with a new formulation of amsacrine (lactate) they demonstrated similar response rates (67% and 33% in Hodgkin's and non-Hodgkin's lymphoma) while using 225 mg/m^2 every 3 weeks. Antitumor activity has also been reported for oral amsacrine 120 mg/m^2/d × 5 days in a single patient with lymphoblastic lymphoma [43].

One of 5 children with non-Hodgkin's lymphoma achieved a partial response after amsacrine treatment in a trial conducted by Tan et al. [44]. These patients were initially treated with total doses of 140–225 mg/m^2 given in divided doses over 2–3 days with dose escalation up to 600 mg/m^2 given over 5 days depending on toxicity.

Diaziquone (aziridinylbenzoquinone, AZQ)

AZQ is a rationally synthesized alkylating agent designed to penetrate the central nervous system by optimizing both lipid and water solubility and having low ionization [45, 46]. It is active in a number of experimental systems including L1210 leukemia, P388 leukemia, colon 26 tumor, and CD8F1 mammary tumor [47, 48]. In animal models significant concentrations of drug have been achieved in the central nervous system and activity has been demonstrated against intracranially implanted L1210 and P388 leukemias when AZQ is given by the intraperitoneal route [47, 48]. Clinical experience with AZQ is limited but it appears to have some inherent activity against lymphomas which can be obscured by prior therapy. Cumulative thrombocytopenia will limit the use of this drug in patients with extensive prior therapy. Future trials will have to pay strict attention to the extent of prior therapy and its impact on the bone marrow reserve.

McLaughlin et al. [49] administered AZQ 30 mg/m^2 every 3–4 weeks to 19 patients and reported one complete response among 9 patients with DHL. This response lasted 6 months. This group of patients had received a median of 3 regimens and 10 antitumor agents prior to treatment with AZQ.

Case and Hayes [50] treated 30 patients using a similar dose and schedule and observed 2 complete and 3 partial responses in 16 patients with DHL, 1 partial response among 8 with NLPD, 1 complete response among 3 with DLPD, one complete response among 3 with Hodgkin's disease, and a single response in a patient with DML. No responses were seen among 2 patients with DLWD and 2 patients with lymphoblastic lymphoma. Cross resistance with prior alkylating agent therapy was suggested by the inverse correlation between responsiveness to treatment and extent of prior therapy and the fact that complete responses occurred only in patients with no more than one prior regimen of treatment. One of 2 patients with solid CNS lesions responded suggesting that therapeutic levels could be achieved in CNS lesions.

In both studies cumulative myelosuppression manifested by thrombocytopenia was dose limiting. Case noted that 50 % of patients given more than 2 cycles of AZQ required dose reductions because of cumulative thrombocytopenia. Other toxicities included nausea, vomiting, alopecia, mucositis and febrile reactions.

The daily × 5 schedule has been used in few patients with lymphomas. Griffin et al. [51] reported no response in single patients with lymphocytic lymphoma and Hodgkin's disease treated on a phase I study. Tan et al. [52] treated patients with 6–9 mg/m^2/day × 5 days and had 2 partial responses in 2 patients with Hodgkin's disease. Myelosuppression was again dose-limiting; vomiting and transient SGOT elevations were also noted.

Mitoxantrone

This drug is a bis substituted anthraquinone [53] which binds DNA tightly [54]. It has excellent activity in animal tumor screens [55] and studies using the human tumor cloning assay suggest little cross reactivity with doxorubicin [56]. Activity in lymphomas has been reported in phase I and confirmed in phase II trials with objective responses observed in all histologic subtypes of lymphoma. Few complete responses have been observed and it is likely that treatment of patients earlier in the course of their lymphoma would produce even higher objective and complete response rates. This level of activity confirms observations in experimental systems of at least a partial lack of cross-resistance with doxorubicin. The future use of this drug in lymphomas will depend on the extent of its contribution to the cardiac toxicity of anthracyclines and how well patients with compromised bone marrow function tolerate myelosuppression from this drug.

A minor response was reported for a lymphoma patient on the daily × 5 schedule in a phase I study [57] and a single partial response was reported in a patient with T-cell lymphoma treated with mitoxantrone 4 mg/m^2/day for 5 days in a second phase I study [58]. In a phase II trial using single doses 12–14 mg/m^2 every 3 weeks a single partial response lasting 6 months was achieved among 3 Hodgkin's disease patients and no response occurred in a single patient with non-Hodgkin's lymphoma [59].

A broad phase II study performed by the EORTC using 12–14 mg/m^2 administered every 21 days was reported by DeJager et al. [60]. They observed response in 1 of 5 patients with Hodgkin's disease and 1 of 2 patients with non-Hodgkin's lymphoma.

Results of two separate phase II trials using mitoxantrone for lymphomas were recently reported by Gams et al. [61] for the Southeastern Cancer Study Group. The first trial treated 32 patients with 5 mg/m^2 on a weekly schedule. Partial responses were seen in 1 of 9 patients with DHL and in single patients with DML and DLPD. No response was observed among 6 patients with Hodgkin's disease, 6 patients with favorable non-Hodgkin's lymphoma and 4 patients with CLL. In a second trial 8 patients were given mitoxantrone as a single dose of 14 mg/m^2 every 4 weeks. Partial responses were seen in 3 of 3 patients with NLPD or NML, 1 of 2 patients with DLPD or DML or nodular histocytic lymphomas, and 1 of 3 patients with DHL. The authors concluded that activity was seen in all histologic subtypes of lymphoma and that the high-dose intermittent schedule appeared to be superior to the lower dose weekly schedule.

Coltman et al. [62] reported results from a Southwest Oncology Group study in which mitoxantrone was given as a single dose of 12 mg/m^2. Response rates were low with only 3 partial responses among 13 Hodgkin's disease patients, and 2 complete and 7 partial responses among 37 patients with non-Hodgkin's lymphomas. Six of the responding patients had response durations greater than 230 days. The patients had been extensively pre-treated with median exposure to 6 drugs prior to mitoxantrone. In this study 5 patients were removed from study because of concerns over cardiotoxicity. All of these patients had prior exposure to anthracyclines.

Both the SEG and SWOG trials reported myelosuppression, nausea, vomiting, and diarrhea as toxic effects of treatment. Observations of cardiac toxicity in patients with prior anthracycline exposure suggest that mitoxantrone could contribute to cardiac toxicity in anthracycline pretreated patients even if the risk from mitoxantrone alone is relatively slight.

Myelosuppressive analogs

Anthracycline analogs

Anthracycline analogs are difficult to evaluate for activity against lymphomas because doxorubicin, the parent compound, is an important part of first and second line treatments. Consequently, nearly all patients eligible for phase II studies will have received doxorubicin first. Phase II trials are likely to demonstrate activity only in analogs with a high degree of non-cross resistance to the parent compound. In addition analogs maybe expected to contribute to anthracycline induced cardiomyopathy and may be unsafe in patients with extensive exposure to doxorubicin.

Aclacinomycin
Clinical trials for this drug began in Japan in 1977. Most trials have used the

weekly or single dose schedule and myelosuppression, manifested by leukopenia and thrombocytopenia was dose-limiting. Other adverse events include nausea, vomiting, diarrhea, and reversible liver function abnormalities. Cardiac conduction abnormalities have been reported [63] and histologic evidence of mild myocardial damage has been found without clinical
signs of congestive heart failure [64]. The available evidence suggests that
aclacinomycin has inherent activity against lymphomas. Unfortunately, the
qualitative pattern of toxicity appears to be similar to that of doxorubicin
and there seems to be significant cross resistance with prior anthracycline
therapy.

Warrell et al. [65] treated 31 extensively pretreated patients using doses of
100 mg/m^2 every 3 weeks and observed PR in 1 of 4 patients with DLPD
and a response in a single patient with lymphoplasmacytoid immunocytoma. No response was seen in 7 patients with Hodgkin's disease, 9 patients
with DHL, 4 patients with NLPD, and 6 patients with mycosis fungoides.
The two objective responses were both brief and occurred in patients with
no prior exposure to anthracyclines. The authors concluded that the low
response rate was probably due to cross resistance with doxorubicin.

Mathé et al. [66] treated 45 patients with acute leukemia or non-Hodgkin's lymphoma using doses of 10–30 mg/m^2/day IV for 6 to 30 days. Two
complete and one partial response occurred in 8 evaluable patients with
lymphoma. Aclacinomycin did not produce alopecia and major cardiac toxicity was not observed although minor EKG abnormalities occurred in 13%
of the entire group. A multicenter phase II trial conducted in Japan was
reported by Oki et al. [63]. One complete and 6 partial responses in 9 lymphosarcoma patients, 2 complete and 3 partial responses in 9 reticulum cell
sarcoma patients, and 1 complete and 2 partial responses in 7 Hodgkin's
disease patients were observed for an overall objective response rate of
60%. A variety of dose schedules were used and details of prior anthracycline exposure were not given (Table III).

Table III. Anthracycline analogs

	Reference	Hodgkin's disease			Non-Hodgkin's lymphoma		
		No.	CR	PR	No.	CR	PR
Aclacinomycin	Warrell [65]	7	0	0	24	0	2
	Mathé [66]				8	2	1
	Oki [63]	7	1	2	18	3	9
4-Demethoxydaunorubicin	Bonfante [68]	3	0	2	1	0	1
	Coonley [69]	6	0	0	16	0	0

4-Demethoxydaunorubicin
This analog of daunorubicin was selected for development because it was less cardiotoxic in animal systems and because it was active by both the parenteral and oral routes in experimental systems. There is evidence for some anti-lymphoma activity but the clinical data base is very limited (Table III).

A phase I study reported by Berman et al. [67] documented leukopenia and thrombocytopenia as the main toxicities. They also demonstrated 32–35% bioavailability for the oral route and higher rates of nausea, vomiting, and alopecia when the drug was given orally. Bonfante et al. [68] reported a partial response in one patient with non-Hodgkin's lymphoma and 2 partial responses among 3 patients with Hodgkin's disease. These patients were treated with 15 or 18 mg/m^2 IV every 3 weeks.

Coonley et al. [69] reported treating patients with 12.5 mg/m^2 IV every 3 weeks with dose escalations if no toxicity was encountered. They observed no response among 6 patients with Hodgkin's disease and 16 patients with non-Hodgkin's lymphoma. These patients had received an average of 3 prior chemotherapeutic regimens containing 8 separate drugs. Minor responses were noted in 3 patients. There was no evidence of cardiac toxicity.

4′ Deoxydoxorubicin
This analog is identical to the parent compound except for the deletion of the hydroxyl group at the 4′ position. It has broad antitumor activity in experimental models and in the rabbit model has less cardiac toxicity. Phase I studies conducted by the EORTC Early Clinical Trials Group showed dose limiting leukopenia along with thrombocytopenia, nausea, vomiting, mucositis, and mild alopecia. Acute cardiac changes are not observed [70]. Phase II studies have been initiated with doses of 30–40 mg/m^2 every 3 to 4 weeks depending on the extent of prior therapy. Results are not available as yet.

Platinum analogs

Carboplatin and iproplatin are among the most exciting new agents currently available for clinical investigation. Both drugs were selected for clinical study because of their reduced potential for nephrotoxicity and antitumor activity similar to cisplatin in experimental systems. *In vitro* studies using the clonogenic assay have shown that cisplatin and carboplatin have very similar patterns of cross-resistance whereas iproplatin appears to be markedly different in its pattern of sensitivity and resistance when compared to the other two drugs. In addition, studies using experimental model systems have shown drug synergy especially for carboplatin and etoposide or iproplatin plus adriamycin. Extensive phase II evaluation of these drugs is currently underway. Significant activity has already been found for carboplatin in ovarian cancer. Iproplatin also appears to have activity against small cell lung cancer, and ovarian cancer and possibly breast cancer as well. Both drugs have dose limiting thrombocytopenia which may hinder their use in patients with significant bone marrow compromise.

Discussion

Identification of new chemotherapeutic agents with useful clinical activity against malignant lymphomas is actively being pursued by many investigators using a wide variety of novel chemotypes and analogs. Although the level of interest is high, as reflected by the large number of studies being conducted, success in identifying and registering new antilymphoma drugs remains very elusive. New antilymphoma agents must have a high degree of inherent activity and have minimal cross resistance with the 6 to 10 drugs most patients enrolled in clinical trials are likely to have received. One added constraint is that the great majority of patients suitable for clinical trials already have markedly diminished bone marrow function. We have consequently classified and reviewed a number of drugs according to whether they are new chemotypes or not and by their myelosuppressive potential, in the belief that new chemotypes would be less likely to be cross resistant with prior therapy and non-myelosuppressive drugs would be less likely to require those dose reductions which make interpreting results, especially negative results, of clinical trials difficult.

Gallium nitrate, mitoguazone and spirogermanium are examples of novel chemotypes with minimal potential for myelosuppression. All three drugs have activity against lymphomas but their lack of myelosuppression did not lead to marked improvements in either safety or therapeutic index. Indeed, dose or schedule adjustments were required for all three drugs to reduce the risk of nephrotoxicity (gallium nitrate), gastrointestinal intolerance or muscle weakness (mitoguazone) and neurotoxicity (spirogermanium). If these early results of activity in lymphoma are confirmed, the lack of myelosuppression for these drugs should allow them to be used at full dose in combination with other drugs in phase III trials.

As examples of non-myelosuppressive analogs, we have reviewed peplomycin and tallysomycin $S_{10}b$. Peplomycin has been shown to have activity against lymphomas but the number of patients studied is small. Tallysomycin $S_{10}b$ is about to enter phase II studies and data in lymphomas should be available within one year. Although one or both analogs may possess antilymphoma activity, the questions which remain unanswered are whether they are non-cross resistant with bleomycin and what would be the therapeutic contribution relative to the parent compound.

Novel myelosuppressive chemotypes include amsacrine, AZQ, and mitoxantrone. These agents may have a lower risk of cross resistance but all are likely to be difficult to use in patients with diminished bone marrow function. Cross resistance with prior therapy appears to be more of a problem for AZQ than for amsacrine or mitoxantrone. Although myelosuppression is prominent for all three drugs, mitoxantrone may also contribute to cardiotoxicity in patients previously exposed to anthracyclines and amsacrine may be cardiotoxic as well. Although these three drugs possess inherent activity against lymphomas, combining them with other agents for phase III trials is likely to be difficult without dose reduction.

Myelosuppressive analogs are likely to have the most difficult time succeeding in the clinic because the probability of cross resistance with the parent compound may be high and attainment of optimal antitumor doses may not be possible in patients with compromised bone marrow function. All of the anthracycline analogs discussed have dose limiting myelosuppression and for aclacinomycin there is also evidence for cardiac toxicity. Clinically useful antilymphoma activity will not be detected for these drugs in early clinical trials unless there is minimal cross resistance with doxorubicin, a drug which virtually all lymphoma patients receive. The platinum analogs, carboplatin and iproplatin, are also myelosuppressive but problems with cross resistance may be less because few lymphoma patients are routinely treated with cisplatin.

New agents will be needed if front-line and salvage regimens are to improve for lymphomas. Some of the difficulties of identifying active new agents in patients with extensive prior therapy have been discussed and these problems will have to be addressed in future trials if we are to enhance the chance of identifying and registering new drugs for lymphoma.

References

1. Adamson RH, Canellos GP and Sieber SM (1975). Studies on the antitumor activity of gallium nitrate (NSC-15200) and other group IIIa metal salts. Cancer Chemother Rep 59:599–610.
2. Winchell HS, Sanchez PD, Watanabe CK et al. (1970). Visualization of tumors in humans using [67]GA-citrate and the Anger whole-body scanner, scintillation camera and tomographic scanner. J Nucl Med 11:459–466.
3. Krakoff IH, Newman RA and Goldberg RS (1979). Clinical toxicologic and pharmacologic studies of gallium nitrate. Cancer 44:1722–1727.
4. Warrell RP, Coonley CJ, Straus DJ and Young CW (1983). Treatment of patients with advanced malignant lymphoma using gallium nitrate administered as a seven-day continuous infusion. Cancer 51:1982–1987.
5. Weick JK, Stephens RL, Baker LH and Jones SE (1983). Gallium nitrate in malignant lymphoma: A Southwest Oncology Group study. Cancer Treat Rep 67:823–825.
6. Keller JW, Johnson L, Raney M and Dandy M (1984). Phase II study of gallium nitrate

(GaNO₃) (NSC #15200) in refractory lymphoproliferative diseases. A Southeastern Cancer Study Group (SCSG) study. Proc Amer Soc Clin Oncol 3:247.

7. Thiele J and Dralle E (1998). Zur Kenntnis des Amidoguanidins. I. Condensations-Produkte des Amidoguanidins mit Aldehyden und Ketonen der Fettreihe. Ann Chemie 302:275–299.

8. Freedlander BL and French FA (1958). Carcinostatic action of polycarbonyl compounds and their derivatives. I. 3-Ethoxy-2-keto-butyraldehyde and related compounds. Cancer Res 18:172–175.

9. Freedlander BL and French FA (1958). Glyoxal-bis (guanylhydrazone) and derivatives. Cancer Res 18:360–363.

10. Freedlander BL and French FA (1958). Hydroxymethylglyoxal-bis (guanylhydrazone). Cancer Res 18:1286–1289.

11. Freedlander BL and French FA (1958). Glyoxal-bis (thiosemicarbazone) and derivatives. Cancer Res 18:1290–1300.

12. Warrell RP and Burchenal JH (1983). Methylglyoxal-bis (guanylhydrazone) (methyl-GAG): Current status and future prospects. J Clin Oncol 1:52–65.

13. Hart RD, Ohnuma T, Holland JF and Bruckner H (1982). Methyl-GAG in patients with malignant neoplasms: A phase I re-evaluation. Cancer Treat Rep 66:65–71.

14. Warrell RP, Lee BJ, Kempin SJ et al. (1981). Effectiveness of Methyl-GAG (methylglyoxal-bis [guanylhydrazone]) in patients with advanced malignant lymphoma. Blood 57:1011–1014.

15. Knight WAT, Fabian C, Costanzi JJ et al. (1983). Methylglyoxal-bis guanyl hydrazone (methyl-GAG, MGBG) in lymphoma and Hodgkin's disease. Investigational New Drugs 1:235–237.

16. Abeloff MD, Slavik M, Luk GD et al. (1984). Phase I trial and pharmacokinetic studies of α-difluoromethylornithine – an inhibitor of polyamine biosynthesis. J Clin Oncol 2:124–130.

17. Janne J, Alhonen-Hongisto L, Seppanen P and Simes M (1981). Use of polyamine antimetabolites in experimental tumors and in human leukemia. Med Biol 59:448.

18. Warrell RP, Coonley CJ and Burchenal JH (1983). Sequential inhibition of polyamine synthesis. A phase I trial of DFMO (α-difluoromethylornithine) and methyl-GAG [methylglyoxal-bis (guanylhydrazone)]. Cancer Chemother Pharmacol 11:134–136.

19. Burchenal JH, Warrell R, Hansen H et al. (1983). Antitumor effects of inhibitors of the polyamine pathway. Froc 13th Int Cancer Congress. P 103.

20. Durie BGM, Salmon SE and Russell DH (1977). Polyamines as markers of response and disease activity in cancer chemotherapy. Cancer Res 37:214.

21. Alhonen-Hongisto L, Seppanen P and Janne L (1980). Intracellular putrescine and spermidine deprivation induces increased uptake of the natural polyamines and methylglyoxal-bis (guanylhydrazone). Biochem J 192:941.

22. Slavik M, Blanc O and Davis J (1983). Spirogermanium: A new investigational drug of novel structure and lack of bone marrow toxicity. Investigational New Drugs 1:225–234.

23. Henry MC and Port CD (1977). Preclinical evaluation of 2-aza-8-germaaspiro (4, 5) decane-2-propanamine, 8, 8-diethyl-N, N-di-methyl-, dihydrochloride in mice and dogs. Final report to the Laboratory of Toxicology, Developmental Therapeutics Program, Division of Cancer Treatment, National Cancer Institute, Bethesda, Md., Feb. 28.

24. Legha SS, Ajani JA and Bodey GP (1983). Phase I study of spirogermanium given daily. J Clin Oncol 1:331–336.

25. Mattsson W (1980). A phase I – study of spirogermanium. Proc Amer Assoc Cancer Res 21:194.

26. Schein PS, Slavik M, Smythe T et al. (1980). Phase I clinical trial of spirogermanium. Cancer Treat Rep 64:1051–1056.

27. Budman DR, Schulman P, Vinciguerra V and Degnan TJ (1982). Phase I trial of spiroger-

manium given by infusion in a multiple-dose schedule. Cancer Treat Rep 66:173–175.

28. Gesme DH, Vogelzang NJ, Ryan M and Kennedy BJ (1982). Phase I-II study of spiroger-manium in advanced neoplastic disease. Proc Amer Soc Clin Oncol 1:676.

29. Espana P, Kaplan R, Robichaud K et al. (1982). Phase II study of spirogermanium (Spiro G) in lymphoma patients. Proc Amer Soc Clin Oncol 1:166.

30. Louie AC, Farmen FH, Gaver RC et al. (in press). Peplomycin and tallysomycin $S_{10}b$, two bleomycin analogs. In: Sikic BI, Carter SK and Rozencweig M (Eds.). Bleomycin: Review and Future Prospects. New York: Academic Press.

31. Mathé G, Armand JP, deVassal F et al. (1982). Phase II trial peplomycin (PEP) in advanced solid tumors and hematosarcomas. Cancer Chemother Pharmacol 9 (suppl):37.

32. Kimura K, Ogawa M, Wakui A et al. (1981). A phase II study of peplomycin on malignant lymphomas. The Gan to Kagakuryoho (Japan) 8:1701–1705.

33. Cain BF and Atwell GJ (1974). The experimental antitumor properties of three congeners of the acridylmethanesulphonanilide (AMSA) series. Eur J Cancer 10:539–549.

34. Cain BF, Seelye RN and Atwell GJ (1974). Potential antitumor agents. 14. acridylmethane-sulfonanilides. J Med Chem 17:922–930.

35. Goldsmith MA, Bhardwaj S, Ohnuma T et al. (1980). Phase I study of m-AMSA in patients with solid tumors and leukemias. Cancer Clin Trials 3:197–202.

36. Weick JK, Jones SE and Ryan DH (1983). Phase II study of amsacrine (m-AMSA) in advanced lymphomas: A Southwest Oncology Group study. Cancer Treat Rep 67:489–492.

37. Case DC (1984). m-AMSA: Phase II trial in advanced lymphoma and leukemia. Amer J Clin Oncol 7:357–360.

38. Warrell RP, Strauss DJ and Young CW (1980). Phase II trial of 4'(9-acridinylamino) metha-nesulfon-m-anisidide (AMSA) in the treatment of advanced non-Hodgkin's lymphoma. Cancer Treat Rep 64:1157–1158.

39. Ahmann FR, Meyskens F, Jones SE et al. (1983). Phase II evaluation of amsacrine (m-AMSA) in solid tumors, myeloma, and lymphoma: A University of Arizona and Southwest Oncology Group study. Cancer Treat Rep 67:697–700.

40. Cabanillas F, Legha SS, Bodey GP and Freireich EJ (1981). Initial experience with AMSA as single agent treatment against malignant lymphoproliferative disorders. Blood 57:614–616.

41. Calabresi F, Conti E, De Nigris A et al. (1981). m-AMSA: Preliminary data on the activity of a new antineoplastic drug. Tumori 67 (2 Supp. A):164 (Abstr).

42. Bajetta E, Viviani S, Valagussa P et al. (1983). Phase II study with amsacrine (m-AMSA, m-AMSA lactate) in resistant malignant lymphomas in Fourth NCI – EORTC Symposium on New Drugs in Cancer Therapy. Dec. 14–17 Brussels, Belgium Abst. 66.

43. DeJager R, Dupont D and Body JJ (1980). Phase I study of oral 4'-(9-acridinylamino) methane sulfon-m-anisidide (m-AMSA, NSC 249992). Proc Amer Assoc Cancer Res 21:146.

44. Tan CTC, Hancock C, Steinberg PG et al. (1982). Phase II study of 4'-(9-acridinylamino) methane sulfon-m-anisidide (NSC 249992) in children with acute leukemia and lymphoma. Cancer Res 42:1579–1581.

45. Khan AH and Driscoll JS (1976). Potential central nervous system antitumor agents. Azir-idinylbenzoquinones 1. J Med Chem 19:313–317.

46. Chou F, Khan AH and Driscoll JS (1976). Potential central nervous system anti-tumor agents. Aziridinylbenzoquinones 2. J Med Chem 19:1302–1308.

47. Clinical Brochure: Aziridinylbenzoquinone (NSC-182986). Bethesda, Maryland. National Cancer Institute. (1979).

48. Driscoll JS, Dudeck L, Congleton G et al. (1979). Potential CNS antitumor agents VI. Aziridinylbenzoquinone 3. J Pharm Sci 68:185–188.

49. McLaughlin P, Cabanillas F, Bedikian AY and Bodey GP (1983). Phase II trials of aziridi-

nylbenzoquinone (AZQ) in patients with refractory lymphoma. Cancer Treat Rep 67:507-508.

50. Case DC and Hayes DM (1983). Phase II study of aziridinylbenzoquinone in refractory lymphoma. Cancer Treat Rep 67:993–996.

51. Griffin JP, Newman RA, McCormack JJ and Krakoff IH (1982). Clinical and clinical pharmacologic studies of aziridinylbenzoquinone. Cancer Treat Rep 66:1321–1325.

52. Tan C, Hancock C, Miller L et al. (1982). Phase I study of aziridinylbenzoquinone (AZQ, NSC-183986) in children with cancer. Proc Amer Assoc Cancer Res 23:120.

53. Zee-Cheng RK-Y and Cheng CC (1978). Antineoplastic agents structure – activity relationship study of bis (substituted aminoalkylamino) – anthraquinones. J Med Chem 21:291–294.

54. Johnson RK, Zee-Cheng RK-Y, Lee WW et al. (1979). Experimental antitumor activity of aminoanthraquinones. Cancer Treat Rep 63:425–439.

55. Wallace RE, Murdock KC, Angier RB and Durr FE (1979). Activity of a novel Anthracenedione, 1, 4-Dihydroxy-5, 8-bis {{2-[(2-hydroxyethyl) amino] ethyl}amino}-9, 10-anthracenedione dihydrochloride, against experimental tumors in mice. Cancer Res 39:1570–1574.

56. Cowan JD, VonHoff DD, Clark CM and Pacque RE (1982). Comparative human tumor sensitivity to adriamycin (A), mitoxantrone (M), and bisantrene (b) as measured by a human tumor cloning assay (HTCA). Proc Amer Assoc Cancer Res 23:187.

57. Wynert W, Harvey H, Lipton A et al. (1981). Phase I study of dihydroxyanthracenedione (mitoxantrone). Proc Amer Assoc Cancer Res 22:352.

58. Estey EH, Keating MJ, McCredie KB et al. (1981). Phase I-II study of dihydroxyanthracenedione (DHAD) in acute leukemia (AL). Proc Amer Assoc Cancer Res 22:490.

59. Earl HM, Amlot PL and Rubens RD (1982). A phase II clinical trial of mitoxantrone in solid tumors and lymphomas. Brit J Cancer 45:636.

60. DeJager R, Cappelaere P, Earl H et al. (1982). Phase II clinical trial of mitoxantrone: 1, 4-dihydroxy-5-8-bis ((2-((2-hydroxyethyl) amino) ethyl) amino) 9, 10 anthracenedione dihydrochloride in solid tumors and lymphomas. Proc Amer Soc Clin Oncol 1:89.

61. Gams RA, Keller J, Golomb HM et al. (1983). Mitoxantrone in malignant lymphomas in XIII International Congress of Chemotherapy. Vienna, Austria. SY 85–11 Part 212/47–51, August 28 to Sept. 2.

62. Coltman CA, McDaniel TM, Balcerzak SP et al. (1983). Mitoxantrone hydrochloride (NSC-310739) in lymphoma. A Southwest Oncology Group study. Investigational New Drugs 1:65–70.

63. Oki T, Takeuchi T, Oka S and Umezawa H (1981). New anthracycline antibiotic aclacinomycin-A. In: Carter SK, Sakurai Y and Umezawa H (Eds.). Experimental Studies and Correlations with Clinical Trials in New Drugs in Cancer Chemotherapy, pp. 21–40 Berlin: Springer-Verlag.

64. Majima H. (1981). Phase I and II Clinical Study of Aclacinomycin-A in Current Chemotherapy and Immunotherapy: Proceedings of the 12th International Congress of Chemotherapy, Vol. II, pp. 1457–1458. Periti P and Grassi GG (Eds.). Florence. Italy.

65. Warrell RP and Kempin SJ (1983). Clinical evaluation of a new anthracycline antibiotic, aclacinomycin-A, in patients with advanced malignant lymphoma. Amer J Clin Oncol 6:81–84.

66. Mathé G, DeJager R, Hulhoven R et al. (1982). L'aclacinomycine-A dans les leucemiques aigues et les lymphomes non-Hodgkiniens leucemiques. Nouv Press Med 11:25–28.

67. Berman E, Wittes RE, Leyland-Jones B et al. (1983). Phase I and clinical pharmacology studies of intravenous and oral administration of 4-demethoxydaunorubicin in patients with advanced cancer. Cancer Res 43:6096–6101.

68. Bonfante V, Bonadonna G, Ferrari L et al. (1982). Phase I study of 4-demethoxydaunorubicin (dm-DNR). Proc Amer Assoc Cancer Res 23:542.

69. Coonley CJ, Warrell RP, Straus DJ and Young CW (1983). Clinical evaluation of 4-deme-

thoxydaunorubicin in patients with advanced malignant lymphoma. Cancer Treat Rep 67:949–950.

70. Rozencweig M, Crespeigne N and Kenis Y (1983). Phase I trial with 4'deoxydoxorubicin (esorubicin). Investigational New Drugs 1:309–313.

8. Autologous stem cell transplant for poor prognosis lymphoma

S. GULATI, B. SHANK, D. STRAUS, B. KOZINER, B. LEE,
R. MERTELSMANN, R. DINSMORE, T. GEE, R. VEGA,
J. YOPP, R. O'REILLY and B. CLARKSON
Memorial Sloan-Kettering Cancer Center, New York, New York, USA

Significant improvements have been made in the treatment of non-Hodgkin's lymphoma. Newer combination chemotherapy using PRO-MACE MOPP [1], M-BACOD [2] and the revised intermediate methotrexate dose m-BACOD [3] results in a high complete remission rate, with significant improvement in disease-free survival. Long term follow-up and confirmation of the initial success with these protocols will be very important.

Recent diagnostic improvements in classification of non-Hodgkin's lymphoma using histopathologic criteria, cell surface markers and biochemical enzyme levels have made it possible to identify patients who have a poor prognosis with increasing reliability. Several institutions have now shown that patients with large cell immunoblastic lymphoma (DHL; diffuse histiocytic lymphoma by Rappaport classification), lymphoblastic lymphoma and small non cleaved (undifferentiated or Burkitt's lymphoma) malignant lymphomas are destined to do poorly especially if the cancer presents with bone marrow involvement or as a large mass (mediastinal and/or abdominal) [4–8]. Patients with DHL who have high serum lactate dehydrogenase levels (greater than 500 units/liter) have a poor long-term response rate on conventional therapy [8].

Since the major dose limiting side effect of chemotherapeutic agents used to treat patients with lymphoma is hematopoietic toxicity, bone marrow transplantation can help circumvent this toxicity and escalated doses of such agents can then be used therapeutically. Allogeneic bone marrow (BM) transplantation has shown significant promise in the therapy of leukemias and lymphomas, but these benefits have been limited to young patients (age below 35 years) with HLA-MLC matched siblings, and graft-versus-host disease has been a significant problem [9–13]. Autologous bone marrow transplantation (ABMT) has wider applicability and the cryopreserved bone marrow can be reinfused after intensive treatment to rescue the patient from hematopoietic toxicity. Several institutions have performed ABMT for patients with lymphoma [14]. Most previous reports involved patients trans-

514

planted at the time of relapse and the best results were in patients with Burkitt's lymphoma [14–18]. Because of generally poor results in heavily pretreated patients, three years ago we decided to assess the role of ABMT in patients with DHL early in the course of their disease who were identified as having a poor prognosis based on their presenting features. In this report we present our initial results which suggest improved therapeutic results in such patients, using total body irradiation (TBI) followed by high-dose cyclophosphamide therapy and hematopoietic rescue by cryopreserved autologous bone marrow.

Materials and methods

From July 1981 to March 1984, untreated patients less than 40 years of age, who had diffuse histiocytic lymphoma (DHL) presenting with bulky mediastinal or abdominal disease (greater than 8×8 cm) and/or a serum lactate dehydrogenase (LDH) level of greater than 500 units/liter, and no or only minimal bone marrow infiltration, were considered for this study. The highest pretreatment serum LDH value was taken for this analysis. In the review of the results of recent trials with combination chemotherapy protocols at our institution, patients with DHL presenting with either one of these features had less than 20% probability of long-term survival [6, 8]. All the protocols used in this study were approved by the Institutional Review Board of Memorial Hospital. The data analysis is as of May 1984.

The initial design of the protocol called for randomization between two arms as described below, but we found most patients preferred to choose one arm over the other and refused randomization. Therefore, patients were allowed to choose which arm they preferred, continuing chemotherapy or induction followed immediately by AMBT.

Arm I

L-17M protocol. L17M is a combination chemotherapy protocol used principally for patients with acute lymphoblastic leukemia (ALL) and lymphoblastic lymphoma (LL) [19]. Induction therapy, usually requiring 35–40 days, consists of cyclophosphamide, weekly vincristine, intrathecal methotrexate $\times$ 4, and doxorubicin. After completion of induction, the bone marrow is evaluated for CFU-c and BFU-e growth and, if this is satisfactory, approximately 1 liter of marrow is taken and cryopreserved for possible use if the patient subsequently relapses. Patients are then continued on the consolidation and maintenance phases of the protocol.

Arm II

Following induction therapy on the L-17M protocol, the bone marrow is cryopreserved. The patients then receive one course of DAT (daunomycin 60 mg/m^2 i.v. day 1-3, cytarabine 20 mg/m^2 bolus, 150 mg/m^2 i.v. as 24 hour infusion day 1-5 and 6-thioguanine 100 mg/m^2 po q 12 h × 5 days) following which they are allowed 2-3 weeks to recover. During this time, CT simulation for radiation therapy, extent of disease work-up and dental evaluations are performed in preparation for ABMT. All but two patients received additional irradiation to the site of the bulky disease (usually 300 rad/day = 4 days). Bactrim ds-po bid day − 8 to − 1 is given as prophylaxis against *Pneumocystis carinii*. Total body irradiation (TBI) with partial shielding of the lungs is given at 120 rad per treatment 4 times a day for 11 treatments on day − 7 to − 4 [20]. On day − 3 and − 2 under adequate hydration and alkalinization of urine, cyclophosphamide 60 mg/kg per day × 2 is given. Two days later the cryopreserved bone marrow is infused. Patients are managed in single rooms during TBI, high dose chemotherapy and subsequent nadir sepsis.

Patients who failed to have complete remissions on the L-17M protocol (Arm I) or who relapsed during the consolidation or maintenance phases were also considered for ABMT and were sub-grouped accordingly. They received the same preparative treatment as patients on Arm II. Four additional patients who had been heavily treated on various conventional protocols were also transplanted. Bone marrow aspiration and biopsy on all patients was evaluated at initial presentation and then 10-14 days prior to bone marrow cryopreservation. The bone marrows were assessed for lymphoma involvement by examination of the smears and surface marker analysis including light chain immunoglobulin clonal excess by flow cytometry [21]. Flow cytometric analysis for RNA-DNA content and chromosomal analysis were also performed when indicated. If there was no evidence of lymphoma involvement of the marrow at presentation the marrow was not purged, but if there was minimal involvement with lymphoma at presentation even though it was no longer detectable after induction therapy at the time of bone marrow cryopreservation the marrow was treated with 4-hydroperoxycyclophosphamide (4-HC) prior to freezing, on the assumption that there might be residual lymphoma cells present [21]. Eight patients (# 5, 6, 7, 10, 17, 19, 20, 22) received 4-HC purged marrow. Case 19 was purged at 60 μM 4-HC and all others were purged at a concentration of 100 μM for 30 minutes at 37 °C. In all cases where purged bone marrow was used, 66 % of the marrow dose infused was cryopreserved untreated to be used in the event that the 4-HC treated marrow did not engraft. All patients receiving untreated and 4-HC purged marrow have so far shown good hematopoietic engraftment although one of the heavily pretreated patients (# 20) had delayed recovery of her platelet count. It has not been necessary to use the untreated reserve marrow in any of the patients who received 4-HC purged marrow.

Results

Only patients with DHL (B-cell) are considered in this report. Table I shows the results of all such patients entered onto the study. The dimensions of the tumor mass at presentation, stage of disease, and highest serum LDH level prior to treatment and at time of ABMT are also shown. Ten patients elected to receive Arm I of the protocol of whom 7 achieved complete remission (CR) and 3 were partial responders (PR). In all of the PR on Arm I and all except case #11 on Arm II, the serum LDH level fell below 250 units per liter on the L-17M, although it later often increased at the time of relapse. The usual reason for designation of PR rather than CR was because of incomplete shrinkage of the mediastinal mass on the chest x-ray. Seven of these patients (4 CR and 3 PR) relapsed 4–17 months after the start of the L-17M therapy. One (case #4) of the seven patients who relapsed on the L-17M therapy did not receive ABMT as he refused to have his bone marrow cryopreserved; this patient subsequently relapsed and died. The other six patients received ABMT after their disease relapsed. Accurate staging in the post transplant period is difficult as often a residual mass persists and surgical confirmation of residual lymphoma is often not possible for months because of the increased risk of infection, as the immunologic recovery is slow. Two of these six patients are alive disease-free at 7+ and 3+ months, two patients relapsed and one of them has died at 9 months (case #7), and the other two patients died of peritransplant complications, one of disseminated Herpes Zoster (before the availability of acyclovir i.v.) and the other of pulmonary complications.

Eight patients elected to have ABMT after completion of the L-17M induction, (Arm II) of whom 2 achieved CR, 5 had PR and one patient's disease progressed (case #18) after induction therapy. The seven patients in CR or PR who were transplanted shortly after the L-17M induction therapy are alive with no known evidence of disease with follow-up of 8+ to 30+ months from initial diagnosis or 5+ to 28+ months from the time of transplant. In one patient (#11) the residual mass excised after completion of ABMT was found to be necrotic and fibrous tissue. This patient is our longest survivor after ABMT. The one patient whose disease progressed after L-17M induction therapy and in whom ABMT was inadvertently delayed for one month died of pulmonary complications associated with his paratracheal lymphoma one month after ABMT.

Four additional patients who relapsed on various conventional lympho-

Table I. Clinical course of patients with poor prognosis lymphoma

Case Number	Age	Sex	Primary site in cm	Bone marrow[a] Initial	Bone marrow[a] ABMT	Stage	LDH Initial	LDH ABMT	Response L-17M (Relapse)[b]	Survival in months from Initial DX	Survival in months from ABMT (Relapse)[b]
ARM I											
Still on L-17M											
1	20	M	Med 14×13	+	–	IV	705		CR	37+	
2	38	M	Med 12×11	±	–	III	254		CR	22+	
3	24	F	Med 12×11	±	–	II	281		CR	19+	
4	37	M	Med >8×8	–	–	IV	251		CR (6)	7	
ABMT at relapse on L-17M											
5	29	M	Med 8×8	–	–	IV	150	380	CR (17)	21+	3+
6	34	M	Med 12×11	±	–	IV	508	352	PR (4)	19+	15+ (6)
7	21	F	Med 10×10	±	–	IV	566	343	CR (5)	16	9 (8)
8	30	F	Med 10×10	–	–	IV	564	304	PR (5)	12+	7+
9	24	M	Rib 12[c]	–	–	IV	160	383	CR (5)	7	1
10	25	F	Med 8×9	±	–	IV	254	322	PR (4)	5	1
ARM II											
ABMT after induction											
11	17	M	Med 11×13	–	–	IV	777	424	PR	30+	28+
12	24	F	Med 12×13	–	–	IV	623	235	CR	27+	22+
13	36	M	Med 10×8	–	–	II	426	225	PR	23+	18+
14	32	F	Med 12×14	–	–	III	834	171	CR	20+	17+
15	34	M	Med 13×14	–	–	IV	182	217	PR	17+	13+
16	28	M	Med 13×14	–	–	III	528	307	PR	16+	13+
17	24	M	Med 18×14	–	–	IV	501	233	PR	8+	5+
18	30	M	Med 16×14	–	–	IV	379	240	Prog.	6	1
ABMT in heavily pretreated											
19	21	M	Med 10×14	±	–	IV	230	401	PR (2)	31+	21+
20	29	F	Med 14×12	±	–	IV	388	144	PR (4)	24+	10+
21	24	F	Med 11×13	–	–	IV	155	927	CR (5)	7	1
22	35	F	Breast 10×12	±	±	II	364	236	PR (15)	21	7

[a] ± = Suspicious by morphology and/or clonal excess, + = definite by morphology and/or surface markers
[b] (Relapse) = Number of months for relapse to occur after start of L-17M or after ABMT
[c] Soft involvement and with multiple lymph nodes. Effusion at relapse

ma protocols were also transplanted. One patient died of peritransplant complications (case 21) and another died of recurrent lymphoma. The other two patients are alive with no evidence of disease at 21+ and 10+ months post ABMT.

All patients who received ABMT showed good hematopoietic engraftment, but one patient had a long delay (6 months) before her platelet count increased over $50,000/mm^3$, (case 20).

Discussion

Initial results indicate that the L-17M protocol, which is effective in treating patients with ALL and LL [19, 22], is also effective for initial therapy of DHL. However, from our experience so far with Arm I of the current protocol, and as was also true with the earlier similar cyclophosphamide L-2 protocol [8], it appears that patients with poor prognosis DHL tend to relapse within the first 6 months after the start of therapy, indicating that the consolidation and maintenance phases of the L-17M protocol are often inadequate to eradicate the lymphoma when it is extensive. The need for more intensive therapy of such patients is supported by the data on patients who received ABMT on Arm II (cases #11–18). Of the eight patients who received transplants after completion of induction therapy, one patient with extensive paratracheal disease that progressed on the L-17M protocol died of pulmonary decompensation. The other seven patients remain free of disease with a median follow-up of 20+ months from initial diagnosis and 17+ months from the time of ABMT.

Fractionated dose TBI [20] plus additional RT to bulky tumor masses and high-dose cyclophosphamide were used to treat the patients on this study. This combination has shown promising results in allogeneic bone marrow transplants for AML [9] and ALL [12], and it is of interest that the same combined therapy also appears to be effective in treating patients with poor prognosis DHL. The results of ABMT when it is performed after the patients have relapsed on the L-17M (Arm I) or in heavily pretreated patients are not as impressive as when ABMT is performed immediately after (L-17M) induction therapy. Perhaps for these two subgroups of patients more aggressive combination chemotherapy will be necessary, if it can be tolerated.

Minimal involvement of the bone marrow by lymphoma in patients with DHL can often be missed by routine morphologic examination. It can be calculated that 2–5% lymphoma cells in the marrow can represent 2 to 5×10^5 tumor cells/ml. In the doses used for purging in this study, 4-HC is probably effective in producing at least 3–4 $\log_{10}$ cell kill of human lymphoma cells [23, 24], but is probably inadequate to eradicate the tumor cells from marrow densely infiltrated with lymphoma. The clinical trial of 4-HC purged bone marrow has therefore been restricted to patients who had minimal bone marrow involvement at presentation and whose bone marrow had no detectable lymphoma at the time of bone marrow cryopreservation; thus the clinical effectiveness of the purging procedure cannot be proven by our studies to date since the induction treatment may have been sufficient to clear the marrow of lymphoma. Eight patients have so far received 4-HC purged ABMT. All patients showed good hematopoietic engraftment with no significant delay except in one case compared to patients receiving untreated marrow.

From the preliminary data presented in this study, it appears that TBI when given with high-dose cyclophosphamide and followed by rescue with cryopreserved marrow is effective therapy for patients with poor prognosis lymphoma especially when the procedure is performed early.

Acknowledgements

This work was supported in part by NIH Grants CA-20194 and CA-23766.

References

1. Fisher RI, DeVita VT, Hubbard SM et al. (1983). Diffuse aggressive lymphomas: Increased survival after alternating flexible sequences of ProMACE and MOPP chemotherapy. Ann Intern Med 98:304–309.
2. Skarin AT, Canellos GP, Rosenthal DS et al. (1983). Improved prognosis of diffuse histiocytic and undifferentiated lymphoma by use of high dose methotrexate alternating with standard agents (M-BACOD). J Clin Oncol 1:91–98.
3. Skarin A, Canellos G, Rosenthal D et al. (1983). Moderate dose methotrexate combined with bleomycin, adriamycin, cyclophosphamide, oncovin and dexamethasone, m-BACOD, in advanced diffuse histiocytic lymphoma. Proc Amer Soc Clin Oncol 2:220.
4. Fisher RI, Hubbard SM, DeVita VT et al. (1981). Factors predicting long-term survival in diffuse mixed, histiocytic, or undifferentiated lymphoma. Blood 58:45–51.
5. Anderson T, DeVita VT, Simon RM et al. (1982). Malignant lymphomas. II. Prognostic factors and response to treatment of 473 patients at the National Cancer Institute. Cancer 50:2708–2721.
6. Koziner B, Sklaroff R, Little C et al. (1984). NHL-3 Protocol. Six-drug combination chemotherapy for non-Hodgkin's lymphoma. Cancer 53:2592–2600.
7. Berard CW, Greene MH, Jaffe ES et al. (1981). A multidisciplinary approach to non-Hodgkin's lymphomas. Ann Intern Med 94:218–232.
8. Koziner B, Little C, Passe S et al. (1982). Treatment of advanced diffuse histiocytic lymphoma. Cancer 49:1571–1579.
9. Dinsmore R, Kirkpatrick D, Flomenberg N et al. (1984). Allogeneic bone marrow transplantation for patients with acute nonlymphocytic leukemia. Blood 3:649–656.

520

10. Sullivan KM, Shulman HM, Storb R et al. (1981). Chronic graft-versus host disease in 52 patients: Adverse natural course and successful treatment with combination immunosuppression. Blood 547:267–276.

11. Kersey JH, Ramsay NKC, Kim T et al. (1982). Allogeneic bone marrow transplantation in acute nonlymphocytic leukemia. A pilot study. Blood 60:400–403.

12. Dinsmore R, Kirkpatrick D, Flomenberg N, et al. (1983). Allogenic bone marrow transplantation for patients with acute lymphoblastic leukemia. Blood 62:381–388.

13. Appelbaum FR, Clift RA, Buckner CD et al. (1983). Allogeneic marrow transplantation for acute nonlymphoblastic leukemia after the first relapse. Blood 61:949–953.

14. Appelbaum FR and Thomas ED (1983). Review of the use of marrow transplantation in the treatment of non-Hodgkin's lymphoma. J Clin Oncol 7:440–447.

15. Phillips G, Herzig R, Lazarus H et al. (1984). Treatment of resistant malignant lymphoma. N Engl J Med 310:1557–1561.

16. Gorin NC, David R, Stachowiak J et al. (1981). Dose chemotherapy and autologous bone marrow transplantation in acute leukemias, malignant lymphomas and solid tumor. Brit J Cancer 17:557–568.

17. Appelbaum FR, Deisseroth AB, Graw RG et al. (1978). Prolonged complete remission following high dose chemotherapy of Burkitt's lymphoma in relapse. Cancer 41:1059–1063.

18. Douer D, Champlin RE, Ho WG et al. (1981). High-dose combined-modality therapy and autologous bone marrow transplantation in resistant cancer. Am J Med 71:973–976.

19. Clarkson B, Gee T, Arlin Z et al. (1984). Current status of treatment of acute leukemia in adults: An overview. In: Buchner Th (Ed.). Acute Leukemia Therapy. Berlin, Heidelberg, New York: Springer-Verlag. (In Press).

20. Shank B, Hopfan S, Kimm JH et al. (1981). Hyperfractionated total body irradiation for bone marrow transplantations. I. Early results in leukemia patients. Int J Radiat Oncol Biol Phys 7:1109–1115.

21. Grebhard D, Czeczotka V, Sirotina A and Koziner B (1982). Quantitative comparison of surface membrane immunoglobulin (SMIG) in normal and neoplastic B-lymphocytes by flow cytometry and calibrated fluoresceinated microbeads. Blood 60:72a (#217).

22. Clarkson B, Arlin Z, Gee T et al. (1983). Improved treatment of acute lymphoblastic leukemia (ALL) in adults. Proc Amer Soc Clin Oncol 2:180.

23. Sharkis SJ, Santos GW and Colvin M (1980). Elimination of acute myelogenous leukemic cells from marrow and tumor suspensions in the rat with 4-hydroperoxycyclophosphamide. Blood 55:521–523.

24. Gulati S, Gandola L, Vega R et al. (1984). Chemopurification of bone marrow in vitro and its clinical application. Proc Am Assoc Cancer Res 25:201.

9. *In vitro* purging with 4-hydroperoxycyclophosphamide and its effects on the hematopoietic and stromal elements of human bone marrow

S. SIENA, H. CASTRO-MALASPINA, S. C. GULATI, L. LU, R. J. O'REILLY, B. D. CLARKSON and M. A. S. MOORE
Memorial Sloan-Kettering Cancer Center, New York, New York, USA

The use of a combination of high-dose chemoradiotherapy and transplantation of 4-hydroperoxycyclophosphamide (4-HC) purged autologous bone marrow is a promising approach to the treatment of leukemia [1] and lymphoma [2, 3]. The rationale supporting this therapeutic modality was provided in 1980 by Sharkes et al. who showed that 4-HC can selectively purge murine acute leukemia cells from marrow suspensions in a dose-related manner without affecting the viability and self-renewal capacity of the non-leukemic pluripotential hematopoietic stem cells (CFU-s) [4].

The studies reported here, were aimed at evaluating the effects of 4-HC on the hematopoietic and stromal elements of human bone marrow. With regard to hematopoietic cells, evidence is presented demonstrating that multipotential (CFU-Mix), and erythroid (BFU-E) colony-forming cells are more 4-HC sensitive than granulomonocytic (CFU-GM) progenitor cells. In contrast, marrow stromal cells are relatively resistant to 4-HC and not functionally affected by the doses currently used for purging autologous bone marrow.

Materials and methods

4-Hydroperoxycyclophosphamide and incubation procedure

The 4-HC (MW 292) was prepared by Dr. M. O. Colvin (The Johns Hopkins Oncology Center, Baltimore, MD) as described elsewhere [5]. The 4-HC powder was dissolved in Ca-Mg free PBS, sterilized by filtration and utilized within 30 minutes. Normal marrow buffy coat cells were incubated at 37 °C for 30 minutes with 4-HC and medium control. After 2 washings at 10 °C, the cells were assayed for colony-forming cells or inoculated for long-term culture as detailed below. Viability was not remarkably changed by the incubation procedure.

Colony assays

The assay for multipotential hematopoietic progenitor cells (CFU-Mix) was carried out according to the method of Fauser and Messner [6] as described [7]. Erythroid burst-forming units (BFU-E) were scored from the same culture dishes. The colony assay for day-7 granulomonocytic progenitors cells (CFU-GM) was as described elsewhere [8] and employed 10% exogenously supplied GM-CSF present in GCT-conditioned medium. The colony assay for marrow fibroblast progenitor cells (CFU-F) was carried out in a liquid culture system [9].

Long-term marrow cultures

Long-term cultures of human bone marrow (LTMC) were established according to the method of Moore at al. [10] as modified by Garner and Kaplan [11]. The supernatant cell counts and CFU-GM numbers per culture flask were determined weekly. Individual LTMCs were examined every 7 days under a phase contrast inverted microscope and the percent of the flask surface covered by a stromal interlocking network was recorded. The heterogeneity of the cells comprising the stromal layers in LTMC was assessed by immunocytochemical techniques to detect fibroblasts (Type III collagen and fibronectin positive), endothelial cells (factor VIII-R antigen positive), adipocytes (oil-red-0 positve) and macrophages [9, 12].

Results

Bone marrow buffy-coat cells from normal volunteers were treated with 25–500 µM 4-HC at two different final cell concentrations, i.e. 10 and 20×10^6 cells per ml. The percentages of recovery of CFU-F, CFU-Mix, BFU-E, and CFU-GM are detailed in Table 1. The values (mean ± sem) of medium-treated controls were as follows: CFU-F 91 ± 11 per 5×10^6 cultured cells; CFU-Mix 10.3 ± 0.9 per 10^5 cells; BFU-R 98 ± 26 per 2×10^5 cells; CFU-GM 79 ± 23 per 10^5 cells. The calculated doses of 4-HC inhibiting 50% of colony formation (ID_{50}) are presented in Table II. When 25 µM 4-HC treated marrow cells were mixed at different ratios with autologous untreated marrow buffy-coat cells, the observed number of colonies corresponded to the expected values calculated on the basis of dilution of CFU-GM, BFU-E and CFU-Mix in the cell mixtures (data not shown).

Human bone marrow treated with 100 and 300 µM 4-HC and then cultured in a LTMC system, were ultimately capable of giving rise to an interlocking adherent stromal layer of heterogeneous composition which was

Table I. Effect of 4-hydroperoxycyclophosphamide on human marrow, stromal and hematopoietic progenitor cell growth *in vitro*

Colony assay	# cells/ml [a]	4 Hydroperoxycyclophosphamide (μM)						
		25	50	100	150	200	300	500
CFU-F	20	102$\pm$9	96$\pm$3	83$\pm$7	72$\pm$8	53$\pm$12	22$\pm$3	0.5$\pm$0.4
	10	n.d.	79$\pm$6	37$\pm$15	30$\pm$12	7$\pm$3	2$\pm$1	0
CFU-GM	20	79$\pm$7	52$\pm$5	34$\pm$6	20$\pm$2	4$\pm$2	1$\pm$0.5	0
	10	n.d.	41$\pm$19	13$\pm$5	4$\pm$2	1$\pm$0.5	0	0
BFU-E	20	62$\pm$5	27$\pm$3	3$\pm$1	0	0	n.d.	n.d.
CFU-Mix	20	44$\pm$7	8$\pm$0.5	0	0	0	n.d.	n.d.

Results are expressed as mean percentage $\pm$ sem of medium-treated controls from 5 (CFU-F), 4 (CFU-GM), and 3 (CFU-MIX, BFU-E) separate experiments. Values of medium-treated controls are reported in the text. n.d. = not determined
[a] Final concentration ($\times 10^6$) of normal marrow buffy-coat cells during treatment with 4 HC

comparable to controls. These *in vitro* marrow stromal cells were comprised of fibroblasts, endothelial cells, adipocytes, and macrophages, all demonstrated by immunocytochemical techniques. At initial stages of culture, week 1–3, the extent of the control stromal layers was more extensive. However, in the following weeks when confluence was already reached in the control groups, the stromal layers derived from 100 μM 4-HC treated marrow became progressively confluent and similar to controls. At the same time the stromal layers derived from 300 μM 4-HC treated marrow were about 20% less confluent than controls. In contrast, treatment of the same marrows with 400 μM 4-HC impaired their capacity to establish a LTMC. The detailed data on the LTMCs derived from 4-HC treated marrows are shown in Table III.

Table II. Dose of 4-hydroperoxycyclophosphamide inhibiting fifty percent (ID_{50}) of stromal and hematopoietic progenitor colony formation *in vitro*

Cell concentration [a]	ID_{50} (μM 4-HC)			
	CFU-F	CFU-Mix	BFU-E	CFU-GM
20	235	31	41	89
10	115	n.d.	n.d.	22

Numbers represent the calculated ID_{50} from 5 (CFU-F), 4 (CFU-GM), and 3 (CFU-Mix) separate experiments
[a] Final cell concentration ($\times 10^6$) during 4-HC treatment; n.d. = not determined

Table III. Extent and composition of the stromal layers of 5-week old long-term cultures derived from 4-hydroperoxycyclophosphamide treated human bone marrow

4-Hydroperoxycyclophosphamide

	100 μM					300 μM					400 μM				
	Cvrg	F	EC	A	M	Cvrg	F	EC	A	M	Cvrg	F	EC	A	M
Exp. #1	100	++++	+	++	++	75	++++	+	++	++	<10	±	n.d.	−	−
Exp. #2	100	+++	+	++	+++	75	++++	−	++	+	<10	±	−	−	−
Exp. #3	5	++++	+	++	++	100	+++++	+	++	+	<10	−	n.d.	−	−
Exp. #4	100	++++	+	++	++										

Cvrg = percent coverage of culture flask surface. F = fibroblast. EC = endothelial cell
A = adipocyte. M = macrophage. n.d. = not determined
− = 0%. + = <10%. ++ = 10–25%. +++ = 26–75%. ++++ = >75%

The numbers of total CFU-GM generated in primary LTMCs derived from control and 4-HC treated marrows are summarized in Table IV. Although in the first 2 weeks of culture the decline of the total adherent cell numbers was slower in the 4-HC treated groups (data not shown), this trend did not reflect the production of a new 'wave' of CFU-GM. However, CFU-GM could be detected in the nonadherent fraction of the 100 µM 4-HC treated group for 5 weeks. In the 300 µM 4-HC treated group, while the primary inoculum was virtually depleted of all CFU-GM, a modest generation of these committed stem cells was found on week 1 and 2 of culture. Treatment with 400 µM 4-HC abolished CFU-GM growth in LTMC.

To assess the functional capacity of stromal layers established from 4-HC treated marrow to sustain hematopoiesis *in vitro*, primary LTMC were totally depleted of all suspension cells after 5 weeks when the total CFU-GM produced per culture was reduced to 45 ± 21. Five groups of cultures were then initiated using a second addition of autologous non-adherent low-density (NAL) cells. The total cell counts and CFU-GM numbers per flask were determined weekly. No impairment in the weekly production of CFU-GM was seen in the group involving the coculture of NAL cells with stromal layers from 4-HC treated marrow as compared to stromal layers derived from untreated marrow. In flasks inoculated with NAL cells without any stromal support, there were low numbers of short-term growth of CFU-GM. In contrast, no growth of CFU-GM was found in the flasks depopulated of all buoyant cells and not reinoculated with fresh NAL cells.

Table IV. Primary long-term cultures derived from control and 4-hydroperoxycyclophosphamide treated human bone marrow

| Week | Total CFU-GM per culture | | | |
| | Medium control [a] | 4 HC (µM) [b] | | |
		100	300	400
0	$9,164 \pm 497$	$2,610 \pm 301$	0.16 ± 0.2	0
1	$4,133 \pm 275$	$1,312 \pm 387$	13 ± 7	0
2	$1,828 \pm 321$	364 ± 98	1.1 ± 0.5	0
3	370 ± 21	116 ± 36	0	0
4	159 ± 87	38.3 ± 19	0	0
5	45 ± 21	3.3 ± 3	n.d.	n.d.
6	3.3 ± 3		n.d.	n.d.

Mean $\pm$ sem of 4 (100 µM 4-HC) and 3 (300 and 400 µM 4 HC) separate experiments. All cultures were incubated at 33 °C and subjected to removal of half the growth medium and nonadherent cells at weekly intervals. n.d. = not determined

[a] primary inoculum 2×10^7.
[b] primary inoculum 4×10^7

Discussion

The dose of 4-HC employable in clinical marrow purging is limited by its toxicity on hematopoietic stem cells. This has been indirectly estimated by assaying the frequency of granulomonocytic progenitor cells (CFU-GM) in the harvested marrows before and after 4-HC treatment [13]. Interestingly, clinical transplantation data have shown that 4-HC purged autologous grafts, despite CFU-GM depletion, retain their capacity to reconstitute the hematopoietic system of transplant patients pretreated with myelo-ablative chemoradiotherapy [1, 3]. This lack of correlation between *in vitro* CFU-GM recovery and *in vivo* marrow repopulating ability, suggests that survival of this committed stem cell does not parallel the survival of primitive pluripotential stem cells. We therefore studied the 4-HC sensitivity of CFU-Mix as this progenitor cell, whose self-renewal characteristics have been studied [14–16], has been considered the putative primitive stem cell. Our results demonstrate that CFU-Mix is even more sensitive to 4-HC than CFU-GM and BFU-E. However, the fact that 100 and 300 μM 4-HC treated bone marrow (i.e. depleted of CFU-Mix, BFU-E, and CFU-GM) can reinstitute full hematopoietic function in supralethally irradiated patients [1–3] suggests that CFU-Mix may not represent the stem cell responsible for hematopoietic reconstitution in the transplanted host.

The successful engraftment of transplanted bone marrow requires, besides intact primitive hematopoietic stem cells, a functional microenvironment or stroma in which hematopoietic stem cells can self-replicate and differentiate [17, 18]. In humans, the marrow stromal cell (MSC) population is comprised of fibroblasts, adipocytes, endothelial cells, and macrophages [19, 20]. Recent studies have shown that the stromal cells forming the *in vitro* microenvironment in human Dexter-type long-term cultures generated from marrow aspirates of allogeneic marrow transplant recipients are of donor origin and that the percentage of donor cells contributing to the culture stromal microenvironment progressively increases in marrow aspirates taken at greater times after transplantation [21]. Although no evidence has been provided that the proliferation of donor MSC *in vivo* is necessary to support grafted hematopoietic cells, it is conceivable that transplantation of MSC constitutes a factor of critical functional significance [22]. Our results show that the progenitors of MSC are affected by 4-HC treatment in a dose and cell-concentration related manner. However, in comparison to hematopoietic progenitors, MSC are shown to be relatively resistant to the *in vitro* action of 4-HC. In fact, higher 4-HC doses (i.e. 400 versus 100 μM) are required to abolish the formation of colonies by CFU-F as well as the capacity of 4-HC treated marrow suspensions to give rise to functional stromal layers in Dexter-type LTMC.

CFU-Mix and BFU-E are shown to be even more 4-HC sensitive than

CFU-GM and therefore these assays are also unsuitable tools for predicting the engraftment capability of 4-HC purged grafts. Human marrows treated with 4-HC doses up to 300 µM and cultured in Dexter-type LTMC show a low degree of nonadherent cell proliferation and differentiation with relatively normal stromal development. These data taken together with the clinical observations concerning the engraftment of CFU-GM depleted marrows, indicate that MSC and pluripotential stem cells (which appear not to be represented by CFU-Mix), are relatively resistant to 4-HC treatment. Since MSC appear to be transplantable and play an essential role *in vitro* and possibly *in vivo* in hematopoiesis [23–25], generation of LTMC from 4-HC treated marrow may be an appropriate means for the examination of the toxicity of such agents to MSC population. If improved culture conditions are found in the future for the human Dexter-type LTMC, the regeneration of committed stem cells in this culture system may be a better indicator of *in vivo* events than is presently the case.

Acknowledgements

This investigation has been supported by the grants ACS-CH 201 from the American Cancer Society, CA-08748, CA-17353, CA-20194 from the National Cancer Institute, by the Gar Reichman Foundation and by the Shenker Foundation for Cancer Research.

Dr. S. Siena is a Fellow of the Associazione Italiana per la Ricerca sul Cancro and American-Italian Foundation for Cancer Research.

References

1. Kaizer H, Stuart RK, Brookmeyer R et al. (1983). Autologous bone marrow transplantation in acute leukemia: A phase I study of *in vitro* treatment of marrow with 4-hydroperoxycyclophosphamide to purge tumor cells. Blood 62:224a.
2. Gulati S, Gandola L, Vega R et al. (1984). Chemopurification of bone marrow *in vitro* and its clinical application. Proc Amer Ass Cancer Res 25:201.
3. Yeager A, Braine H, Kaizer H et al. (1984). Treatment of refractory non-Hodgkin's lymphoma with intensive chemoradiotherapy and autologous bone marrow transplantation. Proc Amer Soc Clin Oncol 3:239.
4. Sharkis SJ, Santos GW and Colvin M (1980). Elimination of acute myelogenous leukemia cells from marrow and tumor suspensions in the rat with 4-hydroperoxycyclophosphamide. Blood 55:521–523.
5. Takamizawa A, Matsumoto S, Iwata T et al. (1973). Studies on cyclophosphamide metabolites and their related compounds. II. Preparation of an active species of cyclophosphamide and some related compounds. J Amer Chem Soc 95:985–986.
6. Fauser AA and Messner HA (1979). Identification of megakaryocytes, macrophages and eosinophils in colonies of human bone marrow containing neutrophilic granulocytes and erythroblasts. Blood 53:1023–1027.

7. Lu L and Broxmeyer HE (1983). The selective enhancing influence of hemin and products of human erythrocytes on colony formation by human multipotential (CFU-GEMM) and erythroid (BFU-E) progenitor cells *in vitro*. Exp Hematol 11:721–729.

8. Pike BL, Robinson WA (1970). Human bone marrow colony growth in agar gel. J Cell Physiol 75:77–84.

9. Castro-Malaspina H, Gay RE, Resnick G et al. (1980). Characterization of human marrow fibroblast colony-forming cells (CFU-F) and their progeny. Blood 56:289–301.

10. Moore MAS, Broxmeyer HE, Sheridan APC et al. (1980). Continuous human bone marrow cultures: Ia antigen characterization of probable pluripotential stem cells. Blood 55:682–690.

11. Gartner S, Kaplan HS (1980). Long term culture of human bone marrow cells. Proc Nat Acad Sci USA 77:4756–4759.

12. Castro-Malaspina H, Saletan S, Gay RE et al. (1981). Immunocytochemical identification of cells comprising the adherent layer of long-term human bone marrow cultures. Blood 58:107a.

13. Korbling M, Hess AD, Tutscka PJ et al. (1982). 4-Hydroperoxycyclophosphamide: A model for eliminating residual human tumor cells and T-lymphocytes from the bone marrow graft. Brit J Haematol 52:89–96.

14. Messner HA and Fauser AA (1980). Culture studies of pluripotential hemopoietic progenitors. Blut 41:327–333.

15. Ash RC, Detrick RA and Zanjani ED (1981). Studies on human pluripotential hemopoietic stem cells (CFU-GEMM) *in vitro*. Blood 58:309–316.

16. Humphries Rk, Eaves AC and Eaves CJ (1981). Self-renewal of hemopoietic stem cells during mixed colony formation *in vitro*. Proc Nat Acad Sci 78:3629–3633.

17. Wolf NS (1979). The haematopoietic Microenvironment. Clin Haematol 8:469–500.

18. Werts ED, Gibson DP, Knapp SA and De Gowin RL (1980). Stromal cell migration precedes hemopoietic repopulation of the bone marrow after irradiation. Radiat Res 81:20–26.

19. Beckstead JH and Bainton DF (1980). Enzyme histochemistry of bone marrow biopsies: Reactions useful in the differential diagnosis of leukemia and lymphoma applied to 2-micron plastic sections. Blood 55:386–394.

20. Burgio VL, Magrini U, Ciardelli L and Pezzoni G (1984). An enzyme histochemical approach to the study of the human bone marrow stroma. Acta Haematol 71:73–80.

21. Keating A, Singer JW, Killen PD et al. (1982). Donor origin of the *in vitro* haematopoietic microenvironment after marrow transplantation in man. Nature 298:280–283.

22. Dexter TM (1982). Is the marrow stroma transplantable? Nature 298:222–223.

23. Kaneko S, Motomura S and Ibayashi H (1982). Differentiation of human bone marrow-derived fibroblastoid colony forming cells (CFU-F) and their roles in haemopoiesis *in vitro*. Brit J Haematol 51:217–225.

24. Blackburn MJ and Goldman JM (1981). Increased haematopoietic cell survival induced by a human marrow fibroblast factor. Brit J Haematol 48:117–125.

25. Gordon MY, Kearney L and Hibbin JA (1983). Effects of human marrow stromal cells on proliferation by human granulocytic (GM-CFC), erythroid (BFU-E) and mixed (Mix-CFC) colony forming cells. Brit J Haematol 53:317–325.

10. Treatment of refractory non-Hodgkin's lymphoma with intensive chemo-radiotherapy and autologous bone marrow transplantation

H. G. BRAINE[1], H. KAIZER[2], A. M. YEAGER[1], R. K. STUART[1], W. H. BURNS[1], R. SARAL[1], L. L. SENSENBRENNER[1] and G. W. SANTOS[1]

[1] *The Johns Hopkins Oncology Center, Baltimore, Maryland and*
[2] *The Bone Marrow Transport Center, Rush-Presbyterian-St. Luke's Medical Center, Chicago, Illinois, USA*

The observation that syngeneic marrow transplantation following supralethal cytoreductive therapy can produce relatively long-term disease-free survival in a significant fraction of patients with acute leukemia [1] and non-Hodgkin's lymphoma [2, 3] suggests that cure of these diseases may be achieved with marrow transplantation without the hazards of graft-versus-host disease that accompany allogeneic marrow transplants.

Although it is rare for a patient to have a monozygotic twin, their remission marrow (autologous marrow) is a source of syngeneic stem cells. The problem that precludes the more general use of autologous marrow for purposes of transplantation is the concern that such marrow may contain occult clonogenic tumor cells, particularly in the case of the acute leukemias and possibly (although less worrisome) in some cases of non-Hodgkin's lymphoma. Previously we have reviewed the rationale, preclinical studies and preliminary results regarding the use of antibody and complement or chemotherapeutic means of 'purging' marrow of suspected occult clonogenic tumor cells [4]. In this communication we wish to report our preliminary results with the transplantation of autologous marrow 'purging' by antibody and complement or by 4-hydroperoxycyclophosphamide (4HC) following supralethal cytoreductive therapy in patients with non-Hodgkin's lymphoma who had failed other cytoreductive therapy.

Materials and methods

Patients

We have considered patients 2–55 years of age to be eligible for therapeutic protocol if they had a histologically confirmed diagnosis of diffuse non-

Hodgkin's lymphoma including Burkitt's and T-cell lymphoblastic lymphoma but excluding well differentiated lymphoblastic lymphoma and chronic lymphocytic leukemia. Patients had failed prior treatment. Criteria for failure were less than 50% tumor reduction with each cycle of induction treatment course and/or relapse within six months of stopping induction treatment. Attempts were made to induce a second remission with second-line therapy. Patients were considered eligible if they attained a complete remission or if they achieved a partial remission or showed no evidence of bone marrow involvement (bilateral iliac biopsies and aspiration) at the time of entry on this study. All patients were required to have an Eastern Cooperative Oncology Group performance score of 0, 1 or 2. Patients were excluded from the study if they had cardiac, pulmonary, hepatic, or renal insufficiency. For those patients who received hyperfractionated total body irradiation (TBI) an additional requirement was that previous or residual bulky disease had to be 'portable' with the field-within-a-field radiation therapy technique. Finally, all patients with T-cell lymphoma were required to have had evidence that the monoclonal antibodies used were cytotoxic to cell samples of the individual patient's tumor.

Seven patients met the criteria for autologous marrow transplantation with T-cell lymphoma and eleven patients met the criteria for autologous bone marrow transplantation in the diffuse non-Hodgkin's lymphoma category. Characteristics of these patients are described in Table I.

Marrow harvesting and purging

Bone marrow was harvested from the iliac crest under general anesthesia and preparation of a single cell suspension was carried out as described by Thomas and Storb [5]. All blood transfusions given in the week prior to harvesting the bone marrow intraoperatively or subsequently were first irradiated with 1500–3000 rad. Every attempt was made to obtain at least 4×10^8 nucleated cells per kg of patient body weight for the treated marrow with 2×10^8 nucleated cells per kg as the reserve marrow.

The harvested blood-marrow mixtures were separated by centrifugation in blood transfer bags (Fenwal 4R203) on a Sorvall RC-3B centrifuge at 2900 rpm (HG-4L head) for ten minutes. The plasma and buffy coat layers were transferred to seaprate bags, residual red cell pellet and plasma were remixed, and a second buffy coat was extracted. The buffy coat fractions were pooled and the volume was adjusted with autologous plasma and tissue culture medium (TC-199) to obtain a final concentration of 2×10^7 nucleated cells/ml in 80% TC-199 and 20% plasma. The monoclonal antibodies leu-1 and leu-9 were kindly provided by R. Levy of Stanford University School of Medicine. For incubation with monoclonal antibodies, the

Table I. Characteristics of patients with non-Hodgkin's lymphoma

UN	Age/Sex	Diagnosis/Date	Prior Treatment	Status at BMH/BMT	Date of transplant
241	6/M	T-cell/12–15–77	1) PO,CY + MED XRT 2) TEST XRT	CR2/CR2	10–3–80
315	28/M	T-cell/5–20–80	1) CY, NM, VINC, MED XRT 2) BACOP X 2 3) PRED 4) CAV X 3	PR2/PR2	10–23–81
336	12/M	T-cell/12–14–79	1) CHOP X 2 2) Test RXT + Main Chemo 3) Cranial XRT + IT MTX 4) IV MTX (retroperitoneal node relapse)	CR4/CR4	2/19/82
378	29/M	T-cell/1–8–80	1) CHOP 2) L-ASP + cranial XRT 3) CHOP X 4 + MTX, 6MP 4) CHOP X 1, L-ASP	CR2/CR2	10–1–82
414	16/F	T-cell/8–8–82	1) Chest XRT 2) LSA2-L2	CR2/CR2	3–25–83
452	12/F	T-cell/3–15–82	1) CHOP X 3, cranial XRT [(VM-26 + MTX) (maint)] 2) VINC, PRED, DRN, L-ASP	CR2/CR2	9–2–83
482	10/M	T-cell/10–6–82	1) CY, ADR, IT MTX, VINC, 6MP, cranial XRT 2) Repeat of 1	CR2/CR2	1–6–84
73	7/M	Burk/10-14-76	1) CY, MTX, VINC, IT MTX	PR1/PR1	2–4–77
320	15/F	Burk/12–11–80	1) COMP X 2 2) CY, ADR	CR1/CR2	11–27–81
282	15/M	LCL/3–15–80	1) CHOP, IT MTX, + Hydrocortisone, cranial XRT 2) IT MTX 3) XRT brain, spine	CR5/CR5	5–15–81
305	14/F	LCL/4–23–81	1) CY, VINC, DRN, MTX, abd XRT 2) VINC, PRED, CY, XRT axilla, paraaortic, abd, mantle 3) CY	CR2/PR3	9–4–81
306	3/M	LCL/2–15–81	1) Med, XRT CHOP 2) ADR, Hi-dose MTX	CR2/CR3	9–11–81

Table I. Characteristics of patients with non-Hodgkin's lymphoma (continued)

UN	Age/ Sex	Diagnosis/Date	Prior Treatment	Status at BMH/BMT	Date of trans- plant
341	18/M	LCL/8-28-81	1) COPA X 8, mantle XRT 2) MTX, L-ASP	PR1/PR1	4-2-82
455	39/M	MCL/12-10-82	1) CHOP X 2	PR2/PR2	9-16-83
481	19/F	LCL/1-3-83	1) XRT, arm BACOP 2) Local XRT	PR2/PR2	12-30-83
493	5/M	PDLL/8-1-81	1) CY, VINC, MTX, PRED 2) LSA 2 L-2 3) XRT, facial 4) ARA- C/L-ASP X 3	CR2/CR2	2-10-84
495	19/M	PDLL/5-19-81	1) VINC, PRED, ADR, CY, CCNU 2) IT MTX, cranial XRT 3) VELBAN 4) VP16 5) L-ASP + VINC	CR2/CR2	2-10-84
505	19/M	PDLL/3-2-81	1) CHOP 2) L-ASP + ARA-C 3) COMLA	PR2/PR2	4-4-84

Abbreviations: UN = unique patient number; Burk = Burkitt's lymphoma; LCL = large cell lymphoma; MCL = mixed cell lymphoma; PDLL = poorly differentiated lymphoblastic lymphoma; BMH/BMT = bone marrow harvest/bone marrow transplantation; CR = complete remission; PR = partial remission; COPA = CY, ADR, VINC, PRED; COMP = CY, VINC, MTX (IT + IV), PRED; BACOP = BLEO, VINC, ADR, CY, PRED; CAV = CY, M-AMSA, VP16; CHOP = CY, ADR, VINC, PRED; LSA2-L2 = VINC, PRED, CY, DRN, IT MTX; Maintenance = 6TG, CY, HYDROXY, DRN, MTX, BCNU, ARA-C, VINC; Consolidation = ARA-C, 6TG, L-ASP, BCNU; COMLA = CY, VINC, MTX, L-ASP

cells were treated as described previously [6]. For incubation with 4HC, a freshly prepared stock solution of 10 mg/ml of 4HC in phosphate buffered saline was then added to the cell suspension to achieve the desired drug concentration. The cells were incubated at 37 °C for 30 minutes, cooled to 4 °C and centrifuged at 2900 rpm for ten minutes. The cell pellet was resuspended at a concentration of 4×10^7 cells/ml in 45% TC-199, 45% autologous plasma and 10% dimethyl sulfoxide (DMSO). Fifty ml aliquots were transferred to polyolefin bags (Del-med Corp., Halbrook, MA # 2030-2) and frozen in a Cryo-med model 100 freezer (Cryo-med Corp., St. Clemens, MI) at 1 °C/minute to −50 °C and then at 10 °C/min to −70 °C. The bags were stored in the liquid phase of a liquid nitrogen freezer. At the time of transplant, each bag was thawed rapidly in a 37 °C waterbath and infused rapidly without further processing and removal of DMSO.

Pre-transplant preparative regimens

The day of autologous marrow infusion is designated as day 0 and the timing of the pre-transplant regimen is denoted by an appropriate negative day number. Three different preparative regimens were employed as follows:
1. Doxorubicin 30 mg/m²/day for days −11, −10, and −9; Cyclophosphamide 50 mg/kg/day for four days, −8, −7, −6, and −5; total body irradiation, 300 rad/day for days −4, −3, −2, and −1 (ADR, CY, TBI).
2. The same protocol as number 1 but without the doxorubicin (CY, TBI).
3. Cyclophosphamide 50 mg/kg/day for days −8, −7, −6, and −5; TBI 180 rad bid plus local field irradiation 120 rad bid (CY, HFTBI).
In all cases of TBI the lungs were shielded for the third day.

Informed consent

The protocols were reviewed and approved by the Joint Committee on Clinical Investigation of the Johns Hopkins Medical Institutions, and appropriate informed consent was obtained from the patient.

Results

Table II displays the results of autologous marrow transplantation in seven patients with T-cell lymphoma as of May 15, 1984. Three patients survive in continuous disease-free remission for 131⁺, 816⁺, and 1320⁺ days following transplantation and three survive for 242⁺, 403⁺ and 578⁺ days following relapse at 91, 48 and 405 days, respectively. One patient relapsed at 75 days following transplantation and died of progressive tumor at 97 days following transplantation. Kaplan-Meier plots indicate a two-year survival of 80% and a two-year probability of remission of 40%.

Data for patients transplanted for diffuse non-Hodgkin's lymphoma are represented in Table III. Except for patient UN 73, all patients received autologous marrow incubated with 4HC. As of May 15, 1984 seven of eleven patients survive in complete continuous remission for 39–2657 days following marrow transplantation. One patient survives for 95 days after a relapse at 53 days. Three patients died with progressive tumor at 384, 85

Table II. Autologous marrow transplantation in T-cell lymphoblastic lymphoma: treatment of marrow with monoclonal antibody

UN	Status at BMH/BMT	Marrow treatment	Preparative regimen	Relapse in days	Survival in days	Present status
241	CR2/CR2	Leu-1	ADR,CY, TBI	–	1320+	Alive in remission
315	PR2/PR2	Leu-1	CY, TBI	75	97	Dead, progressive tumor
336	CR4/CR4	Leu-1	CY, TBI	–	816+	Alive in remission
378	CR2/CR2	Leu-1+9	CY, HFTBI	405	578+	Alive in relapse
414	CR2/CR2	Leu-1+9	CY, HFTBI	48	403+	Alive in relapse
452	CR2/CR2	Leu-1+9	CY, HFTBI	91	243+	Alive in relapse
482	CR2/CR2	Leu-1+9	CY, HFTBI	–	131+	Alive in remission

and 137 days after relapses at 33, 60 and 65 days, respectively, following transplantation. Kaplan-Meier plot analysis revealed a two-year probability of survival of 60% and a probability of remission of 65%.

When all T-cell and diffuse non-Hodgkin's disease patients are taken together as one group of 18 patients, 14 survive for 39–2657 days with a median survival of greater than 322 days. Ten of 18 patients survive in continuous remission for 39–2657 days with a median disease-free survival of 528 days. Kaplan-Meier plot analysis revealed a probability of two-year

Table III. Autologous marrow transplantation in non-Hodgkin's lymphoma

UN	Status at BMH/BMT	4HC marrow treatment (ug/ml)	Preparative regimen	Relapse in days	Survival in days	Present status
73	PR1/PR1	0	ADR, CY, TBI	–	2657+	Alive in remission
320	CR1/CR2	40	ADR, CY, TBI	–	864+	Alive in remission
282	CR5/CR5	60	ADR, CY, TBI	33	384	Dead, progressive tumor
305	CR2/PR3	60	CY, TBI	60	85	Dead, progressive tumor
306	CR2/CR3	60	ADR, CY, TBI	–	895+	Alive in remission
341	PR1/PR1	100	CY, HFTBI	65	137	Dead, progressive tumor
455	PR2/PR2	100	CY, HFTBI	–	242+	Alive in remission
481	PR2/PR2	100	CY, HFTBI	–	137+	Alive in remission
493	CR2/CR2	100	CY, HFTBI	53	95+	Alive in relapse
495	CR2/CR2	100	CY, HFTBI	–	95+	Alive in remission
505	PR2/PR2	100	CY, HFTBI	–	39+	Alive in remission

disease-free survival of 73% and a two-year probability of remission of 50%.

In general the treatments were well tolerated, considering that all patients received supralethal cytoreductive therapy prior to autologous marrow transplantation. The cause of death in all patients who died was progressive recurrent tumor; there were no deaths in the immediate post-transplantation period.

Peripheral blood cell recovery was similar in both groups of patients. The median time and (range) of time in days to reach granulocyte levels of $> 500/mm^3$, reticulocyte levels of $> 1\%$, and platelet levels of $> 50 \times 10^3/mm^3$ were 21 (12–60), 26 (7–53) and 34 (17–61), respectively.

Discussion

The preliminary results reported here are encouraging and at the moment appear as promising as that seen following syngeneic or allogeneic marrow transplantation in non-Hodgkin's lymphoma [2, 3].

Whether or not marrow purging is a requirement in transplantation in lymphomas (as illustrated by one of our patients with Burkitt's lymphoma) is not resolved or indeed addressed by the present or other studies currently reported in the literature. We, however, have found that the prior treatment with the above described monoclonal antibodies and 4HC has not jeopardized engraftment nor caused unexpected toxicities. It is also noteworthy that all deaths were related to recurrent progressive tumor rather than lethal consequences of the preparative therapy.

Time and expansion of the number of patients entered on this form of treatment are required before we can more solidly confirm our initial encouragement and routinely place this therapy in the treatment flow of patients with T-cell and diffuse non-Hodgkin's lymphoma.

Acknowledgements

Supported by grants CA-15396 and CAO-6973 awarded by the National Cancer Institute, Departments of Health and Human Services.

References

1. Santos GW (1984). Allogeneic and syngeneic marrow transplantation in acute leukemia with minimal residual disease. In: Lowenberg B and Hagenbeek A (Eds.). Minimal Residual Disease in Acute Leukemia pp. 323–332. Boston, Martinus Nijhoff Publishers B.V.

536

2. Appelbaum FR, Fefer A, Cheever MA et al. (1981). Treatment of non-Hodgkin's lymphoma with marrow transplantation in identical twins. Blood 58:509–513.
3. Appelbaum FR and Thomas ED (1983). Review of the use of marrow transplantation in the treatment of non-Hodgkin's lymphoma. J Clin Oncol 1:440–447.
4. Santos GW and Kaizer H (1984). *In vitro* chemotherapy as a prelude to autologous marrow transplantation in hematologic malignancy. In: Lowenberg B and Hagenbeek A (Eds.). Minimal Residual Disease in Acute Leukemia, pp. 165–181. Boston, Martinus Nijhoff Publishers B. V.
5. Thomas ED and Storb R (1970). Technique for human marrow grafting. Blood 36:507–515.
6. Kaizer H, Levy R, Brovall C et al. (1982). Autologous bone marrow transplantation in T-cell malignancies: A case report involving *in vitro* treatment of marrow with a pan T-cell monoclonal antibody. J Biol Resp Modif 1:233–243.

11. Transplantation with anti-B₁ monoclonal antibody and complement treated autologous bone marrow for relapsed B-cell non-Hodgkin's lymphoma

L. M. NADLER, T. TAKVORIAN, P. MAUCH,
K. C. ANDERSON, J. RITZ, S. HELLMAN, G. P. CANELLOS
and S. F. SCHLOSSMAN
*Divisions of Tumor Immunology and Medical Oncology,
Dana-Farber Cancer Institute and Department of Medicine, Brigham
and Women's Hospital; Joint Center for Radiation Therapy, and
the Departments of Medicine and Radiation Therapy, Harvard
Medical School, Boston, Massachusetts, USA*

Despite significant advances in the treatment of non-Hodgkin's lymphoma (NHL), the majority of patients still succumb to the disease [1–6]. For the poor prognosis (high grade) large cell lymphomas, the cure rate with intensive chemotherapeutic regimens appears to be in the range of 30–50% [1, 2, 4–6]. In contrast, patients with relapsed NHL are rarely, if ever, cured by second-line therapeutics. To improve survival, one promising approach is the use of intensive multi-modality therapy which has the limiting toxicity of myelosuppression. To protect against myelotoxicity, infusion of isologous or autologous bone marrow has been used. Several small series have suggested that this approach can induce long lasting remissions in approximately 25% of patients with relapsed NHL [7–11].

One major obstacle to the more generalized use of autologous bone marrow support in the treatment of relapsed NHL is the high frequency of bone marrow involvement with lymphoma [12–17]. A number of studies in both animals and man have indicated that one can selectively eliminate small numbers of tumor cells with antibody and complement without inhibiting subsequent hematopoietic engraftment [18–22]. The development of B-cell specific monoclonal antibodies reactive with virtually all B-cell lymphomas, coupled with the development of *in vitro* techniques for the selective elimination of tumor cells from bone marrow have provided the basis for developing a new treatment regimen for relapsed NHL using high dose chemotherapy and autologous bone marrow transplantation (ABMT) [23–26]. We have chosen to utilize the anti-B1 monoclonal antibody which has been shown to be reactive with greater than 95% of normal B-cells and is also expressed on the overwhelming majority of leukemias and lymphomas of B-cell origin [23, 25, 27]. In the present study, anti-B1 antibody and complement have been used to remove the residual tumor cells from the bone marrows of eight patients with relapsed NHL prior to intensive chemoradiotherapy and ABMT.

Materials and methods

Methods

B1 Monoclonal antibody and complement source
The method for generation, and phenotypic and biochemical characterization of the B1 monoclonal antibody (murine IgG2a), which recognizes a B-cell restricted antigen within the hematopoietic system, has been described in detail [27]. The B1 antigen is strongly expressed on the leukemic cells from 50% of patients with non-T cell ALL or lymphoid blast crisis of CML, on 100% of tumor cells isolated from patients with B-cell CLL and from 100% of patients with B-cell non-Hodgkin's lymphoma [23, 25]. The B1 antigen has not been detected on tumors of T or myeloid lineage. Approximately 5% of normal bone marrow also expresses the B1 antigen, however, myeloid precursors (CFU-C, BFU-E, CFU-E, CFU-GEMM or long term myeloid cultures) do not express the B1 antigen [28, 29].

Anti-B1 antibody was obtained from ascitic fluid of BALB/C mice which had been primed with 0.5 ml of pristane (Aldrich Chemical, Milwalkee, WI) followed by intraperitoneal inoculation with 10^6 B1 hybridoma cells. Ascitic fluid was collected under sterile conditions and the cells were removed by centrifugation. B1 ascitic fluid was then heated to 56 °C for 30 minutes, fibrin clots and aggregates were removed by ultracentrifugation at 100,000 g for 20 minutes and fluid was successively passed through 0.45 µ and 0.22 µ filters. This heat inactivated ascites containing anti-B1 antibody was stored at − 70 °C.

Samples of B1 ascites were tested for reactivity *in vitro* by indirect immunofluorescence and complement mediated cytotoxicity of B1 + target cells. Samples were also tested for sterility and for the presence of endotoxin with a limulus amoebocyte lysate test (Microbiologic Associate, Walkerville, MD). The B1 antigen was lytic on B-cell lines and tumor cells isolated from patients at a 1:100,000 dilution. Rabbit complement (new born rabbit complement, Pel-Freeze, AR) was absorbed with AB positive erythrocytes prior to use.

In vitro treatment of bone marrow
Marrow was harvested from anterior and posterior iliac crests under general anesthesia. The cells were collected in RPMI 1640 media with preservative free heparin, filtered through stainless steel mesh, washed and treated with

an IBM cell washer. Our method for *in vitro* treatment of bone marrow is based on our studies to determine the optimum conditions for lysis of small numbers of B1+ tumor cells in the presence of large excess of normal marrow cells. *In vitro* treatment under these conditions does not selectively eliminate myeloid precursors from normal marrow. Mononuclear cells isolated on Ficoll-Hypaque gradients were treated three times with anti-B1 antibody and rabbit complement according to the following protocol. Cells were suspended at a concentration of 2×10^7 cells/ml. Each treatment consisted of 30 minutes incubation with antibody (1:100 dilution) at 20 °C, followed by incubation at 37 °C for 30 minutes with complement (1:10 dilution). ^{51}Cr labelled B1+ Daudi Burkitt's lymphoma cells were added to a separate specimen of bone marrow mononuclear cells and treated in the same way as bulk marrow to assess the efficacy of *in vitro* lysis of B1+ cells.

After three treatments, cells were cryopreserved in medium containing 10% dimethyl sulfoxide and 90% autologous serum at −196 °C in the vapor phase of liquid nitrogen. Before infusion, the cryopreserved marrow was rapidly thawed and cells were diluted in medium containing 25 IU/ml/DNAase to minimize clumping. The viability of the specimens of marrow were determined and cells were also cultured to test sterility.

Clinical protocol

Patients less than 60 years of age with non-Hodgkin's lymphomas which had relapsed after standard chemotherapeutic regimens and whose lymphoma cells expressed the B1 antigen were eligible for this protocol. These patients were treated with a variety of chemotherapeutic regimens and local radiotherapy to achieve optimal clinical remission. Attainment of a nearly complete clinical regression of disease was required for entry. Prior to ABMT bone marrow was evaluated for lymphoma cells by bilateral trephine biopsy using both cytologic and flow cytometric analysis. All patients admitted to this study had histologically normal bone marrow prior to transplantation.

After induction of maximal clinical remission, bone marrow cells were harvested from the patient under general anesthesia. These mononuclear cells were treated with B1 antibody and newborn rabbit complement (Pel-Freeze), as described, and cryopreserved. Cyclophosphamide at 60 mg/kg was given intravenously on days 1 and 2 in all patients. Total body radiation was administered at 5 rad/min either as a single total dose for a total of 850 rad (patients 1 and 2) or fractionated at 200 rad/fraction twice a day on days 3, 4, and 5 (patients 3–8). Approximately 12 hours after completion of TBI, cryopreserved treated marrow was rapidly thawed and reinfused through a central venous catheter.

Evaluation of hematopoietic reconstitution
After bone marrow infusion, daily peripheral blood counts were taken to evaluate hematopoietic reconstitution. Phenotypic analysis was conducted on mononuclear cells purified from peripheral blood by Ficoll-Hypaque density sedimentation. A panel of characterized monoclonal antibodies including I-2 [30], B1 [23, 27], T3 [31], T4 [31], T8 [31], T11 [31], T12 [31], and 901 [32] was used to stain the cells by indirect immunofluorescence. Cells were analyzed by flow cytometry. In addition, quantitative immuno-electrophoresis was undertaken to determine circulating IgM and IgG levels.

Patients

Patient clinical characteristics (Table I)
Of the eight patients, six were male and ages ranged from 30 to 57 years (median 46). Seven of eight patients had poor prognosis diffuse lymphomas, and 5 of 8 patients had evolved to a more aggressive histologic variant at the time of relapse. At diagnosis, only one patient had detectable tumor cells in the bone marrow. At relapse, 6 of 8 patients had gross tumor involvement of the marrow.

Disease status at relapse and following induction
As seen in Table I, patients 1, 2, 3, 6, 7, and 8 had multiple relapses following intensive multimodality therapy, whereas patients 4 and 5 had only a

Table I. Patient clinical characteristics

Patient	Age	Sex	Lymph node histology[a]		BM infiltration at relapse[b]	No. of relapses prior to induction
			At diagnosis	At relapse		
1	50	M	DM	DM	5%	3
2	44	M	DPDL	DLC	30%	2
3	57	M	DLDP	DLC	50%	5
4	43	M	DPDL	DLC	75%	1
5	30	M	NPDL	DLC	5%[c]	1
6	46	F	DPDL	DPDL	50%	2
7	41	F	DM	DLC	30%	2
8	39	M	DPDL	DPDL	70%	2

[a] DM: diffuse mixed; DLDP: diffuse poorly differentiated lymphocytic; NPDL: nodular poorly differentiated lymphocytic; DLC: diffuse large cell
[b] Approximately maximum % of bone marrow infiltration during relapse
[c] Patient 5 had gross marrow involvement at diagnosis

single relapse. At the time of relapse, 6 of 8 patients had bulky (5–10 cm) peripheral and abdominal lymphadenopathy and two patients had extranodal relapses in the lung (patient 2) or the kidney and peripheral blood (patient 4). In contrast, patient 5 had a scalp nodule of 3–4 cm and patient 7 had involvement of the cervix. Prior to ABMT, all patients were retreated to a minimal disease state with no detectable tumor masses greater than 3–5 cm with systemic chemotherapy and/or local irradiation. Moreover, bone marrow involvement of greater than 5% was not detectable by morphologic evaluation. Selection of re-treatment programs varied depending on prior therapy and sites of relapse. Systemic therapy alone (patients 4, 6, 7, 8), radiotherapy alone (patients 1 and 5), and a combination of systemic therapy and radiotherapy (patients 2 and 3) were employed.

Results

Hematologic and immunologic reconstitution (Table II)

The first evidence of marrow engraftment occurred on day 10 with the appearance of the first polymorphonuclear leukocytes (PMN). By day 22, 5 of 8 patients demonstrated greater then 500 PMN/µl. A sustained platelet count greater than 20,000/µl occurred as early as the 20th day and as late as the 60th day post ABMT.

Reconstitution of B-lymphocytes was reflected by the number of B1+ cells in peripheral blood as well as by serum immunoglobulin levels. As seen in Table II, the first B1+ cells in peripheral blood were detected between 35 and 57 days post-transplant. However, normal numbers of B1+ mononuclear cells (approximately 5%) could be consistently detected only after 2–3 months. Normal circulating immunoglobulin levels occurred considerably later than the appearance of B1+ cells. Circulating IgM and IgG levels, which dropped to less than 25% of normal after transplantation, slowly returned to normal within 3–6 months without passive immunization.

In all patients, T-lymphocytes which co-expressed the T3, T11, T12, and Ia antigens were the first to appear. Although T-cells from peripheral blood also normally co-express T3, T11, and T12, the Ia antigens are normally seen on cells after activation. In all patients the ratio of the number of T-cells which express the T8 antigen (cytotoxic/suppressor) and the T4 antigen (helper/inducer) was reversed. In fact, approximately 2/3 of the T-cells express the T8 antigen. This abnormality has persisted for over 6 months in all patients and has gradually returned to normal by the end of the first year. Of interest is the number of cells which express the 901

Table II. Autologous bone marrow transplant and reconstitution

| Patient | No. of cells (X 10⁷/kg) | Hematologic reconstitution post-ABMTX (days) | | | | B-cell reconstitution (days) | | | |
| | | Polymorphonuclear granulocytes | | | Platelets | B1 + cell in blood | | Normal Ig serum levels | |
		1st	500/µl	1,000/µl	20,000/µl	1st	5%	IgM	IgG
1	2.8	10	37	47	35	47	94	150	120
2	4.2	10	21	27	24	49	77	217	245
3	7.3	10	19	29	28	35	67	–	–
4	8.5	10	18	30	20	38	59	93	93
5	7.6	10	22	27	27	45	87	120	97
6	4.8	10	31	43	49	57	74	108	152
7	5.0	10	33	57	60	71	–	–	–
8	5.1	8	12	14	18	–	–	–	–

antigen which is restricted in its expression to natural killer cells. The 901 antigen was found on approximately 10–15% of peripheral blood mononuclear cells in the first 3 weeks post-ABMT.

Toxicity, anti-tumor effect and disease free survival

The acute toxicity following ABMT was minimal. All patients suffered weight loss up to approximately 10% of their body weight. Patients 2–8 developed low grade fever of unknown cause which was treated with antibiotics. Patient 7 had an episode of hypotension associated with fever. Seven of the eight patients developed transient stomatitis and in patient 1 Herpes simplex was cultured from the oral ulcers which promptly responded to Acyclovir therapy. Late toxicities have been seen in 2 of 7 patients followed for over 3 months. Patient 1 suffered from mild pneumonia of unknown cause at biopsy at 3 ½ months post-transplant. Patient 1 also suffered an episode of herpetic conjuntivitis at 7 months post transplant which rapidly responded to local adenosine arabinoside therapy. Patient 2 had localized cutaneous Herpes Zoster which responded to intravenous Acyclovir. Otherwise no late toxicities have been noted. All patients had complete disappearance of disease following ABMT.

Six patients (1, 2, 5, 6, 7, and 8) are in continuous unmaintained remission at 18+, 17+, 8+, 6+, 3+, and 1+ months, respectively. In contrast, patient 3 relapsed 3 months post-transplant in all sites of prior bulk disease (including the bone marrow) and expired 1 month later. Patient 4 relapsed in the site of a previous abdominal mass after a 6 month disease-free interval. At the time of relapse he had no evidence of bone marrow involvement on bilateral trephine biopsies. He is still alive at 11+ months post-transplant on palliative chemotherapy regimens.

Discussion

Autologous bone marrow support has been employed to reverse the aplasia induced by the administration of lethal doses of chemotherapy and/or radiotherapy. Several recent reports have suggested that high-dose chemoradiotherapy with ABMT may be useful to induce long-term remissions in patients with relapsed B-cell NHL [7–10]. These studies clearly demonstrate that relapsed lymphomas are sensitive to higher doses of chemoradiotherapy although they are resistant to conventional doses. Bone marrow cells in these trials were obtained from either an identical twin or from a patient whose marrow was histologically considered to be free of tumor. However, recent evidence from our own and other laboratories suggests that histologically normal bone marrows may frequently be contaminated by occult lymphoma cells [33, Nadler, unpublished observations].

We have undertaken an initial investigation to determine the feasibility of treating autologous bone marrow with anti-B1 monoclonal antibody and complement *in vitro* to eradicate occult lymphoma cells. Based upon our experience in treating bone marrow specimens from patients with relapsed non-T cell acute lymphoblastic leukemia with anti-J5 (CALLA) and complement [22], we devised an *in vitro* strategy to 'clean up' marrow cell suspensions from patients with relapsed B-cell NHL prior to ABMT. Entry onto the study was restricted to patients induced into a minimal disease state with histologically tumor-free bone marrow. Marrow was harvested and treated *in vitro* with anti-B1 and complement. Eight patients have thus far undergone ABMT with anti-B1 treated autologous bone marrow. In all instances the patients achieved complete clinical response with high-dose chemoradiotherapy. Complete hematologic engraftment occurred by eight weeks post marrow infusion and no severe untoward side effects, either acute or chronic, have thus far been observed due to the prompt reconstitution of granulocytes and platelets. These results suggest that anti-B1 treated bone marrow can effectively reverse aplasia induced by intensive combined modality therapy.

The evidence that anti-B1 and complement treated autologous bone marrow engrafted in all patients suggests that this may be an important approach to the treatment of relapsed B-cell NHL. The kinetics of reconstitution was almost identical to that seen with autologous bone marrow which was not manipulated *in vitro* or cryopreserved [34]. Although patients suffered with stomatitis and 10% body weight loss, these toxicities were self limited and rapidly resolved with the appearance of greater than 500 granulocytes/μl.

Immunologic reconstitution lagged significantly behind hematologic reconstitution. The reconstitution of circulating B1 positive cells occurred at 2 to 4 months. During this time, immunoglobulin levels gradually decreased and by 3 months they were at their nadir. Following the reappearance of B1 positive cells in the circulation, the Ig levels began to rise. Nonetheless it was 6 months post-transplant before they achieved normal levels. With the return of normal Ig levels the titer of anti-tetanus antibody returned to pretransplant levels without reimmunization. No infections which might be attributed to hypogammaglobulinemia have so far been observed. The reconstitution of B-cells clearly confirms earlier observations indicating that the B1 antigen is not expressed on the B-progenitor cell [28, 29]. As has been observed with the anti-CALLA autologous bone marrow transplants, T-cells return to the circulation by 2–3 weeks post-transplant. The number of cells expressing the suppressor cell phenotype (T8) is at least twice the number which express the inducer cell phenotype (T4). In addition, it should be noted that preliminary *in vitro* studies demonstrate that irrespective of phenotype the cells isolated are for the most part functionally incompetent. This reversed T4/T8 ratio persists for up to one year post-transplant and may provide one explanation for the propensity of these patients to contract herpes infections.

Although exciting advances have been made in the primary treatment of NHL, the treatment of relapsed NHL has led to few long-term survivors. Previous attempts utilizing intensive combined modality therapy with autologous marrow support have been largely unsuccessful. Patients with obvious tumor masses were treated with no attempt to reduce tumor volume prior to autologous transplantation. The initial success of our trial may be due to the requirement that patients must be in or near a clinical remission prior to ABMT. The first two patients have remained disease-free for almost one and one-half years post-transplant and have returned to normal activity. Prior to ABMT conventional chemotherapy was unable to control their disease. It is important to note that unmaintained second remissions lasting over 12 months are unusual in NHL and, therefore, suggests that this approach may be of therapeutic benefit.

In summary, we have demonstrated that autologous bone marrow transplantation for relapsed B-cell NHL is feasible after *in vitro* treatment with anti-B1 monoclonal antibody and complement. Initial results suggest that some patients with relapsed, extensively pretreated disease may achieve long-term disease-free survival. Efficacy of this program is likely to be enhanced if a second clinical remission can be effected prior to transplantation. In the future, this approach may be attempted in the first remission for patients who are at high risk for early relapse.

Acknowledgements

The authors greatfully acknowledge the outstanding technical assistance of Carol Reynolds, Bruce Slaughenhoupt, David Fisher, Michael Bates, and Darlene Zankowski. We would also like to greatfully acknowledge the help of Felice Coral (DFCI, Tumor Immunology) and Barbara Gargone (DFCI, Blood Component Laboratory). We would also like to recognize the invaluble support of the nursing service of the Medical Intensive Care Unit of the Brigham and Women's Hospital. This work was supported by NIH grant CA 34183-01, Project B6.

References

1. Cadman E, Farber L, Bend D et al. (1977). Combination therapy for diffuse histiocytic lymphoma that includes antimetabolites. Cancer Treat Rep 61:1109–1116.

2. Skarin AT, Rosenthal DS, Moloney WC et al. (1977). Combination chemotherapy of advanced non-Hodgkin's lymphoma with bleomycin, adriamycin, cyclophosphamide, vincristine and prednisone (BACOP). Blood 49:759–768.

3. Portlock CS and Rosenberg SA (1979). No initial therapy for Stage III and IV non-Hodgkin's lymphomas of favorable histologic types. Ann Intern Med 90:10–13.

4. Sweet DL, Golomb HM, Ultmann JE et al. (1980). Cyclophosphamide, vincristine, methotrexate with leucovorin rescue, and cytarabine (COMLA) combination sequential chemotherapy for advanced diffused histiocytic lymphoma. Ann Intern Med 92:785–796.

5. Skarin AT, Canellos GP, Rosenthal DS et al. (1983). Improved prognosis of diffuse histiocytic and undifferentiated lymphoma by use of high dose methotrexate alternating with standard agents (M-BACOD). J Clin Oncol 1:91.

6. Fisher RI, DeVita VT Jr, Hubbard SM et al. (1983). Diffuse aggressive lymphomas: Increased survival after alternating flexible sequences of ProMACE and MOPP chemotherapy. Ann Intern Med 98:304–313.

7. Appelbaum FR, Herzig GP, Ziegler JC et al. (1978). Successful engraftment of cryopreserved autologous bone marrow in patients with malignant lymphoma. Blood 52:85–95.

8. Appelbaum FR, Fefer A, Cheever MA et al. (1981). Treatment of non-Hodgkin's lymphoma with marrow transplantation in identical twins. Blood 58:509–521.

9. Appelbaum FR and Thomas ED (1983). Review of the use of marrow transplantation in the treatment of non-Hodgkin's lymphoma. J Clin Oncol 1:440–447.

10. Gorin NC, David R, Stachowiak J et al. (1981). High dose chemotherapy and autologous bone marrow transplantation in acute leukemias, malignant lymphomas and solid tumors. Eur J Cancer 17:557–568.

11. Philip T, Biron P, Maraninchi D et al. (1984). Role of massive therapy and autologous bone marrow transplantation in non-Hodgkin's malignant lymphoma. Lancet 2:391.

12. Castellani R, Bonadonna G, Spinelli P et al. (1978). Sequential pathologic staging of untreated non-Hodgkin's lymphomas by laparoscopy and laparotomy combined with marrow biopsy. Cancer 40:2322–2329.

13. Chabner BA, Johnson RE, Young RC et al. (1976). Sequential nonsurgical and surgical staging of non-Hodgkin's lymphoma. Ann Intern Med 85:149–154.

14. Coller BS, Chabner BA, Gralnick HR (1979). Frequencies and patterns of bone marrow involvement in the non-Hodgkin's lymphomas: Observation on the value of bilateral biopsies. Amer J Hematol 3:105–119.

15. Dick F, Bloomfield CD and Brunning CD (1974). Incidence, cytology, and histopathology of non-Hodgkin's lymphomas in the bone marrow. Cancer 33:1382–1398.

16. Goffinet DR, Warnke R, Dunnick NR et al. (1977). Clinical and surgical (lapartomy) evaluation of patients with non-Hodgkin's lymphomas. Cancer Treat Rep 61:981–992.

17. McKenna RW, Bloomfield CD and Brunning RD (1975). Nodular lymphoma: Bone marrow and blood manifestations. Cancer 36:428–440.

18. Bast RC, Ritz J, Lipton JM et al. (1983). Elimination of leukemic cells from human bone marrow using monoclonal antibody and complement. Cancer Res 43:1389–1394.

19. Economou JS, Shin HS, Kaiser H et al. (1978). Bone marrow transplantation in cancer therapy: Inactivation by antibody and complement of tumor cells in syngeneic marrow transplants. Proc Soc Exp Biol Med 198:449–459.

20. Feeney M, Knapp RC, Greenberger JS et al. (1981). Elimination of leukemic cells from rat bone marrow using antibody and complement. Cancer Res 41:3331–3335.

21. Kaizer H and Santos GW (1983). Autologous bone marrow transplantation in the treatment of cancer: Current status. In: Ariel (Ed.). Progress in Clinical Science. New York: Grune & Stratton. (In press).

22. Ritz J, Sallan SE and Bast RC Jr (1982). Autologous bone marrow transplantation in cALLA positive acute lymphoblastic leukemia after in vitro treatment with J5 monoclonal antibody and complement. Lancet 2:60–63.

23. Nadler LM, Stashenko P, Ritz J et al. (1981). A unique cell surface antigen identifying lymphoid malignancies of B-cell origin. J Clin Invest 67:134–194.
24. Nadler LM, Stashenko P, Hardy R et al. (1981). Characterization of a human B-cell specific antigen (B2) distinct from Bl. J Immunol 126:1941–1947.
25. Anderson KC, Slaughenhoupt B, Bates MP et al. Expression of human B-cell associated antigens on leukemia and lumphomas: A model of human B-cell differentiation. Blood (in press).
26. Nadler LM, Anderson KC, Marti G et al. (1983). B4, a human B-cell associated antigen expressed on normal, mitogen activated, and malignant B-lymphocyte. J Immunol 131:244–250.
27. Stashenko P, Nadler LM, Hardy R and Schlossman SF (1980). Characterization of a human B-lymphocyte specific antigen. J Immunol 125:1678–1685.
28. Lipton JM, Greenberger JS, Nadler LM et al. (1982). Distribution of B1, cALLA, Beta 2 microglobulin and Ia on hematopoietic progenitors and hematopoiesis supporting cells (HSC) in short- and long-term cultures. Blood 60 (suppl. 1):170A.
29. Greenberger JS, Rothstein L, DeFabritis P et al. Effects of monoclonal antibody and complement treatment of human marrow on hematopoesis in continuous bone marrow culture (submitted).
30. Nadler LM, Stashenko P, Hardy R et al. (1981). Monoclonal antibodies defining serologically distinct HLA-D/DR related Ia-like antigens in man. Hum Immunol 1:77–90.
31. Reinherz EL, Meuer SC and Schlossman SF (1983). The delineation of antigen receptors on human T-lymphocytes. Immunol Today 4:5–8.
32. Griffin JD, Linch D, Sabbath K and Schlossman SF. A monoclonal antibody reactive with normal and leukemic human myeloid progenitor cells. Leuk Res (in press).
33. Benjamin D, Magrath IT, Douglass EC and Corash LM (1983). Derivation of lymphoma cell lines from microscopy normal bone marrow in patients with undifferentiated lymphomas: Evidence of occult bone marrow involvement. Blood 61:1017–1019.
34. Takvorian T, Parker LM, Hochberg FH and Canellos GP (1983). Autologous bone marrow transplantation: Host effects of high dose BNCV. J Clin Oncol 1:610–620.

12. The immunobiology of B-cell lymphoma. Studies with anti-idiotype antibodies

R. LEVY, T. MEEKER, J. LOWDER, D. MALONEY,
K. THIELEMANS, J. GRALOW, R. A. WARNKE, R. A. MILLER,
M. L. CLEARY and J. SKLAR
*Department of Medicine and Pathology, Stanford University,
Stanford, California, USA*

Human B-cell lymphomas are considered to be monoclonal cell populations which are derived from a single transformed cell. This notion is based on analyses of karyotypes [1, 2], X chromosome-linked enzymes [3, 4] and immunoglobulin expression of the tumor cell population. Assuming that these tumors are monoclonal, we produced antibodies directed against the idiotypic determinants of the cell surface Ig of several cases of human B-cell malignancy. We have used these antibodies as diagnostic monitoring reagents, as therapeutic agents, and as probes for the biology of the disease. Each tumor was idiotypically unique but, in addition, some patients had tumor cells representing more than one clone. Diagnostic and therapeutic trials show that anti-idiotypic antibodies have clinical utility. However, their role in the management of these diseases remains to be defined.

Materials and methods

Patients

Patients selected for this study had lymphoid malignancies that contained cell surface immunoglobulin, tumor tissue accessable for biopsy, no evidence of serum paraprotein, and a projected life expectancy of greater than one year. Biopsies were performed to obtain tumor tissue and cells for immunologic analysis [5, 6] and for the production and screening of anti-idiotype antibodies. At least one monoclonal anti-idiotype antibody was produced for each patient. While antibodies were being prepared, patients were clinically monitored. Prior to inclusion in therapeutic trials, patients were re-evaluated. Objectively measurable disease was required. Repeat biopsies were obtained to ascertain the continued reactivity of the tumor with the anti-idiotype antibodies.

Production of antibodies

Two different strategies were developed for the production of these antibodies. One involved the hybridization of human tumor cells to either mouse myeloma cells [7] or to human lymphoblastoid cell lines [8]. Such hybrids secreted the tumor-derived Ig, which could be isolated in pure form and used to immunize mice. The other strategy involved the immunization of mice directly with human tumor cells. In both cases hybridomas that secreted antibodies were produced from the immunized mice and screened for anti-idiotypic specificity. With the first procedure (immunization with pure protein), the frequency of anti-idiotype producing hybridomas was approximately 15%. With the second procedure (immunization with whole tumor cells), the frequency was approximately 1% [9]. The antibodies were used in immunofluorescence and immunoperoxidase procedures on tumor cells and tissues, and in immunoassays to measure idiotype protein in the serum of the patients. For therapeutic trials, the antibody producing hybridoma cells were injected into mice and large quantities of antibody were purified from the resulting ascites fluid [10].

Analysis of immunoglobulin DNA

High molecular weight DNA was purified from 10^6 to 10^7 cells. DNA was digested with the appropriate restriction enzymes and the resulting fragments separated by electrophoresis in agarose gels. These fragments were transferred activated nylon membranes [11], which were hybridized with ^{32}P radiolabeled DNA fragments specific for the heavy chain joining region (JH), the heavy chain constant region (C mu), and the constant region of the kappa (C kappa) and lambda (C lambda) light chain genes [12].

Antibody therapy

Patients were pre-medicated with acetaminophen and diphenhydramine. Antibody doses of less than 10 mg were diluted in 250 ml of 5% albumin. Larger doses of antibody were diluted in normal saline. Antibody infusions were performed over 4 to 24 hours. During periods of therapy, patients were evaluated with physical examination, blood cells counts, chemistry screening panel, urinalysis and creatinine clearance. Serum samples were collected immediately before, immediately after, one hour after, and four hours after each dose. Appropriate x-rays were repeated as indicated. Accessible tumor samples (blood, bone marrow, lymph nodes, or pleural effusions) were obtained to document tumor penetration by antibody.

Results and discussion

The individuality of B-cell tumors

During the screening of hybridomas, culture supernatants were first tested for reactivity against the same human Ig which had been used for immunization. Positive clones were then tested on an extended panel of five different human myeloma proteins or tumor-derived idiotypic proteins. The clones which reacted only with the immunizing protein, but none of the unrelated panel, were chosen. Subsequent testing was performed on tissue sections and cell suspensions of normal tonsil and on the individual patient's tumor. In some, antibodies that seemed specific when tested on isolated proteins reacted with cells in the normal tonsil. In others, antibodies that were specific on isolated proteins failed to react with the same protein on cell membranes. Both of these types of antibodies were discarded.

Fifteen different anti-Id antibodies were used to search for idiotypic cross-reaction among lymphoma patients. Each of these 15 antibodies reacted only with its respective tumor and not with any of the other 14. To expand the power of the analysis, the 15 antibodies were pooled and used to screen a prospective series of 100 additional lymphoma cases. The 15-fold dilution resulting from pooling did not diminish the reactivity of any of the antibodies with its respective tumor target. This pool of antibodies gave no reaction with normal tonsil cell populations. When this pool of 15 was tested on 100 additional lymphoma patients by flow cytometry on cell suspension and by immunoperoxidase on frozen tissue sections, no positive reactions were detected. Therefore, we conclude that the frequency of idiotypic identity among B-cell tumors from different patients must be extremely low. It is still possible, however, that antibodies could be selected by a less rigid screen which would allow for cross-reaction between different tumors.

Idiotype protein in the serum of lymphoma patients

The sera of eight patients with 'non-secreting' B-cell lymphomas were tested for the presence of circulating Id protein. None of these patients had elevated levels of total serum IgG or IgM as determined by radial immunodiffusion. No paraproteins could be detected by immunoelectrophoresis. A two-sided ELISA assay was designed which had a sensitivity limit of 10 ng/ml. Several patients displayed a wide spectrum of serum idiotype levels (Table I). These levels showed no correlation with the histologic type of lymphoma. However, within a given patient, serial measurements mirrored

Table I. Circulating idiotype protein

Patient	Micrograms/Milliliter
BC	243.
CG	0.01
RD	0.10
PE	140.
EV	256.
FS	560.
RB	0.01
TG	0.01
BJ	0.02
CL	2.20

tumor burden as judged by standard clinical evaluations. In selected patients, we isolated idiotypic Ig from the sera by immunoabsorption on anti-Id covalently linked to a solid phase. With this procedure, we calculated that, for the patients with the highest serum Id levels (BL, FS and PE), as much as 60% of the total circulating IgM was derived from their malignant clone.

Clinical trial

Eight patients were selected for therapeutic trials of monoclonal anti-idiotype antibody (Table II). All had disease which was objectively evaluable. Six had follicular lymphoma, one had diffuse poorly differentiated small and large cell lymphoma and one had prolymphocytic leukemia. Seven of these patients had failed multiple courses of chemotherapy and radiotherapy. One patient had received only interferon. No steroids or cytotoxic agents were administered to any patient from one month before therapy until the trial and follow-up were complete.

Plasmapheresis was used to reduce serum idiotype levels in Patients PK, FS and BL. Patients FS and BL had serum idiotype levels in excess of 200 micrograms/ml; both had three whole-volume plasma exchanges on successive days that resulted in a reduction of serum idiotype to 10–20% of initial levels. No further reduction was obtained by continued plasmapheresis, and cessation of the procedure led to a return of serum idiotype to baseline over several days. These two patients were maintained on plasmapheresis during the entire trial of antibody administration. The dose of anti-idiotype antibody required to achieve an excess in the serum varied with each patient according to the level of idiotype protein, the tumor burden and the sites of tumor involvement. During the course of therapy, four of the eight

Table II. Anti-idiotype therapy

Patient	Pre-therapy serum Id (µg/ml)	Mouse isotype	Highest single dose (mg)	Peak serum mouse level (µg/ml)	Total dose (mg)	Duration of therapy (days)	Anti-mouse	Binding to tumor	Response	Toxicity
PK	5	IgG2b	120	14	400	27	−	LN+	CR	None
FS	400	IgG1	560	50	1,530	17	+	PBL+	PR	Fever, chills, myalgias
BL	243	IgG1	900	50	2,101	18	−	PBL+ LN−	NR	Fever, chills, SOB, thrombocytopenia
RD	0.10	IgG1	600	330	1,993	57	−	Not done	PR	None
BJ	0.02	IgG2b	800	107	2,292	29	+	LN+	MR	Fever, chills, late in treatment course
CJ	2.20	IgG1	700	136	3,079	40	+	PBL+	PR	Fever, rigor (correlated with serum Id)
CP	.01	IgG1	730	300	3,080	21	+	LN+	NR	Fever,rigor, rash, neutropenia with anti-mouse response
CG	.01	IgG1	600	300	3,173	38	−	LN+	PR-MR	Mild chills with first dose

patients developed an antibody response against the mouse immunoglobulin. This occurred from 10–30 days after the initiation of therapy. This response was most dramatic in Patient CP, the only patient who had not received prior immunosuppressive therapies. After anti-mouse antibody was present, significant levels of mouse antibody could not be achieved and clinical responses were not seen. In the absence of an immune response or serum idiotype, there was very little toxicity observed. In the presence of either, fever, chills and dyspnea were regularly seen. These symptoms usually subsided on slowing and temporarily stopping the infusion.

The most dramatic anti-tumor effect occurred in the first patient who has remained in unmaintained complete remission for three years with no evidence of return of serum idiotype or idiotype-positive cells in bone marrow or blood. Four other patients had clinically significant, but partial and/or temporary, responses. All responses began between eight and 16 days after initiation of therapy. Two patients have received a second course of therapy with stabilization of growing disease, but no regression. Causes for the different results in these patients can only be speculated at the present time, but they may include differences in antibody class, antibody affinity, idiotype targets, serum idiotype levels, host responses, and tumor heterogeneity.

Genetic heterogeneity in malignant B-cell populations

During the course of these studies, we unexpectedly identified several patients whose lymphomas contained two cell populations, each with a different idiotype (Table III). The heterogeneity of these tumor populations

Table III. B-Cell lymphoma genetic heterogeneity

Patient	Reasons for detection	Prior treatment	Genotype
DH	Kappa plus lambda population	Chemotherapy	Different heavy chains Different light chains
LH	Partial reactivity with anti-Id	None	Same heavy chain Different light chains
LK	Partial reactivity with anti-Id	Chemotherapy	Different heavy chains Different light chains
DS	Loss of reactivity with anti-Id	None	Different heavy chains Different light chains
CJ	Loss of reactivity with anti-Id	Chemotherapy Anti-Id	Same heavy chain Same light chain
CG	Loss of reactivity with anti-Id	Chemotherapy Anti-Id	Same heavy chain Same light chain

became apparent in different ways. Patient DH was immediately suspected of having more than one cell populations because he had both kappa and lambda positive cells. In Patient LH and LK, tissue immunoperoxidase and cell fluorescent analysis disclosed that the anti-idiotype antibody made for each of them reacted with a sub-populations of the tumor cells, even though the entire tumor population expressed IgM kappa.

In Patient DS, a biopsy after one year showed that an initial tumor population, completely reactive with the anti-idiotype antibody, had been replaced by a cell population that did not react with the antibody, even though both populations expressed IgG lambda – an unusual phenotype. The genetic basis of the heterogeneity in these cases was proved by cell separation studies and DNA analysis. Anti-idiotype antibodies were used with the fluorescence activated cell sorter to divide the cells into reactive and unreactive populations. DNA was isolated from each population, cut with restriction endonuclease, and analyzed by the Southern blotting procedure with probes for the heavy and light chain genes. In each of these cases the two cell populations had rearranged different immunoglobulin genes. The two clones in Case LH appeared to have a common origin, as they had the same heavy chain gene rearrangement but different light chain gene rearrangement.

Cases CJ and CG were detected during therapy with anti-idiotype antibody. Subsequent biopsies showed tumor cell populations that no longer reacted with the antibodies even though the cells expressed the same type of heavy and light chain products in the same density on the cell surface. In these cases, DNA analysis showed that the new cell populations were derived from the original clone as they had rearranged the same heavy and light chain genes. Presumably, subtle mutations in the V regions had occurred and were selected for growth under the influence of the antibody treatment. This hypothesis will be tested by determining the nucleotide sequence of the V region genes in these two cases.

Clearly, both types of genetic variation seen here – biclonality and clonal evolution – can complicate attempts to use anti-idiotype antibodies for therapy. Neither is insurmountable, however. For instance, for Patient LK we have produced a second anti-idiotype antibody which reacts with the idiotype of his second clone. More interesting is the implication of these findings for the biology of these tumors. Do these separate clones have their origin in a common stem cell or do they represent a multi-hit induction of malignancy? Are they separate clones or evolved descendants controlled or selected by the host immune mechanisms such as idiotype networks? These will be the subjects of future investigation.

556

Acknowledgements

Supported by Grants IM 114 and NP 376 from the American Cancer Society and CA 34233 and CA 33399 from the National Institutes of Health, USPHS.

References

1. Rowley JD and Fukuhara S (1980). Chromosome studies in non-Hodgkin's lymphoma. Semin Oncol 7:255–266.
2. Klein G (1983). Specific chromosomal translocations and the genesis of B-cell-derived tumors in mice and man.. Cell 32:311–315.
3. Friedman JM and Fialkow PG (1976). Cell marker studies of human tumorgenesis. Transplant Rev 28:17–33.
4. Fialkow PJ, Klein E, Klein G et al. (1973). Immunoglobulin and glucose-6-phosphate dehydrogenase as markers of cellular origin in Burkitt lymphoma. J Exp Med 139:89–102.
5. Warnke R and Levy R (1980). Detection of T- and B-cell antigens with hybridoma monoclonal antibodies. A biotin- avidin-horseradish peroxidase method. J Histochem Cytochem 28:771–776.
6. Loken MR and Herzenberg LA (1975). Analysis of cell populations with a fluorescence activated cell sorter. Ann NY Acad Sci 254:163–171.
7. Levy R and Dilley J (1978). Rescue of immunoglobulin secretion from human neoplastic lymphoid cells by somatic cell hybridization. Proc Nat Acad Sci 75:2411–2415.
8. Handley HH and Royston I (1982). A human lymphoblastoid B-cell line useful for generating immunoglobulin-secreting human hybridomas. In: Mitchell MS and Oethgen HF (Eds.) Hybridomas in Cancer Diagnosis and Treatment pp. 125–132. New York, NY: Raven Press.
9. Thielemans K, Maloney DG, Meeker T et al. Strategies for production of monoclonal anti-idiotype antibodies against human B cell lymphomas. J Immunol (in press).
10. Miller RA, Maloney DG, Warnke R and Levy R (1982). Treatment of B-cell lymphoma with monoclonal anti-idiotype antibody. N Engl J Med 306:517–522.
11. Southern EM (1975). Detection of specific sequences among DNA fragments separated by gel electrophoresis. J Molec Biol 98:503–517.
12. Cleary ML, Chao, Warnke R and Sklar J (1984). Immunoglobulin gene rearrangement as a diagnostic criterion of B-cell lymphoma. Proc Nat Acad Sci 81:593–597.

13. Therapeutic use of monoclonal anti-idiotype antibodies against B-cell lymphoma

A. HEKMAN, E. M. RANKIN, R. SOMERS
and W. TEN BOKKEL HUININK
Netherlands Cancer Institute, Antoni van Leeuwenhoek Huis, Amsterdam, the Netherlands

Human malignant B-cell tumors arise from a proliferation of a single clone of cells [1]. The immunoglobulin (Ig) which is expressed by the tumor cells is limited to the expression of one single V_H and V_L region, and to a single light chain. The unique variable region of the Ig, the idiotype, thus forms a specific tumor marker and a potential target for immunotherapy. Levy and colleagues [2] used a monoclonal anti-idiotype antibody to treat a patient with a nodular poorly-differentiated lymphocytic lymphoma, and achieved a complete remission which has lasted so far for 29 months. This group has treated seven more patients with anti-idiotype antibodies but no complete remissions have been obtained [3]. Polyclonal anti-idiotype antibodies raised in sheep have been given to one patient with promyelocytic leukemia [4] and to three patients with lymphoma [5]. There were transient reductions in the level of circulating lymphocytes, but no long-lasting anti-tumor effect was seen.

This paper describes the treatment of two patients with advanced non-Hodgkin lymphoma, with monoclonal antibodies against the idiotype of their tumor cells. Details of the production and characterization of the anti-idiotype antibodies will be published elsewhere (Rankin and Hekman, submitted for publication). Briefly, the specificity of the antibodies was proven by the lack of reaction with a variety of normal cells, 14 cell lines representing different stages of lymphoid and myeloid cell differentiation and 30 non-Hodgkin's lymphomas. The reaction of the antibodies with determinants on the membrane Ig was demonstrated in two ways: each antibody precipitated Ig heavy and light chains from surface-labelled homologous tumor cell lysates, and their target antigens were capped by anti-light chain antibodies. Both antibodies belonged to the IgG2a subclass.

The antibodies were purified from ascitic fluid by precipitation with 40% saturated ammonium sulphate or by ion exchange chromatography on DEAE Sephadex A59. Antibody preparations were dialyzed against 0.14 M NaCl, centrifuged at 100,000 × g to remove aggregates, passed through a

0.22 μm filter and stored at 4 °C. Preparations were tested for sterility and absence of pyrogens. For administration, the antibodies were diluted to the desired concentration with 0.14 M NaCl with 5 % human serum albumin.

Before each antibody infusion a skin test for immediate hypersensitivity to mouse protein was performed with 2 μg mouse antibody. Allopurinol was given throughout the treatment period in case of massive cell lysis. Patients were carefully monitored for any evidence of anaphylaxis or complications of cell destruction such as hypotension, fever, or disseminated intravascular coagulation.

The study Protocol was approved by the Ethical Committee of the Netherlands Cancer Institute. Both patients gave written informed consent.

Patient top

This 71-year-old woman was found in July 1980 to have Stage IV poorly differentiated diffuse non-Hodgkin lymphoma with involvement of lymph nodes, spleen, bone marrow and peripheral lymphocytosis. She was treated with chemotherapy and splenic irradiation without success. The spleen was removed in December 1982. Tumor cells obtained from the spleen were used to prepare the monoclonal anti-idiotype antibody, T2. When anti-idiotype therapy began in October 1983, there was massive abdominal disease with ascites and generalized lymphadenopathy. No systemic treatment had been given for two years. The white cell count was $19 \times 10^9/l$ with 66 %

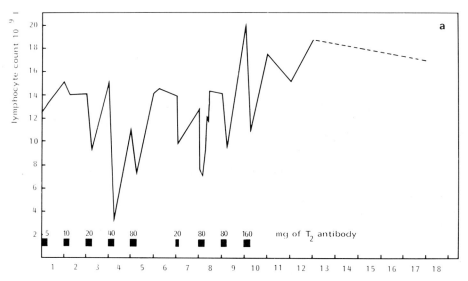

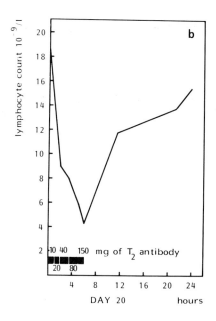

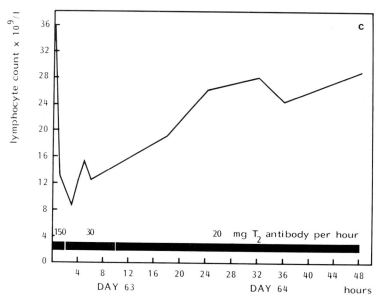

Figure 1. The effect of the administration of antibody T2 on the level of circulating lymphocytes.

a. Schedule 1: doubling the dose daily.

b. Schedule 2: hourly doubling doses.

c. Schedule 3: 300 mg antibody in 2 hours, followed by a continuous infusion of 1000 mg over 46 hours.

lymphocytes; 80 % of the lymphocytes were B-cells with κIgM, IgD and IgG membrane immunoglobulin. All B-cells stained with the anti-idiotype antibody T2, although, as with anti-Igs, there was a considerable variation among cells in the strength of the fluorescent reaction. A peripheral blood smear showed that the lymphocytes were morphologically abnormal. Serum biochemistry, liver function and renal function were normal. There was no paraprotein band in the serum and no excess of monoclonal light chains in the urine. Free (non-cell bound) idiotype was only barely detectable by fluorescence inhibition or enzyme immunoassay.

The anti-idiotype antibody T2 was administered in three different schedules, the effect of which was determined by monitoring the level of circulating lymphocytes. Binding of the antibody *in vivo* was demonstrated by incubating cells taken during or after treatment with FITC-labelled goat anti-mouse Ig. The patient's serum was tested after each dose for the presence of unbound T2 antibodies by immunofluorescence or enzyme immunoassay on cryopreserved cells collected before treatment.

Schedule 1

An escalation schedule, doubling the dose daily, was chosen in order to establish the toxicity of the antibody given as an infusion over 6 hours. The effect of this schedule on the peripheral lymphocytes is seen in Fig. 1a. The number of cells in the circulation fell rapidly with every dose of 20 mg or more, but returned to pretreatment level within 24 hours. Rapid coating of the peripheral lymphocytes by the antibody occurred after the infusion of as little as 10 mg of antibody. These coated cells were still detectable up to 24 hours after the end of the 160 mg infusion. No free mouse immunoglobulin was detected at any time during this first period of treatment. Apart from a single short episode of fever near the end of one infusion no side effects were seen.

Schedule 2

Our next approach was to increase the antibody dose rapidly in order to produce a sustained fall in the lymphocytes. The dose was escalated from 10 mg per hour to 150 mg per hour; a total of 300 mg T2 antibody was given over 6 hours on day 20 (Fig. 1b). The number of circulating lymphocytes fell continuously throughout the period of infusion, with the steepest fall in the first hour. The lymphocytes began to rise again when therapy was stopped, but did not reach the pretreatment level at 24 hours. Sufficient antibody had been given to attain an excess of 12 µg of anti-idiotype antibody per ml in the serum. The free antibody had disappeared 24 hours later. Binding of the antibody to cells in the blood was demonstrated by reaction with fluoresceinated goat anti-mouse antibody. As with schedule 1, the fluorescent staining increased during 24 hr after the end of treatment. Tumor lymphocytes obtained by aspiration biopsy of a cervical lymph node were also coated with antibody, but were not fully saturated with the anti-idiotype. Again, there were no side effects during or following the treatment.

Schedule 3

We attempted to prolong the reduction of circulating lymphocytes, and obtain a sufficient excess of antibody to reach all tumor sites, by rapid administration of a large amount of antibody followed by continuous low-dose infusion. This schedule was applied three times, with comparable results. The fall in circulating lymphocytes, though dramatic, was only transient even when treatment was continued for 48 hours (Fig. 1c). Free T2 antibody was detectable in the serum, after 150 mg of T2, at a level of 1.5 μg/ml. Seventy-two hours later, free T2 was still present. Homing of the antibody to the tumor cells in the lymph node and bone marrow was demonstrated; both sites were saturated with T2 *in vivo*. The ascitic fluid contained antibody-coated tumor cells at the end of the last infusion. Three days later, they were still present.

There was no clinically detectable response, and the peripheral lymphocyte count was rising inexorably; treatment with anti-idiotype antibody was stopped. Two weeks later the lymph nodes were smaller, but not yet half of their original size.

The patient was closely monitored throughout the treatment period. Apart from one short febrile episode no adverse reactions were observed. Specifically, there were no chills, bronchospasm or hypotension. There was no hematologic toxicity and no disturbance of liver or renal function. There was no evidence of activation of the complement pathway, or of disseminated intravascular coagulation. No antibodies to the mouse protein were detectable by passive hemagglutination at any time up to one month after the last treatment was given.

Changes of tumor cell populations

Before treatment, tumor cells in the circulation showed considerable variation in the intensity of the fluorescent staining with anti-Ig antisera and with the T2 antibody. During treatment, the size of idiotype-positive cells, and the intensity of fluorescent staining fluctuated. This was not due to partial

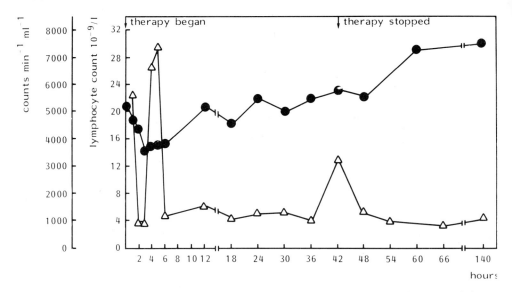

Figure 2. Comparison between the level of circulating Indium-111 labelled lymphocytes and the total number of lymphocytes in the blood duduring treatment with T2 anti-idiotype antibody.

△ Indium-111 labelled lymphocytes, cpm/ml blood.

● total number of lymphocytes in the blood, counted with a coulter counter.

modulation, because weakly staining cells cultured *in vitro* without antibody for 24 hours showed no increase in fluorescence intensity. Shifts of tumor cell populations differing in antigen density seemed to occur as a result of antibody treatment.

Circulation pathways of the tumor cells were investigated, using lymphocytes labelled with Indium-111 oxine. These experiments will be reported in detail elsewhere (Rankin et al., manuscript submitted). [111]In labelled lymphocytes consisting of ca. 80% idiotype positive cells were injected at the beginning of antibody administration. A comparison of the total number of lymphocytes and labelled cells is shown in Fig. 2. It is clear that the rebound in cell numbers bears no relation to the labelled cells and represents the appearance of a new population. Gamma camera scans showed that the labelled cells accumulated in the liver.

To study whether the circulation was repopulated as a result of cell division or by migration of cells from an extravascular reservoir into the blood, the percentage of S phase cells was determined [6] (kindly performed by Dr. L. Smets, Dept. of Exp. Cytology). The blood contained 2% S phase cells, before and after treatment. Similarly, there was no increase in ^{3}H-thymidine incorporation while the cell rebound was occurring at a maximal rate. In the lymph node the percentage of S phase cells changed from 7.5% before treatment to 2% at the end of treatment and 14% four hours after the end of the

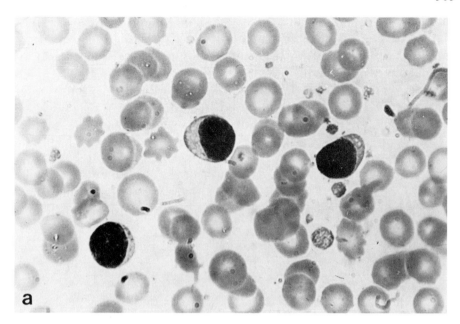

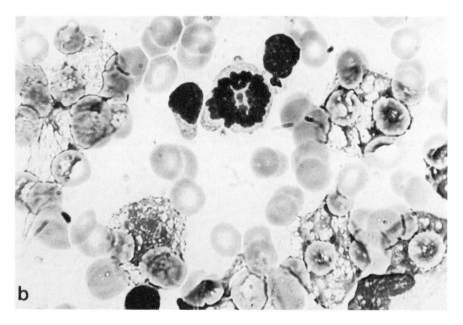

Figure 3. Cytological smears from punch biopsies of the lymph node of patient Top.
a. Before treatment began. Three tumor cells can be seen with large nuclei, dense nucleoli and small amounts of cytoplasm.
b. At the end of the treatment period. Bizarre cells in various stages of lysis can be seen. One cell is undergoing mitosis.

infusion. However, since most of these cells were in early S phase and a substantial part of the repopulation of the blood had already occurred by that time, it seems unlikely that repopulation was a result of the increased proliferation of lymph node cells.

Direct evidence of cell kill was obtained by serial biopsy of the lymph nodes (kindly performed by Dr. P. van Heerde). During the period of anti-idiotype therapy, the percentage of cells showing lysis (Fig. 3) increased from 1% to 20%. The increased amount of S phase cells can thus be explained as a compensatory response to the necrosis induced by T2 [7]. These data indicate that tumor cells in blood and lymph node were killed, and that the blood was repopulated by cells already present in an extravascular compartment.

Patient Kos

This 62-year-old man presented in October 1979 with a Stage IV non-Hodgkin lymphoma. Cervical node biopsy showed a nodular well-differentiated pattern whereas bone marrow examination revealed a diffuse poorly differentiated lymphoma. Partial remission lasting 6 months was obtained by chemotherapy. In March 1983, a node biopsy showed a change to a higher grade malignancy with a diffuse poorly-differentiated pattern. Chemotherapy had no effect on the tumor. The anti-idiotype antibody, K1, was made using lymph node cells. When treatment with anti-idiotype antibody began in December 1983, the patient had rapidly advancing disease with diffuse lymphadenopathy including massive involvement of the paraaortic and mesenteric groups. The white cell count was $6.5 \times 10^9/l$, of which 37% were lymphocytes. Of the lymphocytes, 16% bore κIgM, and 12% stained with the anti-idiotype antibody K1. The bone marrow contained 31% idiotype bearing tumor cells; in the ascitic fluid, 63% of the cells were idiotype positive. Serum biochemistry, liver function and renal function tests were normal. There was no serum paraprotein band, also no excess of monoclonal light chains in the urine. The patient's poor condition precluded extensive investigation for research purposes. We were concerned that he should have the opportunity to benefit from any therapeutic effect resulting from antibody administration.

The number of circulating malignant cells was too low $(0.3 \times 10^9/l)$ to provide a suitable index for monitoring the effects of treatment, but there was a large amount of free idiotype in the serum. Our plan was to establish as rapidly as possible the amount of antibody required to remove all the free idiotype, in order to produce saturation of the lymph node cells and an excess of antibody in the circulation. It can be seen from Fig. 4 that removal of free idiotype from the circulation correlated with the detection of free K1

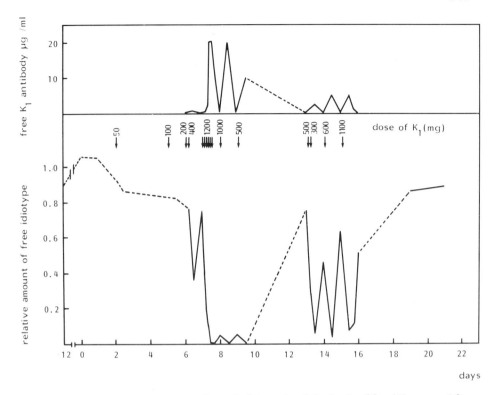

Figure 4. Relation between the dose of K1 administered and the levels of free idiotype and free K1 antibody in the serum.

antibody in the blood. K1 reached a level of 20 µg/ml after administration of a total dose of 1200 mg. This free K1 had not completely disappeared by the following morning, when a very small amount of free idiotype was again identified. At the end of the 1200 mg dose, cells from a lymph node were saturated with K1 antibody *in vivo*. Tumor cells from the ascites, however, were not coated *in vivo* and the ascitic fluid contained no free K1 antibodies.

During a break from treatment over the Christmas period the free idiotype returned almost to the pretreatment level. Three more treatments of 800 mg, 600 mg and 1000 mg of K1 yielded transient falls in the level of free idiotype. Free idiotype returned to much higer levels over 24 hours than in the first treatment period. Free K1 antibody was found in the circulation after therapy, reaching a maximum of 5 µg/ml, but it always disappeared within 24 hours. Lymph node cells were coated but not saturated with K1 on day 14, but after the 1100 mg dose on day 15 no anti-idiotype could be detected on the lymph node cells.

During the period of treatment, there was no evidence of antigen modulation by the antibody or of immunoselection. As with the first patient, treatment was free of toxicity. At no time during or following treatment was there any detectable antibody response to the large amount of mouse protein administered. Serial biopsies showed that there was no significant difference in the number of necrotic cells in the lymph nodes before and after antibody treatment.

A decrease in the size of the femoral and iliac lymph nodes was documented clinically and confirmed by the CAT scan, but it was less than a 50% response. No change in the intra-abdominal tumor was seen on tomography. Treatment with anti-idiotype antibody was stopped, since increasingly high doses of antibody were required for the same effect.

Discussion

Despite the presence in the circulation of large numbers of tumor cells in the case of patient Top, and of a high level of free idiotype in the case of patient Kos, the antibodies were found to reach tumor cells in blood, lymph node and bone marrow and, less reliably, in ascites. In both patients, a decrease in size of involved lymph nodes was seen, but the overall tumor response was minimal (< 50%). Treatment was noticeably free of side effects, in contrast to some published reports [8–12]. Considerable quantities of soluble tumor antigen were removed from patient Kos without disturbance of renal function. Neither patient produced antibodies against the mouse protein.

The phenomenon of transient falls in the circulating tumor cells resulting from antibody treatment is well documented [4–13]. The rapid repopulation of the blood by tumor lymphocytes, which has also been seen after leukopheresis [4], reflects the presence of an extravascular pool of accessible tumor cells. The low level of DNA synthesis in the blood cells suggest that mature, non-proliferating cells migrated into the blood [14].

The mechanisms by which anti-idiotype antibodies exerted their antitumor effects are not clear. Complement-mediated lysis is unlikely, because the antibodies did not fix human complement *in vitro*. The indium labelling studies suggested that the reticulo-endothelial system was responsible for the removal of circulating tumor cells, a finding in accord with that of others [8, 9, 12]. This would explain the persistence of antibody-coated cells in the ascitic fluid. It is known that macrophages mediate the killing of tumor cells *in vitro*, in the presence of murine IgG2a monoclonal antibody to the tumor [15]. Both antibodies T2 and K1 were of the IgG2a subclass. The limited effect of the treatment could be due to an 'effector cell shortage' caused by the large number of tumor cells to be removed. We have no indications that tumor cells escaped by antigenic modulation.

Miller et al. [2] reported a complete remission in a patient whose lymph node biopsy before treatment showed infiltration by reactive T-cells. A biopsy of the regressing lymphoma lesions after therapy showed that there were large numbers of macrophages and activated T-cells present [16]. In our patients, no change in the low number of T-cells in the node was seen after treatment.

To investigate the potential of anti-idiotype antibodies for treatment of lymphoma, patients with a low tumor burden and at a relatively early stage of the disease would be suitable candidates for further Phase I trials. Additional approaches may be required for maximum effect, for instance coupling the antibody to cytotoxic drugs, toxins or radiopharmaceuticals.

References

1. Fialkow PJ, Klein E, Klein G and Singh S (1973). Immunoglobulin and glucose-6-phosphate dehydrogenase as markers of cellular origin in Burkitt lymphoma. J Exp Med 138:89–102.
2. Miller RA, Maloney DG, Warnke T and Levy R (1982). Treatment of B-cell lymphoma with monoclonal anti-idiotype antibody. N Engl J Med 306:517–522.
3. Lowder JN, Meeker TC, Maloney DG et al. (1984). Anti-idiotype monoclonal antibody therapy of human B-lymphocytic malignancy. Proc Amer Soc Clin Oncol 3:250.
4. Hamblin TJ, Abdul-Ahad AK, Gordon J et al. (1980). Preliminary experience in treating lymphocytic leukaemia with antibody to immunoglobulin idiotypes on the cell surfaces. Brit J Cancer 42:495–502.
5. Macbeth FR, Stevenson FK, Stevenson GT and Whitehouse JMA (1983). Anti-idiotype antibody therapy of patients with non-Hodgkin's lymphoma. Proceed 2nd Eur Conf Clin Oncol Cancer Nursing. Amsterdam, p. 75.
6. Smets LA, Taminiau J, Hahlen K et al. (1983). Cell kinetic responses in childhood acute non lymphocytic leukaemia during high-dose therapy with cytosine arabinoside. Blood 61:79–84.
7. Mauer AM, Murphy SB, Hayes AB and Dahl GV (1977). Scheduling and recruitment in malignant cell populations. In: Drewinko B and Humphrey EM (Eds.). Growth Kinetics and Biochemical Regulation of Normal and Malignant Cells, pp. 855–864. Baltimore: Williams & Wilkins.
8. Miller RA, Maloney DG, McKillop J and Levy R (1981). In vivo effects of murine hybridoma monoclonal antibody in a patient with T-cell leukaemia. Blood 58:78–86.
9. Nadler LM, Stashenko P, Hardy R et al. (1980). Serotherapy of a patient with a monoclonal antibody directed against a human lymphoma-associated antigen. Cancer Res 40:3147–3154.
10. Cosimi AB, Burton RC, Colvin RB et al. (1981). Treatment of acute renal allograft rejection with OKT3 monoclonal antibody. Transplantation 32:535–540.
11. Miller RA, Oseroff AR, Stratte PT and Levy R (1983). Monoclonal antibody therapeutic trials in seven patients with T-cell lymphoma. Blood 62:988–995.
12. Dillman RO, Shawler DL, Sobol RE et al. (1982). Murine monoclonal antibody therapy in two patients with chronic lymphocytic leukaemia. Blood 59:1036–1045.
13. Ball ED, Bernier GM, Cornwell GG et al. (1983). Monoclonal antibodies to myeloid differentiation antigens: In vivo studies of three patients with acute myelogenous leukaemia. Blood 62:1203–1210.
14. Zimmerman TS, Godwin HA and Perry S (1968). Studies of leukocyte kinetics in chronic lymphocytic leukaemia. Blood 51:277–191.

568

15. Stepslewski Z, Lubeck MD and Koprowski H (1983). Human macrophages armed with murine immunoglobulin G-2a antibodies to tumours destroy human cancer cells. Science 221:865–867.
16. Levy R and Miller RA (1983). Tumor therapy with monoclonal antibodies. Fed Proc 42 2650–2656.

14. Radioimmunodetection of human B-cell lymphomas with a radiolabeled tumor-specific monoclonal antibody (Lym-1)

A. L. EPSTEIN [1], A. M. ZIMMER [2], S. M. SPIES [2], D. MILLS [3], G. DENARDO [3] and S. DENARDO [3]

[1] *Department of Medicine and the Cancer Center and* [2] *Department of Nuclear Medicine, Northwestern University, Chicago, Illinois and* [3] *Department of Nuclear Medicine, University of California at Davis, Sacramento, California, USA*

A newly developed murine monoclonal antibody, designated Lym-1, has been produced by the fusion of Raji Burkitt's lymphoma-primed spleno-cytes and NS-1 mouse myeloma cells. The monoclonal antibody is of the IgG2a heavy chain subtype and may be obtained in milligram quantities by mass cell culture methods or ascites production in pristane-primed syngene-ic mice. Extensive characterization of Lym-1 (unpublished data) has reveal-ed that the monoclonal antibody binds to the cell surface of approximately 60% of human lymphomas as well as B-cell zones in hyperplastic lymph nodes. Using a panel of frozen tissues from representative human organs, we have found Lym-1 binds to lymph node B-cells and histiocytes, dendritic cells of the thymus, and surface colonic epithelium. Radioimmunoassay experiments with ^{125}I radiolabeled Lym-1 have shown that the antigen recognized by this monoclonal antibody is not shed or modulated from the surface of the lymphoma cells. Because of its highly specific reactivity to B-cell lymphomas, its stability after radiolabeling procedures, and the ap-parent absence of antigen in normal tissues, we attempted to study the imaging capabilities of Lym-1 in an animal model system and in volunteer cancer patients. The results of these studies have shown that Lym-1 is a promising reagent for the immunodetection of metastatic B-cell lymphoma. Based upon these results, Lym-1 may be a useful radioimmunotherapeutic reagent for the treatment of these tumors.

Materials and methods

Purification of Lym-1 and preparation of F(ab) fragments

Lym-1 was obtained from the ascites fluid of pristane primed Balb/c mice as described [1]. The monoclonal antibody was purified by 50% ammonium sulfate precipitation followed by Protein-A sepharose affinity chromatography. Lym-1 was eluted from the Protein-A sepharose column at pH 4.3, dialyzed overnight in PBS, ultracentrifuged at 30,000 rpm for 1 hr, and stored in 1 ml samples containing 1 mg/ml at −80 °C. F(ab) fragments were prepared by papain digestion and separated from Fc fragments by Sepharose-CL-6B column chromatography.

Immunoperoxidase staining procedures

Frozen tissue sections of involved lymph nodes from lymphoma patients were stained with Lym-1 supernatant, using the avidin-biotin complex immunoperoxidase staining procedure as described by Hsu et al. [2], to verify the presence of antigen in the tumors.

Radioiodination procedures

For the animal studies, purified Lym-1 was radiolabeled by a solid phase system using 1, 3, 4, 6-tetrachloro-3a, 6a diphenylglycoluril (Iodogen, Pierce Chemical, Rockford, IL) [3]. In a typical reaction, Iodogen (0.5–2.0 μg) was plated into test tubes using methylene chloride. A mixture of the monoclonal antibody (0.1–1.0 mg/ml) and ^{131}I-sodium iodide (50–500 uCi) (Union Carbide, Tuxedo, NY) was added to the tubes containing Iodogen and incubated at 0–2 °C for 15 minutes. The reaction was terminated by decanting the solution. The radiolabeled monoclonal antibody was purified using gel exclusion chromatography with Biogel P-10, 50–500 mesh (Bio-Rad Labs., Richmond, CA).

For the patient studies, Lym-1 and F(ab) fragments were radiolabeled with ^{123}I-using a modified chloramine-T method [4]. ^{123}I-Lym-1 was evaluated by cellulose acetate (pH 8.6) electrophoresis and by HPLC-TSK 3000 chromatography.

Antibody binding assay

Radioimmunoreactivity of the radiolabeled monoclonal antibody was determined using a live cell assay consisting of 10^6 Raji Burkitt's lymphoma cells. CEM cells from a T-cell acute lymphoblastic leukemia cell line were used to assess the extent of non-specific binding. Purified radiolabeled Lym-1 was added to one ml of the respective cell suspension at antigen excess and incubated at room temperature for 60 minutes. The cell suspension was then centrifuged and washed three times with phosphate buffered saline. The cells were counted using appropriate gamma scintillation spectrometry to assess the degree of binding.

Radioimaging of tumor-bear mice

Athymic nude mice, each bearing, in their right thigh, a human lymphoma induced by an intramuscular injection of 10^7 Raji Burkitt's lymphoma cells, were given Lugols solution orally 24 hours prior to initiation of the study. Between 150–400 µCi of ^{131}I-Lym-1 was then injected intravenously into the heterotransplanted nude mice. Posterior gamma scintillation images (100,000 counts) were obtained up to 7 days after injection using a gamma scintillation camera with a pinhole collimator interfaced to a computer system. Immediately after animal imaging, an appropriate ^{131}I-standard was counted with the same geometry to quantitate the animal data. At 7 days after injection, the animals were sacrificed and organ biodistribution was studied using appropriate gamma scintillation counting.

Radioimaging of cancer patients

Volunteer breast cancer and lymphoma patients were injected with 1–5 MCi ^{123}I-labeled Lym-1 or Lym-1 F(ab) fragments. Serum samples obtained at 5 min, 30 min, 1 hr, 2 hr, 6 hr, 18 hr, 24 hr, and 48 hr post-injection were evaluated by HPLC-TSK 3000 to assess the size of the circulating radiolabeled molecules. Urine samples were also taken to determine the total ^{123}I excreted over 24, 48, and 72 hours post-injection. On selected urine samples, HPLC-TSK 3000 analysis was performed to examine the size of the ^{123}I molecules being excreted. Planar images of the head, chest, and anterior and posterior abdomen were obtained for 750,000 counts with a medium energy collimeter [5] at 0.2 hr, 4–6 hr, and 18–24 hr post-injection. Single photon emission tomographic images were obtained at 2–4 hr and 24 hr post-injection over the chest and abdomen (64 views on an 128×128 matrix). Computer reconstruction and attenuation corrections were performed on these images and uptake was compared to ^{123}I calibration pin phantom [5].

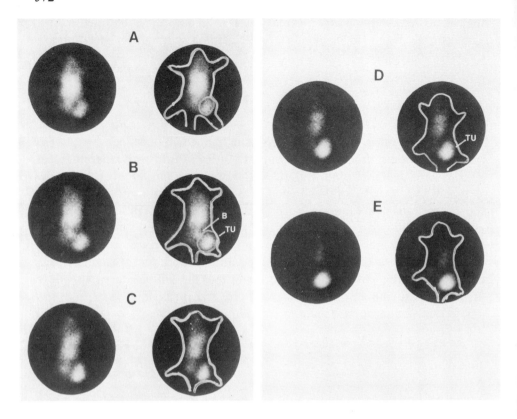

Figure 1. Posterior gamma scintillation images of ^{131}I-Lym-1 in athymic nude mice bearing a right thigh human lymphoma. (A) 24 hrs post-injection; (B) 48 hrs post-injection; (C) 3 days post-injection; (D) 5 days post-injection; (E) 7 days post-injection.

Results

Animal studies

The imaging results for ^{131}I labeled Lym-1 in heterotransplanted nude mice are shown in Fig. 1 and 2. Initially, blood pool activity was observed at 24 hours after injection. By 5 to 7 days after injection, however, the tumor was well visualized with minimal soft tissue activity. Computer analysis (Fig. 2) showed relatively slow whole body clearance of the radiolabeled monoclonal antibody with approximately 22 % of the injected dose retained at 7 days post-injection. High tumor uptake (8 % of injected dose) was observed at 24 hours and remained constant throughout the remainder of the study. The constant tumor activity coupled with decreasing whole body retention resulted in increasing tumor/whole body ratios.

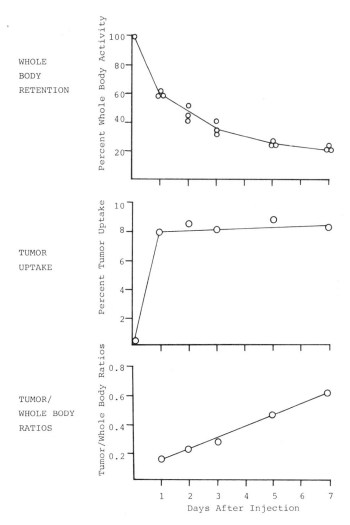

Figure 2. Whole body retention, tumor uptake, and tumor/whole body ratio of ^{131}I-Lym-1 in athymic nude mice bearing right thigh human lymphoma.

The biodistribution data obtained 7 days after antibody administration is shown in Table I. High tumor uptake (8.2% of injected dose) was confirmed. The radioactivity in all other organs measured was relatively low (less than one percent of injected dose), and when compared to tumor activity, resulted in high tumor/organ ratios.

Patient studies

A summary of the patient radioimaging studies using ^{123}I-Lym-1 whole

Table I. Biodistribution of ^{131}I labeled Lym-1 in athymic nude mouse bearing right thigh Raji lymphoma seven days after injection

Organ	% Injected dose	% Injected dose/gm	Ratio tumor/gm organ/gm
Blood	—	1.441	2.7
Heart	0.048	0.355	11.0
Lung	0.088	0.335	11.7
Liver	0.403	0.296	13.2
Spleen	0.044	0.720	5.4
Kidney	0.159	0.383	10.2
Muscle	—	0.165	23.8
Tumor	8.216	3.919	—

antibody or F(ab) fragment is shown in Table II. No significant organ or tumor uptake was observed in the breast cancer patients. These results confirm the histopathologic studies performed on a panel of normal human organs by the immunoperoxidase procedure. Four B-cell lymphoma patients showed significant Lym-1 binding of the lymphoma cells by immunoperoxidase staining of biopsy specimens. All of these patients gave positive imaging results with ^{123}I-Lym-1 as shown by planar and single photon emission tomographic studies. Of interest, positive images of normal lymph nodes or other hematopoietic tissues were not obtained. Metastatic lesions in the lymph nodes, spleen, liver, stomach, and bone marrow were successfully imaged by 2–4 hours after injection. HPLC-TSK 3000 analysis of purified radiolabeled Lym-1, plasma, and urine samples from the lymphoma pa-

Table II. Summary of radioimaging studies on patients with ^{123}I–Lym-1

Patient	Diagnosis	Sites of known tumor	Imaging
E.T.	Breast carcinoma	Abdomen, chest	Negative
G.B.	Breast carcinoma	Chest, liver	Negative
J.W.	Breast carcinoma	Chest	Negative
M.L.	Breast carcinoma	Chest	Negative
K.T.	B-lymphoma	Abdominal mass	Positive
		Lymph nodes	Negative
R.F. [a]	B-lymphoma	Abdominal mass	Positive
C.C. [a]	B-lymphoma	Abdominal mass	Positive
		Mediastinal nodes	Positive
M.E. [a]	B-lymphoma	Bone marrow	Positive
		Spleen	Positive

[a] Fab fragment used

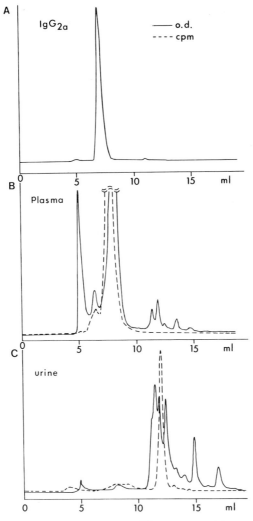

Figure 3. HPLC-TSK 3000 analysis of (A) purified ¹²³I radiolabeled Lym-1; (B) plasma sample 4 hours after injection; and (C) urine sample of lymphoma patient injected with ¹²³I-Lym-1.

tients revealed that the radiolabeled Lym-1 remained as a free molecule in the plasma and that the major route of elimination by the patients was via the kidneys where the monoclonal antibody was broken down into fragments of lower molecular weight (Fig. 3).

Patient K.T., a 63-yr old woman with long-standing chronic lymphocytic leukemia and a 2-month history of B-cell lymphoma, had histologically confirmed lymphoma of the stomach. Immunoperoxidase studies of the gastric lymphoma showed Lym-1 to be strongly reactive with the tumor. CT scans demonstrated extensive involvement of the gastric wall with a large

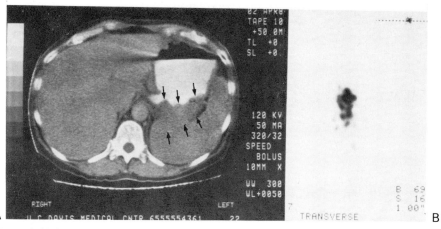

Figure 4. Abdominal scans of patient K.T. with gastric lymphoma. (A) CT scan of abdominal section showing gastric mass; (B) Single photon emission computerized tomogram of transverse section through gastric mass showing active ^{123}I-Lym-1 uptake.

mass posterior to the stomach (Fig. 4). No other areas of involvement were clinically evident. This patient received intravenously 75 µg of labeled Lym-1 containing 4 mCi ^{123}I. HPLC evaluation of the radiopharmaceutical demonstrated a single 150,000 dalton ^{123}I labeled species. Solid phase immunoreactivity using Raji membranes demonstrated 90% reactivity compared to the standard. Plasma samples run on HPLC-TSK 3000 demonstrated that a small percent of the radiolabeled species had a molecular weight greater than 150,000 dalton. However, neither circulating antigen nor human anti-mouse antibodies could be demonstrated in the plasma from pre- or post-injection samples. Imaging studies, using both planar and tomographic images, demonstrated radiopharmaceutical uptake in the gastric lesion at 24 hours (Fig. 4).

Discussion

The data generated by the animal and patient studies have clearly demonstrated the utility of Lym-1 as a radioimaging reagent. High tumor uptake coupled with low normal organ binding resulted in tumor localization using either whole antibody or F(ab) fragment radiopharmaceuticals. The use of F(ab) fragments labeled with ^{123}I, which has a half-life of 13 hours, facilitated the procurement of images in 2–4 hours. Urinary excretion of the radiolabeled Lym-1 significantly reduced the blood pool of unbound antibody and minimized soft tissue retention. From these data, Lym-1 appears to be a promising reagent for the radioimmunodetection of human B-cell lymphomas. In view of high binding reactivity, mode of excretion, and biodistribution in patients, it may act as a vehicle in delivering lethal doses of radiation to metastatic lymphoma.

References

1. Hoogenraad N, Helman T and Hoogenraad J (1983). The effect of pre-injection of mice with pristane on ascites tumor formation and monoclonal antibody production. J Immunological Methods 61:317–320.
2. Hsu S-M, Raine L and Fanger H (1981). Use of avidin-biotin-peroxidase complex (ABC) in immunoperoxidase techniques: A comparison between ABC and unlabeled antibody (PAP) procedures. J Histochem Cytochem 29:577–580.
3. Fraker PJ and Speck JC Jr (1978). Protein and cell membrane iodination with a sparingly soluble chloramide, 1, 3, 4, 6-tetracholor-3a, 6a-diphenyl glycoluril. Biophys Res Comm 83:849–857.
4. Mills SL, DeNardo SJ, DeNardo GL et al. (1984). Chloramine-T radioiodination of monoclonal antibodies with NaI-123. J Nucl Med 25:123.
5. Macey DJ, DeNardo GL, DeNardo SJ and Hines HH (1984). A calibration phantom for absolute quantitation of radionuclide uptake by spect. J Nucl Med 25:105.

15. Treatment of cutaneous T-cell lymphomas with biologic response modifiers: Recombinant leukocyte A interferon and T101 monoclonal antibody

P. A. BUNN Jr.[1], K. A. FOON[2], D. C. IHDE[1], D. LONGO[1],
R. SCHROFF[2], J. D. MINNA[1], J. CARRASQUILLO[3], A. KEENAN[3],
S. LARSON[3] and E. GLATSTEIN[1]
[1] Clinical Oncology and [2] Biologic Response Modifiers Programs,
National Cancer Institute, and [3] Nuclear Medicine Department,
Clinical Center, National Institutes of Health, Bethesda, Maryland,
USA

Mycosis fungoides and the Sezary syndrome are collectively referred to as the cutaneous T-cell lymphomas (CTCL) because of the universal infiltration of the skin by malignant T-lymphocytes [1, 2]. While the clinical and histopathologic features of the cutaneous lesions were well described between the original case description in 1806 and the description of the Sezary syndrome in 1939, the lymphomatous nature of the malignant cells was not proven until 1970 [2, 3]. The cells were subsequently shown to have both functional and phenotypic properties of the helper subset of T-lymphocytes [4–6].

Initially, CTCL was thought to involve only the skin. Infiltration of lymph nodes and other organs, which generally occurred late in the natural history, was usually ascribed to the development of a second malignant process (usually Hodgkin's disease or a diffuse non-Hodgkin's lymphoma) [7]. Pathologic studies in the 1970s demonstrated that extracutaneous lesions were frequent in autopsied cases (approximately 75%) and were always related to the initial cutaneous lymphoma [8]. They were not second neoplasms.

More recent studies from the National Cancer Institute demonstrated that unsuspected malignant cells were almost universally present in extracutaneous sites (peripheral blood, lymph nodes, and/or visceral organs) by the time a diagnosis was established [9]. These studies confirmed that the natural history of CTCL patients was indolent and similar to patients with 'low grade' B-cell non-Hodgkin's lymphomas [10].

The inability of therapies directed at cutaneous lesions (topical nitrogen mustard, psoralen plus ultraviolet A light [PUVA], local or total skin electron beam irradiaton) to cure patients has been ascribed to early systemic dissemination [10]. Unfortunately, systemic chemotherapy has also proven noncurative, at least in patients with advanced stages of disease. Thus, new systemic therapeutic modalities are clearly needed.

The use of serotherapy with anti-T-cell antibodies was a logical extension of studies demonstrating the T-cell nature of these malignancies. Clinical studies with heterologous antithymocyte globulin (ATG) demonstrated antitumor responses but severe toxicities prevented sustained therapy [11]. The development of monoclonal anti-T-cell antibodies opened the way for treatment studies with potentially more potent and less toxic serotherapy, and preliminary studies from Stanford University provided encouraging results [12].

Impure interferon preparations were demonstrated to have considerable antitumor activity in indolent B-cell non-Hodgkin's lymphomas [13]. Phase I clinical trials with purified recombinant leukocyte A, clone alpha interferon (rIFNαA) demonstrated that 50×10^6 units/m^2 was the maximally tolerated dose on a three times weekly schedule [14]. The goals of this study were to evaluate T101 and rIFNαA in patients with advanced, refractory CTCL.

Materials and methods

All patients had histologically confirmed cutaneous T-cell lymphoma refractory to two or more standard therapies. Patient characteristics are provided in Table I. For each treatment group, the median age was in the mid-50s and the majority of patients were white and male. Patients in each treatment group had advanced stages. None of the patients in either group had limited plaque skin lesions and the vast majority had cutaneous tumors or

Table I. Patient characteristics

	rIFN$_a$A = 20	T101 N = 11
Median Age	59	52
Male/Female	13/7	9/2
White/Black	16/4	7/4
Cutaneous Lesions		
Plaques (T2)	5	3
Cutaneous tumors (T3)	10	4
Erythroderma (T4)	5	4
Extracutaneous Lesions	16	8
Peripheral blood	7	6
Lymphadenopathy	20	8
Lymph node involvement	8	7
Visceral organ involvement	2	3

Table II. Prior therapy

Prior Therapy	rIFN$_a$A = 20	T101 = 11
Top/Sys corticosteroids	20	11
Topical HN$_2$	18	9
PUVA	13	7
Total skin electron beam RT	14	5
Systemic chemotherapy	16	7
Other systemic therapy	6	2

erythroderma. The great majority of patients had palpable lymphadenopathy. Lymph node and visceral organ biopsies were not required for protocol entry, but extracutaneous disease was present in these sites and/or in the peripheral blood in the majority of patients.

Both groups of patients were heavily pretreated (Table II). All had previously failed topical and/or systemic corticosteroids. Nearly all patients in both groups had previously received topical nitrogen mustard and the majority had received PUVA and total skin electron beam irradiation. In addition, a large majority of patients had failed systemic therapies. Systemic chemotherapy had previously been given to 16/20 patients in the rIFNαA study and 7/11 in the T101 study.

The treatment programs are outlined in Table III. The rIFNαA, provided by Hoffmann-LaRoche, Nutley, New Jersey, was given in a dose of 50×10^6 units intramuscularly three times weekly. Therapy was planned for three months. Patients in complete or partial response at three months were continued on therapy indefinitely until disease progression, while therapy was discontinued at three months in patients with mixed or minor responses or stable disease. If there was progression during the first three months, therapy was discontinued. Protocol guidelines provided dose reductions to 50% of the initial dose for severe toxicity and a further reduction to 10% of the initial dose for persistent severe toxicity.

Table III. Treatment programs

rIFN$_a$A:	50×10^6 units/m^2 I.M. thrice weekly	20 patients
T101:	1 mg. i.v. over 2 hrs. twice weekly × 4 weeks	2 patients [a]
	10 mg. i.v. over 2 hrs. twice weekly	3 patients [a]
	50 mg. i.v. over 2–24 hrs	3 patients[a]
	100 mg. i.v. over 8 hrs. twice weekly × 1 week	
	200 mg. i.v. over 8 hrs. twice weekly × 1 week	3 patients
	500 mg. i.v. over 8 hrs. twice weekly × 1 week	

[a] 3 additional patients in each of these groups received a single i.v. infusion of [111]Indium labeled T101 over 2–24 hours followed by serial imaging studies.

The T101 monoclonal antibody is an IgG_{2a} murine monoclonal antibody provided by Hybritech, La Jolla, California [13]. It binds to a 65,000 dalton antigen present on >95% of peripheral blood T-cells and >95% of T-cell malignancies but is not present on normal monocytes, B-cells, granulocytes, red blood cells, or platelets. There was a dose escalation scheme for groups of three patients if no severe toxicities were encountered. The antibody was given as an intravenous infusion over two hours twice weekly for four weeks. If there was stable disease after four weeks, the dose could be escalated to the next level. Patients receiving ≥ 50 mg infusions developed acute side effects (vide infra) during the two-hour infusions so that the infusion rate was lengthened to 8–24 hours. The three patients receiving the highest doses each received two 100 mg infusions, followed the next week by two 200 mg infusions, and by two 500 mg infusions in the third week. In addition, serial imaging studies were performed after single intravenous infusions of [111]Indium bound to T101-DTPA conjugates [14] in nine patients according to the dose schedule shown in Table III.

Standard response criteria were used. Complete response required complete resolution of all clinical and pathologic evidence of CTCL, including repeat skin biopsy, lasting at least one month. A partial response required a 50% or greater reduction in the product of perpendicular diameters of measurable lesions lasting at least one month. Progression was defined by the presence of new lesions or a greater than 50% increase in the product of the perpendicular diameters of measurable lesions.

Results

rIFNαA response

Treatment results in the 20 CTCL patients treated with rIFNαA are summarized in Table IV. There were no pathologically documented complete responses. Partial responses were documented in nine patients (45%, 95% confidence intervals 25–69%). There was no association of response with stage of disease or type of prior therapy. Cutaneous lesions improved dra-

Table IV. Treatment results

Response	$rIFN_{\alpha}A$	T101
Partial response	9	0
Mixed/minor response	5	2
Stable disease	3	9
Progression	3	0

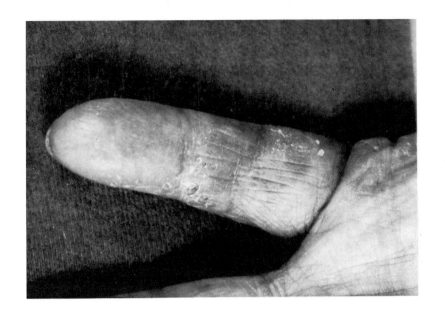

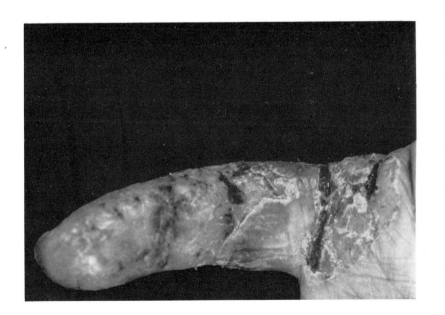

Figure 1. Photomicrographs of plaque lesions on a patient's finger before and three months after rIFNαA therapy. Marked healing of all his generalized plaque lesions as well as disappearance of generalized lymphodenopathy had occurred by this time. The response lasted 9.5 months.

matically in all nine responding patients. An example of the impressive response to interferon is shown in Fig. 1. The patient had generalized plaque lesions, many of which were ulcerated, and generalized lymphadenopathy. Within three months, his skin lesions had completely healed and his adenopathy also disappeared; but repeat skin biopsy showed a few persistent atypical cells.

Responders with extracutaneous lesions responded in these sites as well. Of the 16 patients with biopsy proven extracutaneous disease, eight had a partial response including these areas. Similarly, eight of the 16 patients who had previously failed systemic chemotherapy responded. Thus, eight of the nine responders had previously failed chemotherapy.

The partial responses lasted a median of 5.5 months with three responses lasting three months, two responses lasting five to six months, one lasting 9.5 months, and three responses continuing 11+ to 24+ months.

There were mixed or minor responses in five patients who were not scored as partial responders and who had therapy discontinued after three months. In two of these patients, some skin lesions improved while others worsened; in one, skin lesions improved while lymphadenopathy progressed; and, in two, there was less than a 50% improvement in skin lesions.

There was no improvement or worsening in three patients who were scored as stable disease, and three patients progressed in the first three months of treatment. Two of these patients worsened while receiving interferon and one progressed while off therapy. This patient was removed from the study after the initial injection, because he developed a palpable purpura which was judged to be a possible severe allergic reaction.

T101 response

The treatment summary for T101 is also shown in Table IV. None of the patients had partial or complete responses. There were minor responses (improvement in skin lesions and circulating blood counts of < 50%) in two patients. There was neither improvement nor worsening (stable disease) in nine patients, six of whom had therapy discontinued because of toxicity (vide infra) rather than progressive disease. Each of these patients had received at least four antibody infusions when the treatment was discontinued.

rIFNαA toxicity

Treatment toxicity of rIFNαA in this study was similar to other high-dose series (Table V). The most frequent and dose-limiting toxicity was a consti-

Table V. Treatment toxicities

Toxicity	rIFN$_a$A	T101
Flu-like Syndrome	19	0
Fever	20	3
Hepatic enzyme elevations	2	0
Myelosuppression	2	0
Allergic reactions	1	4
Hives	0	3
Purpura/Serum sickness	1	1
Pulmonary (Shortness of breath)	0	3
Nephrotic syndrome	1	0

tutional flu-like syndrome consisting of malaise, myalgias, anorexia, and depression. This syndrome developed in all 19 patients who received more than one dose of therapy. Associated with this syndrome was a mean fall in performance status of 30 and a mean weight loss of 12 pounds. Febrile responses were noted in all patients with a median peak febrile reaction of 103.9°F. Fever became less of a problem after the first several injections, suggesting a tachyphylaxis developed to this toxicity. Hematologic toxicity was mild and non-dose-limiting. None of the patients developed severe granulocytopenia ($< 1000/\mu l$). Two patients (with initial thrombocytopenia) developed platelet counts $< 50,000/\mu l$, but neither required platelet transfusions. Elevations of hepatic enzymes of 50% or more occurred in two patients, but enzyme levels returned to normal following dose reduction. One previously noted patient developed palpable purpura, a possible allergic reaction, but there were no other allergic reactions. One patient developed reversible nephrotic syndrome and renal failure due to minimal change glomerular lesions ascribed to the interferon [15].

Dose reductions due to the constitutional syndrome were required in all 19 patients who received more than one dose. These symptoms were alleviated by a 50% dose reduction in eight patients, while 11 patients required a further reduction to 10% of the initial dose before symptoms abated. The dose of rIFNαA was later re-escalated in 10 patients who had some, but less than 50%, worsening of lesions while the dose was reduced. After re-escalation, the flu-like symptoms never recurred, suggesting a tachyphylaxis to this toxicity. Clinical improvement after re-escalation was noted in four of these patients.

T101 toxicity

Toxicity after T101 was mild, but clearly dose-related. There were no episodes of bone marrow, liver, or renal toxicity. Mild fevers were noted in three patients. Possibly allergic reactions occurred in four patients including three who developed hives and one who developed palpable purpura. Therapy was continued after institution of antihistamines in the patients with hives, whereas therapy was discontinued in the patient with purpura. Pulmonary symptoms of chest tightness and shortness of breath without wheezing occurred in three patients. Symptoms cleared spontaneously within minutes of stopping T101 infusion, and were associated with spontaneously clearing abnormalities on lung scan (one patient) and chest x-ray (one patient). These symptoms occurred with doses of 10–50 mg over two hours but did not develop in patients with a slower rate of infusion (< 5 mg/hr). Patients receiving the highest doses, even in prolonged infusions of 6–24 hours, often experienced severe side effects including chills, jitteriness, a sense of impending doom, chest tightness, and, in one instance, hypotension. The last treatment at the 500 mg dose had to be terminated in 2 of 3 patients due to these toxicities.

Biologic studies

The mechanism of action of rIFNαA in producing antitumor responses is uncertain. The responses were not related to the degree or extent of febrile reactions or other toxicities. There was no correlation with monitored changes in immune function including natural killer cell activity, monocyte cytostasis, or lymphoproliferative responses to antigens and mitogens. Similarly, there was no correlation between response or response duration and the development of anti-interferon antibodies. Further definition of the mechanism of antitumor response awaits further studies.

While T101 proved ineffective in tumor cytostasis, biologic information obtained from the study will provide the groundwork for future studies with drug, toxin, and radiation particle immunoconjugates. Saturation of tumor binding sites was related to antibody dose, rate of administration, and site of the tumor cells. T101 binding sites on circulating cells were saturated at 10 mg but not at 1 mg. Saturation of tissue bound tumor cells occurred only at doses ≥ 50 mg and was inhomogeneous. Tumor cells in highly vascularized areas stained more heavily than those in poorly vascularized areas. Free T101 in serum was detected only at doses ≥ 50 mg. Antigen modulation occurred promptly and was demonstrated in all tumor bearing sites (Fig. 2). Expression of antigen returned to baseline 24–48 hours after the antibody was discontinued. Low levels of polyclonal antimurine antibodies developed in 80% of patients, but were not associated with clinical problems. Anti-idiotypic antibodies were not detected.

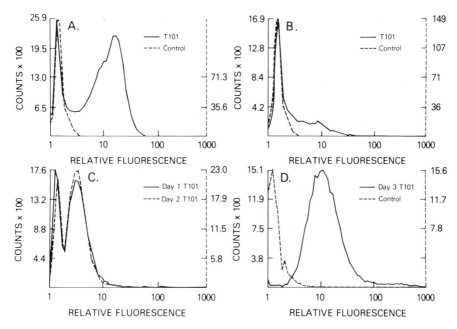

Figure 2. FACS analysis of T101 reactivity of peripheral blood mononuclear cells before *in vivo* administration of T101 (A), at the end of the T101 infusion (B), 24 and 48 hours after the infusion (C), and T101 reactivity of lymph node mononuclear cells 72 hours after infusion (D). Expression of antigen is lost (modulated, down regulated) by the end of the infusion, and antigen expression returns toward baseline over the following 72 hours.

T101 imaging studies

Imaging studies were performed after administration of [111]Indium (In) labeled T101-DTPA conjugate [14]. The total antibody dose was 1 mg in three patients, 10 mg in three patients, and 50 mg in three patients. In each instance, 5 mCi of ^{111}In was administered and serial scans were obtained. At all antibody doses, the blood pool was most heavily labeled at the end of the antibody infusion. There was rapid clearance from the blood pool and specific uptake was noted in tumor bearing areas of skin and lymph nodes from one day through seven days post-infusion (Fig. 3). Specific tumor localization was most impressive 3–7 days after antibody infusion when nonspecific background had cleared from the blood pool and other sites. Tumor localization was optimal with 10–50 mg infusions. The 10-mg infusions were better tolerated by the patients. Tumor localization in lymphatic and cutaneous areas was striking in all patients. Non-specific uptake of radiotracer was noted in the liver and spleen of all patients.

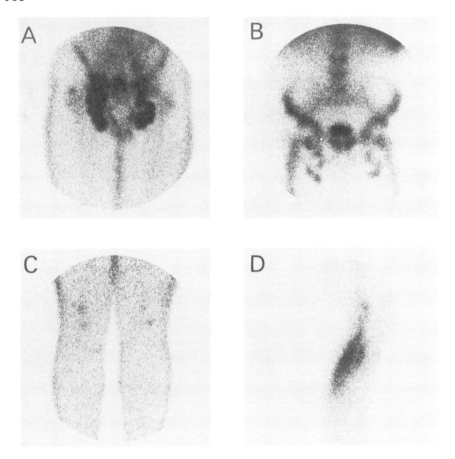

Figure 3. ^{111}In-T101 scan of 4 patients obtained 72 hours after the intravenous infusion of T101. Fig. 3A shows striking tumor localization in skin and inguinal and femoral lymph nodes in a patient with the Sezary syndrome. Fig. 3B shows localization in inguinal and femoral lymph nodes in a patient with mycosis fungoides who had no skin lesions in this region. Note the absence of skin uptake compared to A. Fig. 3C shows lymph node and cutaneous uptake in a patient with the Sezary syndrome and Fig. 3D shows localization in a large tumor mass in the lower leg of a patient with mycosis fungoides.

Discussion

The biologic response modifiers T101 and rIFNαA hold considerable promise for improving the outcome of patients with malignant lymphomas [16, 17]. This study has shown that rIFNαA is highly active in patients with advanced CTCL refractory to most standard agents, including chemotherapy. The 45% response rate we observed was considerably higher than the response rate we have observed with experimental chemotherapeutic agents in similar patients. Most therapeutic agents have considerably greater activity in untreated patients with early stage disease than in those with advanced disease refractory to multiple treatment modalities. Thus rIFNαA will need to be evaluated in untreated patients. It will also be important to evaluate other dose schedules in an attempt to reduce toxicity and improve the complete response rate. Since rIFNαA produces a similar response rate in advanced, indolent B-cell lymphomas [16] parallel studies in untreated patients with these lymphomas should also be performed.

T101 or similar antibodies are unlikely to be useful when given alone. However, radiolabeled T101 holds great promise as a useful imaging modality for staging CTCL patients [18]. Scans performed 3–7 days after 5 mCi T101 (10 mg) identify all areas of clinically palpable lymphadenopathy as well as nonpalpable sites. Nonspecific uptake in liver and spleen remains a problem. Our future studies will evaluate ^{131}Iodine T101 conjugates as well as radiolabeled Fab and F(ab')$_2$ fragments of T101. We also plan to evaluate alternative routes of antibody administration (eg. intralymphatic, subcutaneous).

T101 conjugates with drugs, toxins, or radiolabeled particles also hold great promise. We have shown that radiolabeled iodine has significant cytotoxic effects against T-cell lymphoma lines *in vitro*. We plan to evaluate iodine-labeled T101 *in vivo* in high doses in future experiments. Conjugates of T101 with doxorubicin and vindesine are being prepared and will also be evaluated in the near future.

References

1. Lutzner M, Edelsen R, Schein P et al. (1975). Cutaneous T-cell lymphomas: The Sezary syndrome, mycosis fungoides and related disorders. Ann Intern Med 83:534–552.
2. Broder S and Bunn PA Jr (1980). Neoplasms of T-cell origin. Immunological aspects and therapy. Semin Oncol 7:310–331.
3. Crossen PE. Mellor JEL, Finley AG et al. (1971). The Sezary syndrome: Cytogenetic studies and identification of the Sezary cell as an abnormal lymphocyte. Amer J Med 50:24–34.
4. Brouet JC, Flandrin G and Seligmann (1973). Indications of the thymus derived nature of the proliferating cells in six patients with the Sezary syndrome. N Engl J Med 289:341–344.
5. Broder S, Edelson RL, Lutzner MH et al. (1976). The Sezary syndrome: A malignant proliferation of helper T-cells. J Clin Invest 58:1297–1306.
6. Haynes BF, Metzgar RS, Minna JD and Bunn PA (1981). Phenotypic characterization of cutaneous T-cell lymphoma. N Engl J Med 304:1319–1323.
7. Epstein EH Jr, Levin DL, Croft JD Jr and Lutzner MA (1972).Mycosis fungoides, survival, prognostic features, response to therapy and autopsy findings. Medicine 51:61–72.
8. Rappaport H and Thomas LB (1974). Mycosis fungoides: The pathology of extracutaneous involvement. Cancer 34:1198–1229.
9. Bunn PA Jr, Huberman MS, Whang-Peng J et al. (1980). Prospective staging evaluation of

patients with cutaneous T-cell lymphoma: Demonstration of a high frequency of extracutaneous dissemination. Ann Intern Med 93:223–230.

10. Winkler CF and Bunn PA (1983). Cutaneous T-cell lymphomas: A review. CRC Critical Review in Oncology/Hematology 1:49–92.

11. Edelson RL, Raafat J, Berger CL et al. (1979). Antithymocyte globulin in the management of cutaneous T-cell lymphoma. Cancer Treat Rep 63:675–680.

12. Miller RA, Oseroff AR, Stratti PT and Levy R (1983). Monoclonal antibody therapeutic trials in seven patients with T-cell lymphoma. Blood 62:988–995.

13. Royston I, Majda JA, Baird SM et al. (1980). Human T-cell antigens defined by monoclonal antibodies: The 65,000 dalton antigen of T-cells (T65) is also found on chronic lymphocytic leukemia cells bearing surface immunoglobulin. J Immunol 125:725–731.

14. Sherwin SA, Knost JA, Fein S, et al. (1982). A multiple dose phase I trial of recombinant leukocyte A interferon in cancer patients. JAMA 248:2461–2466.

15. Averbuch SD, Austin HA, Sherwin SA et al (1984). Acute interstitial nephritis with nephrotic syndrome following recombinant leukocyte A interferon for mycosis fungoides. N Engl J Med 310:32–35.

16. Foon KA, Sherwin SA, Abrams PG et al. Recombinant leukocyte A interferon: An effective agent for the treatment of advanced non-Hodgkin's lymphoma. (Submitted).

17. Bunn PA Jr, Foon KA, Ihde DC et al. Recombinant leukocyte A interferon: An active agent in advanced cutaneous T-cell lymphomas. Ann Intern Med (in press).

18. Bunn PA, Carrasquillo J, Keenan A et al. Successful imaging of malignant non-Hodgkin's lymphoma using radiolabeled monoclonal antibody. (Submitted).

16. Clinical interferon (IFN) studies in leukemia and lymphoma

A. Z. S. ROHATINER and T. A. LISTER
ICRF Department of Medical Oncology, St. Bartholomew's Hospital, London, UK

Studies in murine models of leukemia established that interferon (IFN) had a dose-dependent growth inhibitory effect [1, 2] which was subsequently confirmed for human myeloblasts *in vitro* [3, 4]. IFN has also been shown to be inhibitory to normal and leukemic clonogenic cells, both in terms of primary proliferation and self-renewal [5, 6]. These preliminary observations, together with anecdotal reports of activity in follicular lymphoma [7, 8] chronic lymphocytic leukemia (CLL) [8] and myeloma [9] prompted the investigation of IFN in patients with hematologic malignancy.

Early clinical studies were hampered both by limited supplies and excessive enthusiasm from the media. However, increasing availability and the accrual of larger numbers of patients into the recent trials now allows a preliminary evaluation of their benefit. The earliest studies were all conducted with leukocyte interferon; subsequently, purified lymphoblastoid interferon (IFN-α), and recombinant DNA (IFNα$_2$, IFNαA) have been tested.

Phase I studies

Phase I trials of IFN-α at the Westminster Hospital, London showed that the maximum dose given over a prolonged period, and compatible with a 'normal' ambulatory existence was less than 10^7 IU daily [10]. Even at this dose most patients had chills and fever for the first few days and some gradually developed debilitating fatigue. In contrast it was also demonstrated that very much higher doses could be given over a week, using an approach similar to that applied to the testing of high doses of cytotoxic chemicals. At St. Bartholomew's Hospital, London, 39 patients received escalating doses of human lymphoblastoid IFN (IFN-α) administered by continuous intravenous infusion. A maximum tolerated dose (MTD) of 10^8

units/m^2/day was established, central nervous system (CNS) disturbance, hyperkalemia and hypocalcemia being dose-limiting factors [11]. Further evaluation of the CNS toxicity in 11 patients receiving either IFN-α or recombinant DNA IFN (IFN-α$_2$) revealed reversible EEG changes even in the absence of overt clinical toxicity [12]. Subsequent studies with recombinant IFN-αA revealed broadly similar results.

Phase I and II studies

Leukemias (Tables I-II)

Acute
In 1974, Ahstrom et al. [13], using a relatively impure preparation of leucocyte IFN-α, administered 2.5×10^6 units/day to 6 children with acute leukemia (2 acute myelogenous leukemia AML, 4 acute lymphoblastic leukemia ALL). Treatment was continued for periods ranging from one month to more than a year but no anti-leukemic effect was observed.

Table I. Interferon for acute leukemia

Leukemia	IFN subtype	Dose x 10^6 IU	Route	Schedule	Duration	Number of patients	CR proportion
AML	IFN-α (leu)	2.5 [a]	IV	daily	1–12 months	2	0
ALL	IFN-α (leu)	2.5 [a]	IV	daily	1–12 months	4	0
AML	IFN-α (leu)	0.25–2 [b]	IV	daily	not stated	3	2 *
ALL	IFN-α (leu)	0.25–2 [b]	IV	daily	not stated	5	5 *
CML blast crisis	IFN-α (leu)	0.25–2 [b]	IV	daily	not stated	1	1 *
AML	IFN-α (ly)	100 [c]	IVI	daily	7 days	14	0
AML	rIFN-αA	25–125 [c]	IVI	daily	7–14 days	10	0

* response not defined
[a] total dose
[b] per kilogram
[c] per square meter

Table II. Interferon for chronic lymphatic leukemia

IFN subtype	Dose ×10⁶ IU	Route	Schedule	Duration	Number of patients	CR	PR	CR+PR	Reference
IFN-*a* (leu)	100[a]	IV	daily	7 days	4	4	0	4/4	Rohatiner [18]
IFN-*a* (leu)	3[b]	IM	daily	>4 weeks	4	0	1	1/4	Gutterman [8]
rIFN-*a*A	50[a]	IM	×3/week	>3 months	8	0	3	3/8	Sherwin [21]
IFN-*a*₂	2–30[a]	IV/SC	daily	not stated	3	0	0	0/3	Ozer [22]
IFN-*a* (leu)	1.5–6[b]	SC	10 day cycles or for 3 months	up to 3 months	9	0	2	2/9	Misset [30]
				Total	$\overline{28}$	$\overline{4}$	$\overline{6}$	$\overline{10/28}$	

[a] per square meter
[b] total dose

Subsequently, using a higher intravenous dose of IFN-α, responses were reported in 5 patients with ALL, 2 out of 3 patients with AML and one patient with blastic transformation of chronic myeloid leukemia (CML). However, these results are difficult to interpret since the nature of the responses was not specified [14].

In vitro studies conducted on the blast cells from the patients treated in the Phase I study at St. Bartholomew's Hospital showed that the maximum tolerated dose of 10^8 IU/m^2/day for seven days was inhibitory at the 50% level [4, 15]. In the light of these observations, 14 patients with AML who had either failed to enter remission with conventional therapy or had relapsed following such therapy received IFN-α at the MTD for 7 days. Although leukemic blast cells temporarily cleared from the peripheral blood, no complete remissions were achieved and there was no correlation between serum IFN levels, *in vitro* growth inhibition and clinical response [14]. Ten patients with AML treated with recombinant leukocyte A IFN at doses ranging from $25–125 \times 10^6$ units/day also showed no response [16].

Chronic

Chronic myeloid leukemia (CML). A clear demonstration of the anti-proliferative activity of IFN-α (leukocyte) has been made in patients with CML. In a study currently in progress at the MD Anderson Hospital, Houston, 25 patients have been treated with partially pure leukocyte IFN-α, $3–9 \times 10^6$ units daily, administered by intramuscular (IM) injection. Peripheral blood parameters returned to normal in 22 patients and a decrease in splenomegaly was observed in 14 out of 15 patients. Bone marrow (BM) cellularity decreased from a mean value of 98% to 72% and this change was associated with a reduction in the percentage of Philadelphia chromosome positive cells in the BM from 100% to a median of 65%. Such responses have been maintained [17].

In contrast high-dose therapy resulted only in a transient reduction in the peripheral white cell count. Four patients at St. Bartholomew's Hospital received $50–100 \times 10^6$ units/m^2 of IFN-α$_2$ by continuous intravenous infusion for 7–14 days. Although the peripheral white blood count decreased temporarily, there was no change in the degree of splenomegaly or in the morphological appearance of the BM [18].

Hairy cell leukemia (HCL) Low dose chronic administration has also been shown to have activity in HCL. Sixteen patients, thirteen of whom had undergone splenectomy, and all of whom had evidence of progressive disease were treated with 3×10^6 IU/day indefinitely. Responses were achieved in 12 out of 16, with the peripheral blood count returning to normal in all, 'complete' bone marrow remission being seen in 3, and partial bone marrow remission in nine. No infectious complications have been seen to date in the responding patients [19, 20].

Chronic lymphathic leukemia (CLL) Almost regardless of dose and schedule, patients with chronic lymphocytic leukemia (CLL) have shown only transient and incomplete responses in terms of lymphadenopathy or a fall in the circulating lymphocyte count (Table II).

Lymphomas (Tables III-IV)

The initial experience with leukocyte IFN-α in small numbers of patients was suggestive of anti-tumor activity in lymphoma of favorable histology but lack of response in high-grade lymphoma [7, 8]. In general, recent studies confim earlier findings. The National Cancer Institute (NCI) conducted a study of recombinant leukocyte A IFN, in which patients received 50×10^6 units/m^2/day by IM injection thrice weekly [21]. Two complete and 14 partial responses were observed in 25 previously treated patients with 'favorable histology' non-Hodgkin's lymphoma (NHL). Three patients showed no response and there was evidence of tumor progression in 6 patients.

Ozer et al. [22] included 21 patients with 'low-grade' lymphoma in a Phase II study of IFN-α$_2$. Doses ranged from $2-30 \times 10^6$ units/m^2/day, administered by either the intravenous or subcutaneous route. Partial responses were noted in 4 out of 10 patients wiht N-PDL lymphoma and 1 out of 11 patients with D-PDL lymphoma.

The Southeastern Cancer Study Group has investigated low and high dose IFN-α (lymphoblastoid) in patients failing conventional therapy with malignant lymphoma. The initial treatment comprised 5×10^6 IU/m^2 thrice weekly for 8 weeks, with those patients who failed to respond proceeding to 30×10^6 IU/m^2 for 10 days. Responses (only 2 complete remissions) were seen in 8 out of 32 patients in equal frequency in the different histologic subtypes at the low dose, with occasional further responses, (more complete) at the higher doses [23].

A Phase II study of low dose IFN-α$_2$ is in progress at the Christie Hospital, Manchester, eighteen patients have received 2×10^6 IU/m^2 thrice weekly for three months. Toxicity was acceptable, and 4 patients achieved remission (1 CR) [24].

In addition to the above studies with IFN-α, IFN-β has also been administered at low doses to patients with favorable histology NHL and CLL. Minimal BM infiltration resolved after 7 months therapy in one patient and a BM response in the absence of lymph node regression was observed in a second patient. Eight patients showed progressive disease [25].

Table III. Interferon for low grade non-Hodgkin's lymphoma

IFN subtype	Dose $\times 10^6$ IU	Route	Schedule	Duration	Number of patients	CR	PR	CR + PR	Reference
IFN-a (leu)	10 [a]	IM	daily	1 month	3	0	3	3/3	Merigan [7]
IFN-a (leu)	3–9 [a]	IM	daily	>1 month	6	2	1	3/6	Gutterman [8]
rIFN-aA	50 [b]	IM	×3/week	>3 months	25	2	14	16/25	Sherwin [21]
IFN-a_2	2–30 [b]	IV/SC	daily	not stated	21	0	15	5/21	Ozer [22]
IFN-a	5 [b]	IM	×3/week	8 weeks or	25	2	4	6/25	Game [23]
IFN-a_2	2 [b]	SC	×3/week	indefinite	18	1	3	4/18	Wagstaff [24]
				Total	98	7	40	37/98	

[a] total dose
[b] per square meter

Table IV. Interferon for high grade non-Hodgkin's lymphoma

IFN subtype	Dose $\times 10^6$ IU	Route	Schedule	Duration	Number of patients	CR	PR	CR + PR	Reference
IFN-a (leu)	10 [a]	IM	daily	1 month	3	0	0	0/3	Merigan [7]
IFN-a (leu)	3–9 [a]	IM	daily	>1 month	1	0	0	0/1	Gutterman [8]
rIFN-aA	50 [b]	IM	×3/week	>3 months	6	0	2	2/6	Sherwin [21]
IFN-a_2	2–30 [b]	IV/SC	daily	not stated	10	0	4	4/10	Ozer [22]
IFN-a	5 [b]	IM	×3/week	8 weeks or	7	0	2	2/7	Gams [23]
IFNa_2	250 [b]	IVI	q21d	24 hours	7	0	2	2/7	Wagstaff [24]
				Total	34	0	10	10/34	

[a] total dose
[b] per square meter

Results in high-grade lymphoma have in the main been disappointing. Merigan et al. [7] originally treated 3 patients with progressive diffuse histiocytic lymphoma and observed no response, in contrast to 3 patients with follicular lymphoma who showed regression of disease. The NCI study [21] included 6 patients with high-grade lymphoma. No complete responses were documented and in 2 patients with lymphoblastic lymphoma, responses were partial and brief. Moreover, 4 out of 12 patients with diffuse histiocytic lymphoma reported by Ozer et al. [22] also showed only transient, partial responses.

Responses have, however, been observed in advanced refractory T-cell lymphoma (CTCL). Twenty patients received 50×10^6 IU/m^2 of recombinant DNA interferon, with more than half (9 out of 17) responding. However, toxicity demanded dose reduction in all patients. Less intensive schedules may be effective [26].

In Hodgkin's disease (HD), activity has also been reported. Transient, partial responses have been noted in 4 out of 12 patients [22, 27].

In evaluating any new therapeutic agent, potential benefit has to be considered not only against the associated toxicity, but also within the context of other available treatment strategies. Thus interferons have not fulfilled their *in vitro* promise and they have not been of therapeutic benefit when administered as primary therapy to patients with acute leukemia. Results of longer follow-up in CML and hairy cell leukemia are awaited with interest. IFN-γ has recently been shown to induce differentiation in a human leukemic cell line (U937) [28] and in blast cells derived from patients with AML and CML [29]. Whether such an approach will have clinical application remains to be established.

The demonstration that approximately fifty percent of patients with low grade NHL who have already received chemotherapy, respond to interferons suggests that they may have a role in the primary treatment of this group of diseases. It remains to be determined whether they should be used alone, in combination with cytotoxic chemotherapy or as an adjuvant.

Acknowledgements

We thank Jane Ashby for typing the manuscript.

References

1. Gresser I, Brouty-Boye d, Thomas M-T and Macieira-Coelho A (1970). Interferon and cell division. I. Inhibition of the multiplication of mouse leukaemia L1210 cells *in vitro* by an interferon preparation. Proc Nat Acad Sci 66:1052–1058.

2. Gresser I, Bourali C, Chouroulinkov I et al. (1970). Treatment of neoplasia in mice with an interferon preparation. Ann NY Acad Sci 173:694–707.
3. Balkwill F and Oliver RTO (1977). Growth inhibitory effects of interferon on normal and malignant haemopoietic cells. Int J Cancer 20:500–505.
4. Rohatiner AZS. Growth inhibitory effects of interferon on blast cells from patients with acute myelogenous leukaemia. Brit J Cancer. (In press).
5. Greenberg PL and Mosny SA (1977). Cytotoxic effects of interferon *in vitro* on granulocytic progenitor cells. Cancer Res 37:1794–1799.
6. Taetle R, Buick RN and McCulloch EA (1980). Effect of interferon on colony formation in culture by blast cell progenitors in acute myeloblastic leukaemia. Blood 56:549–552.
7. Merigan TC, Sikora K, Breeden JH et al. (1978). Preliminary observations on the effect of human leukocyte interferon in non-Hodgkin's lymphoma. N Engl J Med 299:1449–1453.
8. Gutterman JU, Blumenschein GR, Alexanian R et al. (1980). Leucocyte interferon-induced tumor regression in human metastatic breast cancer, multiple myeloma and malignant lymphoma. Ann Intern Med 93:399–406.
9. Mellstedt H, Bjorkholm M, Johansson B et al. (1979). Interferon therapy in myelomatosis. Lancet 1:245–247.
10. Priestman TJ (1980). Initial evaluation of human lymphoblastoid interferon in patients with advanced malignant disease. Lancet 2:113–118.
11. Rohatiner AZS, Balkwill FR, Griffin DB et al. (1982). A phase I study of human lymphoblastoid interferon administered by continuous intravenous infusion. Cancer Chemother Pharmacol 9:97–102.
12. Rohatiner AZS, Prior PF, Burton AC and Lister TA (1983). Central nervous system toxicity of interferon. Br J Cancer 47:419–422.
13. Ahstrom L, Dohlwitz A, Strander H et al. (1974). Interferon in acute leukaemia in children. Lancet 1:166–167.
14. Hill NO, Pardue A, Khan A et al. (1981). High-dose human leukocyte interferon trials in leukaemia and cancer. Med Pediat Oncol 9:82.
15. Rohatiner AZS, Balkwill FR, Malpas JS and Lister TA (1983). Experience with human lymphoblastoid interferon in acute myelogenous leukaemia. Cancer Chemother Pharmacol 11:56–58.
16. Leavitt RD, Duffey P and Wiernik PH (1983). A Phase I/II study of recombinant leukocyte A interferon in previously treated acute leukaemia. Blood 62,1:205a.
17. Talpaz M, McCredie KB, Keating MJ and Gutterman JU (1983). Clinical investigation of leukocyte IFN (HuIFN-*a*) in chronic myelogenous leukaemia. Blood 62,1:209a.
18. Rohatiner AZS, O'Brien H, Horton M et al. (1983). Experience with IFN-*a*₂ in chronic myeloid and chronic lymphocytic leukaemia. Proc 13th Int Congress Chemother Vienna, 9–15.
19. Quesada JR, Reubn J, Manning JT et al. (1984). Alpha interferon for induction of remission in hairy cell leukaemia. N Engl J Med 310:15–18.
20. Quesada JR, Hersh EM and Gutterman JU (1984). Treatment of hairy cell leukaemia with alpha interferon. Proc Amer Soc Clin Oncol 3:207.
21. Sherwin S, Foon K, Bunn P et al (1983). Recombinant leukocyte A interferon in the treatment of non-Hodgkin's lymphoma, chronic lymphocytic leukemia and mycosis fungoides. Blood 62,1:215a.
22. Ozer H, Leavitt R, Ratanatharathern V et al. (1983). Experience in the use of DNA alpha interferon in the treatment of malignant lymphomas. Blood 62,1:214a.
23. Gams R, Gordon D, Guaspari A and Tuttle R (1984). Phase II trial of human polyclonal lymphoblastoid interferon (Welferon) in the management of malignant lymphoma. Proc Amer Soc Clin Oncol 3:65.
24. Wagstaff J and Crowther D (1984). Human *a*₂ interferon on the non-Hodgkin's lymphomas. A report of two phase II studies. 2nd International Conf Lymphoma, Lugano, 99.

600

25. Siegert W, Theml H, Fink V et al. (1982). Treatment of non-Hodgkin's lymphoma of low-grade malignancy with human fibroblast interferon.Anticancer Res 2:193–198.
26. Bunn P, Foon K, Ihde D et al. (1984). Recombinant leukocyte A interferon in the treatment of refractory cutaneous T-cell lymphomas. Proc Amer Soc Clin Oncol 3:52.
27. Rapson CR, Scholnik AP, Stoutenborough KA and Schwartz KA (1983). Treatment of lymphoproliferative malignancy chemotherapy failures with human leukocyte interferon. Blood 62,1:214a.
28. Ralph P, Harris PE, Punjabi CT et al. (1983). Lymphokine inducing terminal differentiation of the human monoblast leukaemia line U937: A role for interferon. Blood 62:1169–1175.
29. Perussia B, Dayton ET, Fanning V et al. (1984). Immune interferon and leukocyte conditioned medium induce normal and leukemic myeloid cells to differentiate along the monocytic pathway. J Exp Med (in press).
30. Misset JL, Mathe G, Gastiaburu J et al. (1982). Traitement des leucémies et des lymphomes par les Interferons: II Essai phase II de traitement de la leucémie lymphoïde chronique par l'interferon humain. Biomedicine 36:112–116.

VIII. Treatment of childhood lymphomas

1. Current status of the curability of children with Hodgkin's disease: An assessment of the risk: benefit ratio of modern therapy

S. B. MURPHY
St. Jude Children's Research Hospital, Memphis, Tennessee, USA

There is no compelling evidence to suggest that Hodgkin's disease (HD) in children differs materially from the disease in adults. Just as adults in recent years have benefited from the introduction of a comprehensive multidisciplinary approach to management, the survival of children with HD has greatly improved in association with the sequential introduction of improved clinical and surgical staging techniques, and application of both megavoltage extended field irradiation and combination chemotherapy, first for generalized disease and more recently electively as part of the initial management in combined modality regimens. Historical results of treatment of children with HD in the decades prior to 1960 demonstrated an overall 5–10 year survival rate in the range of 25–33%, providing a standard against which current results may be measured [1–3]. Current data on the status of pediatric HD trials, late consequences of treatment, and an assessment of the risk: benefit ratio associated with modern therapy of HD in children form the basis for this review.

Current status of pediatric Hodgkin's disease trials

The impact of modern multidisciplinary management on extended disease-free and overall survival of children with HD is reflected by the compilation of recent results listed in Table I, summarizing the experience of numerous centers and cooperative groups over the past decade. Treatment policy has generally rested upon scrupulous pathologic staging and high-dose extended field radiotherapy for Stages I-III, generally with combination chemotherapy reserved for Stages IIIB and IV. The best results reported, however, have resulted from the combined use of chemotherapy and comparatively low-dose radiation therapy in all stages of disease, resulting in 5-year disease-free survival rates in the range of 90%, often avoiding laparotomy and splenectomy [5, 7, 12, 13].

Table I. Results of modern treatment of Hodgkin's disease in children [a]

Source	No.	Stages	Overall 5-yr survival/DFS	Treatment modalities	Reference
Roswell Park Memorial Institute 1965–1973	37	I–IV	86%/86%	IA, IIA RT alone IIB, III Both modalities IV MOPP (plus Vbl, CCNU)	[2]
Memorial Sloan-Kettering Cancer Center 1970–1975	45	I–IV	80%/Not stated	I, II IF or EF RT III TNI IIIB-IV (ACOPP)	[4]
Toronto 1969–1973	52	PS I–IV	89%/54%	PSI-IIIA EF RT (3500 r) IIIB and IV EF RT + MOPP	[5]
1973–1977	41	I–IV	89%/85%	CSI-IV (except favorable CSIA) MOPP × 3 → EF RT (2000–2500 r) → MOPP × 3	
Stanford University 1962–1972	79	PSI-IV	89%/66%	PSI-III EF, TNI, (3500–4400 r) IV MOPP	[6]
1972–1982	48	PSI-IV	96%/93%	EF RT (1500–2500 r) + MOPP × 6	[7]

[a] Abbreviations used:
DFS = disease-free survival, CS = clinical stage, PS = pathologic stage, RT = radiotherapy, IF = involved field, EF = extended field, TNI = total nodal irradiation, r = rad, MM* = mediastinal mass
Vbl = vinblastine
MOPP = nitrogen mustard, oncovin, procarbazine, prednisone
COP = cyclophosphamide, vincristine, procarbazine
COPP = as COP plus prednisone
A = doxorubicin
ABVD = doxorubicin, bleomycin, vinblastine, DTIC

Table I. Results of modern treatment of Hodgkin's disease in children [a] (continued)

Source	No.	Stages	Overall 5-yr survival/DFS	Treatment modalities	Reference
Children's Hospital of Philadelphia 1977–1983	16	Stages IA-IIA	100%/86%	PSIA-IIA pubertal and post-pubertal EF RT (3600–4400 r)	[8]
	32	Stages IIB-IVB	86%/60%	CSIA-IVB pre-pubertal and CSIIA (MM [b])-IVB post-pubertal COPP × 3 → (2000 r) IF → COPP 3	
National Cancer Institute 1964–1973	38	Stages I-IV	63%/not stated	CSI-II EF or TNI (3500–4000 r) CSIIIA TNI CSIIIB-IVB MOPP	[9]
Joint Center for Radiation Therapy 1968–1977	83	Stages IA-IIIB	95%/77%	IA-IIA EF (3600–4000 r) IIB, IIIA, IIIB TNI or EF RT + MOPP	[10]
St. Jude Children's Research Hospital 1967–1972	54	I-IV	80%/75%	I-II EF RT (3500–4000 r) + CO III-IV TNI (3500–4000 r) + COP	[11]
German Cooperative Group 1978–1981	170	I-IV	92%/96% [b]	I-IV 2 cycles of OPPA + IF (3600–4000 r) then either 3600–4000 r to EF or 1800–2000 r to EF, then IA, IB, IIA No further therapy IIB, III, IV 4 additional cycles COPP	[12]
Istituto Nazionale Tumori Milan 1979–1982	34	I-III	100%/97% [b]	I-IIA ABVD × 3 + EF (2500–3500) IIIA, or B Symptoms ABVD × 3 → EF RT → ABVD × 3	[13]

[a] Abbreviations used:
  DFS = disease-free survival, CS = clinical stage, PS = pathologic stage, RT = radiotherapy, IF = involved field, EF = extended field, TNI = total nodal irradiation, r = rad, MM* = mediastinal mass
  Vbl = vinblastine
  MOPP = nitrogen mustard, oncovin, procarbazine, prednisone
  COP = cyclophosphamide, vincristine, procarbazine
  COPP = as COP plus prednisone
  A = doxorubicin
  ABVD = doxorubicin, bleomycin, vinblastine, DTIC
[b] Reported results from 3–4 years follow-up (not 5)

Adverse consequences of treatment of Hodgkin's disease in children

Since 9 out of 10 children carefully staged and treated for their HD will be long-term survivors, the practitioner must closely consider both the acute toxicity and the adverse long-term late consequences of treatment, the goal being to retain high rates of curability with maximal freedom from side effects. Table II lists the recognized complications of treatment of HD in children with radiation therapy, combination chemotherapy, or both modalities. A number of recent publications review these complications in greater detail [5, 8, 10, 11, 14]. Both the frequency and the severity of the complications seen in children treated for HD is greater with combined modality approaches than with either radiation therapy or chemotherapy alone.

Therapeutic decision making. Assessment of the risk: benefit ratio of modern therapy

Considering the outstanding disease control achieved in pediatric HD patients with combined modality therapy in all stages of disease [5, 7, 12, 13], one could ask whether or not there exists any patient subgroups appropriately treated either with radiation alone or chemotherapy alone, recognizing that the use of either modality alone is associated with a lower complication risk but a higher relapse rate.

In order to answer this question, it is necessary to examine the reported relapse hazard of children with HD treated with radiation therapy alone and the subsequent rate of successful salvage. Cham et al. treated a total of 20 children with pathologically staged I and II HD with involved field radiation therapy only and reported relapse in 8 of 20 patients with short follow-up, i.e., 3-year disease-free survival rate of only 57% [14]. Even with extended fields, Young et al. reported 10 relapses of 21 clinically staged children with Stages I and II disease treated with wide field radiation therapy [9]. Similarly, Jenkin and Barry reported only 54% disease-free survival in a group of 41 pathologically staged patients treated from 1969 to 1972 in

Table II. Complications of treatment of HD in children [5, 8, 10, 11, 14]

---

* Growth retardation
* Hypothyroidism
* Infertility
* Cardiopulmonary complications
* Infectious complications
  (*Herpes zoster,* bacterial sepsis)
* Second malignant neoplasms

Toronto with 3500 rad in extended fields [5]. This high relapse rate in clinically localized disease following radiotherapy alone appears unacceptable, since it is unlikely that any subsequent salvage therapy can consistently cure HD a second time in all the patients. It is necessary to assume that relapse in HD is a bad prognostic sign in children. For this not to be true would require 100% success of salvage therapies, an intrinsically unlikely event considering what is currently known regarding the development of somatic mutations in cancer cells and development of drug resistance. Furthermore, reported results of salvage approaches in relapsed HD patients do not approximate this level of success. For instance, Jenkin has reported a median duration of second complete remissions of HD of only 3 years in the group of 22 children relapsing after initial treatment, and more than half of the children with a first relapse experienced multiple relapses [5]. There is, furthermore, often greater total morbidity associated with salvage approaches entailing prolonged therapies, reflected by increased cardiopulmonary complications, hematopoietic toxicity, poor marrow tolerance with a concomitant increase in infectious complications, preleukemic states and second malignancies. The most successful approach to salvage is to prevent relapse.

Hence, it would appear prudent to adopt a strategy incorporating both radiation therapy and combination chemotherapy for all children with HD in whom the risk for relapse following radiation therapy alone (or chemotherapy alone) is substantial, i.e., Stage IIA with bulky mediastinal and hilar involvement, Stage IIB, Stages IIIA and IIIB, and Stage IV. The only children for whom radiation therapy alone appears to be the treatment of choice include those with localized favorable Stages IA or IIA disease. However, prepubertal patients, even in this favorable group, should be considered for combined modality approaches incorporating low dose (2,000 rad) radiotherapy, in view of the quite significant adverse effects on axial skeletal growth produced by high-dose extended-field radiation treatments. Postpubertal patients with Stages I and IIA favorable disease could be considered for radiotherapy alone in view of the preservation of reproductive functioning desirable in this age group. With the increasingly widespread use of chemotherapy in the majority of children with HD, it appears logical to omit staging laparotomy and splenectomy prior to treatment, unless the results of the surgical staging procedure will influence the determination of radiation volume, as in the Stanford program [7].

Future trials for pediatric HD patients should aim at a further optimization of the risk: benefit ratio, exploring further reductions in both the dose and volume of radiation therapy, introduction of alternative non-cross-resistant drug combinations and schedules of equal effectiveness and lesser toxicity. Considering the effectiveness of combination drugs in the treatment of HD, consideration of elimination of radiation therapy altogether for certain subgroups should be given. Preliminary experience already suggests that this is feasible [16, 17], but this experience must be confirmed by well controlled clinical trials. The experience with alternating combinations of MOPP/ABVD, in particular in combination with radiation therapy, has so far been scanty in children. Preliminary results indicate the approach is probably better tolerated and more effective than MOPP alone, or MOPP plus radiation [18], but the long-term adverse consequences of delivery of this therapy to the child or adolescent with HD are essentially unknown.

Acknowledgements

Work was supported in part by a grant from NIH (CA 21765) and by ALSAC.

References

1. Teillet F and Schweisguth O (1969). Hodgkin's disease in children. Clin Pediat 8:698–704.
2. Shah NK, Freeman AI, Friedman M et al. (1976). Hodgkin's disease in children. Med Pediat Oncol 2:87–98.
3. Jenkin RDT, Peters MV and Darte JMM (1967). Hodgkin's disease in children. Am J Roent Radiol Nuclear Med 100:222–226.
4. Tan C, D'Angio GJ, Exelby PR et al. (1975). The changing management of childhood Hodgkin's disease. Cancer 535:808–816.
5. Jenkin RDT and Barry MT (1980). Hodgkin's disease in children. Semin Oncol 7:202–211.
6. Donaldson SS, Glatstein E, Rosenberg SA and Kaplan HS (1976). Pediatric Hodgkin's disease. II. Results of therapy. Cancer 37:2436–2447.
7. Donaldson SS (1982). Hodgkin's disease. Treatment with low-dose radiation and chemotherapy. Front Radiat Ther Oncol 16:122–133.
8. Lange B and Littman P (1983). Management of Hodgkin's disease in children and adolescents. Cancer 51:1371–1377.
9. Young RC, DeVita VT and Johnson RE (1973). Hodgkin's disease in childhood. Blood 42:163–174.
10. Mauch PM, Weinstein H, Botnick L et al. (1983). An evaluation of long-term survival and treatment complications in children with Hodgkin's disease. Cancer 51:925–932.
11. Wilimas J, Thompson E and Smith KL (1980). Long-term results of treatment of children and adolescents with Hodgkin's disease. Cancer 46:2123–2125.
12. Breu H, Schellong G, Grosch-Worner I et al. (1982). Graduated chemotherapy and reduced radiation dose in Hodgkin's disease in children: A report on 170 patients in a cooperative study HD-78. Klin Paediat 194:233–241.
13. Fossati-Bellani F, Kenda R, Lombardi F et al. (1984). ABVD combined with low dose limited field radiotherapy for Stage I, II, III childhood Hodgkin's disease. Proc Amer Assoc Cancer Res 25:195.
14. Donaldson SS and Kaplan HS (1982). Complications of treatment of Hodgkin's disease in children. Cancer Treat Rep 66:977–989.

15. Cham WC, Tan CTC, Martinez A et al. (1976). Involved field radiation therapy for early stage Hodgkin's disease in children. Preliminary results. Cancer 37:1625–1632.

16. Behrendt H and van Bunningen BFM (1984). Treatment of childhood Stage I and II Hodgkin's disease without radiotherapy. In: Cavalli F, Bonadonna G, and Rozencweig M (Eds). Malignant Lymphomas and Hodgkin's Disease: Experimental and Therapeutic Advances, pp 611–615. Boston: Martinus Nijhoff.

17. Ekert H and Waters KD (1983). Results of treatment of 18 children with Hodgkin's disease with MOPP chemotherapy as the only treatment modality. Med Pediat Oncol 11:322–326.

18. Bonadonna G, Viviani S, Bonfante V et al. (1984). Alternating chemotherapy with MOPP/ABVD in Hodgkin's disease. Proc Amer Soc Clin Oncol 3:254.

2. Treatment of childhood Stages I and II Hodgkin's disease without radiotherapy

H. BEHRENDT [1] and B. F. M. VAN BUNNINGEN [2]
Werkgroep Kindertumoren, [1] Emma Kinderziekenhuis and [2] Antoni van Leeuwenhoekziekenhuis, Amsterdam, the Netherlands

Introduction of the MOPP combination has significantly improved the prognosis of Hodgkin's disease (HD), especially in patients with extended disease [1]. For those with localized disease, however, radiotherapy remains the main treatment modality in most therapy protocols. Although this strategy is satisfactory in adult patients, resulting in disease-free survival rates of 80–90% for Stages I and II disease [2], radiotherapy has some disadvantages for children. Radiotherapy delivered during the period of growth and development frequently causes growth retardation of normal tissues and hypothyroidism. Moreover, sterility may develop after irradiation of the gonads and the incidence of second malignancies may be increased [3]. To avoid some of these sequelae, we started a treatment protocol in which MOPP was the major component. Radiotherapy was used only as adjuvant treatment for children having large tumor masses at entry. The treatment results are reported here.

Materials and methods

From 1975 to 1982, 31 consecutive untreated patients were entered. There were 5 girls and 26 boys, aged 5–15 years.

Patients were divided into two groups, i.e.:

1. Patients with only *small* lymph nodes (less than 4 cm). These patients were treated with MOPP chemotherapy only.
2. Patients with *large* lymph nodes (in excess of 4 cm). These children received bimodal treatment consisting of six MOPP cycles and involved field (IF) radiotherapy.

Clinical Stage (CS) was determined with the usual stage screening methods, including lymphangiography and bone marrow biopsy. No patient underwent laparotomy with splenectomy. The MOPP combination consisted of nitrogen mustard 6 mg/m^2 and vincristine 2 mg/m^2 both intra-

612

venously on days 1 and 8, procarbazine $80\,mg/m^2$ and prednisolone $40\,mg/m^2$ both orally on days 1–14. These courses were repeated at least six times at monthly intervals.

Sixteen patients with *small* tumors received MOPP chemotherapy without radiotherapy. Seven had CS I, three had CS II, and six had CS III disease. Lymphocytic predominance subtype was present in two, nodular sclerosis in nine, mixed cellularity in four and lymphocytic depletion in one. None of the seven Stage I patients had B-symptoms. These were seen in one Stage II and three Stage III patients. Fifteen patients received six MOPP cycles whereas one, who had Stage III disease, received twelve cycles.

Fifteen patients with *large* tumors received six MOPP cycles plus additional IF radiotherapy, 25 Gy, during 3 weeks. Only tumor masses in excess of 4 cm were irradiated. Radiotherapy was given between the third and the fourth MOPP cycle. Six patients had CS I, seven has CS II and two children had CS III disease. Seven had nodular sclerosis histology and eight had the mixed cellularity subtype. One patient with CS I, two with CS II, but none with CS III disease had B-symptoms.

Results

All patients achieved complete remission (Tables I and II) and four relapses have occurred so far (Fig. 1 and 2). All three relapses in Stage III patients were successfully retreated and these patients are still alive with no evidence of disease. One CS II patient relapsed after 26 months and died from progressive HD despite aggressive treatment. Of the relapsed patients, three

Table I. Small tumors

Stage	No.	CR	Rel	Months DFS (Med)
I	7	7	0	17^+–91^+ (45)
II	3	3	0	58^+–113^+ (82)
III	6	6	2	11^+–108^+ (57)

Table II. Large tumors

Stage	No.	CR	Rel	Months DFS (Med)
I	6	6	0	17^+–93^+ (57)
II	7	7	1	16^+–67^+ (44)
III	2	2	1	33–39^+ (36)

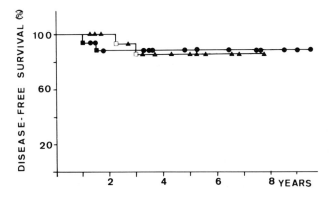

Figure 1. Disease-Free-Survival (DFS) in 31 consecutive children with Hodgkin's disease, all stages. DFS rate for children with small tumors (▲, □ = relapse) = 87%, for children with large tumors (●, ■ = relapse) = 86%.

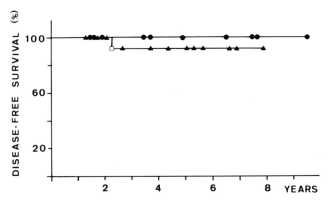

Figure 2. Disease-Free Survival (DFS) in 23 consecutive children with Stages I and II Hodgkin's disease. DFS rate for children with small tumors: 100%, for patients with large tumors: 92%. Symbols = see Fig. 1.

had nodular sclerosis and one had the mixed cellularity subtype. Only one of the relapsed patients had initially B-symptoms.

Special attention must be given to the 23 patients with CS I and II disease. In 10 patients with *small* lymph nodes, no relapse occurred after MOPP alone. Disease-free survival ranges from 17+ to 91+ months (median 45 months) for CS I patients and from 58+ to 113+ months (median 82 months) for those with CS II disease. Among 13 children with *large* lymph nodes treated with MOPP + IF radiotherapy, a single patient, who had initially CS II disease, relapsed after 26 months.

Discussion

There are only few studies concerning the treatment of HD in children with chemotherapy alone. In 1978, Olweny reported results of 48 Ugandan children who were treated with MOPP chemotherapy only [4]. Of 18 children with early stage disease (Stages IA-IIIA), all achieved complete remission and four relapsed. Of 30 late stage patients, 24 attained complete remission and seven of these relapsed. Actuarial survival was 75% for children with Stages I-IIIA disease and 60% for those with more advanced stages. Ekert reported on 18 children with HD treated with MOPP alone [5]. All but one had complete remission after a median follow-up time of 28 months; the actuarial disease-free survival was 80% and total survival was 92%.

In our study, complete remission was obtained in all children. Of 31 patients, 16 were treated with MOPP only, because they were arbitrarily categorized as having 'small tumors'. In this group, two patients with Stage III disease relapsed while no relapses occurred in the children with Stages I and II disease. From the 15 patients who received additional radiotherapy because they had 'large tumors', two patients relapsed, one with Stage II and one with Stage III disease. These results indicate that the relapse rate is more influenced by stage of disease than by size of lymph node invasion.

Because relapse-free survival rates in the two treatment groups are similar, we conclude that additional IF low-dose (25 Gy) radiotherapy is of no benefit for patients who are primarily treated with MOPP chemotherapy. Furthermore, our study indicates that all children with HD can be successfully treated with MOPP chemotherapy alone, without any decrease in the high survival rates obtained with radiotherapy with or without additional chemotherapy.

The advantages of primary chemotherapy in the treatment of children with HD are the avoidance of growth disturbances and hypothyroidism. Furthermore, it obviates the need for staging laparotomy and splenectomy. On the other hand, much attention must be given to the risk of infertility and second malignancies caused by the MOPP combination. The probability of developing sterility is highest among post-pubertal boys and the probability of recovering spermatogenic function is low. With respect to second malignancies, patients who receive bimodal treatment with MOPP plus radiotherapy have the highest risk [3].

We prefer combination chemotherapy as primary treatment for all children with HD. Drug combinations which have the same curative properties as MOPP but without its potential for long-term complications should be explored in large-scale trials.

References

1. DeVita VT, Serpick A and Carbone PP (1970). Combination chemotherapy in the treatment of advanced Hodgkin's disease. Ann Intern Med 73:881–895.

2. Tubiana M, Henry-Amar M, Hayat M et al. (1984). The EORTC treatment of early stage of Hodgkin's disease: The role of radiotherapy. Int J Radiat Oncol Biol Phys 10:197–210.
3. Donaldson SS and Kaplan HS (1982). Complications of treatment of Hodgkin's disease in children. Cancer Treat Rep 66:977–989.
4. Olweny CLM, Katongole-Mbidde E, Kiire C et al. (1978). Childhood Hodgkin's disease in Uganda. A ten year experience. Cancer 42:787–792.
5. Ekert H and Waters KD (1983). Results of treatment of 18 children with Hodgkin's disease with MOPP chemotherapy as the only treatment modality. Med Pediat Oncol 11:322–326.

3. Combined modality treatment with reduced chemotherapy and radiotherapy, and selective splenectomy, in children with Hodgkin's disease

G. SCHELLONG[1], S. STRAUCH[1], A. K. WAUBKE[1],
W. BRANDEIS[2], J. PAWLOWSKY[3], E. W. SCHWARZE[4],
H. RIEHM[5], H. J. LANGERMANN[6] and M. WANNENMACHER[7]
[1] Department of Pediatrics, University of Münster and [2] Heidelberg,
FRG, [3] St. Anna Hospital Wien, Austria, [4] Institute of Pathology,
University of Kiel, [5] Department of Pediatrics, Medizinische
Hochschule Hannover, [6] University of Berlin, and [7] Department of
Radiotherapy, University of Freiburg, FRG

Our therapeutic approach to childhood Hodgkin's disease (HD) has been guided by concerns of long-term complications associated with aggressive combined modality treatments [1]. The risk of developing secondary leukemia appears related to the extent and duration of therapy as well as the type of chemotherapeutic agents [2–4]. Repeated intensive treatment for recurrent disease seems to increase this risk noticeably [2, 4]. Various observations suggest that alkylating agents are especially responsible for both leukemogenesis and infertility [4].

Staging without laparotomy may frequently result in overtreating children with Stages I and IIA diseases [5, 6]. However, whether splenectomy is necessary remains a matter of controversy. Interest in the information derived from this diagnostic procedure must be weighed against increased likelihood of severe bacterial infections.

We have undertaken two consecutive trials with the overall objective of minimizing radiotherapy and chemotherapy as much as possible. Specifically, we aimed at reducing radiotherapy to involved fields, using the lowest dose necessary, with the rationale that appropriate chemotherapy could be sufficient to eradicate occult microfoci in adjacent lymphatic areas. The number of courses of chemotherapy and exposure to alkylating agents were limited and depended upon the stage of the disease.

Our purpose was also to reappraise the need for splenectomy and to define a staging policy which provided adequate evaluation of intra-abdominal disease so that overtreatment in early disease could be avoided. A detailed analysis of our staging findings in the first trial, in which conventional exploratory laparotomy and splenectomy were performed, allowed us, in a second study, to restrict splenectomy to selected cases with a high probability of splenic involvement [7, 8].

618

Protocol DAL-HD 78

This study examined whether the radiation dose to the extended fields could be halved when radiotherapy was combined with chemotherapy (Fig. 1) [7]. Patients were stratified according to Pathologic Stages (PS I and IIA versus PS IIB, III and IV). All were administered induction chemotherapy with two cycles of OPPA, i.e., vincristine (1.5 mg/m^2 i.v. on days 1, 8, and 15; maximal single dose 2.0 mg), procarbazine (100 mg/m^2 p.o. on days 1 to 15; maximal daily dose 150 mg), prednisone (60 mg/m^2 p.o. on days 1 to 15) and doxorubicin (40 mg/m^2 on days 1 and 15). Following these two courses of induction chemotherapy, all children received 35–40 Gy to the involved regions. In addition, they were randomly allocated to receive extended field radiation therapy with a dose of either 36–40 Gy or 18–20 Gy. No additional treatment was given for Stages I-IIA disease. In more advanced stages, radiotherapy was followed by adjuvant chemotherapy with four cycles of COPP, i.e., cyclophosphamide (500 mg/m^2 i.v. on days 1 and 8), vincristine (1.5 mg/m^2 on days 1 and 8; maximal single dose 2.0 mg) and procarbazine (100 mg/m^2 on days 1 to 14; maximal daily dose 150 mg) plus, in the first and fourth cycles, prednisone (40 mg/m^2 p.o. on days 1 to 14).

Exploratory laparotomy and splenectomy were required per protocol. Only children under the age of 5, and a few patients with Stage IV disease, did not undergo staging laparotomy. To reduce the risk of developing overwhelming bacterial infections, all children were given cotrimoxazol during chemotherapy and radiotherapy, followed by prophylactic penicillin for at least two years. Most patients received pneumococcal vaccination prior to splenectomy.

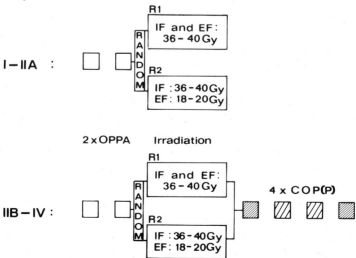

Figure 1. Protocol DAL-HD 78: Outline of the study. IF: involved field; EF: extended field; OPPA and COPP, see text.

Table I. Protocol DAL-HD 78: Sex and age distribution

Sex	Total	No. of patients by age (years)			
		< 5	5–10	10–15	> 15
M	109 (64%)	9	40	52	8
F	61 (36%)	2	12	45	2
	170 (100%)	11 (6%)	52 (31%)	97 (57%)	10 (6%)

Results

A total of 170 patients enrolled in the study between June 1978 and November 1981 at 47 centers [7]. The male to female ratio was 1.79 and the median age was 12.2 years with a range of 2.4 to 16.3 years (Table I). Pathologic Stage according to the Ann Arbor classification was determined in 164 patients (Table II). Six were not laparotomized.

In one-third of the patients (56/164), stage was altered after laparotomy and splenectomy; 23% were restaged as more severe disease, 11% as less advanced disease. There were 73 patients (42.9%) with disease in Stages I and IIA and 97 patients (57.1%) with more advanced stage disease. Of 154 splenectomized children, 60 (39%) had splenic involvement, 50 of whom also had abdominal lymph node involvement. Nine patients had nodal involvement in the abdomen without infiltration of the spleen. We evaluated the individual significance of 16 clinical and surgical findings for predicting splenic involvement (Table III). A statistically significant association to splenic involvement was established for only 6 (3 clinical and 3

Table II. Protocol DAL-HD 78: Distribution of stage according to the Ann Arbor classification

Stage	No. of patients
I A	37 (3) [a]
I B	4
II A	32
II B	17
III A	32 (1)
III B	35
IV A	4
IV B	9 (2)
	170 (6)

[a] ( ) = No. of patients in whom only clinical stage was obtained

Table III. Protocol DAL-HD 78 (154 patients): Significance of clinical variables and operative findings for predicting splenic involvement

Parameter	*p* value
Age	ns [a]
Sex	ns
B-Symptoms	0.003
Palpable enlargement of spleen	0.03
Site of lymph node involvement	
cervical (left)	ns
cervical (right)	ns
pharyngeal	ns
axillary (left)	ns
axillary (right)	ns
mediastinal	0.03
inguinal (left)	ns
inguinal (right)	ns
Nodular changes of splenic surface	<0.0001
Enlargement of lymph nodes	
splenic hilus/tail of pancreas	<0.0001
upper abdomen (other)	0.02
lower abdomen	ns

[a] Not significant

operative) of these variables. None, however, provided satisfactory discrimination between patients with and without splenic involvement, when considered singly. A multivariate analysis with the Cox linear logistic regression model indicated that changes in the splenic surface and enlargement of lymph nodes at the splenic hilus/tail of pancreas were most informative (Table IV) whereas the other parmeters could be disregarded. Three risk-groups were defined accordingly (Table V) and it was believed that splenectomy could be avoided in the lowest risk category.

Table IV. Protocol DAL-HD 78 (154 patients): Factors associated with splenic involvement (Cox linear logistic regression model)

Parameter	x^2	*p* value
Changes of splenic surface	32.94	<0.00001
Enlargement of lymph nodes at hilus of spleen/tail of pancreas	22.19	<0.00001
Mediastinal involvement	0.88	0.35
B-Symptoms	0.32	0.57
Enlargement of other upper-abdominal lymph nodes	0.27	0.63
Enlargement of spleen	0.22	0.64

Table V. Protocol DAL-HD 78 (154 patients): Risk groups according to splenic involvement

Group	Changes in splenic surface	Enlargement of lymph nodes at hilus of spleen/tail of pancreas	Incidence of splenic involvement
1	+	+/−	19/20 = 95%
2	−	+	22/36 = 61%
3	−	−	19/98 = 19%

One child with Stage IVB disease and severe clinical symptoms died on the 10th day of treatment. Two patients had progression in the lungs and/or skeleton during therapy. Complete remission occurred in 167/170 patients (98.2%), three-fourths of them before irradiation. Seven died in continuous remission 5 to 17 months after initiation of treatment, three due to pneumonia, two due to septicemia, one each due to varicella and GvH reaction after granulocyte transfusion. These seven patients had advanced stages of disease and had received high-dose extended field irradiation. As of March 1, 1984, six patients have relapsed, three in each of the two randomization groups. The remaining 154 complete responders have been in continuous first remission for 26 to 68 months. There are 160 patients still living. So far, no second malignancies have been observed.

The probability for disease-free survival after more than five years is 90% for the overall group; 94; for Stages I and IIA and 88% for Stages IIB to IV (Fig. 2). Poorer results in advanced stages (the difference is not significant)

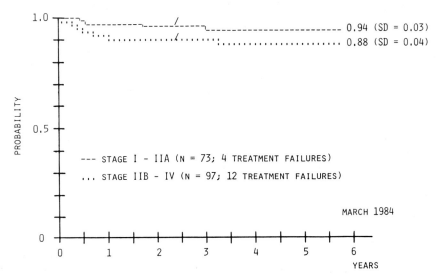

Figure 2. Protocol DAL-HD 78: Probability of disease-free survival by stage. Life table analysis according to Cutler and Ederer [9]. / = last patient of the group.

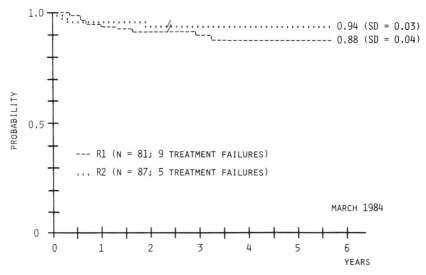

Figure 3. Protocol DAL-HD 78: Probability of disease-free survival by extended field radiation dose, R1 = high-dose; R2 = low dose (see Fig. 1). Life table analysis according to Cutler and Ederer [9]. / = last patient of the group.

are due to the seven deaths that occurred in patients in first remission. The difference in disease-free survival between the two randomization groups is also minimal with 5-year probabilities of 88% and 94%, respectively (Fig. 3).

Protocol DAL-HD 82

In this study, all patients receive chemotherapy followed by radiotherapy (Fig. 4). In Stages I-IIA patients, chemotherapy consists of two courses of OPPA. Those with more advanced disease also receive two courses of this regimen plus two (Stages IIB-IIIA) or four courses (Stages IIIB-IV) of COPP. Radiotherapy is limited to involved fields. The radiation dose is selected according to the number of cycles of chemotherapy: 35 Gy after two cycles, 30 Gy after four cycles, and 25 Gy after six cycles. This dose reduction was derived from favorable reports from Stanford [10] and Toronto [11].

Splenectomy is performed according to specific findings at laparotomy based on the previously mentioned analysis (Tables IV and V). The surgical procedure is as follows (Fig. 5). First, the splenic surface is examined by palpation and inspection. If the surface is nodular, indicating a high probability of splenic involvement, splenectomy is performed (approximately 13% of all patients). If, however, the surface is inconspicuous, the lymph

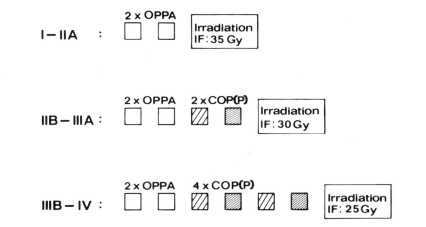

Figure 4. Protocol DAL-HD 82: Outline of the study. Abbreviations: see Fig. 1 and text.

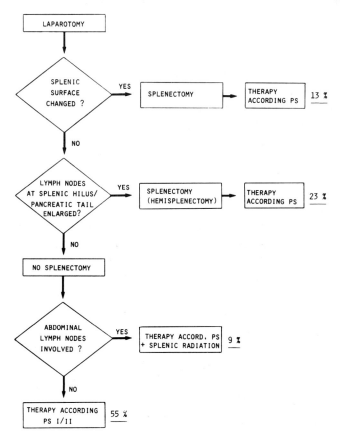

Figure 5. Protocol DAL-HD 82: Flow diagram for selective splenectomy.

nodes at the spleen and the tail of the pancreas are examined. If one or more lymph nodes of this group are enlarged, the probability for splenic involvement is approximately 60%, and splenectomy therefore is performed. This group includes approximately 23% of all patients. If both criteria are negative, splenectomy is not necessary. This applies to approximately 64% of all patients. If abdominal lymph nodes are involved in nonsplenectomized children, radiation therapy includes the spleen, since the probability of splenic involvement in such cases is about 70%. This affects approximately 9% of all patients. Splenic involvement is undetected in an additional 6%. Our strategy of selective splenectomy, therefore, can be used only in combination with chemotherapy.

Results

Between December 1981 and May 1984, 49 centers contributed 163 patients between 3 and 16 years of age to the study. Laparotomy according to our new strategy of selective splenectomy was done in 138 children. Performance of laparotomy and/or splenectomy diverged from our protocol outlines in the remaining 25 patients. Fifty-two patients (38%) were splenectomized and 38 (73%) removed spleens were involved (Table VI). These results correspond very closely to expectations. In 4 of 138 children, the spleen was irradiated. Among the 78 children with Stages I/IIA disease, 86% did not undergo splenectomy.

All patients achieved complete remission (Table VII). As of May 1984, with a median observation period of 16 months, only one child had a relapse in the lungs and this child had presented initially with pulmonary involvement. Two patients with Stage IIIB disease died of infection during disease remission and both were splenectomized. At this time, none of the 122 patients in the other two risk groups have relapsed or died. Therefore, the probabilities for disease-free survival after 2.5 years, as calculated with the life table method, are 100% for Stages I/IIA as well as for Stages IIB/IIIA and 89% for Stages IIIB/IV disease.

Table VI. Protocol DAL-HD 82: Results of selective splenectomy

	Percentage	
	Actual	Expected
Splenectomy/laparotomy	38 (52/138)	36
Splenic involvement/splenectomy	73 (38/52)	73

Table VII. Protocol DAL-HD 82: Interim therapeutic results (May 1984)

	No. of patients			
	Total	I, II A	II B, III A	III B/IV
Entered	163	78	44	41
Complete remission	163	78	44	41
Alive in first remission	160	78	44	38
Death during first remission	2	0	0	2
Recurrent disease	1	0	0	1

Discussion

Compared to conventional approaches, staging laparotomy, chemotherapy, and radiotherapy, can be appreciably reduced in the treatment of children with Hodgkin's disease if combined appropriately. Our preliminary results indicate that our strategy accurately identifies those patients for whom splenectomy is unnecessary for diagnosis and treatment of Hodgkin's disease.

In the second study, almost two-thirds of the patient population did not require splenectomy, according to our guidelines. In most children with Stages I/IIA, i.e., approximately one-half of the patients, an excellent outcome may be expected with laparotomy without splenectomy, two OPPA cycles, and involved field irradiation with 35 Gy. Our reduced combination modality treatment prevents relapses in those few children with undetected splenic microfoci. It may be hoped that this strategy will also favorably affect the incidence of long-term sequelae, but much longer follow-up is needed to assess this aspect of our treatment program.

References

1. Longo DL, Young RC and DeVita VT Jr (1982). Chemotherapy for Hodgkin's disease: The remaining challenges. Cancer Treat Rep 66:925–936.
2. Cadman EC, Capizzi RL and Bertino JR (1977). Acute non-lymphocytic leukemia. A delayed complication of Hodgkin's disease therapy: Analysis of 109 cases. Cancer 40:1280–1296.
3. Unger PF, Auclerc G, Weil M and Jacquillat C (1981). Tumeurs solides apres traitement pour maladie de Hodgkin. Nouv Presse Med 10:1463–1467.
4. Valagussa P, Santoro A, Fossati Bellani F et al. (1982). Absence of treatment-induced second neoplasma after ABVD in Hodgkin's disease. Blood 59:488–494.
5. Jenkin RDT, Freedman M, McClure P et al. (1979). Hodgkin's disease in children. Treatment with low dose irradiation and MOPP without staging laparotomy. Cancer 44:80-86.

6. Berkowicz M, Rath P, Aghai E et al. (1978). Selective splenectomy in Hodgkin's disease, Stages I and II. Israel J Med Sci 14:1275–1282.

7. Breu H, Schellong G, Grosch-Wörner I et al. (1982). Abgestufte Chemotherapie und reduzierte Strahlendosis beim Morbus Hodgkin im Kindersalter. Ein bericht über 170 Patienten der kooperativen Therapiestudie HD 78. Klin Pädiat 194:233–241.

8. Schellong G, Waubke AK, Langermann HJ et al. (1982). Bedeutung klinischer und intraoperativer Befunde für die Voraussage eines Milzbefalls beim Morbus Hodgkin im Kindesalter. Eine retrospektive statistische Analyse bei 154 Patienten der Therapiestudie HD 78. Klin Pädiat 194:242–250.

9. Cutler SJ and Ederer F (1958). Maximum utilization of the life table method in analyzing survival. J Chronic Dis 8:699–712.

10. Donaldson SS (1981). Pediatric Hodgkin's disease: Focus on the future. In: Eys JV and Sullivan MP (Eds.). Status of the Curability of Childhood Cancer, pp. 235–249. New York: Raven Press.

11. Jenkin RDT and Berry MP (1980). Hodgkin's disease in children. Semin Oncol 7:202–211.

4. Strategies for management of childhood non-Hodgkin's lymphomas based upon stage and immunopathologic subtype: Rationale and current results

S. B. MURPHY

St. Jude Children's Research Hospital, Memphis, Tennessee, USA

Treatment of children with non-Hodgkin's lymphoma (NHL) with intensive combined modality regimens, incorporating combination chemotherapy, involved field radiotherapy and prophylaxis of the central nervous system, reproducibly cures the majority, as demonstrated by a number of reports [1–4]. Cure of a majority of cases ought not to mask however the considerable heterogeneity characteristic of NHL, either in adult or pediatric age groups. While virtually all lymphomas in children are high grade malignancies, significant differences in the relapse hazard with modern therapy are related to the primary site, stage and immunopathologic subtype (T or B). A rational strategy for success in management of childhood NHL therefore requires consideration of these factors. The review will outline such a strategy, rationale and recent results.

Table I. A clinical staging classification for childhood NHL

Stage	Criteria for extent of disease
I	A single tumor (extranodal) or single anatomic areas (nodal), with the exclusion of mediastinum or abdomen.
II	A single tumor (extranodal) with regional node involvement. Two or more nodal areas on the same side of the diaphragm. Two single (extranodal) tumors with or without regional node involvement on the same side of the diaphragm. A primary gastrointestinal tract tumor, usually in the ileocecal area, with or without involvement of associated mesenteric nodes only, grossly completely resected.
III	Two single tumors (extranodal) on opposite sides of the diaphragm. Two or more nodal areas above and below the diaphragm. All the primary intra-thoracic tumors (mediastinal, pleural, thymic). All extensive primary intra-abdominal disease, unresectable. All paraspinal or epidural tumors, regardless of other tumor site(s).
IV	Any of the above with initial CNS and/or bone marrow involvement.

Staging

Table I outlines a clinical staging classification for childhood NHL. When coupled with information regarding the primary site of tumor, it provides a clear system for reporting and comparing end results of treatment. A number of reports have demonstrated the prognostic utility of such a system [1, 4], and other series confirm the good prognosis characteristic of children with localized disease (excluding mediastinum) [2, 3]. A more detailed discussion of this staging system, in comparison to others, and reasons for eschewing use of the Ann Arbor system for childhood NHL, has been published elsewhere [5].

Strategy of management

Following clinical staging, a useful strategy for management of children with NHL is shown in Fig. 1.

Identification of children with localized favorable presentations of disease (Stages I and II) permits recognition of a subgroup of children (approximately 30% of all cases) who are highly curable regardless of histopathologic subtype. Since 85–90% of these cases are cured by modern therapy [1–4], it is appropriate to test a reduction in the intensity of their treatment (see below).

The majority of childhood NHL cases are in non-localized unfavorable anatomic sites at diagnosis, often involving the marrow and/or central nervous system (Stages III and IV). These cases clearly require further subclassification into two major groups: either lymphoblastic, T-cell derived or non-lymphoblastic, B-cell derived; and each group properly requires development of an effective treatment based upon differences in natural history, relapse patterns, and drug sensitivity. Investigators of the Children's Cancer Study Group have shown that treatment success for patients with disseminated disease is influenced both by the histologic subtype of disease and the therapeutic regimen followed. A 10-drug treatment program was more effective than a 4-drug regimen for patients with disseminated lymphoblastic disease (76% vs 26% 2-year disease-free survival), whereas the 4 drug regimen was more effective than the 10-drug program for non-lymphoblastic disease (57% vs 28%, respectively) [3].

This strategy outlined in Fig. 1 is generally applicable to roughly 95% of cases of childhood NHL, but exceptions exist and deserve individual consideration. These exceptions include: nodular lymphomas (2% of all childhood NHL) [6], mediastinal non-lymphoblastic tumors (3%) [7], large cell lymphomas, primary in skin (< 1%), and 'true' histiocytic neoplasms (1%). Whether it is either feasible or clinical relevant to further subdivide the

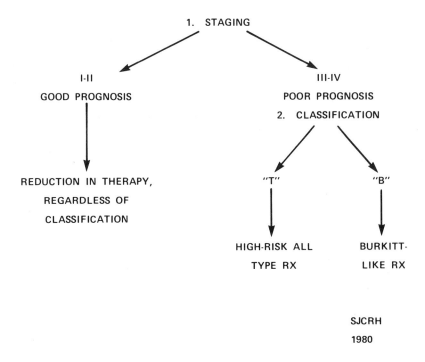

Figure 1. Childhood NHL strategies for management.

categories of Stages III-IV non-lymphoblastic lymphomas (large cell, immunoblastic, versus small, non-cleaved, Burkitt or non-Burkitt's pleomorphic) is doubtful, but requires further study.

Recent results

Stages I and II NHL

Recognizing the frequency and severity of both the acute toxicity and long-term adverse consequences of intensive combined modality therapy administered to the growing child, in 1978 we began testing the feasibility of reducing the intensity of treatment. Results in 28 children with Stages I or II NHL treated at our center from 1978–1982 have recently been published [8]. The two-year disease-free survival rate was 85.7%, not significantly different from other more intensive regimens. Results provide encouragement for further controlled trials in more children with localized lymphomas.

Consequently, the Pediatric Oncology Group is prospectively testing the contribution (if any) of involved field radiotherapy to a multiple drug regimen of moderate intensity and short duration (six months) by randomizing Stages I and II patients to receive either drug treatment alone or drugs plus radiotherapy. A preliminary report of this trial has appeared, and results so far are excellent [9], with a 100% CR rate and no relapses to date, in over thirty children.

Stages III-IV (T) lymphoblastic NHL

In view of the numerous clinical and biologic similarities between lymphoblastic T-NHL and T-acute lymphoblastic leukemia, and the frequency of marrow involvement and leukemic evolution of T-NHL cases in childhood, it is rational to approach the two disorders with the same therapeutic strategy. In this context, it should be noted that the LSA_2-L_2 therapy which has proven so effective for management of lymphoblastic lymphomas, particularly with mediastinal presentations [2, 3], was developed originally at Memorial Sloan-Kettering Cancer Center as leukemia therapy.

Since 1979 at St. Jude Children's Research Hospital, we have treated Stages III-IV lymphoblastic NHL on the same protocol (Total Therapy X-High Risk) as high-risk forms of acute lymphoblastic leukemia. The background, rationale and schema for the early and intermittent use of the combination of the epipodophyllotoxin VM-26 and cytosine arabinoside, imposed on a conventional anti-leukemia regimen (vincristine, prednisone, asparaginase, methotrexate, mercaptopurine, and CNS prophylaxis), has been described elsewhere [10], and preliminary results of the successful application of this treatment to children with advanced stages of lymphoblastic NHL have been reported [11]. Since 1979, we have treated a total of 22 children with Stages III-IV lymphoblastic NHL and have obtained a 95% complete response rate, with only 3 relapses occurring so far, with a median follow-up of two years from diagnosis [12]. These results represent a significant improvement, compared to our previous institutional experience [1] and provide evidence supporting the incorporation of VM-26 and cytosine arabinoside into future therapeutic trials for lymphoblastic lymphomas. Notably, the results were achieved with a regimen completely lacking anthracyclines, cyclophosphamide, high dose methotrexate, or mediastinal radiotherapy.

Others have also recently demonstrated improvements in the outcome of patients with advanced stage lymphoblastic NHL, and the challenge for future therapists will be to reduce the toxicity of these multiple drug therapies, whilst retaining cure of the majority of children.

Stages III-IV (B) non-lymphoblastic NHL

This group of children, composed of locally advanced or disseminated cases of diffuse undiffereniated, Burkitt's-type or immunoblastic NHL, constitute the most difficult to treat, characterized by a high frequency of metabolic complications related to massive tumor cell burdens, frequent failures to attain remission, and early relapse.

Since 1979 at St. Jude Children's Research Hospital we have adopted a treatment based upon appreciation of rapid tumor growth kinetics, consisting of high dose fractionated cyclophosphamide treatments (300 mg/m^2 q12 h × 6 doses) followed by vincristine and doxorubicin, alternating with continuous infusions of high doses of methotrexate and cytosine arabinoside. Rationale for this approach, drug doses and schedule of treatment, and results in 29 children with advanced B-cell disease treated at our center from 1979–83 have been presented in detail elsewhere [13]. Results with this approach are encouraging, particularly for Stage III cases (100% complete remission, with 10 of 11 remaining disease-free) but further improvements in the outcome for children with advanced disease initially involving the bone marrow and/or CNS are still necessary.

Intensive chemotherapy schedules have likewise been introduced for treatment of advanced stages of B-cell disease in children in Europe and have been used with notable success, particularly the French LMB-01-02 protocols and the German BFM-81-83, as reviewed recently by Lemerle [14].

Acknowledgements

Work was supported in part by a grant from NIH (CA 21765) and by ALSAC.

References

1. Murphy SB and Hustu HO (1980). A randomized trial of combined modalities therapy of childhood non-Hodgkin's lymphoma. Cancer 45:630–637.
2. Wollner N (1982). LSA$_2$ – L$_2$ in childhood non-Hodgkin's lymphoma. In: Rosenberg SA and Kaplan H (Eds.). Malignant Lymphomas, pp. 603–626. New York: Academic Press Inc.
3. Anderson JR, Wilson JF, Jenkin DT et al. (1983). Childhood non-Hodgkin's lymphoma. The results of a randomized therapeutic trial comparing a four drug regimen (COMP) with a ten drug regimen (LSA$_2$ – L$_2$). N Engl J Med 308:559–565.
4. Magrath IT, Janus C, Edwards BK et al. (1984). An effective therapy for both undifferentiated (including Burkitt's) lymphomas and lymphoblastic lymphomas in children and young adults. Blood 63:1102–1111.

632

5. Murphy SB (1980). Classification, staging and end results of treatment of childhood non-Hodgkin's lymphomas: Dissimilarities from lymphomas in adults. Semin in Oncology 7:332–339.
6. Frizzera G and Murphy SB (1979). Follicular (nodular) lymphoma in childhood: A rare clinical pathologic entity. Cancer 44:2218–2235.
7. Bunin N, Hvizdala E, Link M et al. (1984). Mediastinal non-lymphoblastic lymphomas in children: Clinical pathologic features. Proc Amer Soc Clin Oncol 3:240.
8. Murphy SB, Hustu HO, Rivera G and Berard CW (1983). End results of treating children with localized non-Hodgkin's lymphomas with a combined modality approach of lessened intensity. J Clin Oncol 1:326–330.
9. Link M, Donaldson S, Berard C and Murphy S (1984).Effective therapy with reduced toxicity for children with localized non-Hodgkin's lymphoma. Proc Amer Soc Clin Oncol 3:251.
10. Rivera G, Dahl GV, Murphy SB et al. (1983). The epipodophyllotoxin VM-26 in treatment of high-risk acute lymphoblastic leukemia: Rationale and early results. In: Murphy SB and Gilbert JR (Eds.). Leukemia Research: Advances in Cell Biology and Treatment, pp. 213–220. Elsevier Science Publishing Co.
11. Dahl G, Murphy S, Abromowitch M et al. (1983). VM-26 plus ara-C as initial and intermittent treatment for Stage III-IV lymphoblastic lymphoma and acute lymphoblastic leukemia with a mediastinal mass. Proc Amer Soc Clin Oncol 2:216.
12. Dahl GV et al. (in preparation).
13. Murphy SB, Bowman WP, Hustu HO and Berard CW (1984). Advanced stage (III-IV) Burkitt's lymphoma and B-cell ALL in children: Kinetic and pharmacologic rationale for treatment and recent results (1979-1983). In: O'Conor GT and Lenoir G (Eds.). Burkitt's Lymphoma. IARC-WHO Publications (in press).
14. Lemerle J (1984). The treatment of B-cell non-Hodgkin's malignant lymphomas of childhood in Europe – recent and ongoing studies. In: O'Conor GT and Lenoir G (Eds.). Burkitt's Lymphomas. IARC-WHO Publications (in press).

5. BFM trials for childhood non-Hodgkin's lymphomas

St. MÜLLER-WEIHRICH[1], G. HENZE[2], E. ODENWALD[3]
and H. RIEHM[3]

*Departments of Pediatrics: [1] Technische Universität München,
München, [2] Freie Universität Berlin and
[3] Medizinische Hochschule Hannover, FRG*

A total of 215 patients with highly-malignant non-Hodgkin's lymphoma (NHL) were treated in two consecutive studies of the German BFM Multicenter Study Group, 116 from 1975 to 1981 and 99 from 1981 to 1983. All were less than 18 years of age, had no or minor pretreatment and less than 25% bone marrow blasts. The Murphy's staging system was used [1]. However, in the 81/83 study, Stage II NHL of immuno-histologic B-type was subdivided into resectable (Stage 'II-R') and unresectable disease (Stage 'II-NR'). The former consisted mostly of abdominal disease and was treated much less intensively. Histologic classification was performed according to the Kiel classification.

B-type NHL included Burkitt-type lymphoblastic, lymphoblastic B-non-Burkitt, centroblastic and most immunoblastic lymphomas. Whenever possible, the classification as B- or non-B-NHL was confirmed by immunologic methods. A small number of primarily intra-abdominal lymphomas were considered of the B type despite inconclusive histology, immunology or both since a primary site in the abdomen is highly specific for B-type lymphomas.

Treatment in the study 1976/81

In the 1976/81 study, all patients were treated, irrespective of immunohistologic subtype, with a chemotherapeutic regimen that had demonstrated high effectiveness against childhood acute lymphoblastic leukemia (Fig. 1) [2]. Induction chemotherapy (Protocol I) was administered for 8 weeks following an initial course of high-dose cyclophosphamide. High-risk patients defined as those with primary CNS-involvement and/or disseminated intra-abdominal disease also received a 6-week reinduction program (Protocol II).

Protocol I consisted of two consecutive 4-drug regimens (Fig. 2). It also

634

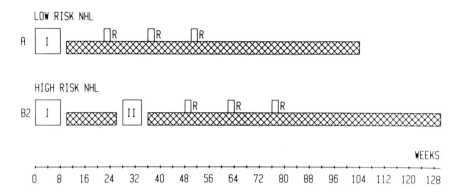

Figure 1. Therapy study BFM NHL 1975/81: study design. I: Protocol I; II: Protocol II; R: prednisone/vincristine reinduction pulses; shadowed areas: Continuation therapy with oral 6-mercaptopurine and methotrexate.

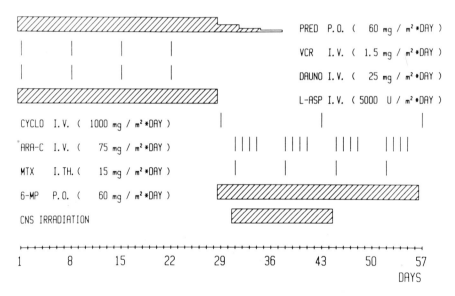

Figure 2. Protocol I of BFM NHL studies 1975/81 and 1981/83.
PRED: prednisone; VCR: vincristine; DAUNO: daunorubicine;
L-ASP: L-asparaginase; CYCLO: Cyclophosphamide;
ARA-C: cytosine-arabinoside; MTX: methotrexate;
6-MP: 6-mercaptopurine.
Study 1975/81: One single dose of CYCLO (1000 mg/m^2) five days before Protocol I
Study 1981/83: Cytoreductive prephase before Prot. I; Two doses of CYCLO only in Phase 2,
    Protocol I Age dependent doses of intrathecal MTX (see Fig. 5).

635

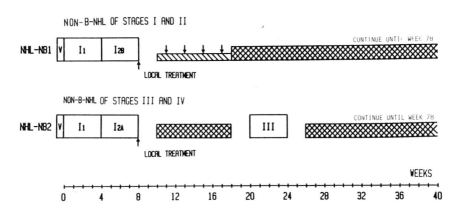

Figure 3. Therapy study BFM NHL 1981/83: study design for non-B-NHL.
V: Cytoreductive prephase; I_1: Protocol I, Phase 1;
I_{2A}: Protocol I, Phase 2 with CNS irradiation
I_{2B}: Protocol I, Phase 2 without CNS irradiation
III: Protocol III, arrows: MTX intrathecally and 24-hr parenteral infusion (500 mg/m^2) with leucovorine rescue after 48 hr; shadowed areas: oral 6-MP and MTX.

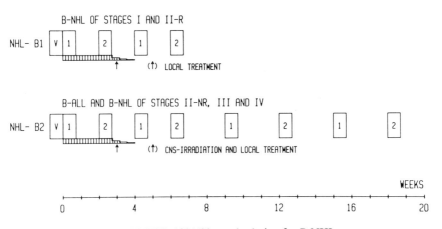

Figure 4. Therapy study BFM NHL 1981/83: study design for B-NHL
V: cytoreductive prephase; 1: block 1; 2: block 2;
shadowed area: prednisone 60 mg/m^2 daily.

included CNS-prophylaxis with intrathecal methotrexate and cranial irra-diaton. Protocol II, involved only slightly different agents as compared to Protocol I. Localized tumors were irradiated with about 30 Gy. Results were excellent in non-B-type NHL, but highly unsatisfactory in disseminated B-type lymphomas. In 1981, our treatment policy for NHL was adapted to clinical stage and a new approach to B-type NHL was investigated.

636

Treatment in the study 1981/83

Non-B-NHL was treated according to Protocol I (Fig. 2 and 3) after a cyto-reductive prephase with cyclophosphamide and prednisone. In localized stages, cranial irradiation was omitted; intrathecal and intermediate i.v. doses of methotrexate were given for CNS-prophylaxis and additional systemic therapy. Patients with disseminated non-B-lymphomas received a 4-week reinduction therapy (Protocol III) with cytostatic drugs similar to those of Protocol I. Continuation chemotherapy was terminated after 1.5 years. Thymic tumors were not irradiated unless there was evidence of residual tumor after treatment according to Protocol I.

Patients with B-type NHL received two alternating chemotherapy blocks after cytoreductive prephase (Fig. 4 and 5). Four of these therapy blocks were given within 8 weeks to patients with Stage I and II-R and eight blocks

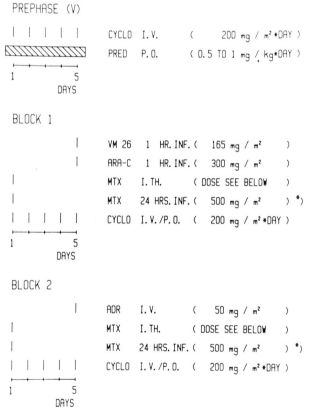

Figure 5. Therapy study BFM NHL 1981/83: therapy elements for B-NHL
* Leukovorine rescue 48 hr after start of MTX-infusion.
Intrathecal MTX doses: under 1 year: 6 mg; 1-2 years: 8 mg; 2-3 years: 10 mg; over 3 years: 12 mg.

within about 20 weeks to those with more advanced stages. No continuation therapy was given. Prophylactic CNS-irradiation was restricted to patients with advanced stages. In disseminated and non-resectable intra-abdominal lymphomas, a second look laparatomy was performed after the second or third therapy block. The abdomen was not irradiated unless residual tumor persisted after second look laparatomy. Since no residual tumor was found at second look laparatomy in a majority of the patients, towards the end of the study, this operation was undertaken only if non-invasive diagnostic procedures showed evidence of persisting tumor.

Patients

In the 81/83 study, 56 patients had B-type NHL and 42 non-B-type NHL. Most had advanced stage disease (Table I). Stage II-R lymphomas were often ileocoecal primaries. Abdominal primary tumors were always B-lymphomas and the vast majority of mediastinal primary tumors were non-B-lymphomas. Other primary sites were much less frequent and not type specific (Table II). Male preponderance was about 3:1 in B- as well as in non-B-NHL.

Therapy results

The probability of continuous complete remission (CCR) was calculated by

Table I. BFM NHL study 1981/83: Stages, initial bone marrow and CNS involvement: primary sites in Stage II-R B-NHL

	All patients (n = 98)	B-NHL (n = 56)	Non-B-NHL (n = 42)
Stage I	14	8	6
Stage II	18	15	3
Stage II-R		11 [a]	
Stage II-NR		4	
Stage III	48	27	21
Stage IV	18	6	12
Bone marrow/CNS manifestation at diagnosis in Stage IV			
Bone marrow	14	3	11
CNS	3	2	1
Bone marrow and CNS	1	1	

[a] Primary tumors in B-NHL, Stage II-R: ileocoecal (8), ileum (1), colon (1), cervical lymph nodes (1).

638

Table II. BFM NHL study 1981/83: Primary sites

	All patients (n = 98)	B-NHL (n = 56)	Non-B-NHL (n = 42)
Abdomen	36	36	—
Mediastinum	30	2	28
Cervical lymph nodes	10	6	4
Peripheral lymph nodes	5	2	3
Nasopharynx	5	3	2
Skeletal system	6	4	2
Other locations	6	3	3

Other locations: B-NHL: skin, cerebrum, ovaries; Non-B-NHL: orbita, testes, mamma

life table analysis [3]. In the 75/81 study, 14 (12.1%) of the 116 highly malignant NHL could not be classified with certainty as B- or non-B-lymphomas. These patients are included in the life table analyses of the total group, but omitted from the type-specific analyses. In B-NHL, the groups analyzed in the stage-specific life tables are not identical for the two studies, since Stage II B-NHL was subclassified, in 1981, according to resectability.

For the entire groups, probabilities of CCR were 64% after 9 years in the 75/81 study, and 80% after approximately 3 years in the more recent trial (Fig. 6). The corresponding figures for the few Stage I or II non-B-NHL patients were 60% and 89%, respectively (Fig. 7). The single relapse in

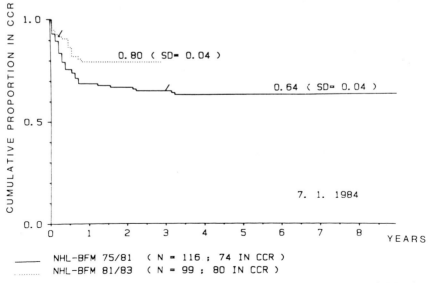

Figure 6. BFM NHL studies 1975/81 and 1981/83: Cumulative proportion of CCR in all patients.

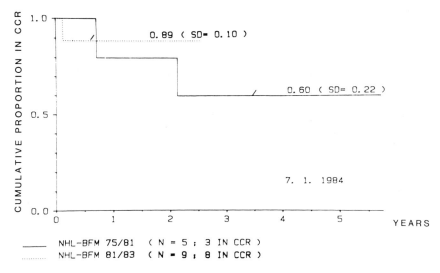

Figure 7. BFM NHL studies 1975/81 and 1981/83: Cumulative proportion of CCR in Stages I and II Non-B-NHL.

localized non-B-lymphomas occurred in a patient who had B-type lymphoma upon relapse and, therefore, might have been misdiagnosed at entry. In advanced stage non-B-lymphomas, the probability of CCR was nearly the same in both studies (Fig. 8), as might have been expected with very similar treatment.

None of the 19 patients with Stage I and II-R B-NHL have relapsed in the 81/83 study, while 5 of 26 patients with Stage I or II B-NHL relapsed in the

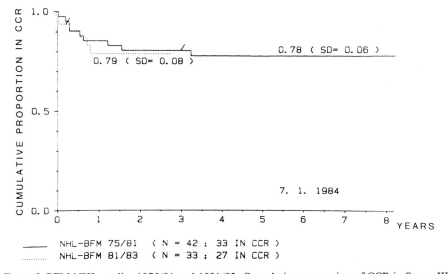

Figure 8. BFM NHL studies 1975/81 and 1981/83: Cumulative proportion of CCR in Stages III and IV Non-B-NHL.

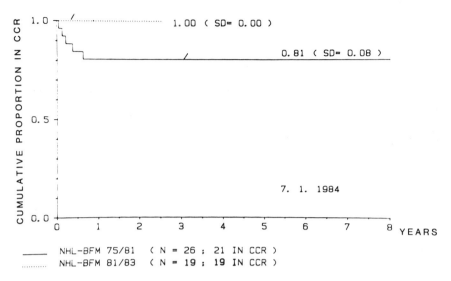

Figure 9. BFM NHL studies 1975/81 and 1981/83: Cumulative proportion of CCR in Stages I and II (study 1975/81) and Stages I and II-R (study 1981/83) B-NHL.

previous study (Fig. 9). Probability of CCR in Stages II/II-NR/IV B-NHL was 34% in the 75/81 study, in contrast to 67% in the 81/83 study (Fig. 10). All 4 patients with Stage II-NR B-NHL in the recent study are in CCR. In B-NHL, relapses occurred exclusively within 7 months after diagnosis in both studies.

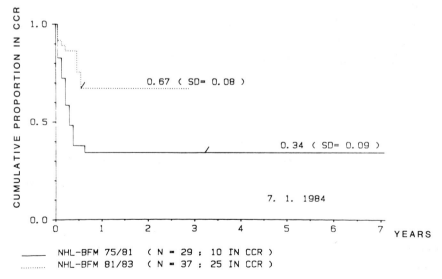

Figure 10. BFM NHL studies 1975/81 and 1981/83: Cumulative proportion of CCR in Stages III and IV (study 1975/81) and Stages II-NR – IV (study 1981/83) B-NHL.

Table III. BFM NHL study 1981/83: Outcome of the patients

Stages	B-NHL		Non-B-NHL	
	I/II-R	II-NR/IV	I/II	III/IV
Patients on study	19	37	9	33
Non-responders	0	1	0	0
Death without relapse	0	3	0	2
Relapses	0	8	1	4
(after months)		(1–6)	(1)	(3–9)
bone marrow	0	0	0	9
CNS	0	3	0	0
local	0	3	1	3
combined	0	2	0	1
In complete continuous remission	19	25	8	27
(after months)	(3–30)	(6–33)	(6–29)	(2–31)

The causes of therapeutic failure (study 81/83) in 12/56 patients with B-NHL and 7/42 patients with non-B-NHL are shown in Table III. One non-responder with primarily intra-cerebral B-NHL and very poor condition at presentation died a few days after initiation of chemotherapy. In advanced stage B-NHL, 3/37 patients died of iatrogenic causes. Four of the eight relapses in this group were CNS relapses, either isolated (three) or combined with local recurrence (one).

Of the 33 patients with Stages III and IV non-B-NHL, two with mediastinal lymphomas died of respiratory or cardiac complications before initiation of chemotherapy. Four patients relapsed either locally (mediastinum, two; peripheral nodes, one) or simultaneously in the bone marrow and lymph nodes (one).

Discussion

During the last decade, several studies have contributed to dramatically improve the prognosis of childhood NHL [4–6]. It is now widely accepted that treatment of these diseases must be adapted to immuno-histologic types [6–10]. In our studies, two entities (B- and non-B-NHL) were defined with characteristic features in terms of histology, immunology, predominant primary site, prognosis, response to chemotherapy, and time to relapse. Our results have been remarkable. In localized stages of both B- and non-B-NHL, virtually all patients of our recent study are alive free of disease. Overtreatment has to be avoided in this group. Though none of the 81/83

642

patients with localized NHL received cranial irradiation, no CNS relapses wee observed in localized disease.

In disseminated non-B-NHL, further effort should be devoted to prevent local relapses which are seen mostly in the mediastinum. In disseminated B-type lymphomas, relapses occur predominantly in the abdomen and the CNS. Second look laparatomy seems indicated at least for patients in whom conventional diagnostic procedures suggest the presence of residual tumor after initial chemotherapy. Abdominal irradiation does not seem very effective. CNS invasion at presentation or upon relapse occurs frequently in disseminated B-NHL, and even more so in childhood acute lymphoblastic leukemia of B-type. In our study, these diseases are treated similarly. Of 22 patients with B-ALL, six died of CNS relapses resistant to cranial irradiation. New strategies for CNS disease are urgently needed, but, unfortunately, promising alternatives are currently lacking.

References

1. Murphy SB (1980). Classification, staging and end results of treatment of childhood non-Hodgkin's lymphomas: Dissimilarities from lymphomas in adults. Semin Oncol 7:332–339.
2. Riehm HJ, Gadner H, Henze G et al. (1983). Acute lymphoblastic leukemia: Treatment results in three BFM studies (1979–1981). In: Murphy SB and Gilbert JR (Eds.). Leukemia Research: Advances in Cell Biology and Treatment, pp. 251–263. Elsevier Science Publishing Co.
3. Cutler SJ and Ederer F (1958). Maximum utilization of the life table method in analyzing survival. J Chron Dis 8:699–712.
4. Kersey JH, Lebien TW, Hurwitz R et al (1979). Childhood leukemia-lymphoma. Heterogeneity of phenotypes and prognoses. Amer J Clin Pathol 72 (Suppl.):746–752.
5. Müller-Weihrich St, Henze G, Jobke A et al. (1982). BFM-Studie 1975/81 zur Behandlung der Non-Hodgkin-Lymphome hoher Malignität bei Kindern und Jugendlichen. Klin Pädiat 194:219–225.
6. Pichler E, Jürgenssen OA, Radaszkiewicz T et al. (1982). Results of LSA$_2$-L$_2$ therapy in 26 children with non-Hodgkin's lymphoma. Cancer 50:2740–2746.
7. Gasparini M, Lombardi F, Fossati-Bellani F et al. (1983). Childhood non-Hodgkin's lymphoma: Prognostic relevance of clinical stages and histologic subgroups. Amer J Pediat Hematol Oncol 5:161–171.
8. Anderson JR, Wilson JF, Jenkin RDT et al. (1983). Childhood non-Hodgkin's lymphoma. The results of a randomized therapeutic trial comparing a 4-drug regimen (COMP) with a 10-drugs regimen (LSA$_2$-L$_2$). N Engl J Med 308:559–565.
9. Wollner N, Exelby PR, Liebermen PH (1980). Non-Hodgkin's lymphoma in children. A progress report on the original patients treated with the LSA$_2$-L$_2$ protocol chemotherapy. Cancer 45:3034–2039.
10. Patte C, Philip T, Bernard A et al. (1984). Improvement of survival of Stage IV B-cell non-Hodgkin lymphoma (NHL) and B acute leukemia (B-ALL). A study of the French Pediatric Oncology Society (SFOP). Proc Second International Conference on Malignant Lymphoma, Lugano, Switzerland-34.

6. Characteristics and results of treatment of non-Hodgkin's lymphoma in young people – Experience of the Pediatric Branch, NCI, USA

I. T. MAGRATH[1], E. SARIBAN[1] and B. EDWARDS[2]
[1] Pediatric Branch and [2] Biometric Research Branch. Division of Cancer Treatment, National Cancer Institute, National Institutes of Health, Bethesda, Maryland, USA

In 1977, a protocol for the treatment of childhood non-Hodgkin's lymphoma, known as 77–04 was initiated at the Pediatric Branch of the National Cancer Institute (NCI), USA. The objective of this protocol was to provide information on prognostic factors in non-Hodgkin's lymphoma in young people. At that time, data on this subject were scanty and, in general, results of therapy were extremely poor with few exceptions [1].

Prior to protocol 77–04, only patients with Burkitt's lymphoma had been treated at the Pediatric Branch (PB) of the NCI, using a drug combination recently selected for the treatment of African patients with Burkitt's lymphoma. The early NCI protocols consisted of only 3 cycles of therapy and produced an overall prolonged disease-free survival of 40–50%.

In Protocol 77–04, all histologic types of non-Hodgkin's lymphoma were to be included and treated with the same drug regimen. In protocols being used at that time in other centers, including the LSA_2-L_2 protocol [1], chemotherapy was administered for a period of about two years. This contrasted dramatically with the three cycles of therapy administered to patients with Burkitt's lymphoma at the NCI. We chose an intermediate duration of therapy for Protocol 77–04 of about one year (estimated as 15 cycles of therapy) except in patients with localized undifferentiated lymphoma or completely resected abdominal disease. Based on data from Africa and the NCI, these groups were expected to do well with much less therapy. We hoped to achieve better results in extensive Burkitt's lymphoma by continuing treatment for the entire period in which patients were at risk to relapse. Since no information was available as to an appropriate therapy duration in lymphoblastic lymphoma, we opted to treat these patients also for 15 cycles.

644

Preliminary information from Bleyer (unpublished data) and Djerassi [2], suggested that high dose of methotrexate (HD-MTX) was effective therapy for childhood lymphomas, and this was substituted for the standard methotrexate dose used previously. Because HD-MTX would provide some therapy to the central nervous system (CNS), no additional prophylactic CNS therapy was initially planned. The occurrence of four isolated CNS relapses among the first 19 patients, however, persuaded us to incorporate an intensive intrathecal prophylactic regimen into the protocol. This was based on a regimen successful in the treatment of overt CNS disease in both African and American patients with Burkitt's lymphoma.

The NCI Pediatric Branch series is unusual in several respects. Although the lymphomas studied are those which occur predominantly in childhood, the age range is 2–35 years, with a median age of 17 years. This has provided an opportunity to assess the influence of age on prognosis. In addition, patients with extensive bone marrow involvement were included, whereas many pediatric non-Hodgkin's lymphoma series are confined to patients with less than 25% of tumor cells in the bone marrow.

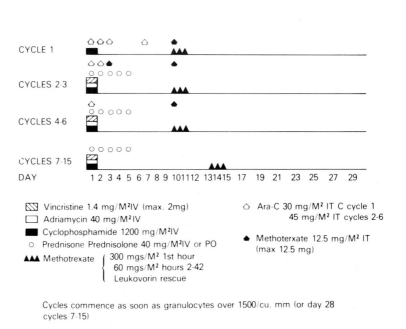

Figure 1. Treatment schema used in Protocol 77–04.

Materials and methods

Treatment

Treatment consisted of a 4-drug regimen (cyclophosphamide, adriamycin, vincristine and prednisone) alternating with a 42-hour methotrexate infusion followed by leucovorin rescue (48 mg/m^2 at hour 42, then 12 mg/m^2 every 6 hours until serum MTX is below 5×10^{-8} M). Doses and the general schema are provided in Fig. 1. In the first cycle, likely to be complicated by renal and metabolic problems resulting from rapid tumor lysis, cyclophosphamide was given alone instead of the 4-drug regimen. Intrathecal prophylaxis using methotrexate and cytosine arabinoside (ara-C) was administered during the first 6 cycles (Fig. 1), with the methotrexate infusion commencing on day 10. Thereafter, in all patients except those with limited or completely resected undifferentiated lymphomas (who received no further theapy) methotrexate administered on day 14, and a further nine cycles of therapy were given.

Radiation therapy was not used except in emergencies such as spinal cord compression (1 patient), SVC obstruction (1 patient) or optic nerve involvement (1 patient). One additional patient with localized bone involvement received radiation in addition to chemotherapy.

Patients

As of May 1984, 85 patients between 2 and 35 years old have been entered into the protocol. Seventy-six presented prior to May 10, 1983, and 75 of these patients have been deemed evaluable as of May 1984. One patient who died within a day of the commencement of chemotherapy has been excluded from the evaluation. The median duration of follow-up is four years.

Table I. Distribution of age and sex by disease

	Total	Lymphoblastic lymphoma		Non-lymphoblastic lymphoma	
		M	F	M	F
16 years or less	37	3	3 (1:1)	25	6 (4:1)
17 years or more	38	7	2 (3:1)	22	7 (3:1)
All ages	75	10	5 (2:1)	47	13 (3.6:1)

Table II. Classification of patients by two clinical staging schemes

St. Jude Stage	Lympho-blastic	PB Stage (non-lymphoblastic)				
		A and AR	B	C	D	Total
I and II	3	10	2	0	0	15 (20%)
III	8	7	2	11	15	43 (58%)
IV	4	0	2	0	10	16 (22%)
Total	15 (20%)	17 (23%)	6 (8%)	11 (15%)	25 (35%)	

Characteristics regarding age and sex are shown in Table I. Fifteen patients had lymphoblastic lymphoma, and 59 non-lymphoblastic lymphoma, either undiffereniated [55] or large cell (4). Forty-four of the 55 with undifferentiated lymphoma were diagnosed as Burkitt's lymphoma. One patient had an unclassifiable lymphoma and, in this analysis, is included only in general tabulations and overall curves of disease-free interval and survival.

The distribution of patients among various clinical stages is shown in Table II, in which the two staging systems used in this study are compared. One, based on a classification devised for African Burkitt's lymphoma [3] and used at the NCI, is applied here only to non-lymphoblastic lymphomas. A second staging system devised by Murphy at St. Jude Hospital [4] for

Table III. Major anatomic sites of involvement at presentation in 74 patients

	Burkitt's	Lymphoblastic	Other [a]
Abdomen	40	1	11
Pleural effusion	10	6	2
Bone marrow	9	3	2
Jaw	6	0	2
Pharynx	6	1	0
Bone (excluding jaw)	4	2	3
CSF/Cranial nerves	4	1	1
Testis	3	0	2
Peripheral lymphadenopathy	3	6	4
Paraspinal	2	0	0
Mediastinal	2	9	1
Total patients [b]	44	15	15

[a] Includes patients with undifferentiated non-Burkitt's or large cell lymphomas
[b] N.B. many patients had multiple sites of involvement
   One patient with generalized lymphadenopathy and indeterminate type of lymphoma is not included here

non-Hodgkin's lymphoma is used here to classify all patients. Stages III and IV together accounted for 80% of the patients. All patients with bone marrow involvement had greater than 50% marrow replacement and are classified as Stage IV in the St. Jude schema, although the original St. Jude staging system excluded patients with greater than 25% tumor cells in the bone marrow.

Major anatomic sites of involvement for patients in each histologic group are shown in Table III. Of interest is the finding that 40 of 44 (91%) patients with Burkitt's lymphoma and 51 of 59 (86%) patients with non-lymphoblastic lymphomas had abdominal tumor at the time of presentation. Only one patient with lymphoblastic lymphoma had abdominal disease, and this consisted solely of hepatosplenomegaly. Nine of 15 patients with lymphoblastic lymphoma (60%) had an anterior superior mediastinal mass.

Results

Sixty-eight of the 75 patients (91%) achieved a complete response (i.e. no clinically or radiologically detectable disease). Seven patients had a partial response (i.e., more than 50% reduction in the tumor diameter). All 7 were males of 16 or more years old. Five had Burkitt's lymphoma and two, large cell lymphomas. Three of the partial responders had bone marrow involvement. Disease-free interval and survival curves (Kaplan-Meier plots) for the entire group are shown in Figs. 2a and b. Two patients who died from infection while disease free are censored from the plots of disease-free interval at the time of death. They are, however, included in the survival curve.

Disease-free interval by histology is shown in Fig. 3. Lymphoblastic lymphoma patients had the best prognosis, and there was no difference between undifferentiated lymphomas of Burkitt's and non-Burkitt's types.

Disease-free interval by NCI stage and in lymphoblastic lymphoma is shown in Fig. 4. Patients with completely resected abdominal, or a single extraabdominal, non-lymphoblastic lymphoma had a very good prognosis, which differed significantly from that of other non-lymphoblastic patient groups. Interestingly, no difference in the survival curves between patients with Stages B, C or D non-lymphoblastic lymphoma were discernable. Disease-free interval according to St. Jude clinical stage is shown in Fig. 5. This demonstrates that patients with CNS and BM involvement at presentation (Stage IV) had a particularly poor prognosis. The negative impact of bone marrow involvement applies to both lymphoblastic and non-lymphoblastic lymphomas as shown in Fig. 6. Indicators of tumor burden – notably elevated serum LDH (> 1000) and uric acid (> 9.0) – were significantly correlated with prognosis in non-lymphoblastic lymphomas. These indices were

648

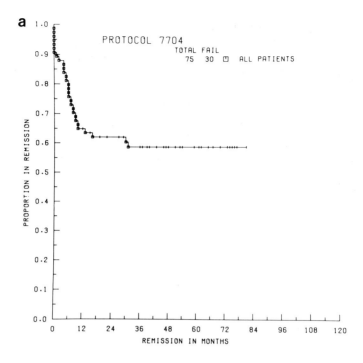

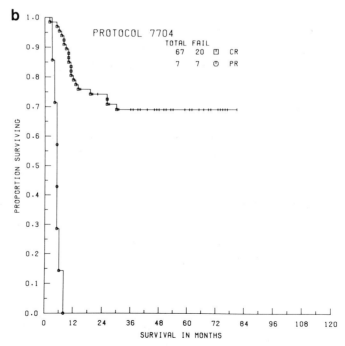

Figure 2. (a) Disease-free interval and (b) survival in complete (CR) and partial (PR) responders in 75 patients with non-Hodgkin's lymphoma.

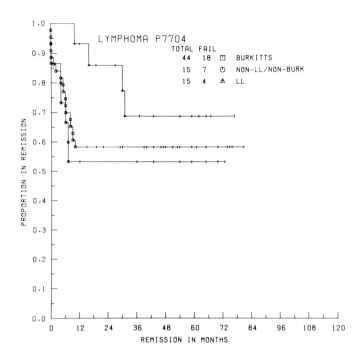

Figure 3. Disease-free interval by histology.

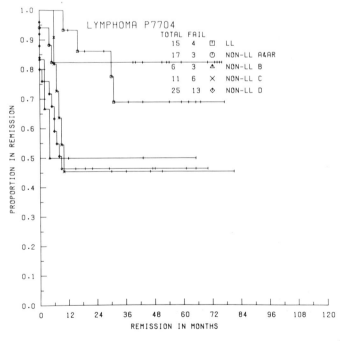

Figure 4. Disease-free interval in lymphoblastic lymphoma, and by Pediatric Branch stage in patients with non-lymphoblastic lymphoma.

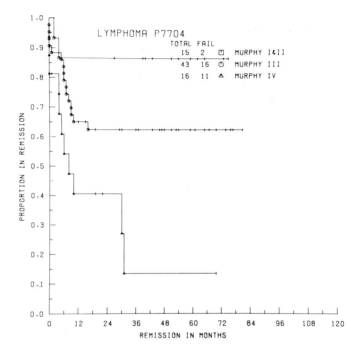

Figure 5. Disease-free interval by St. Jude (Murphy) stage.

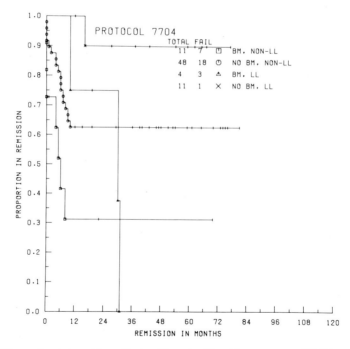

Figure 6. Disease-free interval in patients with and without bone marrow (BM) involvement in lymphoblastic (LL) and non-lymphoblastic (non-LL) lymphomas.

not of prognostic significance in lymphoblastic lymphoma. Age was not a significant prognostic factor in this series, unlike previous series in the Pediatric Branch in which older patients had a worse prognosis. A multivariate analysis has shown that the most important prognostic factors are clinical stage, bone marrow involvement and chemical indices which reflect tumor burden [5].

Sites of relapse

The disease recurred after a period of complete remission (up to 2 years in lymphoblastic lymphoma, or up to 10 months in non-lymphoblastic lymphoma) in 22 of 74 patiens (Table IV). The patient with unclassified lymphoma also relapsed in peripheral blood (but not bone marrow) and lymph nodes. Of note is the high frequency of isolated CNS relapse, which occurred in eight patients with non-lymphoblastic lymphoma, seven of them 16-years old or younger. Four of these patients did not receive intrathecal prophylaxis and two presented with CNS disease. The intrathecal prophylaxis regimen appears to have been successful: 4 isolated CNS relapses occurred in 19 patients (13 non-lymphoblastic) who did not receive it, whereas 2 relapses occurred in 55 (47 non-lymphoblastic) who received prophylaxis. There is a trend towards improved disease-free interval in patients who received CNS prophylaxis (55) compared to those who did not (19) (Fig. 7). Survival at four years in these groups was 67% and 53%, respectively.

Of the five patients with lymphoblastic lymphoma who relapsed, four had presented with marrow involvement and three had marrow involvement as

Table IV. First relapse sites

	Total (74)	16 yrs or less (35)	17 yrs or more (39)
All relapses	22	13	9
Isolated CNS relapse	8	7	1
Spermatic cord	2	1	1
Testis	1	1	0
Abdomen	3	2	1
Bone marrow	5	2 [a]	3
Bone marrow/CNS/abdomen	1	0	1
Mediastinum	2	0	2

[a] Diagnosed in 1 case on the basis of a single clump of tumor cells seen only on clot section. Bilateral aspirates and biopsies were normal

One patient with unclassified lymphoma, not included in this table relapsed with circulating blast cells (but no involvement of marrow) and recurrent lymphadenopathy

652

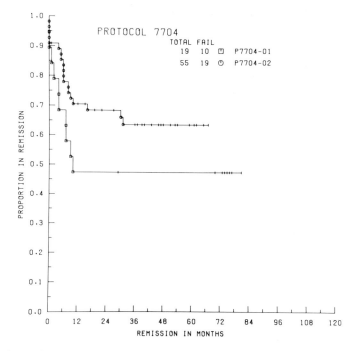

Figure 7. Disease-free interval with (77-04-04) and without (77-04-01) intrathecal CNS prophylaxis.

the initial site of relapse. One patient relapsed in the mediastinum and then the marrow; the fifth patient developed recurrent mediastinal and pleural tumor.

Toxicity

The major toxicities were myelosuppression involving predominantly white cells (median nadir, 1,100 WBC/mm³). Rarely did the platelet count drop below 100,000/mm³. Stomatitis of moderate to severe degree occurred in about half the patients. In three patients methotrexate was withheld completely after 3, 4 and 12 cycles because of esophagitis in one and hepatitis in two. Doxorubicin cardiotoxicity was not seen. Approximately 17% of the cycles were associated with fever during a period of neutropenia, but in less than 5% was bacterial infection documented. One patient died of sepsis.

Discussion

This protocol appears to provide excellent therapy for patients with lymphoblastic lymphomas without bone marrow involvement regardless of tumor burden, although the number of such patients is presently small. In addition, unlike the disease specific regimens used by the CCSG and described recently, this regimen is also highly effective for limited or completely resected non-lymphoblastic lymphomas, and provides good results in patients with extensive non-lymphoblastic lymphomas without bone marrow involvement (Stage III). It represents poor therapy, however, for all patients with marrow involvement regardless of histology.

Of note is that radiation therapy was used in only a small number of patients (4), although this modality is frequently used in other childhood NHL protocols for the treatment of 'bulk' diseaxe. The comparable results in these separate protocols raises questions as to the value of radiation used in this way. Further, patients with completely resected non-lymphoblastic lymphomas received only six cycles of therapy, yet enjoyed an excellent prognosis. It is probable that prolonged therapy even in patients with extensive non-lymphoblastic lymphoma provides little advantage.

The prognosis in this protocol was similar in young adults and children, although partial response occurred more often in the former. Four of the 14 relapses in children were isolated CNS relapses occurring in patients who did not receive prior intrathecal prophylactic therapy. Only one of these 4 patients subsequently survived (disease free at six years). One of the two patients who failed CNS prophylaxis had an L3 form of leukemia. Such patients are at high risk for CNS recurrence even after cranial vault irradiation [6].

References

1. Wollner N, Burchenal JH, Lieberman PH et al. (1975). Non-Hodgkin's lymphoma in children. Med Pediat Oncol 1:235–263.
2. Djerassi I and Kim JS (1976). Methotrexate and citrovorum factor rescue in the management of childhood lymphosarcoma and reticulum cell sarcoma (non-Hodgkin's lymphomas). Cancer 38:1043–1045.
3. Magrath IT, Lwanga S, Carwell W and Harrison N (1974). Surgical reduction in tumor bulk in the management of abdominal Burkitt's lymphoma. Brit Med J 2:308–312.
4. Murphy SB and Hustu HO (1980). A randomized trial of combined modality therapy of childhood non-Hodgkin's lymphoma. Cancer 45:630–637.
5. Magrath IT, Janus V, Edwards BK et al. (1984). An effective therapy for both undifferentiated (including Burkitt's) lymphomas and lymphoblastic lymphomas in children and young adults. Blood 63:1102–1111.
6. Müller-Weihrieh St, Henze G, Odenwald E and Riehm H (1985). BFM trials for childhood non-Hodgkin's lymphomas. In: Cavalli F, Bonodonna G, and Rozencweig M (Eds). Malignant Lymphomas and Hodgkin's Disease: Experimental and Therapeutic Advances, pp 633–642. Boston: Martinus Nijhoff.

Subject index

664

IPT